NEPHROTOXICITY IN THE EXPERIMENTAL AND CLINICAL SITUATION

DEVELOPMENTS IN NEPHROLOGY

Cheigh JS, Stenzel KH, Rubin AL: Manual of Clinical Nephrology of the Rogosin Center. 1981. ISBN 90-247-2397-3

Nolph KD ed: Peritoneal Dialysis. 1981. ISBN 90-247-2477-5

Gruskin AB, Norman ME eds: Pediatric Nephrology. 1981.
ISBN 90-247-2514-3

Schück O ed: Examination of the Kidney Function. 1981.
ISBN 0-89838-565-2

Strauss J ed: Hypertension, Fluid-Electrolytes and Tubulopathies in Pediatric Nephrology. ISBN 90-247-2633-6

Strauss J ed: Neonatal Kidney and Fluid-Electrolytes. 1983.
ISBN 0-89838-575-X

Strauss J. ed: Acute Renal Disorders and Renal Emergencies. 1984
ISBN 0-89838-663-2

Didio LJA, Motta PM eds: Basic, Clinical, and Surgical Nephrology.
1985. ISBN 0-89838-698-5

Friedman EA, Peterson CM eds: Diabetic Nephropathy: Strategy for Therapy. 1985. ISBN 0-89838-735-3

Dzúrik R, Lichardus B, Guder W eds: Kidney Metabolism and Function.
1985. ISBN 0-89838-749-3

Strauss J ed: Homeostasis, Nephrotoxicity, and Anomalies in the Newborn. 1986. ISBN 0-89838-766-3

Oreopoulos DG ed: Geriatric Nephrology. 1986. ISBN 0-89838-781-7

Paganini EP ed: Acute Continuous Renal Replacement Therapy. 1986.
ISBN 0-89838-793-0

Cheigh JS, Stenzel KH, Rubin AL eds: Hypertension in Kidney Disease.
1986. ISBN 0-89838-797-3

Deane N, Wiheman RJ, Benis GA eds: Guide to Reprocessing of Hemodialysers. 1986. ISBN 0-89838-798-1

Ponticelli C, Minetti L, D'Amico G eds: Antiglobulins, Cryoglobulins and Glomerulonephritis. 1986. ISBN 0-89838-810-4

Strauss J ed: Persistent Renal-Genitourinary Disorders. 1987
ISBN 089838-845-7

Andreucci VE, Dal Canton A eds: Diuretics: Basic, Pharmacological and Clinical Aspects. 1987. ISBN 0-89838-885-6

Bach PH, Lock EA eds: Nephrotoxicity in the Experimental and Clinical Situation. 1987. ISBN 0-89838-977-1 (Part 1); 0-89838-980-1 (Part 2)

Nephrotoxicity in the experimental and clinical situation

Part 1

edited by

P. H. BACH
The Robens Institute
University of Surrey
Guildford, Surrey
England

E. A. LOCK
Biochemical Toxicology Section
Imperial Chemical Industries plc
Alderley Park, Macclesfield, Cheshire
England

1987 **MARTINUS NIJHOFF PUBLISHERS**
a member of the KLUWER ACADEMIC PUBLISHERS GROUP
DORDRECHT / BOSTON / LANCASTER

Distributors

for the United States and Canada: Kluwer Academic Publishers, 101 Philip Drive, Assinippi Park, Norwell, MA 02061, USA
for the UK and Ireland: Kluwer Academic Publishers, MTP Press Limited, Falcon House, Queen Square, Lancaster LA1 1RN, UK
for all other other countries: Kluwer Academic Publishers Group, Distribution Center, P.O. Box 322, 3300 AH Dordrecht, The Netherlands

Book information

ISBN-13: 978-94-010-8012-5   e-ISBN-13: 978-94-009-3367-5
DOI: 10.1007/978-94-009-3367-5

British Library Cataloguing in Publication Data

Nephrotoxicity in the experimental and
   clinical situation. --- (Developments in
   nephrology).
   1. Kidneys --- Diseases   2. Toxins
   I. Bach, P.H.   II. Lock, E.A.
   III. Series
   616.6'1   RC902

Copyright

Copyright 1987 Martinus Nijhoff Publishers
Softcover reprint of the hardcover 1st edition 1987

CONTENTS

PREFACE

There are many aspects of renal function and malfunction that we still do not understand. Homeostasis is central to renal function, but its maintenance also serves to mask the earliest features of malfunction. Thus renal dysfunction is buffered and cannot be identified until degeneration has reached a level at which homeostasis is severely compromised. Because of this, diagnosis of the vast majority of nephropathies are often so late as to preclude therapeutic intervention. More importantly, it has been impossible to establish the aetiology of many nephropathies.

The kidney is known to be a frequent target for toxicity, because of its size in relation to the many functions it must perform. All to often in the past there has been a failure to adequately perceive this in the early development of new therapeutic agents, their clinical trials and subsequent drug usage. Industrial and environmental chemicals have also been implicated in several nephropathies, but the causal link with exposure to the offending chemical may not have been immediately established.

These volumes cover the different methods that are used to assess renal function in health and disease. The biology of many model nephropathies that are directly relevant to the clinical situation (especially those where a mechanistic understanding is helping to define the primary lesion and its secondary consequences) and a broader appreciation of the different types of clinical nephrotoxicity and factors that may affect their diagnosis and progression. The objective of NEPHROTOXICITY IN THE EXPERIMENTAL AND CLINICAL SITUATION is to use a multidisciplinary scientific approach as the foundation to better understand nephrotoxicity. The experimental systems will serve to provide a basis for improved screening for potentially nephrotoxic drugs and chemicals, the development of less nephrotoxic drugs, they will improve the approach to the prevention of nephrotoxicity and also provide a rational basis for the more successful clinical management of all nephropathies.

Peter H. Bach, Guildford, Surrey
Edward A. Lock, Alderley Edge, Cheshire

LIST OF CONTRIBUTORS

T. Almén
Department of Diagnostic
   Radiology
Malmö General Hospital
S-214 01 Malmö
Sweden

J. Atkinson
Laboratoire de
   Pharmacologie
Faculté des Sciences
   Pharmaceutiques et
   Biologiques
54000 Université de
   Nancy 1
5 rue Albert le Brun
Nancy
France

P.H. Bach
The Robens Institute
University of Surrey
Guildford
Surrey
GU2 5XH
UK

J.R.J. Baker
Department of Biology
Research Centre
Ciba-Geigy
   Pharmaceuticals
Wimblehurst Road
Horsham
West Sussex
RH12 4AB
UK

D. Baran
INSERM U.28
Hôpital Broussais
96 rue Didot
75674 Paris Cedex 14
France

W.O. Berndt
Department of
   Pharmacology
University of Nebraska
   Medical Center
42nd Street and Dewey
   Avenue
Omaha
NE 68105
USA

R.E. Bulger
Renal Research Laboratory
University of Texas
   Graduate School of
   Biomedical Sciences
PO Box 20708
Houston
TX 77030
USA

K. Cain
MRC Toxicology Unit
Woodmansterne Road
Carshalton
Surrey
SM5 4EF
UK

W.R. Cattell
Department of Nephrology
St Bartholomew's Centre
   for Research
St Bartholomew's Hospital
London
EC1A 7BE
UK

K. Crowshaw
ONO Pharmaceutical
   Company
London Office
St Alphage House
18th Floor
2 Fore Street
London
EC2Y 5DA
UK

P.G. Davey
Department of Clinical
   Pharmacology
Ninewells Hospital and
   Medical School
Dundee
DD1 9SY
UK

A. Dawnay
Department of Chemical
   Pathology
St Bartholomew's Centre
   for Research
St Bartholomew's Hospital
London
EC1A 7BE
UK

J. Diezi
Institut de Pharmacologie
Université de Lausanne
Bugnon 27
CH-1005 Lausanne
Switzerland

D.C. Dobyan
Renal Research Laboratory
University of Texas
   Graduate School of
   Biomedical Sciences
PO Box 20708
Houston
TX 77030
USA

P. Druet
INSERM U. 28
Hôpital Broussais
96 rue Didot
75674 Paris Cedex 14
France

G. Eknoyan
Department of Medicine
Baylor College of
   Medicine
Houston
Texas 77030
USA

J.-P. Fillastre
Department of Nephrology
Hôpital de Bois-Guillaume
2720 route de Neuf-Châtel
76230 Bois-Guillaume
France

B.A. Fowler
National Institute of
   Environmental Health
   Sciences
PO Box 12233
Research Triangle Park
NC 27709
USA

J.R. Glaister
Hazleton Laboratories
   (Europe) Ltd
Otley Road
Harrogate
North Yorkshire
HG3 1PY
UK

P.L. Goering
Center for Services of
    Radiological Health
Division of Life Sciences
Food and Drug
    Administration
12709 Twinbrook Parkway
Rockville, MD 20857
USA

R.S. Goldstein
Department of
    Investigative
    Toxicology
Smith Kline & French
    Laboratories
1500 Spring Garden Street
PO Box 7929
Mail Code L-66
Philadelphia, PA 19101
USA

K. Golman
Department of
    Experimental Research
Malmö General Hospital
S-214 01 Malmö
Sweden

N.J. Gregg
The Robens Institute
University of Surrey
Guildford
Surrey
GU2 5XH
UK

G.C. Hard
Fels Research Institute
3420 N. Broad Street
Temple University School
    of Medicine
Philadelphia, PA 19140
USA

E.S. Harpur
Department of
    Pharmaceutical
    Sciences
Aston University
Aston Triangle
Birmingham
B47 ET
UK

E. Holtz
NYCOMED A/S
Box 4220
0401 Oslo 4
Norway

J.B. Hook
Preclinical Research and
    Development
Smith Kline & French
    Laboratories
1500 Spring Garden Street
PO Box 7929
Mail Code L735
Philadelphia
PA 19101
USA

J.W. Hopewell
CRC Normal Tissue
    Radiobiology Research
    Group
Research Institute
(University of Oxford)
Churchill Hospital
Oxford
OX3 7LJ
UK

C. Jacquot
INSERM U.28
Hôpital Broussais
96 rue Didot
75674 Paris Cedex 14
France

S. Kacew
Department of
    Pharmacology
University of Ottawa
451 Smyth Road
Ottawa
Ontario
K1H 8M5 Canada

D. Kleinknecht
Hôpital de Montreuil
56 bd. de la Boissière
93105 Montreuil Cedex
France

M.M. Lipsky
Department of Pathology
University of Maryland
    School of Medicine
10 South Pine Street
Baltimore
MD 21201
USA

C.L. Litterst
Developmental
    Therapeutics Program
Division of Cancer
    Treatment
National Cancer Institute
Bethesda
Maryland
USA

E.A. Lock
Biochemical Toxicology
    Section
Imperial Chemical
    Industries plc
Central Toxicology
    Laboratory
Alderley Park
Macclesfield
Cheshire
SK10 4TJ
UK

J.I. Lowrie
Department of Anatomy and
    Cell Biology
University of Sheffield
Western Bank
Sheffield
S10 2TN, UK

J.-P. Mery
Department of Nephrology
Hôpital Bichat
170 Bd. Ney
75018 Paris
France

P. Mistry
Department of
    Biochemistry
Brunel University
Uxbridge, Middx.
UB8 3PH
UK

K. Ormstad
Department of Forensic
    Medicine
Karolinska Institute
Box 60400
S-10401 Stockholm
Sweden

G.A. Porter
Department of Medicine
Oregon Health Sciences
    University
3181 S.W. Sam Jackson
    Park Road
L-455
Portland
OR 97201
USA

M.E.C. Robbins
CRC Normal Tissue
    Radiobiology Research
    Group
Research Institute
(University of Oxford)
Churchill Hospital
Oxford
OX3 7LJ
UK

F. Roch-Ramel
Institute de
    Pharmacologie
Université de Lausanne
Bugnon 27
CH-1005
Lausanne
Switzerland

D.P. Sandler
Epidemiology Branch
Division of Biometry and
    Risk Assessment
National Institute of
    Environmental Health
    Sciences
PO Box 12233
Research Triangle Park
NC 27709
USA

P.N. Skelton-Stroud
Ciba-Geigy
    Pharmaceuticals
Stamford Lodge
Altrincham Road
Wilmslow
Cheshire
SK9 4LY
UK

M.D. Stonard
Toxicity Section
Imperial Chemical
    Industries
Central Toxicology
    Laboratory
Alderley Park
Macclesfield
Cheshire
SK10 4TJ
UK

J.B. Tarloff
Department of
    Investigative
    Toxicology
Smith Kline & French
    Laboratories
1500 Spring Garden Street
PO Box 7929
Mail Code L-66
Philadelphia
PA 19101
USA

B.F. Trump
Department of Pathology
University of Maryland
    School of Medicine
10 South Pine Street
Baltimore
MD 21201
USA

E.D. Wachsmuth
Research Department
Pharmaceutical Division
Ciba-Geigy Limited
Basel
Switzerland

R.B. Weiss
Medical Oncology
Walter Reed Army Medical
    Center
Washington DC
USA

M.A. Williams
Department of Anatomy and
    Cell Biology
University of Sheffield
Western Bank
Sheffield
S10 2TN
UK

1

FIXATION OF RENAL TISSUE FOR CYTOCHEMICAL EVALUATION

M.A. WILLIAMS

INTRODUCTION

In many morphological studies of the kidney a major objective is conserving particular chemicals or groups of chemicals. This demands preservation of an activity (e.g. enzymic or antigenic) at or near its in vivo location and it implies conservation of the kidney architecture necessary to permit accurate localization. In this type of study the primary objectives are different from those pursued in morphometric work and the fixation (and embedding) methods differ markedly. Many of the preservation problems are not specific to the kidney and experience from other tissues may be directly applicable. Thus gaps can be filled to allow conclusions to be drawn that are relevant to the kidney.

A.   Categories of chemicals present in kidney tissue

Tissues (both cells and their extracellular matrices) are made up of a bewildering variety of natural chemical constituents. These range from macromolecules (nucleic acids, proteins and sugar-rich polymers), to various classes of micromolecules such as lipids, monosaccharides, oligosaccharides, organic acids, peptides and nucleic acid building materials, to simple cations and anions such as Na^+ and Cl^- and hydrogen and hydroxyl ions.

B.   Objectives in tissue preparation for microscopy

A significant proportion of the tissue architecture must be conserved by immobilization of selected cellular material, and then specifically contrasted by a suitable chromogen, fluorogen or electron dense atom (see Lewis and Knight)[1]. The staining process almost always depends crucially on the fixation process (unfixed tissues are very difficult to stain), the material used for embed-

1

ment and the thickness of sections. Routinely, tissue is infiltrated with wax, epoxy resin, methacrylate or other resinous polymer to provide support for the sectioning process. These embedding processes necessitate gradual replacement of the water in the tissue by the embedment. The whole of the conventional tissue preparation process, fixing through to embedding and sectioning, is summarized in Figure 1. The many ways in which kidney tissue can be prepared for cytochemical examination are summarized in Figure 2.

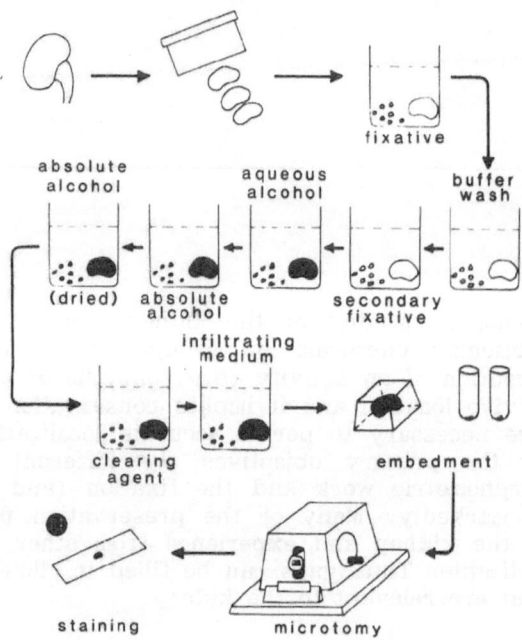

Figure 1 An outline of conventional tissue processing procedures. Immersion fixation is depicted followed by washing, secondary fixation, dehydration, clearing, embedding, sectioning and staining.

II. CONSEQUENCES OF APPLYING CONVENTIONAL TISSUE PREPARATION METHODS

Fixation as outlined above (Figure 1) generally succeeds in immobilizing much of the macromolecular mass of the specimen, which ultimately provides stained sections that reveal the tissue architecture. Whereas conventional light microscopic (LM) images depend very largely on immobilized macromolecules, those of electron microscopy (EM) also depend on the lipidic components of cytomembranes. Specific methods can also be used to image small molecules, ions and biological active groups.

Fixatives are chemically (but selectively) reactive and increase membrane permeability. Thus the conventional ways of

2

preparing tissues for microscopic examination are very unlikely to leave the chemical composition or biological activity within cells un- altered. The number of different tissue processing techniques is very large, as is the number of different tissue components (Table 1). Thus only a simplified consideration of the commonly used stages of tissue preparation will be presented.

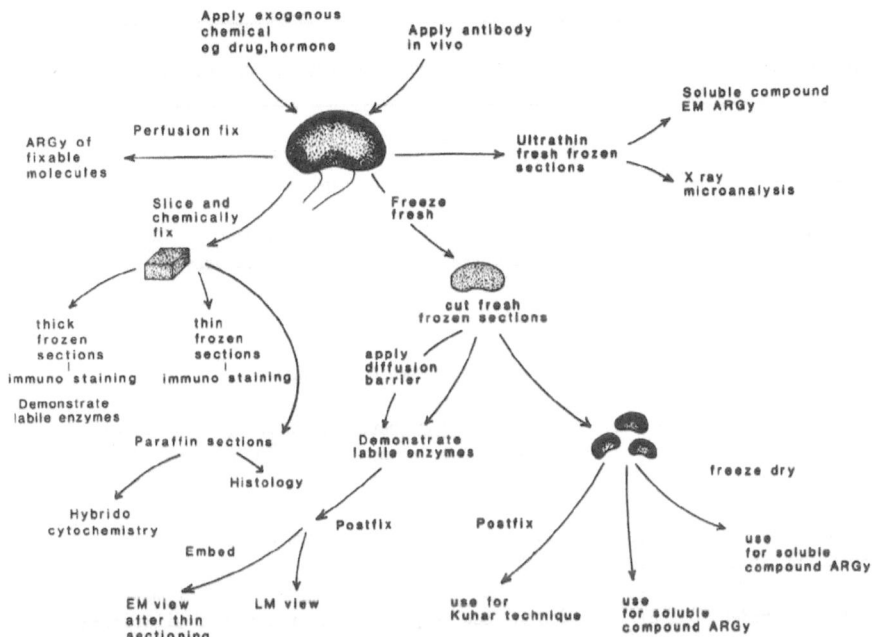

Figure 2 Chart summarizing the major routes of tissue preparation for cytochemical study of the kidney.

Fixatives and their mechanisms of fixation have been reviewed by Horobin[2]. In recent years the use of glutaraldehyde has become widespread for both LM and EM work along with another bifunctional aldehyde, acrolein and the more traditional cross-linker formaldehyde. Other fixatives include the organic denaturants, such as methanol, mercuric chloride and osmium tetroxide, which is generally considered here as a secondary fixa- tive. No attempt is made to distinguish between the use of alcohols and acetones for dehydration, despite the fact that the effects of the two, although similar, are not identical. Embedments include traditional paraffin wax for LM work and the epoxy resins which are widespread in EM work. In addition, the glycol-methacrylate group of resins (for EM and LM) and JB4 resin and epoxy resins (for LM) are all gaining increased popularity.

The interactions between processing agents and cell com- ponents are set out in Table 2. It will be noted that the deleterious effects of processing agents fall under three headings:

1. mobilization leading to movement and possibly to total extraction;
2. chemical modification and loss of biological activity of retained molecules; and
3. reduction of accessibility of retained molecules.

Table 1 Natural constituents of tissues

Tissue component	Preparation method necessary for preservation
Proteins - globular, fibrous nucleic acids	Most chemical fixatives will immobilize them
Mucosubstances	Addition of cetyl pyridinium chloride to fixative; avoid glycol and other water-miscible methacrylates
Polysaccharides	Avoid water-miscible methacrylates
Peptides > 500 mw	Glutaraldehyde fixation necessary
Amino acids, oligopeptides	Freezing, low temperature sectioning or glutaraldehyde fixation (probably not complete preservation)
Nucleosides, nucleotides bases, pyrimidine, purine	Freezing, low temperature sectioning
Monosaccharides, oligosaccharides	Freezing, low temperature sectioning or silicone-epoxy resin embedding
Fatty acids saturated unsaturated	Freezing, low temperature processing and sectioning or osmium tetroxide fixation
Di- and triglycerides, phospholipids	Osmium tetroxide fixation (does not work for saturated fatty acids)
Cholesterol	Creation of digitonide necessary
Other steroids	Freezing, low temperature cutting
Organic acids, e.g. acetate, lactate	Freezing, low temperature cutting
Cations, H^+, Na^+, K^+, Mg^{2+}, Ca^{2+}, etc., anions, Cl^-, OH^-, I^-	Freezing, low temperature cutting ultra low temperature maintenance some precipitation methods available for metallic cations

Table 2 Effects of the standard tissue preparation methods on some tissue chemicals

Process/chemicals	Effects on proteins	Effects on lipids (phospholipids, cholesterol)	Effects on sugars, amino acids	Effects on Na^+, I^-, Cl^- and other ions
Fixative agents formaldehyde glutaraldehyde	Cross-links peptide chains; dimerizes proteins; loss of certain groups; loss of some secondary tertiary structure	Very little solubility unmodified	Amino compounds may be "trapped" others unaffected	Mobilizes and extracts ions
methanol, chloroform mercuric chloride	Denatures proteins; cross-links, reacts with tyrosine and ⁻SH	Dissolves lipids;some reaction	Likely to extract sugars & amino acids	Mobilizes and extracts ions
Fixative vehicle aqueous buffer	Can dissolve some unmodified proteins	Little effect	Most untrapped molecules extracted	Mobilizes and extracts ions
Secondary fixative osmium tetroxide	Complex formation with, addition to, and oxidation of proteins, thus lowers solubility Oxidation of proteins, denatures, splits S-S links, lowers solubility	Reacts with olefin groups, makes many phospholipids insoluble; cholesterol not	Remaining untrapped, molecules extracted	More ions extracted, only tightly bound ions left
Dehydrating agents aqueous alcohol aqueous acetone absolute alcohol absolute acetone glycol methacrylate	May denature	Dissolve unreacted lipids of all kinds, remove them from tissue		
Clearing agent xylene epoxypropane	Could denature but little effect on fixed proteins			
Embedment paraffin wax glycol methacrylate butyl methacrylate, JB4 epoxy resin	Surrounds proteins; little effect on fixed proteins	Dissolves unreacted neutral lipids		

A.   Loss of biological activity

The major objective of most fixation is to immobilize tissue macromolecules, which is achieved using cross-linking (within and between) molecules. Fixation may also precipitate large molecules or greatly disrupt their conformation. It is inevitable, therefore, that the activity of many enzymes[3-5] and antigens will be lost[6-8] as well as specific receptor sites. The literature contains numerous reports of the effects of fixatives on enzymes, but less on deac-

5

tivation of antigens - and even fewer on receptors. The loss of biological activity varies considerably from enzyme to enzyme[9], and much can be gained by trying different fixatives and fixation times to develop a suitable protocol for the enzyme of interest. It is also possible to use a substrate for the protection of the active site[10]. Generally, mitochondrial enzymes are highly sensitive to fixatives[11] whilst lysosomal enzymes are less so[12], and can usually be demonstrated on fixed sections. The brush border enzymes such as alkaline phosphatase activity are quite resistant to fixation[13]. Improved survival of biological activity may be achieved by brief fixation times (down to 15 min, compared with 3-24 hours), at low aldehyde concentrations (down to 0.5%, compared to 1.5-6.0%) or the use of less active hydroxyadipaldehyde. In such experiments the protein may not be fully immobilized[3,8] and subsequent aqueous buffer washes or incubations (to effect cytochemical reactions) may result in the diffusion of the biologically active protein into the medium[14].

Despite the difficulties of inactivation and diffusion, many successful localization studies have proved possible using immunocytochemical staining, including the enzymes tyrosine carboxylase[15], Na^+,K^+-ATPase[16] and carbonic anhydrase[17]. Secondary fixatives such as osmium tetroxide generally abolish biological activity. In most enzyme cytochemical, immunocytochemical or receptor studies the reaction incubation is carried out before[18] or immediately after fixation. In some instances the tissue is post-embedded[19].

Many EM immunocytochemical studies employ a monoclonal primary antibody, followed by colloidal gold particles coated with a secondary antibody. The high specificity of monoclonal antibodies naturally lowers the staining intensity compared to polyclonal antibodies. Thus, if the antigen is present only in small amounts, the monoclonal staining reaction may be only a little above the non-specific background staining, and partial deactivation of antigen by fixative may easily eliminate it. Quantitative tests of the fixation required for antigen survival should be made on cell free systems before EM studies are undertaken.

Alcohols used for dehydrating are likely to have somewhat deleterious effects on biological activity, but aldehyde-fixed molecules may well be less labile to alcohols than unfixed ones. Embedding in epoxy resin eliminates some accessibility, but also causes deactivation (see below). Glycol methacrylate is less damaging from both points of view, especially when employed at low temperature (-20 °C). The main loss of enzyme activity in such circumstances occurs during the previous chemical fixation.

B.   Loss of accessibility of retained molecules

Dewaxed paraffin embedded sections are quite porous and allow almost all low molecular weight staining reagents to reach tissue components. The density of various tissue components varies and the molecular weight of the stain affects the rate of its penetration to particular tissue sites. This factor lies at the root of many differential staining effects[2]. Similarly, the degree of cross-linking fixation with aldehydes affects the penetration of some antibody preparations. By contrast resin sections are generally stained with the embedment in place, and selectivity (e.g. toluidine blue or eosin and light green) depends, in part, on easier penetration of the dye into the material containing less resin. Thus even in well-embedded tissue specimens there are parts of the tissue that do not completely infiltrate with resin. The saccharide-rich basement membranes in the kidney (e.g. Bowman's capsule), do not infiltrate well because they do not dehydrate completely, due to the strong water binding properties of the saccharides. Other tissue components fail to infiltrate well due to their high density, such as the lysosomes of the S_2 segment of the rat kidney and the granules of the juxtaglomerular apparatus. These resin-poor structures stain well with charged dye molecules, whilst the remainder of the tissue (e.g. ground cytoplasm of podocytes or tubule cells) stains poorly[21]. When the more hydrophilic resin glycol methacrylate or JB4 is used, stains can be applied to all parts of kidney cells and differential contrast is thus less. Epoxy resin monomers are able to react with certain chemical groups, such as carboxylates and hydroxyls, which explains the deactivation of the biological activity of proteins. Etching of the plastic section surface with solvents (e.g. acetone, methanol, benzene) or acidified H_2O_2, sometimes renders more tissue accessible. However, this may be the reversing of a 'resealing' process that occurs after sectioning, rather than the disruption of resin-tissue bonding[2].

C.   Hybridocytochemistry

Recent years have seen an explosive growth of the hybridization procedures to study specific DNA sequences of animal cells. Translational activities of mRNAs for various enzymes and non-enzyme proteins may now also be studied. The literature contains numerous references to studies on free kidney cells, but few on kidney tissue. In situ hybridization uses a tritium-labelled cloned DNA fragment obtained by nick translation of tritiated poly-U, or [^{3}H]RNA, as probe and LM autoradiography to localize the probe. This approach is currently valuable in localizing viral DNAs and may be used in tandem with immunocytochemistry, which localizes the relevant antigens. The in situ hybridization approach generally requires that the nucleic acid of interest is preserved intact, that access to it is available for the probe, and that the sequence before and after probe binding is immobilized. Usually 1% formaldehyde fixation for 1-15 min has proved superior to glutaraldehyde or Carnoy fixative[22-24]. Tissues have been embedded in paraffin wax or methacrylate; the latter may become standard.

III.   MOBILIZATION AND EXTRACTION OF TISSUE COMPONENTS BY CONVENTIONAL PROCEDURES

A.   Macromolecule loss

Fixative procedures are primarily chosen to immobilize macromolecules. All those in Table 1 are reasonably efficient at immobilizing proteins and nucleic acids provided the concentration and the duration of fixation are sufficient. Saccharide-rich molecules such as the PAS-positive materials associated with the basal laminae in glomeruli are not well-fixed by perfusion of the kidney with aldehydes, and much PAS-positive material is lost in subsequent aqueous treatment solutions (Mason and Beaven, personal communication). This problem can be remedied by adding cetyl-pyridinium chloride to the fixative[25,26]. Mast cell granules and glycogen are similarly labile, and in the absence of secondary fixatives such as OsO_4 are extracted by glycol methacrylate and perhaps aqueous buffers.

B.   The fixation of peptides and amino acids

Cross-linking aldehydes react strongly with α amino groups and ε-NH_2 groups of lysine to attach small peptides or amino acids to tissue proteins[27]. Based on protein secretion studies[28,29], Peters and Ashley[30] showed that considerable amounts of amino acids could be fixed to tissues with glutaraldehyde. This "parasite labelling" was thought to be serious enough to interfere with the study of protein synthesis, but this has proved to be largely unfounded. The observation is, however, being exploited to study the accumulation and binding of amino acids or small peptides by or in cells. For example, gamma-aminobutyric acid[31] and glutamate[32] have been studied, and the glycine specific synapses[33].

Peptides containing 8-10 or more amino acids are fixed by glutaraldehyde (2-3%) with >90% retention. This makes possible the study, by autoradiography, of insulin and somatostatin and their fragments[34] plus other peptides. This relative ease of immobilizing peptides does not imply that very small peptides and free amino acids would be similarly completely preserved. In some cases no more than 50% of the labelled amino acid would appear to be fixed, and it remains to be investigated which factors most influence the autoradiographic distributions. These could be influenced by the local concentrations of protein in the tissue, membrane permeabilities and frequencies of particular glutaraldehyde-reactive chemical groupings (-SH, -NH_2). Quite evidently, amino acids produced by degrading enzymes, e.g. the aminopeptidase of the kidney proximal tubule microvilli[35], could be incorporated into nascent proteins, and contribute to autoradiographic images by secondary incorporation. Lowrie, Baker and Williams[34] have shown the apparent S_3 segment labelling by amino acids released from peptides degraded in the S_2 segment of the proximal tubule (see also Figures 3-6). The status of the "parasite labelling" effect[30] was considered elsewhere[36] and has changed little since that time.

C.   Preservation of exogenous chemicals in kidney tissue

There are many groups of exogenous low molecular weight chemicals that arrive at and accumulate in the kidneys. Conserving

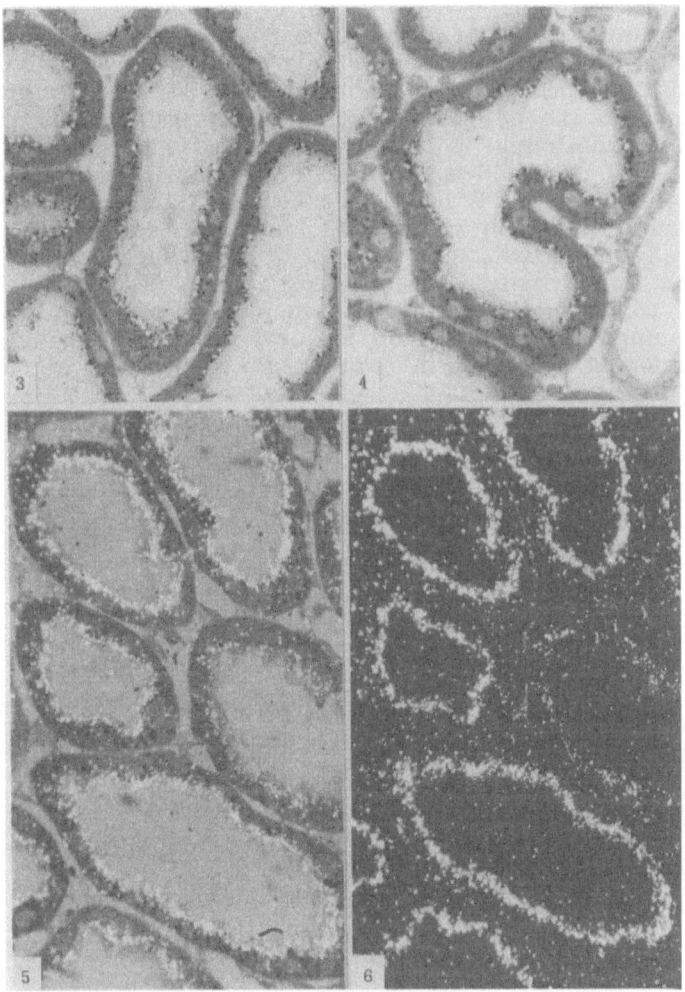

Figures 3-6 Light microscope autoradiographs (x450) showing the retention of a peptide, mini-somatostatin, molecular weight circa 1100, by perfusion with glutaraldehyde followed by secondary osmium tetroxide treatment. **Figure 3**, S_1 tubule; **Figure 4**, S_2 tubule (both seen in bright field). **Figures 5** (bright field) and **6** (incident dark field) showing the more intense labelling of S_2 as against S_1 tubules.

these substances for cytochemistry can be considered in terms of the proportions of tightly bound and diffusible chemical in the cells, fixation and immobilization methods, and detection methods. In addition, the changes in the kidney architecture may be caused by nephrotoxins.

A fraction of most endogenous and exogenous substances that enter kidney cells via the blood stream may become tightly or loosely bound; the remainder being free. Aldosterone, for example, accumulates in the cytoplasm and especially the nucleus[37]. Some cytoplasmic aldosterone is strongly associated with the basal plasmalemma and mitochondria[38], but the remaining material in the nucleus and cytoplasm is not tightly bound. Aldosterone appears to affect nuclear events in kidney cells and toad bladder cells, and it is generally not immediately obvious if the tightly bound fraction represents an important locus of action or not.

By contrast, the tightly binding fraction of noradrenaline in nerve endings is usually taken to represent loci of action. Thus some caution is necessary in relating the distribution of chemicals to their site of action.

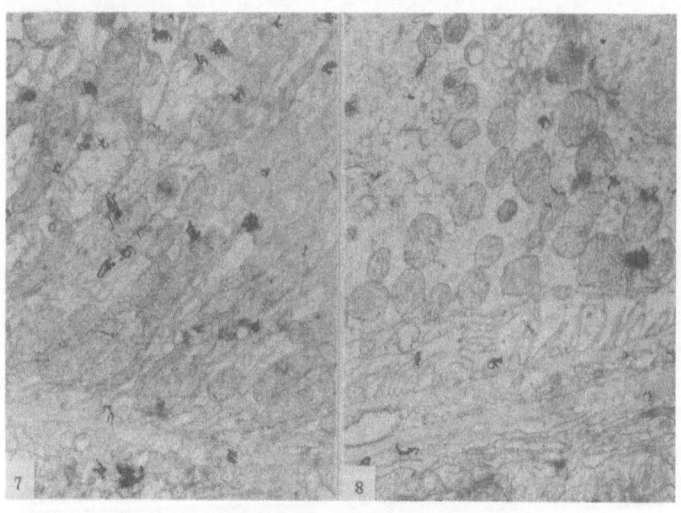

Figures 7 and 8 Electron microscope autoradiographs showing the tight binding of ^{203}Hg chlormerodrin to S_1 (**Figure 7**) and S_3 (**Figure 8**) tubules. Immersion fixation in Palades osmium tetroxide solution (x8150).

Many exogenous chemicals are metabolized, and the retention and localization of the metabolites may be of interest. Some chemicals are easier to study because they are tightly bound to cells at loci of biological effect, thus the mercurial mersalyl is bound to the proximal tubule cells (see the autoradiographs in Figures 7 and 8). Mercurials are known to covalently bond to -SH groups as part of their action. Autoradiography is the method of choice for localizing most exogenous toxic chemicals. However, the particular methodology for autoradiography[40] requires careful consideration and possibilities summarized in Table 3. Protocols A and B are used only to localize tightly bound exogenous molecules, whereas C and D are appropriate for highly diffusible substances. Protocol E[41] gives better morphology than C and D at the LM level and is useful for many organic molecules, but would not be suitable for highly diffusibles like Na^+ or Cl^- ions[42-44]; cf.[39].

Table 3 Some protocols for preparing microautoradiographs

Protocol	Immobilization process	Subsequent histological processing	Emulsion application method	Level*	Reference
A	Chemical fixation in liquid vehicle	Postfixation - dehydration, resin embedding in OsO_4	Layered with, or dipped in emulsion, e.g. NTB2, K2, L4	LM EM	Rogers[42] Williams[43]
B	Chemical fixation in liquid vehicle	Frozen sectioning - air dry	Layered with, or dipped in emulsion, e.g. NTB2, K2, L4 Dry layer L4	LM EM	Williams[43], Kuhar[65] Williams[43], Kuhar[65]
C	Freezing	Frozen sectioning	Pressed to dry emulsion AR10	LM	Appleton[56]
D	Freezing	Frozen sectioning - freeze drying of sections	Pressed to dry emulsion AR10	LM EM	Stumpf and Roth[57] Baker and Appleton[55]
E	Freezing	Freeze drying, vapour fixation resin embedding (plus silicone 200)	Cut on water, dipped in emulsion NTB2	LM	Stirling and Kinter[41]

* LM - light microscopy; EM - electron microscopy.

D.   Preservation of lipids

Lipids comprise a large and assorted collection of molecules, the common properties of which are solubility in organic solvents and (usually) insolubility in water. They range from steroids (cholesterol and many metabolic derivatives) to the numerous species of mono-, di- and triglycerides, phosphatides of choline, ethanolamine and inositol, and fatty acids; and the group also includes carotenoids and many other substances such as cardiolipin.

Unmodified lipids are generally soluble in dehydrating fluids such as alcohols and acetones, and embedding resin monomers of almost all kinds, including those sometimes referred to as "water-miscible resins". (For a comprehensive study and review see Cope and Williams[45-47], Williams[48] and Stein and Stein[49]) Despite the studies on lipid retention during tissue processing there are almost no data on kidney tissue, but there is no reason to assume it behaves differently from other tissue.

Aldehyde fixatives have virtually no effect on most steroids, their esters, phospholipids, fatty acids and neutral glycerides. Consequently the lipids of tissues which are not subjected to secondary fixation with osmium tetroxide or chromate treatment can only be conserved if frozen sections are employed (see Table 3, protocols B-E, and secondary fixation uses protocol A). It should be noted that "wet" fixatives, followed by dehydrating and embedding (Table 2), subject tissue to a wide range of solvent polarities, which ensure that anything that is extractable will be extracted. The water-miscible resins such as glycol methacrylate, hydroxpropylmethacrylate, JB4 and Lowecryl are all excellent lipid solvents. They are essentially "organic" even though they are water-miscible, but low temperature embedding in GMA (see Cope and Williams[47]) or Lowecryl 4HR may conserve some of the lipid; however the degree of preservation is not necessarily satisfactory. If dehydration is attempted, secondary fixation should always be employed. This unfortunately does not conserve cholesterol. Scallen and Dietert[52] have suggested how cholesterol can be conserved, but the efficacy of these approaches is still debated. Darrah et al[50] have indicated that cholesterol is not easily conserved in the lung, but the material left after embedding is probably not relocated. Various attempts to preserve lipids by freeze drying or freeze substitution followed by vacuum embedding have been reported. However, although scintillation counting control measures sometimes indicate high conservation levels, much of the "conserved" label is in the resin rather than in the cells. Staining methods can give some indication of the species of lipid molecule present (see Bayliss-High[51] for details), and have been used to study some kidney pathologies, e.g. nephrotic syndrome and Bright's disease. Frozen sections should ideally be used, and formaldehyde treatment to preserve proteins. The same approaches are useful in studies of intracellular neutral fat in the nephron of some species of experimental animal, e.g. dog and cat. Otherwise, autoradiography using well chosen lipid precursors has great scope when applied to tissues which have been treated to secondary OsO_4 or chromate fixation (see Stein and Stein[49]; Williams[43]). As a rider it should be noted that it may be important to conserve lipids since they are often an accumulation site for exogenous chemicals.

E. Extraction studies

In those studies where the survivals of particular chemicals are important the tissue processing fluids should be analysed. If necessary, special experiments should be set up using radiotracers and appropriate chromatography and radioisotope counting to construct a balance sheet[46,47,49]. Macromolecules may occasionally require such checks to be carried out, but these approaches are especially valuable in the study of exogenous chemicals, tissue lipids and any substances which could be diffusible. It is important to include all tissue processing fluids (even resins) in the balance sheets as lipid-soluble substances may be resin-soluble.

IV. METHODS FOR IMMOBILIZING WATER-SOLUBLE CELL AND TISSUE COMPONENTS

A. Cryofixation

All of the "wet" techniques described so far are likely to seriously disturb the levels and distributions of ions and small molecules such as Na^+ and Ca^{2+}, Mg^{2+} and Cl^- and sugars, amino acids, etc., and this has stimulated efforts to evolve preservation methods for diffusible substances. Freezing cells results in soluble substances being immobilized, but considerable effort is required to produce workable tissue preparations where water is present as an ice "glass". At temperatures above about -120 °C, frozen water grows into crystals, which can cause considerable disruption within the fine organization of the cells. To avoid this, tiny pieces of tissue about 1 mm cube must be frozen extremely rapidly. This may be achieved by quenching in Freon 22 cooled in liquid nitrogen, and storage at a very low temperature. Stumpf and Roth[53] were able to cut semi-thin sections for the autoradiography of soluble compounds. The same method is usable at the LM level for highly diffusible molecules such as iodide and sodium ions, sugars, amino acids and steroids etc. For EM studies greater structural preservation is necessary, and the addition of cryoprotectants[55] is perhaps attended by some risks of translocation. Baker and Appleton[54] have shown in autoradiographic studies of $^{22}Na^+$ that some ultrastructural studies can be effected by use of unmodified frozen kidney tissue. At the LM level, Appleton[56] has pioneered an autoradiographic method using frozen sections, and Stumpf and Roth[57] one using freeze-dried sections. Nagata and Murata[58] have also illustrated the use of fresh frozen ultra-thin sections.

After the rapid freezing of a tissue a number of technical options are available. Freeze drying is one; another is freeze drying followed by resin embedding[41,57,59-61]. A third possibility is cryoultramicrotomy at temperatures between -120 °C and -140 °C. They may be subjected to X-ray microanalysis[39] after freeze drying or with the water still in place. The latter approach has the advantage of permitting the estimation of water content at particular sites, and hence the concentrations of elements.

Freeze-substitution followed by resin embedding has been reviewed by Harvey[62]. A popular substitution fluid is 20% v/v acrolein in diethyl ether, which after a few days may be followed by embedding in epoxy resins or methacrylates at low temperatures. Stirling and Kinter[41] have described osmication and embedding of the freeze-dried tissue in an Araldite mixture containing silicone 200, to localize ouabain binding sites in rabbit kidney tubules[59,60]. This approach is not adequate for ions such as I^-, Cl^- or Na^+, but testosterone has been studied at the EM level[61].

B.   Precipitation reactions

The microscopic localization of cations by low solubility precipitates include Cl^- precipitated gold ions, Ca^{2+} and Pb^{3+} with oxalate and a variety of ions including Na^+, K^+, Zn^{2+} and Ca^{2+} with pyroantimonate[63]. These methods must engender ion translocation and precipitation losses dependent on the type of fixation employed. Baker[64] has found that osmium tetroxide used as a primary fixative is better for preserving Ca pyroantimonate precipitates than glutaraldehyde. In any event the pyroantimonate reaction is not of high specificity, and its stoichiometry is uncertain. The advantage of the methods lies in the microanalytical data obtained, combined with the good image quality yielded by standard fixation and embedding routines.

REFERENCES

1.   Lewis, P.R. and Knight, D.P., Staining methods for sectional material, in Practical Methods in Electron Microscopy, Glauert, A.M., Ed., North Holland Press, Amsterdam, 1976, Ch. 5.

2.   Horobin, R.W., Histochemistry, Gustav Fisher/Butterworth, Stuttgart, New York, London, 1982.

3.   Janigan, D.T., The effects of aldehyde fixation on acid phosphatase activity in tissue blocks, J. Histochem. Cytochem., 13, 476, 1965.

4.   Arborgh, B., Ericsson, J.L.E. and Helminen, H., Inhibition of renal acid phosphatase and aryl sulfatase activity by glutaraldehyde fixation, J. Histochem. Cytochem., 19, 449, 1971.

5.   Hopwood, D., Fixatives and fixation: a review, Histochem. J., 1, 323, 1969.

6.   Kraehenbuhl, J.P. and Jamieson, J.D., Localization of intracellular antigens using immunoelectron microscopy, in Electron Microscopy and Cytochemistry, Wisse, E., Ed., North Holland Press, Amsterdam, 1973.

7.   Hed, J. and Enastrom, S., Detection of immune deposits in glomeruli: the masking effect on antigenicity of formalin in the presence of proteins, J. Immunol. Meth., 41, 57, 1981.

8.   Brantzaeg, P. and Rognum, T.O., Evaluation of tissue preparation methods and pair immuno fluorescence staining for immunocytochemistry of lymphomas, Histochem. J., 15, 655, 1983.

9.   Hanker, J.S., Kusyk, C.J., Bloum, F.E. and Pearse, A.G.E., The demonstration of dehydrogenases and monoamineoxidase by the formation of Osmium Blacks at the site of Hatchetts Brown, Histochemie, 33, 205, 1973.

10.   Prosperi, E. and Raap, A.K., Substrate protection during the fixation of β-glucuronidase: cytochemical model system studies, Histochem. J., 14, 689, 1982.

11.   Pearse, A.G.E., Histochemistry Theoretical and Applied, 3rd Ed., Churchill-Livingstone, Edinburgh, Ch. 2, 1972.

12.   Christie, K.N. and Stoward, P.J., A quantitative study of the fixation of acid phosphatases by formaldehyde and its relevance to histochemistry, Proc.

Roy. Soc. London B, 186, 137, 1974.

13. Janigan, D.T., Tissue enzyme fixation studies. 1: The effects of aldehyde fixation on β glucoronidase, β galactosidase, N-acetyl β glucosamidase and β glucosidase in tissue blocks, Lab. Invest., 13, 1038, 1964.

14. Wachsmuth, E.D., Assessment of immunocytochemical techniques with particular reference to the mixed-aggregation immunocytochemical technique. Trends in enzyme histochemistry and cytochemistry, Ciba Foundation Symposium, 73, Elsevier/North Holland, Amsterdam, 135, 1980.

15. Berod, A., Hartman, B.K. and Piyol, J.F., Importance of fixation in immunohistochemistry: use of formaldehyde solutions at variable pH for the localization of tyrosine hydroxylase, J. Histochem. Cytochem., 29, 844, 1981.

16. Kyte, J., Immunoferritin determination of the distribution of (Na^+K^+) ATPase over the plasma membranes of renal convoluted tubules. I: Distal segment, J. Cell. Biol., 68, 287, II: J. Cell. Biol., 68, 314, 1976.

17. Kumplainen, T., Human carbonic anhydrase EC 4.2.1.1 isoenzyme C effects of some fixatives on the antigenicity and improvement in the method of localization, Histochemistry, 72, 425, 1981.

18. Vogt, A., Bockburn, H., Kosima, K. and Sonsaki, M., Electron microscopic localization of the nephro-toxic antibody in the glomeruli of the rat after intravenous application of purified nephrito-genic antibody-ferritin conjugates, J. Exp. Med., 127, 687, 1968.

19. Graham, R.C. and Karnovsky, M.J., The early stages of absorption of injected horseradish peroxidase in the proximal tubules of the mouse kidney, J. Histochem. Cytochem., 14, 291, 1966.

20. Cope, G.H., Low temperature embedding in water miscible methacrylates after treatment with antifreezes, J. R. Microsc. Soc., 88, 235, 1968.

21. Williams, M.A. and Lowrie, J.I., this volume.

22. Brahic, M., Haase, A.T. and Cash, E., Simultaneous in situ detection of viral RNA and antigens, Proc. Natl. Acad. Sci. USA, 81, 5445, 1984.

23. Myerson, D., Hackman, R.C., Nelson, J.A., Ward, D.C. and MacDougall, J.K., Widespread presence of histologically occult cytomegalovirins, Hum. Pathol., 15, 430, 1984.

24. Jamrich, M., Mahon, K.A., Garvis, E.R. and Gall, J.G., Histone RNA in amphibian oocytes visualized by in situ hybridisation to methacylate-embedded tissue sections, EMBO J., 3, 1939, 1984.

25. Engfelt, B. and Hjertquist, S-O., The effect of various fixatives on the preservation of acid glycosaminoglycans in tissues, Acta Pathol. Microbiol. Scand., 71, 219, 1967.

26. Scott, J.E., Tigwell, M.J. and Sajdera, S.W., Loss of basophilic (sulphated) material from sections of cartilage treated with periodate solution, Histochem. J., 4, 155, 1972.

27. Benditt, E.P., Martin, G.M. and Plattner, H., Application of freeze-drying and formaldehyde vapour fixation to radioautographic localization of soluble aminoacids, in The Use of Radioautography in Studying Protein Synthesis, Leblond, C.P. and Warren, K., Eds., Academic Press, New York and London, 65, 1965.

28. Caro, L.G. and Palade, G.E., Protein synthesis and storage and discharge in the pancreatic exocrine cell. An autoradiographic study, J. Cell. Biol., 20, 473, 1964.

29. Clarke, S.L., The synthesis and storage of protein in isolated lymphoid cells, examined by autoradiography with the electron microscope, Am. J. Anat., 119, 375, 1966.

30. Peters, T. and Ashley, C.A., An artifact in radioautography due to binding

of the amino acids to tissues by fixatives, J. Cell. Biol., 33, 53, 1967.

31. Orkland, P.M. and Kravitz, E.A., Localization of the site of gamma-aminobutyric acid (GABA) uptake in lobster nerve-muscle preparations, J. Cell. Biol., 49, 75, 1971.

32. Faeder, I.R. and Salpeter, M.M., Glutamate uptake by a stimulated insect nerve-muscle preparation, J. Cell. Biol., 46, 300, 1970.

33. Price, D.L., Stocks, J.W., Young, A. and Peck, K., Glycine-specific synapses in spinal cord. Identification by electron microscope autoradiography, J. Cell. Biol., 68, 389, 1976.

34. Lowrie, J.I., Baker, J.R.J. and Williams, M.A., in Renal Heterogenicity and Target Cell Toxicity, Bach, P.H., Ed., Wiley & Sons, New York, 1985

35. Wachsmuth, E.D. and Woodhaus, R., Uniform distribution and concentration of aminopeptidase in proximal tubules of pig kidney, J. Histochem. Cytochem., 21, 685, 1973.

36. Williams, M.A., Electron microscopic autoradiography: its application to protein biosynthesis, in Techniques in Protein Biosynthesis, Campbell, P.N. and Sargent, J.R., Eds., Academic Press, London, 125, Ch. 3, 1973.

37. Bogaroch, R., Studies on the intracellular localization of tritiated steroids, in Autoradiography of Diffusible Substances, Roth, L.J. and Stumpf, W.E., Eds., Academic Press, New York and London, 99, 1969.

38. Williams, M.A. and Baba, W.I., The localization of (^{3}H)-aldosterone and (^{3}H)-cortisol within renal tubular cells by electron microscopic autoradiography, J. Endocrinol., 39, 543, 1967.

39. Chandler, J.A., X-ray microanalysis in the electron microscope, in Practical Methods in Electron Microscopy, Glauert, A.M., Ed., North Holland Press, Amsterdam, Ch. 5, 1977.

40. Baker, J.R.J., this volume.

41. Stirling, C.E. and Kinter, W.B., High resolution autoradiography of galactose-^{3}H accumulation in rings of hamster intestine, J. Cell. Biol., 35, 585, 1967.

42. Rogers, A.W., Techniques of autoradiography, 3rd Ed., Elsevier, Amsterdam, 1979.

43. Williams, M.A., Autoradiography and immunocytochemistry, in Practical Methods in Electron Microscopy, Glauert, A.M., Ed., North Holland Press, Amsterdam, 6, 1977.

44. Williams, M.A., Autoradiography: its methodology at the present time, J. Microsc., 128, 79, 1982.

45. Cope, G.H. and Williams, M.A., Quantitative studies on neutral lipid preservation in electron microscopy, J. Roy. Microsc. Soc., 88, 259, 1968.

46. Cope, G.H. and Williams, M.A., Quantitative studies on the preservation of choline and ethanolamine phosphatides during tissue preservation for electron microscopy, I, J. Microsc., 90, 31, 1969.

47. Cope, G.H. and Williams, M.A., Quantitative studies on the preservation of choline and ethanolamine phosphatides during tissue preservation for electron microscopy, II, J. Microsc., 90, 47, 1969.

48. Williams, M.A., The assessment of electron microscopic autoradiographs, in Advances in Optical and Electron Microscopy, Barer, R. and Cosslett, E.V., Eds., Academic Press, London and New York, 219, Ch. 3, 1969.

49. Stein, O. and Stein, Y., Light and electron microscopic radioautography of lipids: techniques and biological applications, Adv. Lipid. Res., 9, 1, 1971.

50. Darrah, H.K., Hedley-Whyte, H. and Hedley-Whyte, E.T., Radioautography of cholesterol in lung, J. Cell. Biol., 49, 345, 1971.

51. Bayliss-High, O., Lipid histochemistry, Royal Microscopical Society, Oxford

University Press, 69, 1984.

52.   Scallen, T.J. and Dietert, S.E., The quantitative retention of cholesterol in mouse liver prepared for electron microscopy by fixation in a digitonin containing aldehyde solution, J. Cell. Biol., 40, 802, 1969.

53.   Stumpf, W.E. and Roth, L.J., Thin section cut at temperatures of -70 °C to -90 °C, Nature, 205, 712, 1965.

54.   Barnard, T., Ultrastructural effects of the high molecular weight cryoprotectants Dextran and polyvinylpyrrolidone on liver and brown adipose tissue in vitro, J. Microsc., 120, 93, 1980.

55.   Baker, J.R.J. and Appleton, T.C., A technique for electron microscopic autoradiography (and X-ray microanalysis) of diffusible substances using freeze-dried fresh frozen sections, J. Microsc., 108, 307, 1976.

56.   Appleton, T.C., Autoradiographs of soluble labelled compounds, J. Roy. Microsc. Soc., 83, 277, 1964.

57   Stumpf, W.E. and Roth, L.J., Vacuum freeze drying of frozen sections for dry mounting high resolution autoradiography, Stain Technol., 39, 219, 1964.

58.   Nagata, T. and Murata, F., Proc. 5th Int. Congr. Histochem. Cytochem., Bucharest, 1976.

59.   Shaver, J. and Stirling, C.E., Ouabain binding to renal tubules of the rabbit, J. Cell. Biol., 76, 278, 1978.

60.   Ernst, S.A. and Mills, J.W., Autoradiographic localization of ouabain-sensitive sodium pump sites in ion transporting epithelia, J. Histochem. Cytochem., 28, 72, 1980.

61.   Fredericks, P.M., Autoradiography of diffusible substances, Thesis, Erasmus University, Rotterdam.

62.   Harvey, D.M.R., Freeze-substitution. J. Microsc., 127, 209, 1982.

63.   Simson, J.A.V., Blank, H.L. and Spicer, S.S., X-ray microanalysis of pyroantimonate precipitable cations, Scan. Electron Microsc., II, 779, 1979.

64.   Baker, J.R.J., personal communication.

65.   Kuhar, W.S. and Young, M.J., A new method of receptor autoradiography: [^{3}H] opioid receptors in rat brain, Brain Res., 179, 255, 1979.

17

2

THE APPLICATION OF HISTOCHEMISTRY AT THE LIGHT MICROSCOPIC LEVEL TO THE STUDY OF NEPHROTOXICITY

P.H. BACH, N.J GREGG AND E.D. WACHSMUTH

I. INTRODUCTION

Light microscopy continues to represent the major method by which nephropathies are identified in chemical safety assessment[1] and in the clinical situation[2]. While ultrastructural studies provide a very important technique for detailed subcellular investigations, they generally do not contribute to diagnosis or treatment. Furthermore, these specialized methods are both time-consuming and costly. Histochemical techniques at the light microscopic level provide a broad approach to the study of renal injury that cannot, at present, be investigated as conveniently by electron microscopy or any biochemical method. Haematoxylin and eosin (H&E) is the routine histochemical stain used to vizualize cells, cellular structures and changes associated with tissue injury. Once cell changes have been identified by H&E a host of other histochemical techniques can be applied to help interpret the cause(s) of a lesion. There are, however, examples where subtle or specific cellular changes have not been identified by H&E, and hence more sophisticated techniques are needed. This full range of "routine" to highly "specialized" techniques can all be used to address the question of the molecular changes associated with a toxic insult.

There is also a need to understand more about the factors involved in the degenerative changes that follow a primary renal lesion. These often occur in a discrete anatomical region of the kidney, and subsequently lead to the involvement of other areas. Histochemical methods may help to define and inter-relate the cascade of degenerative changes that follow primary injury and provide information on morphology, cell constituents and biochemistry, from which the "final" renal lesion can be understood.

Normal renal morphology at the light microscopic level has been reported by Moffat[3] and Kriz[4] for the rat, Kaissling and

Kriz[5] for the rabbit and by Kriz and Koepsell[6] for the mouse. This chapter will discuss those applications of renal histochemistry that have been useful in identifying, localizing and understanding a variety of chemically induced renal lesions. Both conventional histochemical methods and the specific receptor-mediated techniques (e.g. antibody, lectin, radiolabelled chemicals) will be considered. Where appropriate attention will be focused on how these techniques can be used to help understand the primary lesion.

A.   Nomenclature and inter-relating histochemical and biochemical changes

This chapter will use the term histochemistry to cover those techniques that involve the microscopic assessment of tissue "biochemistry". Immunohistochemistry is a sub-branch which is highly selective and sensitive. The microdissection of material from the different regions of the nephron will not be considered.

There is a great deal of difficulty in inter-relating the findings of histochemistry with those from pure biochemistry. This is not surprising because of the difficulties in analysing materials in a complex environment such as tissue sections. Also the mass of the material available is small and instrumentation to quantify data is extended to its limits. There are a number of analytical constraints using tissue sections that have been exposed to various treatments (e.g. fixation, freeze-drying, embedding, etc.), to conserve morphological features.

Another problem in interpreting histochemistry is the inconsistency in terminology. The often confused nomenclature for complex carbohydrates[7,8] has highlighted the need to exercise caution in naming material assessed by histochemistry in biochemical terms. Similarly, "lipid" material may be a measure of hydrophilicity; the high affinities of a binding site present on an antibody are of little value if the antigen is masked; even a monoclonal antibody may bind to non-specific sites and the binding of lectins may be changed by a number of factors. It is well established that proteolytic or cytolytic processes accompany cell damage, and the associated changes may destroy or unmask reactive sites, or alter the cell's microenvironment. Histochemical methods may, however, cause reproducible artefacts, which are of value for diagnosis and may even lead to the better understanding of the pathomechanism of injury. Validation of each method is needed for the most relevant interpretation of data, and several criteria have been put forward[9]. Thus all data derived from histochemical methods should be interpreted with caution. It is also necessary to understand the potential and limitations of each of the histochemical methods being used.

B.   Frozen or fixed tissue

Different techniques of preparing tissue may affect histochemical methods because of the unique chemical process upon which each functional group or biological activity is based. Increasingly, two or more histochemical methods are used in tandem (either on serial sections or the same section), thus the possibility can arise of an optimal fixation procedure for one method that precludes the use of other techniques.

II.   ENZYMES

Enzymes have been determined in nephron segments by microdissection using fluorimetric or radiochemical assay methods[10-12], or by incubating whole kidney sections with substrates that are specific for the particular enzyme (together with a coupling reagent if necessary)[13-47].

Table 1 Typical enzyme activities that can be shown in the kidney by several different methods

Enzyme	Reference
Acid phosphatase	13-15
Alkaline phosphatase	13,14,16
D-Amino acid oxidase	17
Aminopeptidase	16,18,19
Mg^{2+}-ATPase	14,20
Carbonic anhydrase	21,22
Cytochrome oxidase	23
Diaphorase	24,25
Glucose-6-phosphatase	26
Glucose-6-phosphate dehydrogenase	23
β-Glucuronidase	13
Gamma-glutamyl-transpeptidase	16,27
Glutamic dehydrogenase	28
β-Hydroxybutyric dehydrogenase	24
Inosine 5'-diphosphatase	29
Invertase	30
Lactic dehydrogenase	31
Leucine aminopeptidase	32
Non-specific esterase	13
Succinic dehydrogenase	23,25,33,34

The final reaction product (FRP), gives data on the distribution and relative activity of the enzyme if it has adequate contrast and is localized to the site of formation. Traditionally enzyme histochemistry has been undertaken in fresh frozen or fixed sections, where the range of enzymic activities that have been assayed are very large (Table 1).

Pitfalls in using the enzyme histochemical approach are numerous. For example, lactic dehydrogenase (LDH) isoenzymes type A4 (M-LDH) diffuses approximately six times slower than type B4 (H-LDH) in muscle[35] and since the molar substrate turnover of M-LDH is twice that of H-LDH it will produce more FRP, even if its concentration at the tissue site had been originally smaller. Both of these isoenzymes are present in the different parts of the kidney[31,36], and failure to differentiate between the two could lead to erroneous conclusions. Intracellular peptidases appear to be less affected by pathological changes than brush-border membrane peptidases[37,38], but the difference may not become apparent due to intracellular enzyme diffusion artefacts.

Table 2 The effects of different classes of lytic enzymes on the normal expression of renal membrane bound marker enzymes

	Renal marker enzymes			
	5'-Nucleotidase	ATPase	Alkaline phosphatase	Leucyl-β-naphthylamidase
Lipolytic enzymes				
Phospholipase C	+++	++	0	0
Lipase VII	0	0	0	0
Glycolytic enzymes				
Neuraminidase	++	0	0	0
β-Galactosidase	++	0	0	0
β-Glucosidase	0	0	0	0
Proteolytic enzymes				
Trypsin	++	0	0	++
Papain	+	+	0	++
Protease	++	+	0	+
α-Chymotrypsin	0	0	0	+
δ-Chymotrypsin	0	0	0	+
Collagenase	0	0	0	0

0 = No changes, + = slight, ++ = moderate and +++ = strong decrease in activity compared to controls.

The interpretation of changes in the amount of FRP also presents a problem, where it is often difficult to be certain whether the increased activities represent de novo synthesis, unmasking, or the loss of factors that normally inhibit the reaction. Hardonk et al.[39] described the influence of a variety of lytic enzymes on renal membrane-bound markers. Exposure of normal renal cryostat sections to lipolytic, glycolytic and proteolytic enzymes showed that some renal marker enzyme activities were decreased, while others were unaffected (Table 2). By contrast liver sections showed increased enzyme activities. These data illustrate the complexity in interpreting changes induced by similar enzymes.

Another problem that pervades enzyme histochemistry is that cryostat sections less than 4 μm can rarely be cut from large pieces of tissue, and more often sections are 8-10 μm, as a result of which microscopic resolution may be unsatisfactory. The introduction of the hydrophilic methacrylate-based embedding media has facilitated production of 1 μm sections routinely. Provided mild fixation protocols are followed (see below) an unknown fraction of the original enzymic activity may be maintained, which (if it is more than 10%) suffices for histochemistry. Fixation may, however, totally change enzyme distribution compared to frozen sections. The alkaline phosphatase staining pattern in proximal tubules may be reversed by fixing[45]. Similarly, aminopeptidase is localized to the brush-border when assessed in frozen sections by the localization of FRP and antibodies directed against the enzyme[18,46], but the cytoplasm of low-temperature fixed tissue[41]. Alternatively, other enzymes such as human carbonic anhydrase are not greatly altered[21,47].

A.   Frozen sections

The proximal tubules can be identified by the wide variety of brush-border membrane enzymes, but other nephron segments (such as the distal tubule or the connecting and collecting ducts), have specific immunologically reactive markers (see below). A variety of other oxidative enzymes[48] have been characterized in the kidney, notably the medullary collecting duct and interstitial cells.

LDH has been widely used as a urinary marker of renal injury, and early studies showed that its distribution in the kidney was ubiquitous, although the collecting duct and proximal tubule stain most strongly. This has been of little use in the histochemical identification of the target of renal injury. The addition of 4 M urea to the incubation system inhibits LDH isoenzyme(s) and has allowed the distribution of renal LDH to be defined in terms of its different activities. The thick ascending limb and the distal tubule are rich in H-LDH, whereas the convoluted tubules of the inner cortex, collecting ducts, glomeruli and vasa recta contain largely M-LDII[31], a finding that is consistant with immunohistochemical data[36].

Heterogeneity in histochemistry is also evident in each part of the nephron in different species[34]. Figure 1 illustrates the difference of FRP concentrations of three enzymes in the   rat, rabbit, dog, marmoset and baboon kidney. This comparison shows that none of these enzymes are ideal markers for any nephron segment in these species. GGT appears to be the best general marker to identify proximal tubule segments[49]. In addition to species differences,   sex-linked,   ontogeny and differentiation-dependent differences occur.

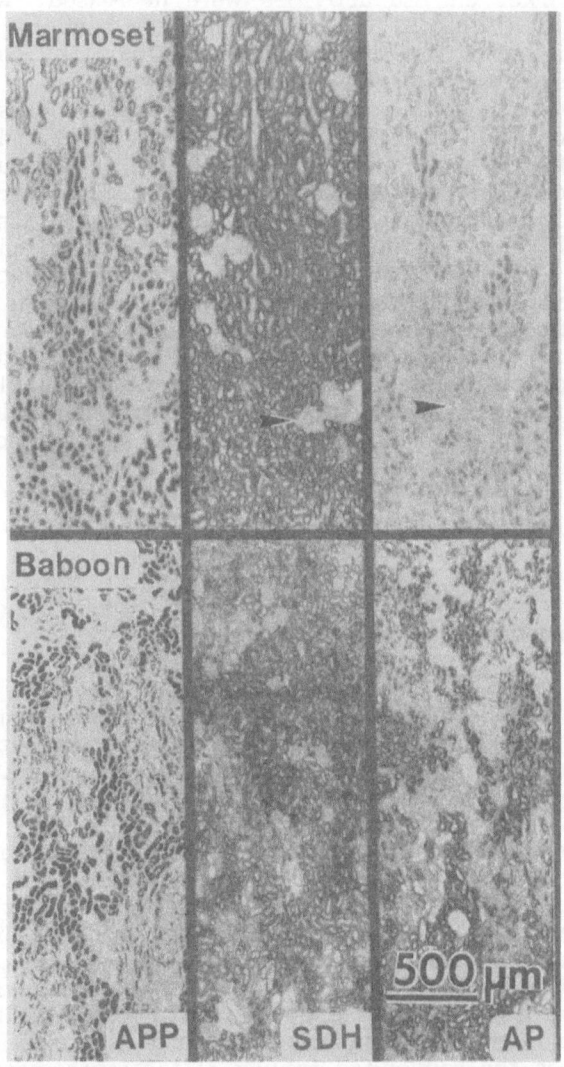

Figure 1 Enzyme histochemistry of normal kidney. The concentration of the FRP of a given enzyme is different in each nephron segment and the distribution is not the same in different species. The FRP pattern also varies with each enzyme. Frozen, acetone-fixed serial sections stained for the brush-border enzymes alkaline phosphatase (APP) and aminopeptidase (AP), and the mitochondrial enzyme succinic dehydrogenase (SDH). Cortex at the top and outer stripe of outer medulla at the bottom of each photograph. Arrow head pointing to arteria arcuata. Same magnification throughout.

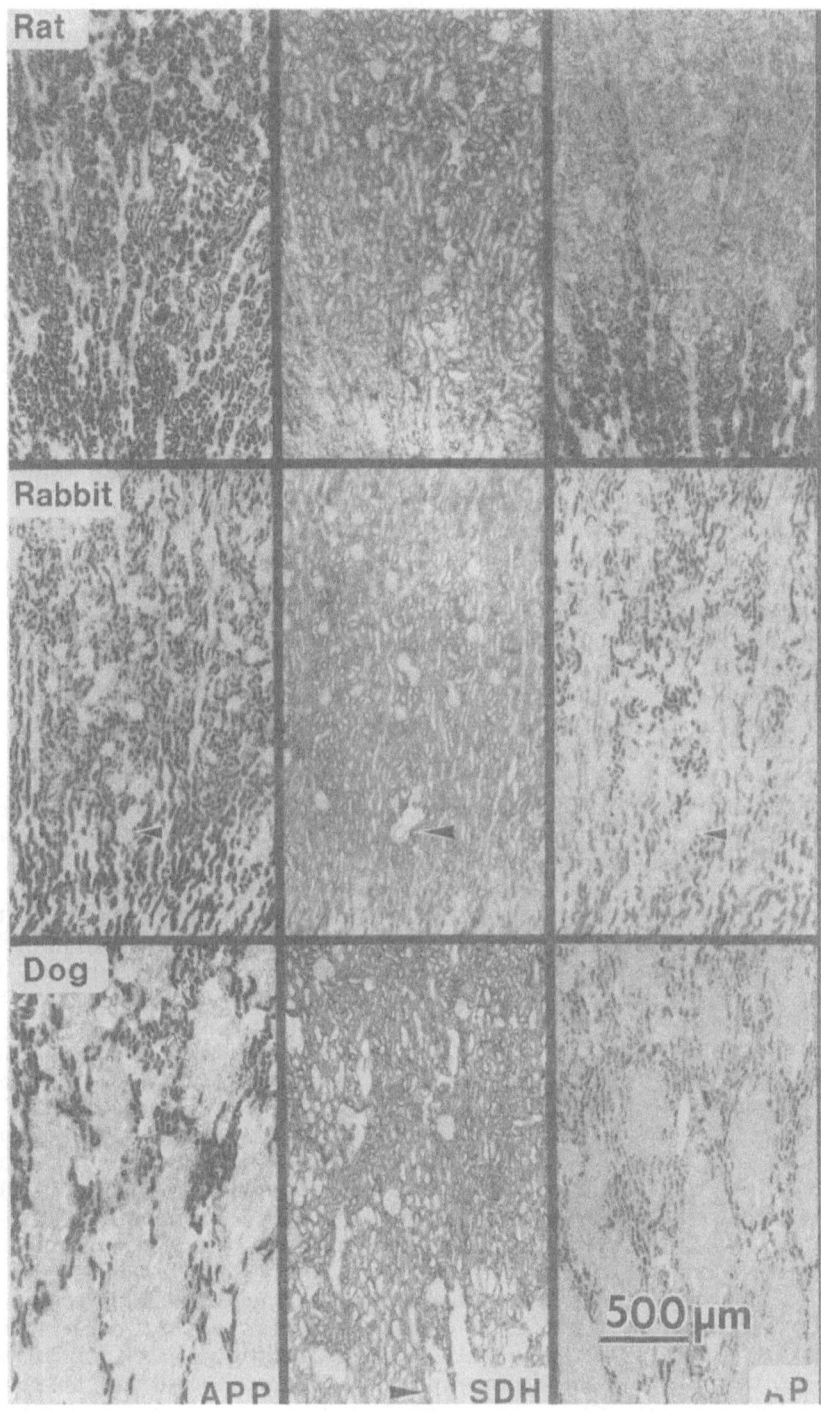

Figure 1 continued

For instance, sex differences in P_1 and P_2 segments of the proximal tubule have been described for various cytoplasmic NAD- and NADP-dependent oxido-reductases and some mitochondrial enzymes in the rat[50-53]. Differential increases of brush-border membrane enzymes and cytoplasmic enzymes during ontogeny have also been demonstrated[51,54,55].

Renal lesions can be detected by changes in renal (enzyme) catalytic FRP following exposure to a variety of chemicals[33] including mercury[14,34,23,26,55,56], D-serine[34] and cephaloridine[57]. In general chemical insults may be vizualized by a reduced FRP in the area of lesion, but it has been very difficult to interpret, particularly in relation to changes in urinary enzymes. Cottrell and co-workers[32] showed that loss of alkaline phosphatase, lactate dehydrogenase and leucine aminopeptidase FRP all closely paralleled the dose- and time-related damage to the renal cortex caused by mercuric chloride and p-aminophenol. By contrast, increased glucose-6-phosphatase FRP, in the inner cortex (where it is normally not detected), following mercuric chloride-induced injury, was taken as evidence for the utilization of glucose needed for energy production during the repair phase[23,26], and supports the concept of cell regeneration. FRP formed by the catalytic activity of succinic dehydrogenase, non-specific esterase, and in particular alkaline phosphatase and aminopeptidase have been shown to be valuable indicators of acute nephrotoxicity after cephaloridine administration to rats and rabbits[58].

FRP concentrations of a well chosen enzyme may be suitable for defining the site and quantifying the severity of renal lesions. In mice, proximal tubules of the outer stripe of the outer medulla contain twice the concentration of aminopeptidase compared to the cortical tubules[59]. Thus the enzyme cannot be used to demonstrate lesions in the proximal tubule or the proximal convoluta in general, whereas alkaline phosphatase, which does not show this difference in mice and rats, has proved useful. So it can be clearly demonstrated by means of alkaline phosphatase FRP that the P_3 segments of rats, but not of rabbits, are affected by cefsulodin[60-62]. By contrast, cephaloridine was shown to affect mainly the P_1 and P_2 segments in both species[57]. This can be automated by means of television image analysis which compares areas with high FRP alkaline phosphatase concentrations (e.g. brush-border membrane) within areas of low FRP concentrations (e.g. proximal tubule cross-sections). The loss of alkaline phosphatase FRP is a measure of the number of proximal tubules with lesions. For instance, the area occupied by the proximal tubular marker decreased with increased doses of cephaloridine in rats and rabbits. Pretreatment with probenecid prevented the lesion, in agreement with the protective effects of this anion transport inhibitor, and the area of FRP was closer to controls[60].

The changes in acid phosphatase and succinic dehydrogenase FRP following a single dose of cis-platin (Figure 2) demonstrate the unsuitability of these two staining techniques for quantification, because the resolution for the different segments is poor, and there is no discrimination on the FRP level between damaged tubules and those with naturally low enzymic activity. In this instance the use of brush-border membrane enzymes is better[49].

26

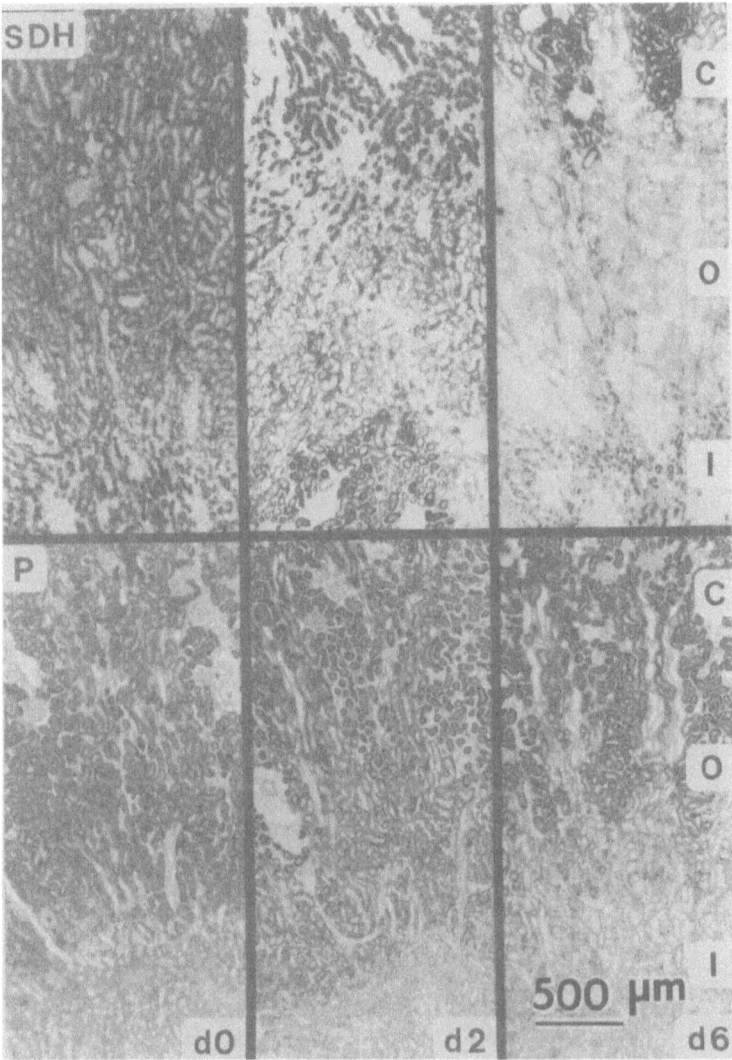

Figure 2 Histochemistry showing the loss of enzymic activity and proximal tubular cell necrosis in the outer stripe of the outer medulla of the male rat kidney over several days after a single i.v. dose of 6 mg/kg cis-platinum. Sections show control (d0), and changes after 2 days (d2) and 6 days (d6). Frozen, acetone-fixed sections stained for the mitochondrial enzyme succinic dehydrogenase (SDH). Baker-fixed frozen sections stained for the lysosomal enzyme acid phosphatase (P). Cortex (C), outer stripe (O) and inner stripe (I) of outer medulla. Same magnification throughout.

27

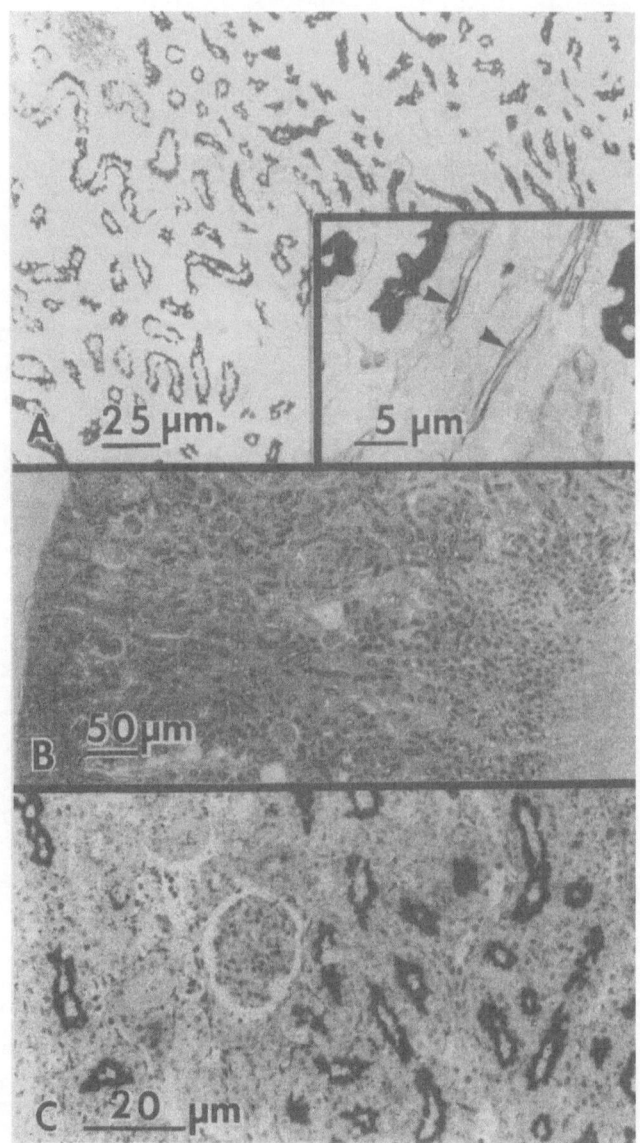

Figure 3 Enzyme histochemistry in semi-thin sections of fixed renal tissue.
A. Alkaline phosphatase staining of proximal tubule brush-borders in a 1 μm section
of control kidney embedded in glycol methacrylate. Methyl green pyronin counter-
stain. Insert shows endothelial staining with alkaline phosphatase (arrowheads).
B. Distribution of adenosine triphosphatase (ATPase) in control kidney proximal
tubule brush border in cortex only, in 1 μm semi-thin section of glycol methacrylate
embedded kidney. Counterstained with methyl green pyronin. **C.** Gamma-glutamyltranspeptidase (GGT) staining of proximal tubule brush border in control kidney embedded in glycol methacrylate, counterstained with haematoxylin.

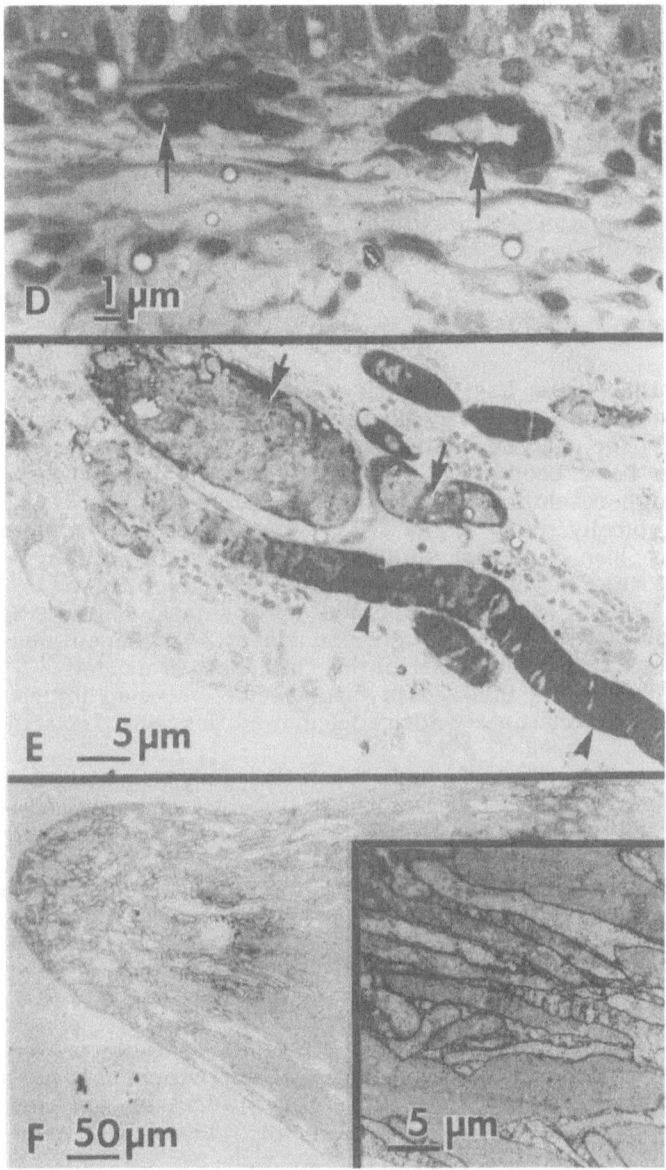

Figure 3 D. Increased ATPase staining of endothelium (arrow) in basal sub-urothelial capillaries 144 h after a single 100 mg/kg i.p. dose of 2-bromoethanamine (BEA). Kidney embedded in glycol methacrylate, 1 μm section counterstained with methyl green pyronin. **E.** Alkaline phosphatase staining of proteinaceous casts in necrotic loops of Henle (arrows) and collecting ducts (arrowheads) in papilla 144 h after single 100 mg/kg i.p. injection of BEA. Kidney embedded in glycol methacrylate counterstained with methyl green pyronin. **F.** GGT staining in necrotic papilla 144 h after single i.p. injection of BEA (100 mg/kg). Kidney embedded in glycol methacrylate 1 μm section counterstained with haematoxylin.

Renal enzymic changes may also be associated with abnormal kidney physiology in the absence of an overt lesion. Ammonium chloride (0.25 mol/l) given to rats in drinking water over 6 days induces acidosis and renal enlargement[28]. Histochemically, increased glutamic dehydrogenase FRP was found in the straight and proximal convoluted tubule, whereas in control rats it was seen in the straight portion. This finding is compatible with nephron adaptation or expression of renal functional reserve following exposure to injury or abnormal demands, such as the increased ammonia production in these NH_4Cl-loaded animals[28].

B. Methacrylate-embedded fixed tissue

Glycolmethacrylate has recently been widely adopted for routine high-resolution microscopy, where it is used particularly advantageously for enzyme histochemistry. A large number of fixation protocols have been used, but the common factors for successful use of high-resolution enzyme histochemistry has been low temperature (typically -25 to +4 °C), low concentration of fixative (typically less than 5% glutaraldehyde, paraformaldehyde and/or calcium:formaldehyde) and the minimal period of fixation[40-44]. Excellent ATPase, acid and alkaline phosphatase, GGT (Figure 3), non-specific esterase, β-glucuronidase, aminopeptidase, and cytochrome C oxidase distribution has been reported[40-44,63] and changes have been followed in target selective renal injuries caused by 2-bromoethanamine, indomethacin, adriamycin, hexachlorobutadiene and polybrene[64-66].

Similarly, the same high-resolution enzyme histochemistry has been used to demonstrate a number of key marker enzymes in normal and diseased human renal tissue. These include α-naphthylacetate esterase (ANAE), acid and alkaline phosphatase, and ATPase, all of which are confined to the tubule and collecting ducts in the normal kidney following paraformaldehyde fixation[67,68,68a]. Whereas severely damaged allographs generally retained this staining pattern, there are histochemical differences in renal malignancies. For example, it was possible to differentiate 90% of renal carcinoma based on reduced reactions for acid and alkaline phosphatase, and ANAE. By contrast 90% of Wilm's tumours were weakly positive for acid phosphatase and ANAE. Other enzyme activities (e.g. 5'-nucleotidase) have also been studied in non-renal human tissue using acetone or periodate-lysine paraformaldehyde fixation for 4 h at 4 °C in calcium:formaldehyde[69].

C. Enzymic changes in parenchymal and urothelial malignancies

Renal cell carcinoma accounts for about 85% of all primary kidney malignancies in man[70], where the histogenesis is thought to be from the epithelium of the proximal tubule. These carcinomas can be induced in experimental animals by the use of N-hydroxyethylnitrosamine (EHEN) and dimethylnitrosamine. Jasmin and Riopelle[71] reported that the enzymic profile of the tumours suggested their proximal tubular origins, although glucose-6-phosphatase, 5'-nucleotidase and alkaline phosphatase stained much less intensely than the normal adjacent epithelial cells. Subsequently, there was little GGT and alkaline phosphatase FRP compared to the adjacent tissue[72,73]. The presence of PAS-positive brush-border on the carcinoma cells also served to confirm their origins[73]. The GGT-FRP is also much reduced in human and rat fetal cells[74,75]. Taken together these data suggest that the EHEN-induced neoplasia represents similar undifferentiated and rapidly dividing cells[72].

The histochemical changes associated with chemically induced urothelial malignancies are also widely studied. Kunze[76-79] and others[80,81] have shown the focal loss of alkaline phosphatase from otherwise apparently histologically normal rat bladder urothelial cells follows carcinogenic doses of di-N-butylnitrosamine, N-butyl-N-(4-hydoxybutyl)-nitrosamine (HO-BBN) or N-[4-(5-nitro-2-furyl)-2-thiazolyl]formamide. The loss of alkaline phosphatase was irreversible and occurred after the discontinuation of the carcinogen; it could not therefore be a direct toxic effect. These alkaline phosphatase-free cells are considered to be preneoplastic, and develop into papillomas and carcinomas (Figure 4).

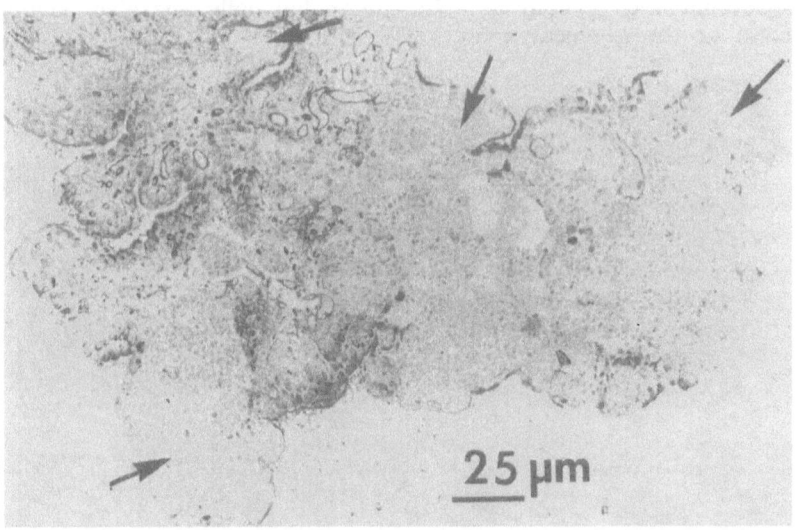

Figure 4 Mosaic pattern of alkaline phosphatase staining in bladder papilloma from animal initiated with HO-BBN then promoted with BEA and sacrificed 18 weeks later. Arrows show "preneoplastic" areas with focal loss of staining. Bladder embedded in glycol methacrylate 1 μm sections counterstained with methyl green pyronin.

Ozono[82] has also shown that a high frequency of GGT-positive cells is present in otherwise normal urothelia after exposure to HO-BBN. GGT-positive cells are already well established as markers for the premalignant changes in other organs[83-89]. It has therefore been generally assumed that the presence of foci of GGT in the urothelia is a sensitive and specific marker of malignancy, especially because these changes are present in nodular hyperplasia and carcinoma that develops after HO-BBN. These enzymic changes may not be pathognomonic indicators of premalignant changes under all circumstances. For example, Vanderlaan et al.[90] suggested that GGT-FRP identifies only advanced carcinoma and large papillomas. Similarly, whereas Kunze[76-79] has reported a variable reduction in NADPH-diaphorase in about two-thirds of the urothelial cells with reduced alkaline phosphatase activity, Vanderlaan et al.[90] found increased NADPH-diaphorase in focal nodular hyperplasia, under similar experimental conditions.

III. CARBOHYDRATES

A number of different types of carbohydrate material predominate in discrete anatomical areas of the kidney, and the histochemistry of each shows their unique localization. The basement membrane of the proximal tubule, and especially the glomeruli, are filled with a mucopolysaccharide (MPS) matrix, the medulla interstitium is very rich in MPS (Figure 5), and the distal tubule is coated with glycoproteins and glycolipids. The urothelial cells are also covered by mucin or the glycocalyx[91].

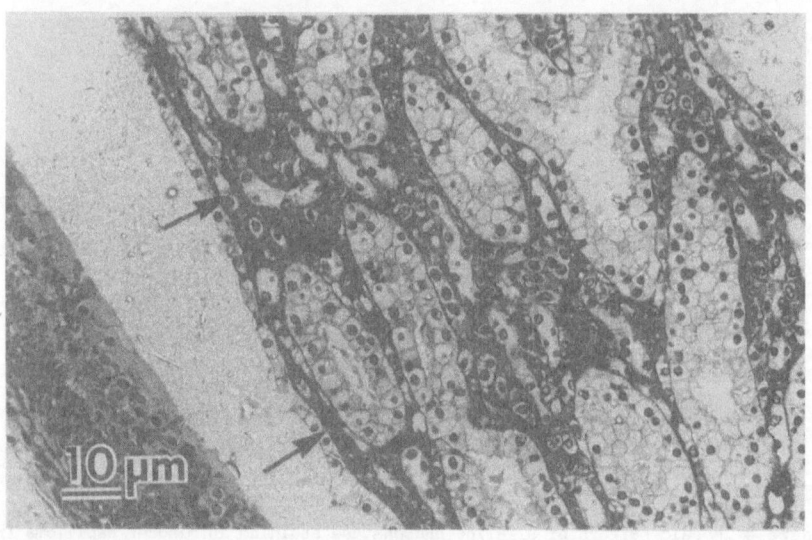

Figure 5 Mucopolysaccharide (MPS) staining of medullary interstitial matrix (arrows) in control kidney embedded in glycol methacrylate 1 μm section, Giemsa.

A. Chemical reactions

The individual classes of carbohydrate may, to some extent, be differentiated by simple histochemistry. For example, basement membrane, proximal tubule brush-border and surface mucin are rich in poly-vic-glycols and give a high-contrast stain with periodic acid and Schiff (PAS) or methanamine silver[91,92]. Some of the complex carbohydrates, such as Tamm-Horsfall glycoprotein, only stain weakly by this method and immunohistochemistry is much more effective (see below).

1.   Mucopolysaccharides

Mucopolysaccharides (MPS), which in biochemical terms are considered to be glycosaminoglycans, and their supramolecular structures, the proteoglycans, are present in:

(i)   the glomeruli, where they form an essential part of the glomerular basement membrane, and (through their poly-anionic nature) impart permselectivity to the glomerular apparatus;

(ii)   the medulla, where the very extensive quantities of MPS represent a tissue of transition for binding water and cations that are in the process of being reabsorbed.

(iii) The binding capacity for both water and cations is very high and if the matrix is disrupted (see below) the homeostasis of water and electrolyte will be markedly altered.

A number of histochemical methods have been used to show the strongly acidic nature of this matrix[92,93]. The histochemical demonstration of these molecules depends to a significant extent on the method used for fixing tissue[94], and it may be preferable to the use of cetylpyridinium chloride to insolubilize MPS[95].

Several early publications reported that the decrease of MPS staining by the addition of magnesium chloride could be used to identify the type of glycosaminoglycan in biochemical terms[96]. This is not the case. On the other hand, selective enzymic digestion[97,98] of MPS reported for non-renal tissue may help define the presence of a specific glycosaminoglycan in a matrix. The autoradiographic distribution of labelled glycosaminoglycan precursors may not help substantiate the presence of MPS[99], because these molecules are also taken up into glycoproteins, and the carbohydrates may be extensively metabolized to other molecules.

(a) Disruption of glomerular carbohydrate. The glomerular basement membrane is thickened in diabetes and nephrotic syndrome when assessed by the PAS stain[100]. The proteinuria associated with a number of chemical insults may be caused by damage to the glomerular basement membrane, altering the foot process and the loss of the polyanionic matrix. This contributes to a loss of permselectivity and the increased leakage of proteins. For example, adriamycin causes a proteinuria that may result from the disruption of the basement membrane-related MPS. Bertani et al.[101] have shown that within 3 h of adriamycin administration the polyanionic sites of the glomerular epithelial cell decrease progres-

33

sively, a change that precedes proteinuria and ultrastructural abnormalities.

(b) Disruption of medullary MPS. The medullary MPS serves as a tissue of transition for water and electrolyte homeostasis, supports the delicate elements of the microvasculature and loops of Henle, and provides some support for the collecting ducts. Loss of medullary MPS histochemical staining has been observed in several instances. For example, McAuliffe[102] has shown that the intensity of the medullary interstitial MPS staining is greatly reduced in the homozygous Brattleboro rat, but returns to near normal if these animals are treated with antidiuretic hormone. Similarly, the interstitial matrix MPS staining is greatly reduced in rodents with lithium-induced nephropathy[103]. Such observations are consistent with lithium blocking the actions of antidiuretic hormone, but appear to be a secondary consequence of the lithium toxicity rather than a cause.

The loss of MPS staining from the medulla has also been reported in association with renal papillary necrosis. Medullary MPS staining has been reported to be both increased[104] and absent[105] in human analgesic abusers. Molland[106] described a dense fibrillary network of PAS-positive material in animals with an aspirin-induced renal papillary necrosis that became irregular with deeply staining fibres and bodies in the interstitium (see below). Using an acute model of renal papillary necrosis it has been possible to establish that shortly after chemical insult there is a marked increase in the staining of the medullary matrix, at the same time as the earliest changes are taking place in the interstitial cells[107,108]. Subsequently, a time-dependent loss of medullary staining occurs in those areas where necrosis develops. About 6 h after a dose of 2-bromoethanamine hydrobromide there is a more intense PAS-positive material at the tip of the papilla, which increased to a maximum at 48 h, at which stage the PAS staining in the mid-medulla was decreased. Even when there is a re-epithelialization of the affected area there is a failure to re-establish the presence of the MPS matrix, probably due to the absence of medullary interstitial cells. The loss of non-specific staining could represent either masking of the functional groups, the loss of those chemical moieties responsible for colour reactions or marked physicochemical changes in the glycosaminoglycan/proteoglycan. Recent biochemical studies[109] have shown that there is a very marked loss of sulphate groups from the medullary matrix and urinary macromolecular carbohydrate turnover showed changes in the molecular weight polydispersion; taken together these data suggest that the matrix is increasingly disrupted, and eventually lost from the medulla.

(c) Epithelial carbohydrate granules. Tucker et al.[110] and Alroy et al.[111] have reported the presence of PAS and Alcian Blue positive granules in the human pelvic epithelial cells, where carcinoma was present in the upper ureter, and in cells that had metastasized from these regions. A series of similar changes have been described by Hukill and Vidone[112] for bladder malignancies. Intracytoplasmic glycogen or intercellular lakes of mucin were common. Similar changes have also been noted associated with renal papillary necrosis induced by aspirin[106] and 2-bromoethanamine (Figure 6)[108]. There is also an accumulation of PAS-positive granules in the cells of the collecting duct and the covering epithelium. These granules appear before cell necrosis, and may therefore represent the autophagic processes. The presence of similar granules in the pelvic and urothelial cells 21 weeks after the induction of an acute papillary necrosis[113] suggests that this change is a long-term aberration of cellular function, especially because they were most marked in those regions where the urothelial dysplasia was greatest.

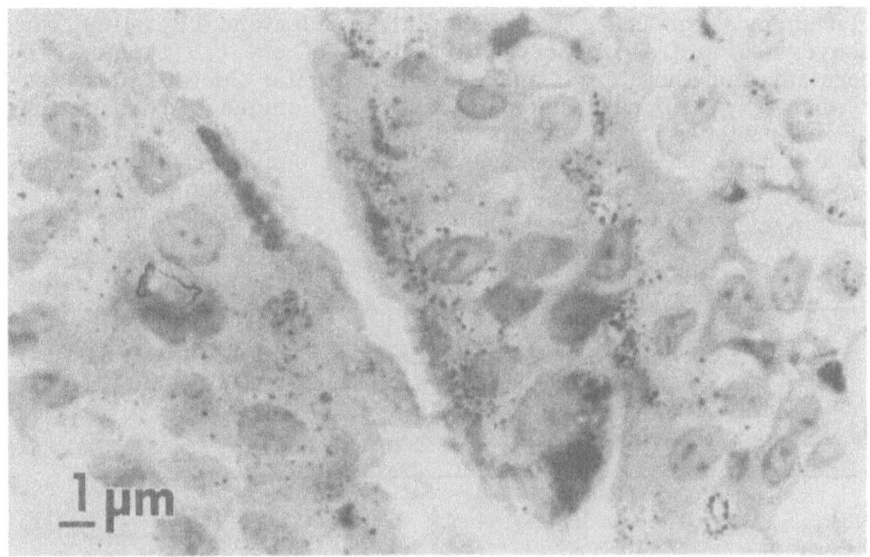

Figure 6 PAS-positive granules in the superficial layer of ureteric urothelium from animal treated with BEA (100 mg/kg). Ureter embedded in glycol methacrylate 1 μm section counterstained with haematoxylin.

The presence of these granules could be related to the glycocalyx, particularly because changes in these complex carbohydrates have been linked to tumorigenesis[114], and cell surface recognition[115]. These changes in carbohydrate staining may therefore represent early or subtle changes in the urothelial cells that predispose them to abnormal growth patterns. On the other hand these changes may not be indicative of malignancy or hyperplasia, because they also occur in rodents with lithium-induced nephropathy[103], where amylase digestion suggested the material was glycogen. The marked changes in the medullary matrix caused by renal papillary necrosis and lithium toxicity may therefore reflect the shunting of simple carbohydrate material (normally used for MPS synthesis) into stored glycogen.

2.   Glycoproteins

There are a number of other anatomical regions of the kidney in which the glycoproteins and/or glycolipids predominate. These will be considered below, under immuno- and lectin histochemistry, although it must be appreciated that some of the less selective stains also demonstrate the presence of these molecules.

B.   Affinity techniques with lectins

Lectins bind to well-defined sugar residues[116] wherever these are available; i.e. they occur on glycoproteins, mucopolysaccharides, glycolipids, etc. The cell surface, intracellular and interstitial carbohydrates in fresh or cryostat sections of one cell type may be constant and therefore visualized with specific fluorescent or enzyme (e.g. peroxidase-linked) lectins. This unique relationship has been reported for both human and animal tissue, where the binding of a number of lectins is associated with one or more renal cell types[117-123] (Table 3).

Table 3 Selective staining of nephron segments by lectins

LECTIN	Soy bean agglutinin		Winged pea agglutinin			Peanut agglutinin		Luex europeaus	Dolichos biflorus
SPECIES	Rat	Rabbit	Rat	Rabbit	Man	Rabbit	Man	Man	Man
Glomeruli	+	+	-	-	-	-	-	-	-
Proximal S$_1$	+	-	-	+	+	-	-	-	-
tubule S$_2$	+	-	-	+	+	-	-	-	-
S$_3$	-	-	-	+	+	-	-	-	-
Henle loop	-	-	-	-	-	+	-	-	-
Distal tubule	+	+	+	-	-	-	+	-	+
Collecting duct	+	+	+	-	-	+	+	-	+
Vascular endothelia	-	-	-	-	-	-	-	+	-

The binding of peanut agglutinin to the intercalated cells (or dark cells) of the collecting and connecting ducts in cryostat sections of rabbit kidneys is particularly noteworthy[119], because there are very few markers for these cells at a light microscopic level. By contrast Stoward et al.[124] reported that peanut lectin bound to the brush-border of the rat proximal tubule and collecting ducts, and it was variable in the distal tubule. Glomeruli only reacted positively after sialidase digestion. In the mouse[125], however, peanut lectin stained Bowman's capsule, the tubules and basement membrane and the collecting ducts, but the lectin from Dolichos biflorus stained only Bowman's capsule and the collecting ducts. Some selectivity also exists in any single species, but this may be different in another species (see Table 4 for differences in soy bean and winged pea agglutinin). Thus a nephron segment specific lectin is not available, nor are there any systematic relationships between species, although the mouse, rabbit and man have similar lectin staining patterns, which differ from the rat[122]. Some lectins such as limulin[126] have not yet been studied in a number of different species, and therefore its binding to sialoglycoproteins of the rat glomeruli, and to a lesser degree both the proximal and the distal tubule, may not preclude its usefulness in studying other species.

Table 4 The differentiation between proximal and distal tubules using lectins

LECTIN	Species where only one tubule type is stained	
	Proximal tubule	Distal tubule
Wheat germ	guinea pig, quail, frog,	0
Ricinus communis	rabbit, guinea pig, frog	0
Soy bean	0	dog, mouse
Peanut	0	dog, rabbit, mouse, man
	guinea pig, rat, frog	0
Ulex europeus	0	dog, rabbit, guinea pig, frog
Dolichos biflorus	0	dog, rabbit, guinea pig, mouse, quail, frog, trout, man

Fixation may drastically alter lectin binding, winged pea agglutinin binds to rat tubular epithelium after fixation in Carnoy solution, whereas only vascular structures were seen after glutaraldehyde[123]. By contrast Faraggiana and co-workers[127] have reported that fixation and wax embedding had little effect on the binding profile of lectin-peroxidase conjugates that were used for human tissue. The lectin from Lotus tetragonolobus bound exclusively to the proximal tubule, while peanut and soy bean lectin were confined to the collecting duct. Wheat germ lectin bound several parenchymal components including the glomerular capillary wall and its podocyte cell coat. These workers also unmasked glycoproteins using sialidase digestion, after which the glomeruli stained with soy bean and peanut lectin. Lectins can also be used on normal semi-thin methacrylate embedded sections, where they have been used coupled to colloidal gold particles[128] or fluorescent probes[129].

It is reasonable to assume that a variety of pathological processes, such as enzymic degradation of carbohydrates, could alter or destroy lectin receptor sites, whereas loss of lipid or protein from complex macromolecules unmasks different binding sites. The main problem with the use of lectins is that their staining pattern can only be related to the availability, masking and unmasking of specific sugar moieties, and that further molecular interpretation is precluded.

IV. ANTIGENS

A. Application of antigen-based histochemistry

There has been an increasing interest in the use of antibodies directed against unique or novel characteristics along the nephron. These antigenic determinants may be present on enzymes, glycoproteins or other molecules, associated with membranes or soluble cytosolic constituents. Many of the monoclonal antibodies so far reported react with one or more regions of the nephron and/or parts of the cell[130,131]. There are some major disadvantages to using antibodies; their production is time-consuming and their specificity may be doubtful, only a few antibodies will detect the same antigen in an unrelated species, and each antibody is a unique entity, the production of which cannot be exactly reproduced. Even when taken from the same source, polyclonal antibodies may vary in titre between batches, and their production depends on the longevity of the animal producing them.

Visualization of the site of antibody binding to the antigenic determination is done by labelled antibody, e.g. labelled with enzymes, fluorescent dyes or radioactive groups. It is evident that proximal tubules can easily and specifically be stained by anti-brush-border membranes, and distal tubules by means of antibodies directed against tonin[132] and Tamm-Horsfall glycoprotein[133]. However, not all enzymic antigens present in the brush border membrane can be demonstrated histochemically, e.g. whereas aminopeptidase binds its antibody[46] alkaline phosphatase does not[134], which may indicate hidden antigenic determinants.

Provided the concentration is sufficiently high, the antibody will act as a native cross-linking agent in frozen, unfixed sections[35,135]. The use of high antibody concentrations may, however, be inappropriate due to the presence of antibodies against undesirable antigens giving rise to misleading staining, if the binding site is not specifically monitored. For example, monospecific anti-renin diluted 1:1000 not only stained the juxtamedullary apparatus in mice, but also stained the epithelial cells of the afferent arterioles and some cells of the proximal tubule and collecting duct. A 10-fold dilution resulted in the loss of proximal tubule and collecting duct staining, whereas an additional 100-fold dilution (i.e. 1:1,000,000) resulted in the disappearance of the arteriole staining. These data were interpreted in terms of the quantity of renin released from the juxtamedullary apparatus and its uptake by pinocytosis, but equally they may represent decreased binding to the biotransformed product angiotensin I[136].

1. Polyclonal antibodies

Antisera raised against purified epithelial cells may be useful to stain particular nephron segments[137], but may contain antibodies with various antigen specificities. If only one of these reacted with

38

antigenic determinants shared by cells of other nephron segments or the interstitium, the staining is not specific. If, on the other hand, the specificity of an antiserum has been established, antigen concentrations can be quantified in sections using antibody concentrations close to saturation levels[18,59]. This approach is different from the conventional one, which aims at the number of antigenic sites by diluting out the antiserum.

2. Monoclonal antibodies

More recently, specific renal antibodies have been produced by cloning techniques[138], and appear to be the most promising technique for detecting specifically defined antigenic determinants in renal sections. The applicability of monoclonal antibodies may be restricted if the density of antigenic determinants is too low.

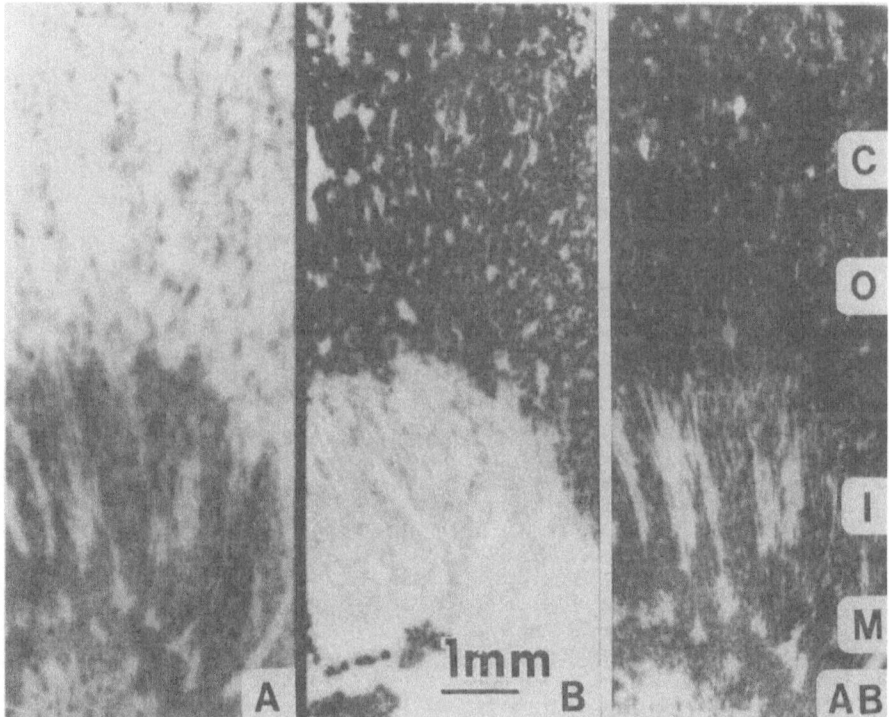

Figure 7 Immunohistochemistry of normal male rat kidney showing the different concentrations of the cytoplasmic isoenzymes aldolase-A and aldolase-B within and between nephron segments. Frozen, acetone-fixed serial sections stained for aldolase (ALD) activity after treatment of sections with antibody against ALD-A and consecutively with antigen ALD-A (A), antibody against ALD-B and antigen ALD-B (B), and both antibodies and antigens (AB). Cortex (C), outer stripe (O) and inner stripe (I) of outer medulla and inner medulla (M).

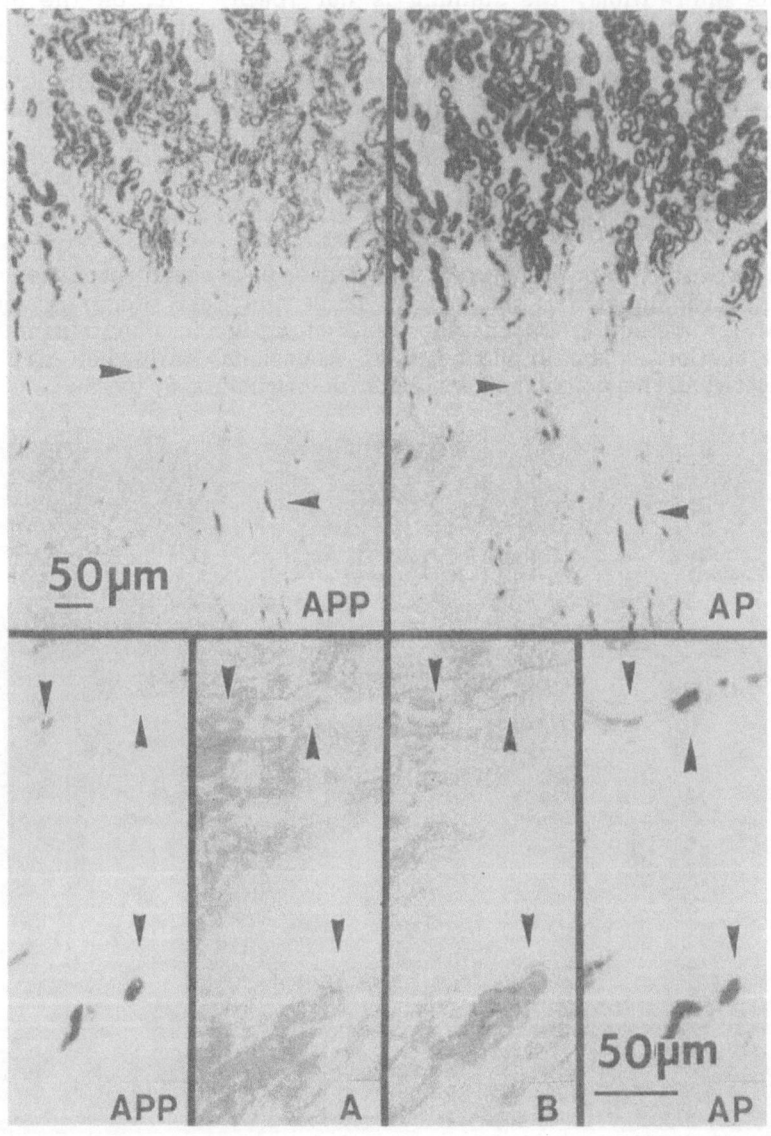

Figure 8 Enzyme- and immunohistochemical changes in rat kidneys 24 h after a single 1.3 g/kg i.v. dose of cephaloridine. FRP of enzymes is normally only present in proximal tubules, but following cephaloridine insult it is also demonstrated in distal tubules where it is associated with hyaline casts. Frozen, acetone-fixed sections stained for the brush-border enzymes alkaline phosphatase (APP) and aminopeptidase (AP), and using immunohistochemistry for the cytoplasmic isoenzymes aldolase-A (A) and B (B). Outer and inner stripe of outer medulla, with stained proximal tubules and casts (top) and serial sections through distal tubules of inner stripe containing FRP of enzymes of the proximal tubule (bottom). Arrowheads point to tubular casts.

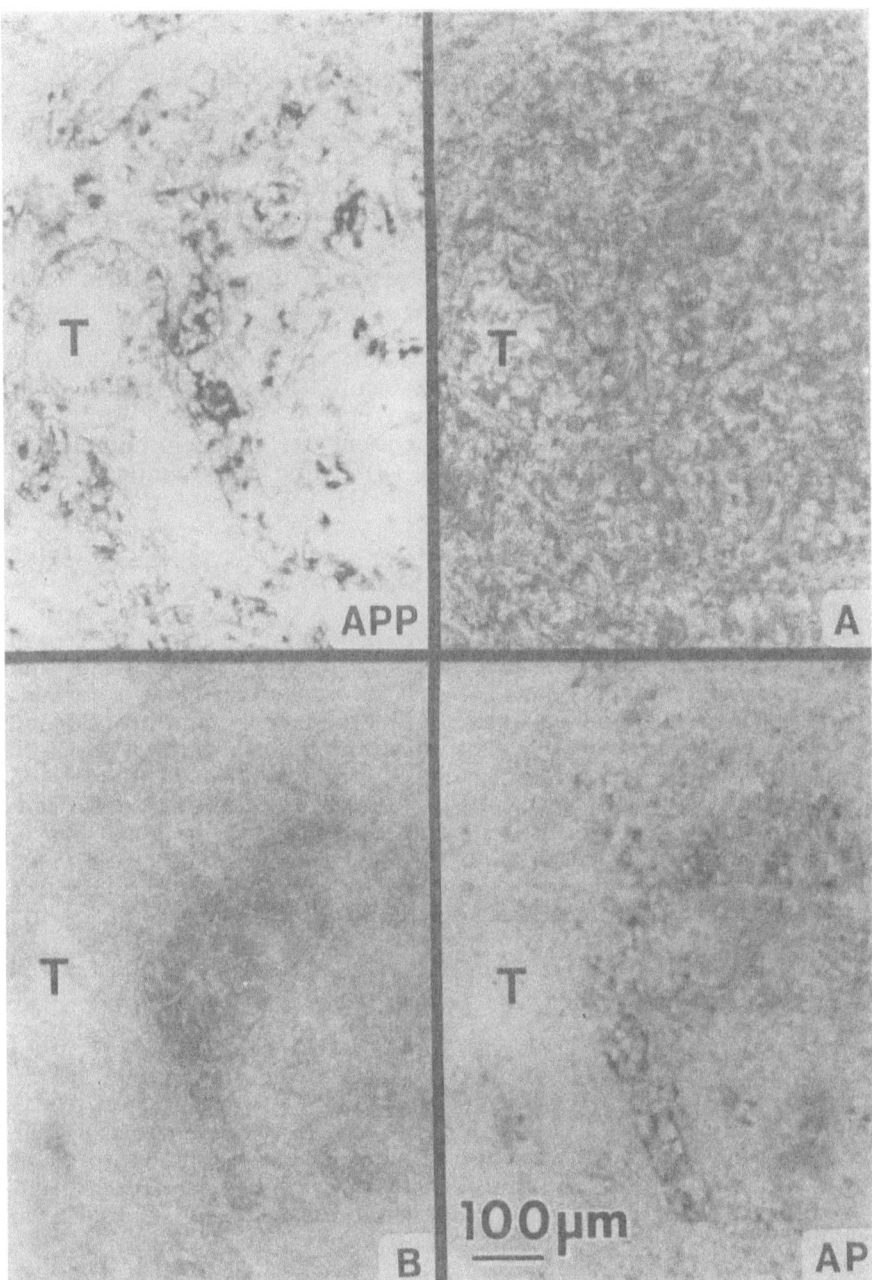

Figure 9 Histochemistry of human hypernephroid carcinoma. The FRP concentration of each enzyme is heterogeneously distributed in the tumour cells. Frozen, acetone-fixed serial sections immunohistochemistry stained for aldolase-A (A) and aldolase-B (B) and using enzyme histochemistry for alkaline phosphatase (APP) and aminopeptidase (AP). Tubular lumen (T).

3.   Antibodies to enzymes

The use of antibodies is also of advantage in the investigation of enzymes with the same catalytic activity, but different molecular properties, i.e. isoenzymes. The mixed aggregation immuno-cytochemical technique[35] has been used to localize and quantify specifically renal isoenzymes of lactate dehydrogenase[36] and aldolase[53] in nephron segments. For instance, during renal matura-tion aldolase-B monomers increase in the proximal tubules of rats, but not in the distal tubules. By contrast, aldolase-A monomers in-crease in the distal tubules, but not in the proximal tubules[53]. It can be concluded that renal casts in adult rats that contain mainly aldolase-B monomers are derived from proximal tubules (Figure 7). Similarly, the presence of proximal tubule markers can be shown in hyaline casts after a nephrotoxic insult (Figure 8). Moreover, isoenzyme determinations may be useful in the study of tumorigenesis (see below) and development[139], and help established tumour cell heterogeneity (Figure 9) with other antisera and lectins[122].

4.   Fixed or frozen sections

Immunohistochemical techniques have been applied to both frozen and fixed sections.   Increasing use is being made of semi- and ultra-thin sections of epon- or methacrylate-embedded materials. Ultra-cryostat sections are also being employed, but are beyond the scope of this chapter.   The literature on the optimal methods to be used is not consistent and depends on the technique and type of molecule being studied.   Generally protease treatment reverses the loss of antigen binding sites caused by a variety of fixation methods[140]. Increasingly, however, short fixation of fresh tissue is becoming popular, especially at low temperatures for the duration of fixing, dehydration and embedding[141].

B.   **Renal immunomarkers**

Immunohistochemical methods have also been used to demonstrate a variety of functional protein epitopes in discrete localizations of the kidney[132,133,137,140-162] (Table 5), but very few of these tech-niques have been applied to help elucidate the mechanisms of neph-rotoxicity. There are a number of macromolecules that are present in the glomeruli[163-165] (Table 6), some of which are also present throughout the tubular basement membrane.   Under pathological conditions a variety of immunodeposits have been observed in a large number of glomerulopathies, and immunofluorescence monitor-ing provides the standard means of diagnosis.   Glomerular immunochanges[166-169] are beyond the scope of this chapter. There are several tubular epitopes that warrant special comment because of their importance in studying target cell toxicity. The use of an-tibodies for assessing arachidonic acid metabolites and the enzymes responsible for their bioconversion is covered below in Section VI.

Table 5 The distribution of structural and functional proteins, exogenous filtered proteins and enzymes in the kidney as assessed by immunohistochemistry

Characteristic	Distribution	Species	References
Albumin	Proximal convoluted tubule basement membrane apical vesicles and lysosomes	Guinea pig	142
Aminopeptidase IV	Proximal tubule brush-border	Rat	143
Na^+,K^+-ATPase	Proximal tubule weak basolateral Distal tubule strong basolateral Absent intercalated cells	Mouse	144
Atrial natriuretic factor	Intercalated cells of the collecting ducts - homogeneous in some and apical in others	Rat	145
Carbonic anhydrase	Weakly in the proximal tubule Strongly in the loop of Henle Strongly in the collecting ducts Distal convoluted tubule - a mosaic of very strong and absent in adjacent cells	Rat	146
Carbonic anhydrase isoenzymes	Only isoenzyme II in the loop of Henle and distal nephron	Rat	146
Cathepsin D	Cortical and medullary collecting ducts Mesangial cells Proximal tubule weakly positive	Rat	147
Clathrin	Apical portion of the proximal tubule	Rat	148
Enoyl-CoA hydratase			
Heat-stable	Proximal and distal epithelial cell mitochondria Absent from glomeruli	Rat	149
Heat-labile	Proximal tubule epithelial cells	Rat	149
Ferredoxin*	Glomerulus and proximal convoluted tubule	Chick	150
α-Glucosidase F_1	Proximal convoluted tubule brush-border and loop of Henle	Human	151
Kallikrein	Distal tubule cytoplasm Sometimes vascular poles glomeruli and collecting ducts Apical regions some distal tubules Reabsorption droplets proximal tubules Some collecting ducts in medulla	Rat Mouse	152,153 153

Table 5 (continued)

Characteristic	Distribution	Species	References
Metallothionein	Epithelia of collecting duct and distal convoluted tubule in controls After Cd loading - strong proximal convoluted and collecting duct epithelia staining in both nuclei and cytoplasm Weak to moderate staining in glomerular mesangial and visceral epithelial cells and vascular smooth muscle cells There was no staining in vascular endothelial cells	Rat	154
Renin	Juxtamedullary apparatus Epithelioid cells of the juxtamedullary apparatus	Mouse Rabbit Dog Mouse	155 156 156 157
	Epithelioid cells of the afferent arteriole in the juxtamedullary apparatus	Human	158,159
Cu-Zn superoxide dismutase	Thick ascending limb of the loop of Henle Proximal convoluted tubule	Dog Rat	160 161
Tissue polypeptide antigen**	Strongly positive lining renal pyramid thin segment of loop of Henle collecting ducts Weakly positive parietal cells of Bowman's capsule	Human	140
Trehalase	Proximal tubule brush-border	Rabbit Rat	162 162

* Iron-sulphur part of 25-hydroxy-vitamin-D_3-hydroxylase.
** Also stains most extra-renal tissue.

Table 6 The distribution of structural proteins in the kidney glomeruli as assessed by immunohistochemistry

Structural protein	Distribution	Species	Reference
Collagen type IV	GBM* laminae densa Mesangial matrix	Rat	163
Entactin	GBM peripheral capillary loops Tubular basement membrane	Rat	164
Fibronectin	Strongly mesangial matrix GBM laminae rara at the endothelial- mesangial interface	Rat	163
Glycoprotein GP-2	GBM tubular basement membrane	Guinea pig	165
Laminin	GBM lamina rara Mesangial matrix	Rat	163
	GBM peripheral capillary loops Mesangial matrix Tubular basement membrane	Rat	164

*GBM = Glomerular basement membrane

1.   Cytochrome P-450

The role of oxidative metabolism in the generation of biologically reactive intermediates has received much attention[170,171], and anti-cytochrome P-450 has been used to show the localization to the proximal tubule, particularly the P_2 and P_3 segments, and the induction following exposure to dioxin[172,173].

2.   Ligandin and brush border antibodies

Ligandin or glutathione-S-transferase B is located in the proximal tubule of both animals and man[174-176] and the thick limb of the loop of Henle in man[176,177]. Similarly the distribution of anti-aminopeptidase to the brush-border has been described for several species[18,36,59] and brush-border antigens in rats[178,179].

3.   Tamm-Horsfall glycoprotein and other distal tubular
      macromolecules

Tamm-Horsfall glycoprotein (THG) is localized to the distal nephron, where it plays an essential, but not yet fully understood,
role in urinary concentration[133,180]. The distribution of this
glycoprotein is perturbed by a number of nephrotoxins. Potassium
dichromate[180] caused a biphasic release of THG and deposits along
the luminal borders of the epithelial cells within 12 h, loss from
the distal nephron and an increase in the number and size of casts
from 48 h after dosing. Luminal casts accounted for all of the
THG-positive staining material by 144 h, but distal epithelial THG
increased from 192 h, and the distribution was normal by 14 days.

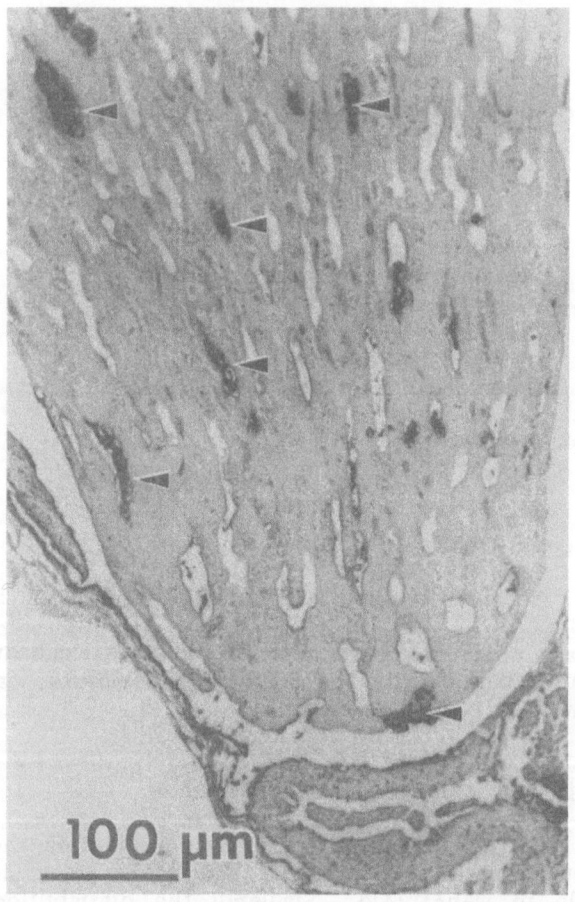

Figure 10 Aggregates of immunohistochemically positive Tamm-Horsfall glycoprotein
hyaline tubular casts present in medullary collecting ducts 7 days after the induction of an acute papillary necrosis using 100 mg/kg i.p. of BEA.

THG is also lost from the distal nephron at an early time point during the course of development of an acutely induced renal papillary necrosis (Figure 10)[181]. Only later when the medullary MPS staining had been lost do large casts of THG positive material deposit, especially in the collecting ducts and ducts of Bellini in the necrosed areas, where they are associated with cellular debris[181]. The nephrons that appear to feed blocked collecting ducts are generally dilated. Some of the THG-positive material is extravasated, and many of the superficial glomeruli thus affected have THG-positive material in Bowman's space. The presence of THG in Bowman's space may be related to glomerular sclerosis[182], following an acutely induced medullary injury. Alkaline phosphatase-, ATPase- and GGT-FRP are present in these casts, which supports the idea that there are proximal tubular changes during the development, or as a result of renal papillary necrosis[108].

There are several examples where the cross-selectivity of antibodies to proteins derived from different species has been useful. For example, much of the research on the changes in animal THG has been based on the use of antibodies raised to human THG. There are also instances where data that are difficult to interpret have been generated from the application of antibodies to tissue other than the one of interest. Pich et al.[183] reported the very strong binding of an anti-human casein antibody to the mammary glands and sweat gland, and also the distal tubule and the collecting duct. The unexpected renal distribution of this protein suggests that it may be involved in the control of electrolyte, water and other fluid movement. Identification of the antigen had not been undertaken and cross-reactivity with other antigens could not be excluded.

THG and the anti-casein positive material are not the only proteins that function in different regions of the body to modulate ion and water permeability and transport. Molin et al.[184] showed that antibodies to the α-subunit of the S-100 protein (originally found in the central nervous system) also stained the thin limb of the loop of Henle, and the connecting and collecting ducts in the rat. No other part of the kidney or urothelium reacted positively to this antibody, and the antibody to the β-subunit of S-100 did not react with the kidney or urothelium. The distribution of S-100 in the kidney closely parallels the distribution of the carbonic anhydrase - isoenzyme C[184]. The S-100 protein has been strongly implicated in calcium binding, and its presence in the distal part of the nephron suggests that it plays some role in modulating Ca^{2+} reabsorbtion, perhaps similar to the role played by THG in Na^+ uptake. A vitamin D-induced calcium-binding protein (first described in the chick intestine) has also been reported in the rabbit, rat and chick kidney[185,185a]. There were some species differences, but in general this calcium-binding protein appeared to be distributed almost identically with that described for the S-100. The potential perturbation of these novel proteins by chemicals, and the resulting disruption of calcium and other electrolyte homeostasis, warrants further investigation. At present there are no data to confirm that the S-100 and vitamin D-dependent calcium-binding protein are the same molecules, and very little is known about the relationship of either of these to THG.

4. Renin and kallikrein distribution

There are a number of other enzymes that play major roles in renal homeostasis, the most important of which are renin[155-159] and kallikrein[152,153]. These two enzymes produce essentially opposite functional effects in the kidney[186]. Renin-secreting cells appear to be on the outer aspects of the vessel wall, and immunoreactive angiotensin II is present in high concentrations with renin granules and is therefore assumed to be excreted with them[187]. Ørstavik and Inagami[188] showed that the localization of the individual mediators is separate; whereas kallikrein is localized in the thick ascending limb of the loop of Henle (up to the distal tubule), renin was always associated quite separately in the epithelioid cells of the afferent arteriole. Renin is also localized to this position in the normal human kidney[158,159]. More importantly, in those kidneys with ischaemic injury[158,159] or Bartter's syndrome[158] the renin-positive epithelial cells showed increased staining intensity, and in afferent arterioles that were some distance from glomeruli. The pattern of staining was normal in localized parenchymal areas where ischaemic injury had not occurred[159] and in other types of nephropathy, even when plasma renin levels were high[158]. This novel observation needs to be confirmed in the experimental situation, where this abnormal distribution may help identify those injuries where chemicals cause a direct or indirect anoxia of the renal parenchyma. It may also give some indication of the mechanisms involved and the consequences of renal ischaemic injury.

5. α_{2u}-Globulin distribution in the kidney

The development of renal carcinoma in only male rats exposed to branched-chain light hydrocarbons[189] has heightened interest in the hepatic synthesis and renal excretion of α_{2u}-globulin[190]. In the proximal tubule the reabsorption of this low molecular weight protein gives rise to the hyaline droplet that is the characteristic feature of "old rat" and light hydrocarbon nephropathy. Roy and Raber[191] used a rhodamine-linked anti-α_{2u}-globulin to show the distribution in the liver (cytoplasmic in the parenchymal cells) and the kidney, where it was localized to the cells of the proximal tubule, the loops of Henle and the distal tubule. The distribution of rhodamine-labelled α_{2u}-globulin showed the presence of the protein along the length of the nephron. More recently, Simpson et al.[192] used an indirect immunoperoxidase assay and showed that the presence of α_{2u}-globulin was not confined to the hyaline droplets, but was also present in the cytoplasm and lumen of the proximal tubule of male rats treated with the branched-chain hydrocarbon 2,2,4-trimethylpentane. α_{2u}-Globulin is also synthesized by the duct cells of the submaxillary gland, where it is not under sex hormone control, although the protein is immunologically identical to that produced by the liver[193].

6. Tumour antigens

Cordon-Cardo et al.[194] used a variety of human urothelial and renal cancer cell lines to produce monoclonal antibodies which were then shown to be selectively associated with different parts of the nephron. Each of these antibodies was novel and did not cross-react with other previously identified antigens such as THG, fibronectin, laminin, etc. There has been some interest in the potential use of these regio-specific markers to identify areas of renal necrosis using the presence of urinary excreted antigens from damaged cells as a measure of injury.

Monoclonal antibodies raised to cytokeratin polypeptides have been shown to react with various renal sites, including the proximal and distal tubule and the urothelia[195]. More importantly, the pattern of renal carcinoma and type I and II carcinoma were each unique and different from the rest of the kidney and urothelial tract[195]. Wang and Krueger[196] also reported an antibody that is selective for rapidly proliferating cells in different regions of the body. The identification of rapidly dividing cells could be used to show the presence of proliferative bursts of activity that were indicative of repair, hyperplasia or malignancy, especially if combined with other methods.

The ABO isoantigens normally associated with blood groups have also been used to differentiate between normal and non-invasive transitional urothelia carcinoma (which stains for the tissue isoantigen) from invasive carcinoma which frequently did not stain[197].

There is also limited clinical data to suggest that anti-ligandin reacts with renal adenocarcinoma, but not with undifferentiated carcinoma, papillary adenoma, well-differentiated papillary adenocarcinoma and Wilm's tumours in man[177]. Immunoreactive renin-containing cells are present in most renal tumours where they are also intimately associated with blood vessels[187]. Another series of markers in a very large number of renal tumours is the co-presence of the intermediate-sized filaments of cytokeratin and vimentin. While cytokeratin is present in other parts of the normal kidney, it is never present with vimentin. This suggests that vimentin is expressed as part of the neoplastic transformation[198].

C. High-resolution immunohistochemistry

Most of the immunohistochemical methods decribed make use of wax sections. Generally these are 5 μm or thicker (often 7-10 μm), but the use of special techniques may facilitate semi-thin sections. For example Clyne et al.[199] reported the immunohistochemical tubular localization of albumin in those patients with proteinuria, where the tissue was freeze-substituted, paraffin-embedded and cut at 0.5 μm.

The use of low-density methacrylate resins has also opened the potential of undertaking immunohistochemistry on semi-thin sections, which provides vastly improved resolution and precise localization of the antigen labelling[67]. There is loss of antigenicity as a result of the processes involved in embedding material in glycol methacrylate resin. Hemming et al.[200] reported that cryosections used an antibody titre that was 1000 more dilute than that necessary for semi-thin sections, but the superior morpholgical detail seen in the methacrylate material made it most useful. Several of the technical difficulties associated with low-temperature embedding of tissue have been made more simple by the device reported by Wells[201].

The most important criterion for successful immunohistochemistry in methacrylate material is the use of low-temperature fixation and processing to preserve both morphology and antigenicity[67,141,168,200,202-207]. Protease treatment helps to improve the availability of antigens[67,168], but these tend to be the extracellular binding sites, and etching the resin may be necessary to detect intracellular antigens. The double antibody technique[208] has been used successfully to contrast antigens in glycol methacrylate, where the secondary antibody has included immunogold[207], fluorescent labels[168,206] avidin-biotin-peroxidase[67] and peroxidase-anti-peroxidase[200]. In general, the most successful application of immunohistochemical methods to glycol methacrylate has been with those antigens that are most resistant to fixation[67,168,209-211].

V. LIPIDS

There are many aspects of lipid histochemistry that require more extensive or renewed evaluation, because of the subtle differences that may be introduced by fixation and staining properties of the different lipid stains. Thus fixation procedures have been evaluated for their ability to unmask lipid from lipoproteins[212] or to stabilize membranes[213], and several of the approaches have been compared[214]. While it is generally appreciated that dehydration for wax or methacrylate embedding will remove lipid, the remaining vacuoles may be interpreted as structures in their own right[215]. Some lipids are also water-soluble and may be leached out of tissue that has been subjected to prolonged fixation[94]. The other important aspect that has to be re-evaluated are the differences between adipose fat globlets, fat droplets, the different types of lipid material such as membranes, free neutral and fatty acids, sterols; the more complex lipids such as lipoproteins, glycolipids and also the question of cytoplasmic "lipid domains", which show varying degrees of lipophilicity[212-216]. Depending on the stain used any one or more of these different characteristics can be shown[216-218] and various artefacts have been described[215]. Berg[216] used the now-established carcinogen 3,4-benzpyrene (benzo[a]pyrene) and showed that there was a very strong fluorescence associated with the brush-border and basal filaments (probably the mitochondria of the proximal tubule) in formaldehyde-fixed frozen mouse kidney. Sudanophilicity was also present in these epithelial cells. By contrast Oil Red "O" stains the lipid droplets in the interstitial cells of the medulla heavily, but not other parts of the kidney[219]. The medullary interstitial cells have a very high lipogenic potential and the numerous lipid droplets are rich in polyunsaturated fatty acids, especially those with C18 to C24 chain lengths[220]. These lipid droplets are also apparent as osmophilic material in semi-thin sections[219].

A. Abnormalities in lipid distribution following chemical insult

While lipid changes are well described following liver injury there is a paucity of data on nephrotoxicity. The outstanding histo-chemical changes in patients with analgesic abuse-related renal papillary necrosis is the accumulation of very large quantities of Oil Red "O" positive lipid material[221]. Similar changes have also been reported in experimentally induced papillary necrosis following aspirin[222] and a prolonged essential fatty acid-deficient diet[223]. More recent studies have shown that these changes also occur in an acutely induced papillary necrosis (Figure 11), where the earliest changes took place in the capillaries.

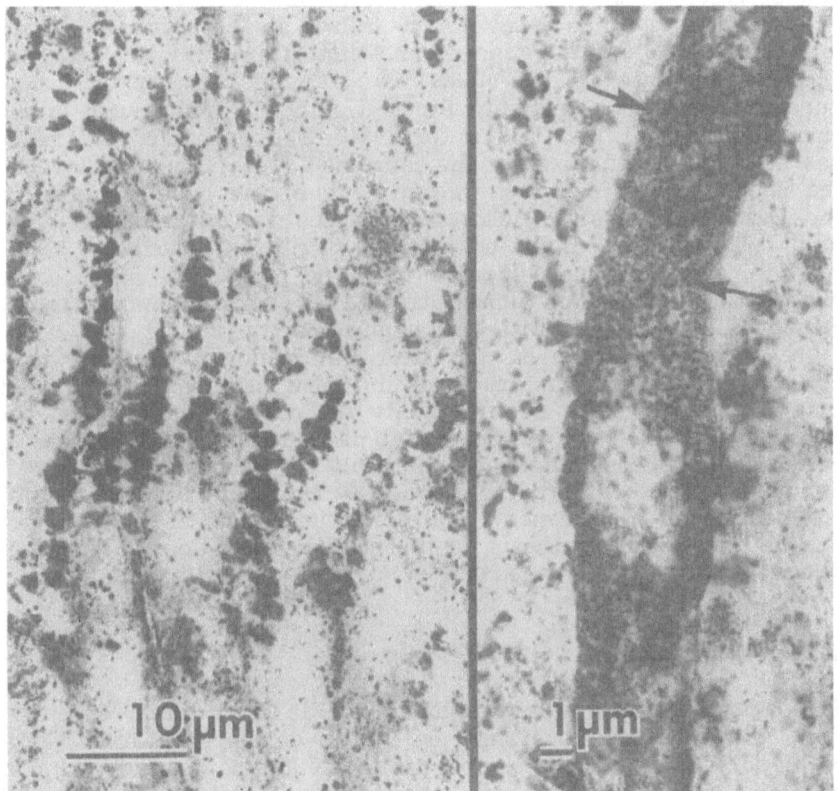

Figure 11 Accumulation of lipid in collecting duct epithelial cells in papilla from rat 48 h after single i.p. injection of BEA (100 mg/kg). Fixed-frozen section stained with Oil Red "O". Insert shows lipid accumulation in proteinaceous casts in loops of Henle and covering epithelium of papilla (arrows).

51

There was also a marked accumulation of lipid in the epithelial cells (normally there is no lipid material in these cells as assessed by Oil Red "O"). The epithelial accumulation of lipid material extended into those areas of the outer medulla which were not affected by the papillotoxin and appeared to be normal by routine H&E staining[219]. A comparison with a variety of other nephrotoxic lesions, such as those caused by hexachlorobutadiene, aminoglycosides, cis-platin and polybrene, suggest that the capillary and epithelial deposits of lipid material are pathognomonic for renal papillary necrosis[224]. Chemical assay of the medullary tissue has recently suggested that these histochemical changes represented a phospholipidosis[225]. The greatly increased levels of lipid material in the hyperplastic urothelia may be pathognomonic of, or associated with, malignant or premalignant changes. These have been described in other malignant tissues[226] and in exfoliating urothelial cells[227].

Other published data suggest that the development of renal lipid changes is associated with specific types of nephrotoxicity. Aminoglycosides cause a proximal tubule phospholipidosis[228], which in common with other renal lesions caused by chromium[229], carbon tetrachloride[230], tetracycline[231] and aflatoxin[232,233] also caused a localized increase in Oil Red "O" staining. Puromycin aminonucleoside targets selectively for the glomeruli and causes an accumulation of Oil Red "O" material[234]. The rubeanic acid method has also been used to show the increased free fatty acid levels in the nephrotic syndrome[235]. Recently, there has been a report that the immunosuppressive cyclosporin causes an accumulation of Oil Red "O" positive lipid material in cultured proximal tubular cells[236], although there appears to be no published evidence from histochemical studies on animals treated in vivo to show that similar changes are associated with this nephrotoxicity.

At present there is very little information to explain the increased staining of lipid material in these damaged cells. In the case of aminoglycoside nephrotoxicity the phospholipidosis has been explained on the basis of decreased degradation and lysosomal accumulation of phospholipids as a result of membrane turnover[237], but obviously other "lipid" changes may represent lipid unmasking, degradation of membranes, and/or accumulation of lipid material due to increased synthesis or decreased utilization in those instances where it is changed[216-238].

VI. PROSTANOIDS

The importance of the prostaglandins (PGs) in normal renal function, and their controversial role in the development of a variety of nephropathies such as nephrotic syndrome, renal papillary necrosis and hydronephrosis, have been widely studied[239,240]. Much of the information on the distribution of prostanoid metabolism has come from biochemical studies on medullary and cortical tissue slices, isolated glomeruli and cultured cells, and by the use of classical microdissection studies. For example, the presence and distribution of NAD- and NADP-15-hydroxyprostaglandin dehydrogenase, and other enzymes related to arachidonic acid metabolism, has been established using tissue fragments from cryostat sections[241]. It is important to stress that the absence of a particular PG or one of the enzymes that metabolize arachidonic acid from any one cell type does not exclude the potential for the cell to produce the arachanoid of interest. Three distinct approaches have been used:

A.   Antibodies raised to the enzyme

Smith and Wilkin[242] used an anti-cyclo-oxygenase to show that the distribution of cyclo-oxygenase was confined to the medullary interstitial cells and the collecting ducts in the rat, rabbit and guinea pig, and in the cow and sheep[242a,243] In the cortex[243] cyclo-oxygenase antigenicity was localized in the endothelial cells of all arteries and aterioles, and the collecting ducts in the rat, rabbit, guinea pig, cow and sheep. This enzyme was also present in glomerular epithelial cells of the rabbit, cow and sheep.

B.   Antibodies raised to the prostaglandins

Mori and Mine[244] used antibodies raised to each of the prostaglandins, and showed the PGE_2 and $PGF_{2\alpha}$ were present in the cortical and medullary collecting ducts, the medullary interstitial cells, both glomeruli, mesangial and epithelial cells and endothelial cells of the arteries and arterioles. By contrast PG-6-keto-$F_{1\alpha}$ (the stable metabolite of PGI_2) was localized in both mesangial and epithelial glomerular cells, and the endothelial cells of arteries and arterioles. The tissue localization of PGA_2 has also been shown to be more marked in the tubular cells of the renal medulla compared to the cortex[245], but there was no discrete localization. These data suggested that PGA_2 was localized to the cell membrane rather than the cytoplasm as appears to be the case for the other PGs.

C.   Substrate oxidation to a chromophore

Janszen and Nugteren[246,247] based their histochemical method on cyclo-oxygenase-mediated arachidonic acid oxidation of diaminobenzidine (using cyanide as a blocking agent for mitochondrial oxidation). They showed intense staining of the secretory epithelia of seminal vesicles, and especially the renal collecting ducts and medullary interstitial cells. It has proved difficult to confirm that this colour change relates to the enzyme PG cyclo-oxygenase, although the distribution parallels were described by Smith[242,243]. Treating animals with analgesics or non-steroidal anti-inflammatory drugs, or the addition of these inhibitors of PG synthesis to the incubation medium, did not alter the intensity or formation of polymerized benzidine reaction product[248-250]. Litwin[248,249] has suggested that the colour reaction represents "total" peroxidative enzyme activity, based on the fact that diaminobenzidine oxidation is blocked by 3-amino-1,2,4-triazole, a well-established inhibitor of catalase and peroxidase. This was supported by the fact that the renal enzymic activity, demonstrated by this method, was the same with hydrogen peroxide and arachidonic acid (there was no reaction with unsaturated fatty acids), it is heat-stable and the pH optima parallel other peroxidases. Also, whereas glutathione abolished the colour reaction, catalase had no effect. The main question that remains to be resolved is which of the several possible different peroxidases can be visualized by this method, especially because of the recent importance that has been accorded the role of metabolic activation by these enzymes[250a]. Litwin[248,249] suggested that the activity was "a special peroxidase related to PG synthesis". This suggests PG hydroperoxidase, which together with cyclo-oxygenase forms PG synthase, or a lipoxygenase. Unfortunately the higher activity in the collecting duct compared to the medullary interstitial cells, and the fact that no activity was reported for glomeruli, does not support the biochemical data already available for these enzymes in the different regions of the kidney[239,240].

D.   Perturbations of prostanoid metabolism in response to nephropathy

Despite the implicated pathophysiological role for these lipids (and their related products) in several nephropathies, and the number of techniques available to study prostanoid metabolism, only very limited published material is available. Smith et al.[251] showed that there was a time-related increase in cyclo-oxygenase staining in the cortical collecting tubule and the loops of Henle of rabbits with surgically induced hydronephrosis. Contrary to expectations there were no vascular or glomerular changes, nor were there any changes in the medullary staining for this enzyme. Hydronephrosis is associated with phospholipidosis[252] and the very marked increase in thromboxane A_2 synthesis[253], which suggests that a full understanding of this change may only come from the application of histochemical, microdissection and other techniques.

VII.   OXIDASES AND ANTI-OXIDANTS

The presence of oxidative enzymes includes a series of mixed functional oxidase systems such as the cytochrome P-450 enzymes, the distribution of which is shown by immunohistochemistry[172,173] (see above). The distribution of cytochrome P-450 can also be shown by direct microspectrophotometric measurement[254], but this approach does not appear to have been applied to the kidney. There are other oxidase systems in the kidney. Large numbers of peroxisomes are localized in the P_3 portion of the proximal tubule, but they are absent from the glomeruli and the distal nephron[255]. There are highly selective methods for their vizualization[255,256], and their origins and development[257,258] in the metanephric kidney have been well documented. The full renal functions of the peroxisomes remain ill-defined. It is generally assumed that urate oxidase is responsible for the conversion of uric acid to urea[257]. In addition to urate oxidase, these organelles also contain catalase, and D-amino acid oxidase[258]. D-amino acid oxidase activity has been demonstrated in fixed and fresh renal proximal tubules using D-proline or D-alanine, peroxidase and diaminobenzidine (among other methods)[17], but the physiological function of the enzyme is far from certain. Reddy[259] has speculated on the role of D-amino acid oxidase in the genesis of the highly localized necrosis to the P_3 region of the nephron following the administration of D-serine. There is also evidence that oxalate and polyamines are oxidized in the proximal tubule peroxisomes[260]. The presence of these two oxidases is particularly important during incipient renal failure when the filtered load of oxalate and polyamines is known to be high.

The level of catalase is greatest in the proximal tubule, less in the distal tubule and very low in the glomeruli (there were no data on the medulla) in Syrian hamsters. Furthermore, the catalase levels in the proximal tubule were reduced at the same time as diethylstilboestrol-induced renal adenocarcinomas. Subsequent progesterone treatment reversed the carcinogenic effect[261] and also restored the catalase levels to normal.

Using the controlled staining of frozen sections with mercury orange, Ashgar et al.[262] showed that glutathione (GSH) was localized to the proximal convoluted tubule. Recently, Chieco and Boor[263] used low temperatures to decrease the diffusion of the mercury glutathione complex, which also reduced the colour intensity, but this decreased sensitivity was partially offset by the fluorescence of the complex. The "Prussian blue" method of Smith et al.[263a] forms much more rapidly that the mercury orange complex and will therefore show better localization. It has been used for determining GSH in liver, but produces an artefactual GSH distribution in the kidney, where the medulla stains very intensely. This probably represents staining of the medullary mucopolysaccharide matrix by colloidal iron[264]. There is little histochemical data on the distribution of other molecules that are likely to protect the cell from the effects of reactive intermediates.

The distribution of superoxide dismutase has recently been established using immunohistochemical techniques, which showed marked species differences in the dog[160] and rat[161] (see above). There are, however, at least three distinct types of superoxide dismutase, and until the distribution of each is defined it will be difficult to relate the absence of enzymic activity to target cell injury in the kidney.

VIII. CATECHOLAMINES

A significant proportion of the control of renal blood flow is resident in the nervous system, and the presence of catecholamine-containing neurons has been shown in many areas of the kidney[265]. These data are generally based on the fluorescence complex formed between formaldehyde and catecholamines using the Falck-Hillarp method[266], but this fails to differentiate between chemically distinct representatives within this group. Recently, Dinerstein et al.[267] showed that norephinephrine-fluorophore fades very rapidly on exposure to HCl vapour, but the dopamine-fluorophore does not. The presence of dopaminergic elements in association with the vascular poles of the glomeruli, supports a role for the neuronal control of renal haemodynamics, the release of renin and the related renal changes[267].

IX. HEAVY METALS

A number of heavy metals are potently nephrotoxic. While autoradiography (see below) has been an important method for studying metal distribution, histochemistry can also be used. Recently the localized renal distribution of mercury to the lysosomes of the proximal tubule has been shown by the silver amplification of the mercury sulphide[268]. This silver amplification technique could also be applied to other heavy metals, including gold. There are also a number of sensitive chromogenic chelating agents, such as benzothiazolylazophenol derivatives that bind cadmium very selectively[269].

Changes in metallothionein levels are a frequent consequence of heavy metal exposure. The distribution of metallothionein has been shown by immunohistochemical methods[154] (see above). There are a number of histochemical methods that have been used to demonstrate the presence of macromolecular thiols. Morselt et al.[270,271] showed a dose- and time-related increase in histochemically stainable macromolecular disulphide granules in the proximal and distal (high dose only) tubules of rats treated with $CdCl_2$. Based on the high disulphide:protein ratio these granules were assumed to be cadmium-thionein. Ultrastructural studies and X-ray microprobe analysis supported high sulphur and cadmium levels and showed that these "granules" were in fact lysosomes.

X.   AUTORADIOGRAPHY

One of the major advantages of autoradiograpy is the wide variety of tracer molecules that are available, the ability to study both water-diffusible and "fixed" molecules, and the fact that the technique can be used in tandem with other histochemical methods. Furthermore, the distribution of a host of potentially nephrotoxic radiolabelled molecules can be assessed at both a whole-body and a microscopic level[272]. The technique can be greatly strengthened by the use of an appropriately labelled precursor, where some degree of certainty can be maintained on the nature of the molecule, and by the selective administration of the label, where localized infusion (rather than the systemic route) will label a tissue of choice. Many of the advantages of autoradiography can be further enhanced by the use of semi-thin sections, particularly because it is then possible to use ^{14}C-labelled material and still maintain very good localization of distribution at the light microscopic level[272a]. The interpretation of autoradiography has been covered in several texts[273,274], but may still need careful controls and intelligent consideration. For example the binding of ^{125}I-insulin to the apical surfaces of the proximal tubule represents the normal handling of filtered peptides and not a hormone receptor[275].

Most of the histochemical techniques have the disadvantage of

dead end-point measurements. In order to obtain kinetic information it is necessary to introduce markers into the animals which
will be incorporated into renal cells, i.e. radioactively labelled
precursors of DNA (mostly ^{3}H-thymidine), and of carbohydrates or
proteins. While there are a large number of studies that have used
the autoradiographic distribution of nucleic acid precursors, it has
not been generally recognized that their incorporation shows some
degree of tissue-specificity, that may depend on the distribution of
enzymes involved in purine salvaging. For example, the incorporation of uridine (as assessed at the whole-body level) has been
reported to be far greater in the kidney than deoxythymidine[276].

It is possible to obtain information on the duration of S-
phase cell cycling in a tissue specimen using the double isotope
pulse-labelling technique[277]. The two DNA-precursors [3]H- and
[14]C-thymidine are pulse-labelled a few hours apart. All the cells in
S-phase at the time of both pulses will be dual labelled, while the
cells that are at the end of S-phase when the first pulse is given
will only be labelled by the first isotope and not the second. Conversely those cells that are in S-phase when the second label is
given will only carry that isotope. The duration of the S-phase can
be estimated from the time between pulses, and the proportion of
cells that have the three different combinations of labelled nuclei.
As yet there are no published data on the use of this technique in
relation to nephrotoxicity, but it would be appropriate to give an
insight into regeneration in different regions of the kidney. Dual
labelling has also been used to study the dynamics of metal-protein
complex handling by the kidney. Murakami and co-workers[278,278a]
showed that while [109]Cd and ^{125}I-labelled metallothionein enter the
cell together, the [109]Cd is lost at a very early stage.

The effect of some polycyclic aromatic hydrocarbons consists
of an inhibition of thymidine incorporation[279] and that following
HgCl$_2$-induced nephrotoxicity the incorporation of amino acids increased, consistent with the morphological criteria of regeneration[280]. Similarly, an increased incorporation of thymidine into
DNA has been described for HgCl$_2$ nephrotoxicity[14]. Using the 1-h
[3]H-thymidine pulse labelling technique it has been possible to show
that the proliferative rate of tubular cells is low in adult rats (8
weeks or older), but about twice this rate in 5-week-old rats. In
both age groups the area of highest proliferative activity is that of
the inner stripe, which is about twice that of the rest of the kidney. Severe proximal tubule damage 24 h after a single dose of
cephaloridine is associated with a slight proliferation, and increases
up to 4 days with repair (Figure 12). Regeneration is fast, and
similar after a single dose or after multiple daily doses. Balazs[281]
has already drawn attention to the resistance of regenerated cells
to further toxic insult. Conventional light microscopy of the
cephaloridine-induced lesion did not show any dose-dependent abnormalities at the end of the chronic study, but hyperplasia could
be assumed on the basis of an increase in organ weight. By contrast chronic dosing with gentamicin produces a dose-related increase in proliferation and severity of the lesion. Thus [3]H-
thymidine pulse labelling allows those nephrotoxic effects where
cells develop resistance to multiple insults to be differentiated from
toxins that repeatedly damage cells. Similar results were obtained

by Laurent et al.[282], using homogenate analyses in a 14-day toxicity studies with gentamicin.

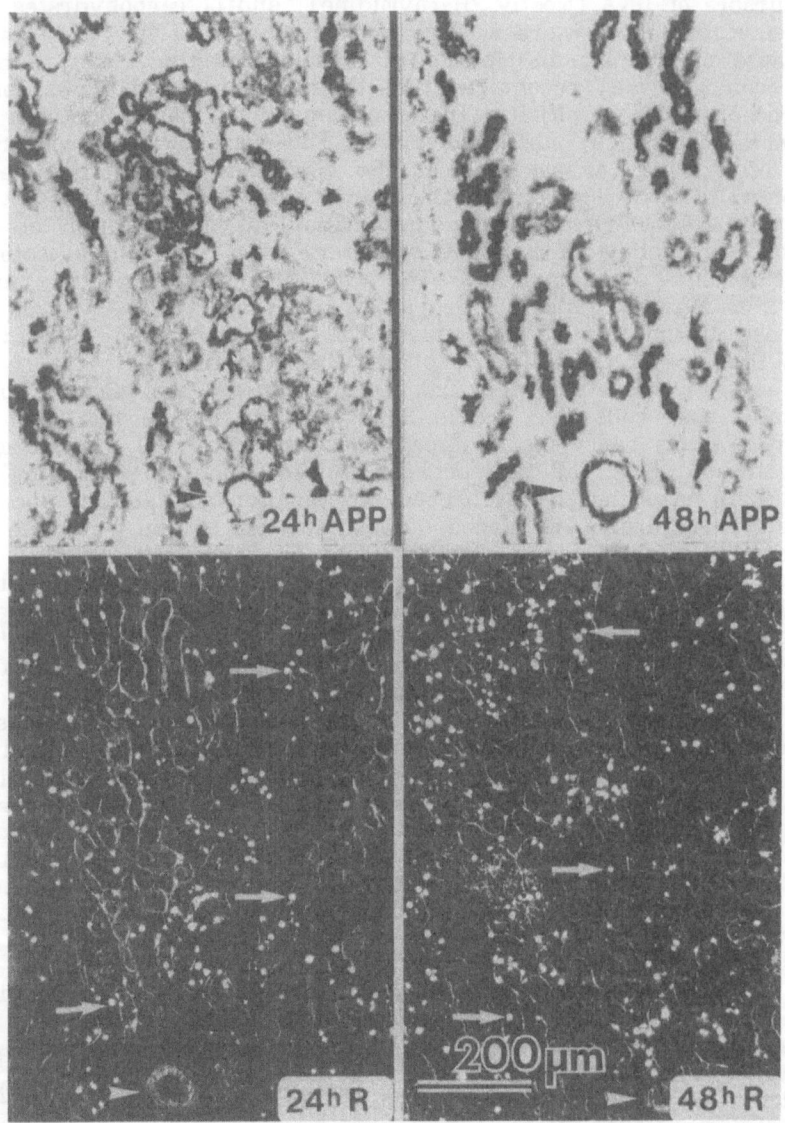

Figure 12 Autoradiography of the rat kidney 24 h and 48 h after a single 0.8 g/kg i.v. dose of cephaloridine and a 1 h i.p. pulse of ^{3}H-thymidine. The number of labelled (proliferating) cells is greatly increased 24 h after the nephrotoxin and is largest in the regenerating tubules by 48 h. Frozen, acetone-fixed sections stained for alkaline phosphatase (APP), Carnoy fixed, PAS-stained autoradiographs in darkfield illumination (R). Arteria arcuata (arrowheads) and some labelled cells (arrows). Note the reduced distribution of FRP in necrotic tubules at 24 h, which is increased in the regenerated tubules at 48 h.

While pulse labelling gives information of the extent of proliferative change at a single time point, it does not give a measure of tissue regeneration. Such information can be obtained by assessing the total number of new cells formed over a period during which ^{3}H-thymidine is continuously infused from a mini-osmotic pump, or other device. Using this technique it is possible to show the marked increase in cell labelling within 24 h of a nephrotoxic insult. More importantly, while there is no recognizable renal pathology 5-8 days after a single dose of cephaloridine, the tremendous labelling of cell nuclei shows that the proximal tubule represents almost totally repaired tissue (Figure 13). Other techniques cannot identify the regeneration of relatively resistant cells and there is a need to establish where similar changes escape conventional techniques used in subchronic and chronic toxicity studies.

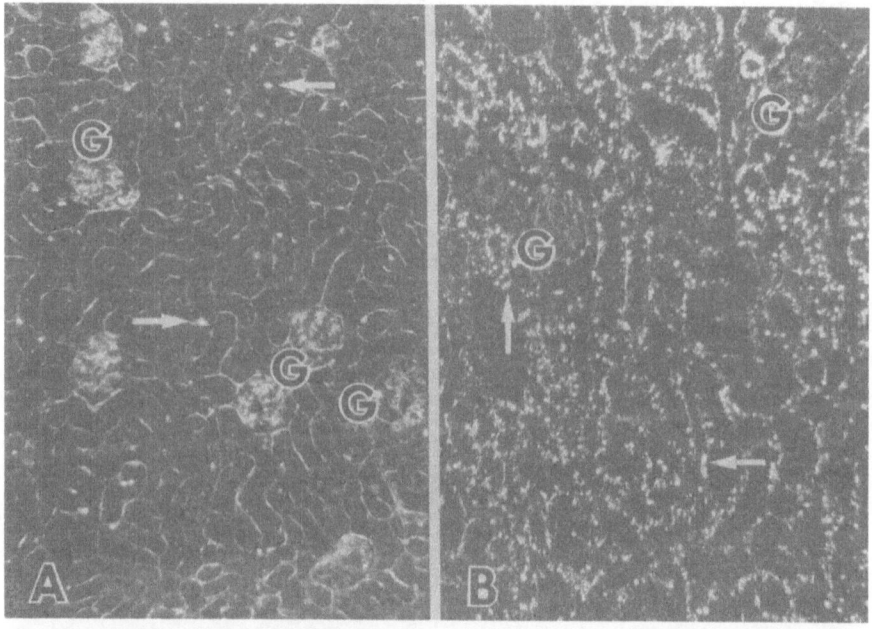

Figure 13 Autoradiography can show the total cell proliferation that has occurred, using ^{3}H-thymidine continuously infused s.c. from a mini-osmotic pump 2 to 5 days after the insult, and the rat killed on day 7. There is limited cell proliferation in control rats (**A**), whereas heavy nuclear labelling occurred after 0.8 g/kg i.v. cephaloridine, (**B**). Darkfield illumination, G shows glomeruli.

It is also possible to study the kinetic response of different renal cell types in response to renal injury. Contralateral hypertrophy (in response to uninephrectomy) is up to 4-fold more marked in the cortex compared to the medulla, and this response to the release of renotropic factor is suppressed by water deprivation[283].

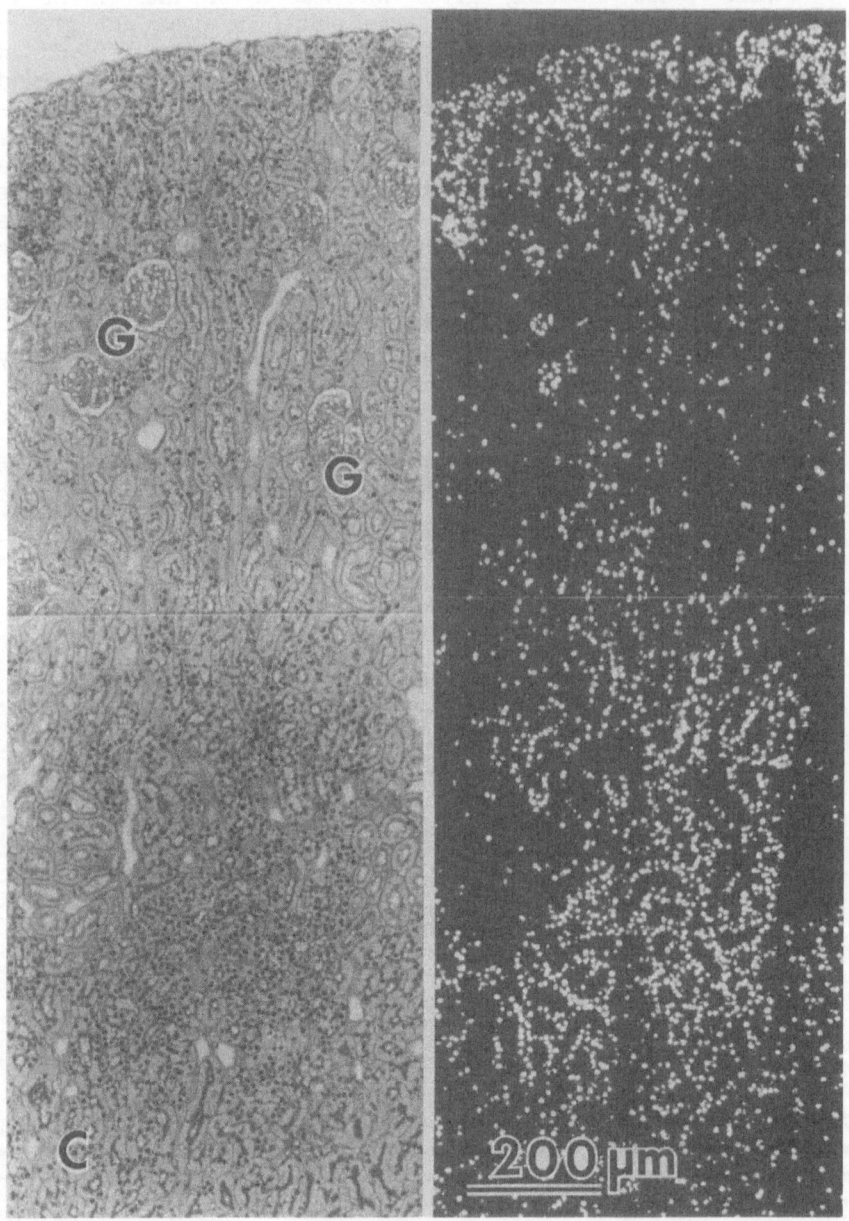

Figure 13 continued (C) Conventional histology fails to identify the presence of regenerated cells (left side) despite the extensive silver grains above regenerated cells (right side). Carnoy fixed, PAS-stained autoradiographs: darkfield photographs of the juxtamedullary junction, showing glomeruli (G), some labelled cells (arrows). Transmitted light for conventional histological evaluation (left side) and the same field in darkfield illumination for demonstration of the labelled nuclei (right side).

Autoradiography of semi-thin, methacrylate-embedded sections showed that normally the turnover of epithelial cells (infusing ^{3}H-thymidine at zero order from an implanted mini-osmotic pump for 144 h) differed in the major regions of the kidney. The cell turnover was similar in the proximal and distal tubules, the urothelia covering the papilla and the adjacent pelvic epithelia. A lower labelling index was observed in the ureter and the collecting duct and the lowest was the pelvic fornix. Following an acutely induced papillary necrosis there was a 6-fold increase in the pelvic fornix adjacent to the papillary injury and a 2- to 3-fold increase in the turnover in all other regions[284].

XI. OTHER HISTOCHEMICAL METHODS FOR ASSESSING THE KIDNEY

A. Renal haemodynamics, glomerular permeability and filtration

Assessment of the renal haemodynamics and glomerular filtration generally includes examination of the whole kidney by blood flow monitoring[285] or gross anatomical distribution of a labelled material[286,287]. These methods measure regional flow or total clearance and give no data on the distribution within the medulla and cortex. They cannot therefore be used to study the subtle and focal changes that may relate to target-selective injury. Several histochemical methods are available to assess these changes, although these have not been used to follow the time course of those renal injuries where such information would be valuable.

1. Nephron perfusion and microvascular control

The subtle control of kidney microvasculature and the shunting of blood to (or from) different regions of the medulla and cortex present a most fundamental process in normal renal function. This may be altered in nephrotoxic lesions that have been linked to is-chaemic injury. The introduction of exogenous particulate material into the renal microvasculature gives some indication of the patency of the vessels and/or the presence of vasoconstriction/occlusion. The morphological methods described below cannot differentiate between stasis and high flow rate areas, nor can they generally identify "leaky" capillaries, an endothelial defect that could play a very important role in disrupting renal compartmentalization.

Colloidal carbon has been used to show the loss of medullary microvascular filling at an advanced stage of ethyleneimine-[288] and aspirin-induced[289] renal papillary necrosis. The introduction of this material for assessing vascular filling may present some difficuties. India ink has been used as the common source of colloidal carbon, a variety of additives (phenols, shellac and fish glue)[290] used to enhance its drawing properties, and the colloidal nature of this material imparts a substantial oncotic pressure, both of which may cause artefacts in assessing microvascular filling. These circumvent using India ink that has been dialysed against isotonic saline[107]. Colloidal carbon prepared thus has been used to follow the time course of microvascular changes in animals treated with 2-

bromoethanamine. There was an early shift (2-4 h after dosing) of microvascular filling from the cortex to the outer medulla, after which the filling of the inner medulla was more pronounced, but at the expense of the outer part of the medullary plexus at 8-26 h. These changes coincided with the development of renal papillary necrosis. By 48 h when necrosis was complete the damaged medulla was avascular. During the course of development of RPN, however, the microvasculature was patent in the medullary tissue beyond the regions in which necrosis had occurred. These data were interpreted as showing that an acute medullary necrosis can occur without capillary occlusion[107]. These observations have also been confirmed by high-resolution microscopy where platelet adherence and microvascular changes did not occur until late in the development of the lesion[108].

The inherent difficulties associated with using colloidal carbon as a suitable particulate material for intravascular filling prompted Joris et al.[291] to use Monastral Blue B (a copper phthalocyanine), the advantages of which are water-insolubility, non-toxicity, uniform size distribution, commercial availability, and high contrast for thin and thick sections. Recently, this method has been used to address the possible role of microvascular occlusion or leakage in the genesis of renal papillary necrosis. The distribution of vascular labelling in semi-thin methacrylate sections showed that glomeruli and pelvic basal epithelia were well labelled (Figure 14). No Monastral Blue B was present in the papillary matrix, data that suggest that the capillary integrity was intact and the leakage of material into the interstitium was not involved in the pathogenesis of renal papillary necrosis[108].

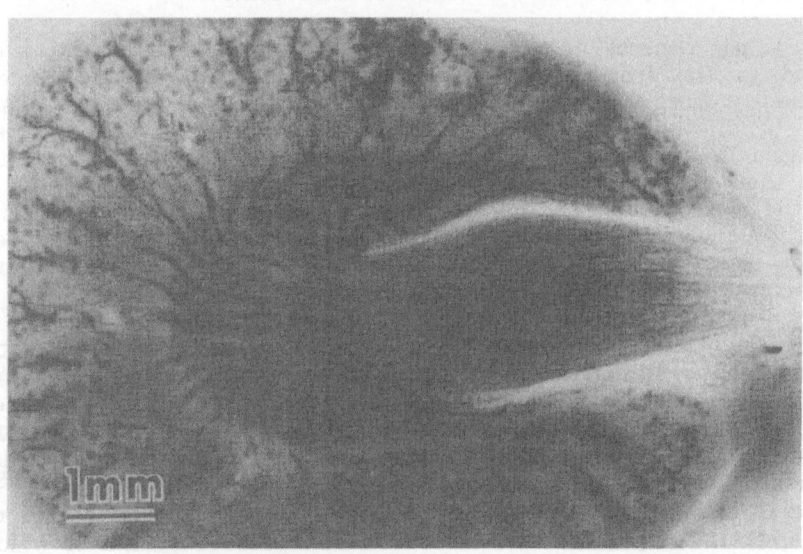

Figure 14 Distribution of Monastral Blue B vascular label throughout kidney. Photomicrograph from en bloc kidney embedded in glycol methacrylate.

Erythrocytes also offer a natural marker for studying vascular filling, and can be isolated, washed, formaldehyde-fixed and tagged with a fluorescent or radiolabelled marker[292], but it has been suggested that labelling the erythrocyte impairs its flexibility, and may alter its normal distribution. It is, however, possible to make use of the endogenous erythrocytes, because of several of their unique staining properties. Early studies made use of the benzidine staining technique, and showed the marked blood filling changes in the kidney following 5-hydroxytryptamine (serotonin) exposure[293], which were consistent with the shunting of blood away from the cortex to the juxtamedullary area. It is generally assumed that this shunting of blood plays an essential role in the development of the ischaemic proximal tubular necrosis that commonly follows high doses of serotonin. The established carcinogenic properties of benzidine preclude its use, but erythrocytes can be contrasted by the presence of enzymes such as esterase, glucose-6-phosphate dehydrogenase, acid or alkaline phosphatase; the high levels of phospholipids shown by the Sudan black method; by a variety of routinely used stains such as Masson's trichrome, Toluidine blue, Giemsa[92,93] and the high macromolecular thiol levels by the diazotized N-(4-aminophenyl)-maleimide method[294].

2. Glomerular filtration

Total glomerular filtration may be unchanged in those nephropathies (e.g. renal papillary necrosis)[182] where single nephron glomerular filtration rates are reduced. While it is possible to measure single nephron glomerular filtration rates in superficial nephrons by micropuncture, this technique is very slow and gives no information on the juxtamedullary nephrons. The "Hanssen technique" makes use of the localization of glomerular filtered ferrocyanide to the tubular lumen (which is not reabsorbed or secreted), that has been precipitated by ferric chloride (in the frozen kidney) as Prussian blue[295-297]. Many workers have then microdissected whole nephron segments and studied the distribution of Prussian blue in relation to nephron length, total glomerular filtration rate and in the diuretic versus normal and/or antidiuretic states[296,297]. This approach has also been quantitated using radiolabelled ferrocyanide[182].

There are few reports using this technique to describe the degree of glomerular filtration in nephrons exposed to chemicals. Normally only 75% of the nephrons are actively filtering[298], an observation that supports the functional reserve that is present in the nephron. The number of non-filtering nephrons increases in animals in which hydronephrosis has been induced by ureter ligation, probably in those nephrons where there is cast formation and tubular dilatation. This does, however, need confirmation using the Hanssen technique and suitable markers for luminal casts. This may be relevant in renal papillary necrosis where the presence of Tamm-Horsfall glycoprotein casts has been linked to tubular dilatation and subsequent glomerular sclerosis and scarring of the cortex[181,182,299].

There is presently interest in the marked hyaline droplet formation that occurs in male rats exposed to branched-chain hydrocarbons[189-192]. These can be shown by Mallory's Heidenhein stain, their eosinophilia or the use of antibodies to α_{2u}-globulin. The heterogeneity of hyaline droplet formation highlights several questions:

(i). which nephrons are filtering, those with or without the protein over-load; and

(ii). is switching off the filtering nephrons a way of giving the resting nephron a chance to remove this material?

Ferrocyanide does, however, bind to protein[300] and therefore will give higher values in male rats (because of the sex hormone related proteinuria), in those circumstances where glomerular permselectivity is altered, as a result of glomerular damage and when the proximal tubule protein reabsorbtive capacity has been decreased.

3.   Changes in glomerular protein filtering and proximal tubule uptake

Glomerular permselectivity and the proximal tubular uptake of a number of filtered proteins is a very important indication of normal renal function. The peroxidative activity of several low molecular weight enzymes (such as horseradish peroxidase, myeloperoxidase and myoglobin) have been used to study glomerular permeability and protein uptake by the proximal tubule[301-303]. The horseradish peroxidase (HRP) is taken up into apical vacuoles or phagosomes in the proximal tubule that merge with lysosomes, and slowly undergoes degradation. The clearance of HRP can be altered by a saline or mannitol diuresis, which decreases cellular uptake. Mannitol in particular produced a large number of vesicles which were assumed to be involved in fluid transport at the expense of HRP uptake[304]. The administration of these exogenous protein markers is not, however, without the adverse effect of vascular leakage, a response that can be inhibited by histamine and serotonin antagonists[305]. There is also some evidence to suggest that arachidonic acid metabolites may be involved in the hypotensive effect caused by the administration of HRP, because this can be prevented by indomethacin and aspirin[306]. Despite the potential value of these methods there appears to be a paucity of published data on their application to studying chemical induced proteinuria.

B.   Fluorescence vizualization of chemicals

Many chemicals with nephrotoxic potential fluoresce strongly (Table 7), and therefore offer the potential to vizualize their distribution at a cellular and subcellular level (an objective most often achieved by autoradiography). Some of these chemicals also show spectral changes as a result of metabolism, a property that ensures that more information can be attained from this method than from autoradiography, which measures total drug-derived material only. One of the major problems with the use of fluorescent monitoring is the significant tissue autofluorescence that may be present. Thus it is essential to screen control tissue to ensure that the choice of filter combinations maximizes the visualization of the chemical of interest.

Table 7 Nephrotoxic chemicals with fluorescent properties

Actinomycin
Aflatoxins
Aminoglycosides
Anthracyclines
Biphenyls
Catecholamines
Tetracyclines

For example, the fluorescence of streptomycin has provided data on its distribution in the inner ear[307], an approach that could also be applied to the kidney. The anthracycline antibiotic adriamycin (doxorubicin) and its analogue daunomycin are rapidly taken up by the kidney and cleared from the cytoplasm to leave only the nuclei showing the presence of these chemicals after 60 min[308]. These data closely paralleled the renal pharmacokinetics of the anthracyclines, but failed to help explain why this compound targets selectively for the glomeruli[101].

XII. CONCLUSION AND FUTURE TRENDS IN THE USE OF HISTOCHEMICAL TECHNIQUES

The applications of histochemistry and immunohistochemistry are many, and the topics we have covered represent only a partial overview of how fundamental questions can be addressed. More importantly, despite the problems that may be experienced from time to time in reproducing these techniques they have several very important advantages:

1. They provide the most cost-effective way of bridging the dichotomy between renal structure and function, and may give information that relates directly to a subcellular or molecular level.

2. Even when the bases for histochemical change are empirical (as many still are), they are discriminatory and help visualize renal heterogeneity and focal lesions.

3.   Microspectrophotometry and fluorimetry, with computer manipulation of the extensive data that have been generated, and the automation of slide scanning, are increasingly providing objective means of handling large quantities of material.

4.   The indication that a "general" histochemical change has occurred (e.g. loss of a carbohydrate matrix or glycoprotein, lipid change, etc.) is a far more logical starting point for specific and specialized studies (e.g. biochemical, immunological assessment, ultrastructural evaluation, etc.) than can currently be rationalized from other experimental protocols.

5.   There are instances where histo- and immunohistochemical methods give information that is usually only otherwise available from ultrastructural studies, but provide markedly larger areas of tissue and offer the potential for more rapid assessments.

6.   Histochemistry gives data on the kinetics of cell damage and its repair, in relation to associated cell types that may not be damaged. Another approach is the determination of proliferative and regenerative capacity of renal cells by means of either the frequency of mitotic figures or counting labelled cells after infusion with ^{3}H-thymidine. Such techniques may be helpful in the detection of specifically affected sites and in the quantifying of pathological changes, and may even shed light on mechanisms of toxicity.

7.   The trend in toxicology has shifted from descriptive pathology to one with a molecular focus that will provide a rational basis for safer drug design, better treatment of disease and more reliable hazard assessment. The transition between "organ toxicity" and the focal lesions of "target cell toxicity" must begin with light microscopic evaluation, and progress to a biochemical level in which the identity of the morphologically damaged cell must be maintained.

Histology is still the basis for defining renal lesions in toxicology, while urine and serum analyses can be of help in determining the sequences of events in individuals. For detection of test compound-related renal lesions in animals with varying background pathology, it is advantageous to supplement the conventional staining techniques. The following problems have to be encountered:

1.   extensive cell injury may have caused the loss of the specific characteristic;

2.   regenerating cells may not yet have acquired the specific characteristic;

3.   the method used may be based on minor differences and may not readily discriminate between cells;

4.   residual compound may interfere with the histochemical reaction;

5.   sampling error may be large, e.g. in the case of focal lesions;

6.   species differences in morphology and reactivity will be encountered;

7.   special investigations have to be arranged as an essential part of the study protocol and can cause logistic problems if used for routine toxicity tests.

ACKNOWLEDGEMENTS

The authors are grateful to Ted Lock for critical comment, and to M. E. van Ek and H. Scott for preparing the manuscript. The authors' research was supported by the Wellcome Trust, the Cancer Research Campaign, the International Agency for Cancer Research, the National Kidney Research Fund, the Commission of the European Communities - Biotechnology Action Programme, and Ciba-Geigy.

REFERENCES

1.   WACHSMUTH, E.D. (1981). The rationality and relative contribution of histochemical approaches to pharmacology and toxicology. Histochem. J., 13, 793-797.

2.   HEITZ, P.U. (1979). Histochemistry as a tool in clinical and experimental pathology. Pathol. Res. Pract., 164, 24-34.

3.   MOFFAT, D.B. (1982). Morphology of the kidney in relation to nephrotoxicity - portae renales. In Nephrotoxicity, Assessment and Pathogenesis. [Eds. P.H. Bach, F.W. Bonner, J.W. Bridges and E.A. Lock]. Wiley, Chichester, 10-26.

4.   KRIZ, W. (1976). Der architektonische und funktionelle Aufbau der Rattenniere. Z. Zellforsch., 82, 495-535.

5.   KAISSLING, B. and KRIZ, W. (1979). Structural analysis of the rabbit kidney. Adv. Anat. Embryol. Cell Biol., Springer, Berlin, 56

6.   KRIZ, W. and KOEPSELL, H. (1974). The structural organization of the mouse kidney. Z. Anat. Entwickl. Gesch., 144, 137-163.

7.   SPICER, S.S., LEPPI, T.J. and STOWARD, P.J. (1965). Suggestions for a histochemical terminology of carbohydrate-rich tissue components. J. Histochem. Cytochem., 13, 599-603.

8.   STOWARD, P.J., BARKER, S.A., KENT, P.W. and PEARSE, A.G.E. (1966). Some British comments on the histochemical nomenclature of mucosubstances. J. Histochem. Cytochem., 14, 681.

9.   STOWARD, P. (1980). Criteria for the validation of quantitative histochemical enzyme techniques. In Trends in Enzyme Histochemistry and Cytochemistry. Ciba Found. Symp. 73, Excerpta Medica, Amsterdam, 11-31

10.   ROSS, B.D. and GUDER, W.G. (1982). Heterogeneity and compartmentation in the kidney. In Metabolic Compartmentation. [Ed. H. Sies]. Academic Press, New York, 363-409.

11.   BONNER, F.W., BACH, P.H. and DOBROTA, M. (1982). The biochemistry of the
       kidney. In Nephrotoxicity, Assessment and Pathogenesis. [Eds. P.H. Bach,
       F.W. Bonner, J.W. Bridges and E.A. Lock]. Wiley, Chichester, 437-459.

12.   GUDER, W.G. and ROSS, B.D. (1984). Enzyme distribution along the nephron.
       Kidney Int., 26, 101-111.

13.   IRINTSCHEFF, A. and DAVIDOFF, M. (1981). Ueber die Verteilung einiger
       Hydrolasen in der Rattenniere. Histochemistry, 71, 463-480.

14.   CUPPAGE, F.E. and TATE, A. (1967). Repair of the nephron following injury
       with mercuric chloride. Am. J. Pathol., 51, 405-429.

15.   MOYAYAMA, H., SOLOMON, R., SASAKI, M., CHI-WEI, L.N. and FISHMAN, W.H.
       (1975). Demonstration of lysosomal and extralysosomal sites for acid phos-
       phatase in mouse kidney tubule cells with p-nitrophenylphosphate lead-salt
       technique. J. Histochem. Cytochem., 23, 439-451.

16.   NEISS, W.F. and KLEHN, K.L. (1981). The postnatal development of rat kidney,
       with special reference to chemodifferentiation of the proximal tubule. His-
       tochemistry, 73, 251-268.

17.   HORIIKE, K., ARAI, R., TOJO, H., YAMANO, T., NOZAKI, M. and MAEDA, T.
       (1985). Histochemical staining of cells containing flavoenzyme D-amino acid
       oxidase based on its enzymatic activity: Application of a coupled peroxida-
       tion method. Acta Histochem. Cytochem., 18, 539-550.

18.   WACHSMUTH, E.D. and WOODHAMS, R. (1973). Uniform distribution and concentra-
       tion of aminopeptidase in proximal tubules of pig kidney. J. Histochem.
       Cytochem., 21, 685-692.

19.   JEDRZEJEWSKI, K. and KUGLER, P. (1982). Peptidases in the kidney and urine
       of rats after castration. Histochemistry, 74, 63-84.

20.   JACOBSEN, N.O., JORGENSEN, F. and THOMSEN, A.C. (1967). On the localisation
       of some phosphatases in three different segments of the proximal tubules in
       the rat kidney. J. Histochem. Cytochem., 15, 456-469.

21.   LÖNNERHOLM, G. (1973). Histochemical demonstration of carbonic anhydrase ac-
       tivity in the human kidney. Acta Physiol. Scand., 88, 455-468.

22.   LÖNNERHOLM, G. (1971). Histochemical demonstration of carbonic anhydrase ac-
       tivity in the rat kidney. Acta Physiol. Scand., 81, 433-439.

23.   BÖTI, Zs., SZTRIHA L. and ORMOS J. (1981). Histochemical studies of
       oxidoreductases in rat kidney regenerating after mercuric chloride injury.
       Exp. Pathol., 19, 247-256.

24.   WALKER, D.G. (1963). A survey of dehydrogenase in various epithelial cells
       in the rat. J. Cell Biol., 17, 255-277.

25.   STERNBERG, W.H., FARBER, E. and DUNLAP, C.E. (1956). Histochemical localisa-
       tion of specific oxidative enzymes: II. Localisation of diphosphopyridine
       nucleotide and triphospho-phyridine nucleotide diaphorases and the succinic
       dehydrogenase system in the kidney. J. Histochem. Cytochem., 4, 266-283.

26.   BÖTI, Zs., KOBOR, J. and ORMOS, J. (1982). Activity of glucose-6-phosphatase
       in regenerating tubular epithelium in rat kidney after necrosis induced with
       mercuric chloride: A light and electronmicroscopical study. Br. J. Exp.
       Pathol., 63, 615-624.

27.   GLENNER, G.G., FOLK, J.E. and McMILLAN, P.J. (1962). Histochemical
       demonstration of a gamma-glutamyl transpeptidase-like activity. J. Histo-
       chem. Cytochem., 10, 481-489.

28.   SEYAMA, S., IIJIMA, S. and KATUNUMA, N. (1977). Biochemical and histochemi-
       cal studies on response of ammonia-producing enzymes for HN_4Cl-induced
       acidosis. J. Histochem. Cytochem., 25, 448-457.

29.   NOVIKOFF, A.B., SPATER, H.W. and QUINTANA, N. (1983). Transepithelial endo-
       plasmic reticulum in rat proximal convoluted tubule. J. Histochem.
       Cytochem., 31, 656-661.

30.   DAHLQVIST, A. and BRUN, A. (1962). A method for the histochemical demonstra-
       tion of disaccharidase activities, application to invertase and trehalase in
       some animal tissues. J. Histochem. Cytochem., 10, 294-302.

31.   McMILLAN, P.J. (1967). Differential demonstration of muscle and heart type
       lactic dehydrogenase of rat muscle and kidney. J. Histochem. Cytochem., 16,
       21-31.

32.   COTTRELL, R.C., AGRELO, C.E., GANGOLLI, S.D. and GRASSO, P. (1976). His-
       tochemical and biochemical studies of chemically induced acute kidney damage
       in the rat. Fd. Cosmet. Toxicol., 14, 593-598.

33.   WACHSTEIN, M. and MEISEL, E. (1954). Influence of experimental renal damage
       on histochemically demonstrable succinic dehydrogenase activity in the rat.
       Am. J. Pathol., 30, 147-159.

34.   WACHSTEIN, M. (1955). Histochemical staining reactions of the normally
       functioning and abnormal kidney. J. Histochem. Cytochem., 3, 246-270.

35.   WACHSMUTH, E.D. (1980). Principles of immunocytochemical assays. Proc. Royal
       Microsc. Soc., 14, 252-255.

36.   WACHSMUTH, E.D. (1973). An immunohistochemical method for localization of
       enzymes in tissue sections: The use of antibody bound to tissue antigen and
       its property of binding cross reactive soluble antigen. Histochemie, 37,
       251-263.

37.   LOJDA, Z. (1979). The histochemical demonstration of peptidases by natural
       substrates. Histochemistry, 62, 305-323.

38.   GOSSRAU, R. and LOJDA, Z. (1980). Study on dipeptidylpeptidase II (DPP II).
       Histochemistry, 70, 53-76.

39.   HARDONK, M.J., MESKENDORP-HAARSMA, T.J. and KOUDSTAAL, J. (1978). A histo-
       chemical study about the influence of lytic enzymes on plasma membrane en-
       zyme activities in rat liver and kidney. Histochemistry, 58, 177-181.

40.   ARBORGH, B., ERICSSON, J.L.E. and HELMINEN, H. (1971). Inhibition of renal
       acid phosphatase and aryl sulfatase activity by glutaraldehyde fixation. J.
       Histochem. Cytochem., 19, 449-451.

41.   ASHFORD, A.E., ALLAWAY, W.G. and McNULLY, M.E. (1972). Low temperature em-
       bedding in glycol methacrylate for enzyme histochemistry in plant and animal
       tissues. J. Histochem. Cytochem., 20, 986-990.

42.   HOSHINO, M. and KOBAYASHI, H. (1971). The use of glycol methacrylate as an
       embedding medium for the histochemical demonstration of acid phosphatase ac-
       tivity. J. Histochem. Cytochem., 19, 575-577.

43.   RUSSO, J. and WELLS, P. (1975). Light microscopic localisation of cytochemi-
       cal reactions in epoxy-embedded material for electron microscopy. J. Histo-
       chem. Cytochem., 23, 921-931.

44.   MAYAHARA, H. and OGAWA, K. (1980). Ultracytochemical localisation of
       ouabain-sensitive, potassium-dependent p-nitrophenyl-phosphatase activity in
       the rat kidney. Acta Histochem. Cytosol., 13, 90-102.

45.   LONGLEY, J. and FISHER, E.R. (1956). A histochemical basis for changes in
       renal tubular function in young mice. Quart. J. Microscop. Sci., 97, 187-
       195.

46.   WACHSMUTH, E.D. (1968). Localisation von Aminopeptidase in Gewebeschnitten
       mit einer neuen Immunofluoreszenztechnik. Histochemie, 14, 282-296.

47.   LÖNNERHOLM, G. (1972). Histochemical demonstration of carbonic anhydrase ac-
       tivity in the human kidney. Acta Pharmacol. Suppl. I, 31, 52-87.

48.   SZOKOL, M. and SOLTESZ, M.B. (1973). Histochemical study on the oxidative
       enzymes of the interstitial cells of the renal medulla in rats. Acta Histo-
       chem., 46, 120-129.

49.   WACHSMUTH, E.D. (1985). Renal heterogeneity at a light microscopic level. In
       Renal Heterogeneity and Target Cell Toxicity. [Eds. P.H. Bach and E.A.

Lock]. Wiley, Chichester, 13-30.

50. SCHIEBER, T.H. and MUHLENFELD, E. (1960). Ueber geschlechts-spezifische Un-
     terschiede im Fermentmuster der Ratte. Anat. Anz. Erg. Heft., 120, 41-48.

51. MUEHLENFELD, W.E. (1969). Ueber die Entwicklung und Chemodifferenzierung de
     Rattenniere unter besonderer Beruecksichtigung der Geschlechtsunterschiede.
     Histochemie, 18, 97-131.

52. JACOBSEN, N.O. (1975). Enzyme histochemical observations on the segmentation
     of the proximal tubules in the kidney of the female rat. Histochemistry, 43,
     11-32.

53. WACHSMUTH, E.D. and STOYE, J.P. (1976). The differentiation of proximal and
     distal tubules in the male rat kidney: The appearance of aldolase isozymes,
     aminopeptidase and alkaline phosphatase during ontogeny. Histochemistry, 47,
     315-337.

54. CORDER, C.N., COLLINS, J.G., BRANNAN, T.S. and SHARMA, J. (1977). Aldolase
     reductase and sorbitol dehydrogenase distribution in rat kidney. J. His-
     tochem. Cytochem., 25, 1-8.

55. ZALME, R.C., McDOWELL, E.M., NAGLE, R.B., McNEIL, J.S., FLAMENBAUM, W. and
     TRUMP, B.F. (1976). Studies on the pathophysiology of acute renal failure.
     Virchows. Arch., 22, 197-216.

56. BÖTI, ZS., IVANYI, B., KOBOR, J. and ORMOS, J. (1979). Histochemical studies
     on peroxisomes in regenerating proximal tubules of the kidney. Br. J. Exp.
     Pathol., 60, 620-4.

57. WACHSMUTH, E.D. and THOMANN, P. (1982). Testing for renal tolerability. Cef-
     sulodin in rats and rabbits. In Nephrotoxicity, Assessment and Pathogenesis.
     [Eds. P.H. Bach, J.W. Bridges and E.A. Lock]. Wiley, Chichester, 498-503.

58. WACHSMUTH, E.D. (1981). Nephrotoxicity of cefotiam (CGP 14221/E) in rats and
     rabbits. Arch. Toxicol., 48, 135-156.

59. WACHSMUTH, E.D. (1976). Quantitation of enzymes in tissue sections by es-
     timation of hydrolytic activity and antigenic determinants. Acta Histochem.,
     Suppl.-Bd., 16, 221-231.

60. WACHSMUTH, E.D. (1981). Quantification of nephrotoxicity in rabbits by
     automated morphometry of alkaline phosphatase stained kidney sections. His-
     tochemistry, 71, 235-248.

61. WACHSMUTH, E.D. (1982). Quantification of acute cephaloridine nephrotoxicity
     in rats: Correlation of serum and 24 hr urine analyses with proximal tubule
     injuries. Toxicol. Appl. Pharmacol., 63, 429-445.

62. WACHSMUTH, E.D. (1982). Adaptation of nephrotoxic effects of cephaloridine
     in subacute rat toxicity studies. Toxicol. Appl. Pharmacol., 63, 446-460.

63. HOSHINO, M. and KOBAYASHI, H. (1972). Glycol methacrylate embedding in im-
     munocytochemical methods. J. Histochem. Cytochem., 20, 743-745.

64. BURNETT, R. (1982). A study of enzymatic and structural renal damage induced
     by nephrotoxic agents in the rat. M. Phil. thesis, University of Nottin-
     gham.

65. GREGG, N.J. and BACH, P.H. (1986) Unpublished data.

66. KIRBY, G., GREGG, N.J. and BACH, P.H. (1986) Unpublished data.

67. BECKSTEAD, J.H. (1985). Optimal antigen localization in human tissues using
     aldehyde-fixed plastic-embedded sections. J. Histochem. Cytochem., 33, 954-
     958.

68. ALPERS, C.E. and BECKSTEAD, J.H. (1984). Enzyme histochemistry of normal and
     neoplastic transitional epithelium. Am. J. Clin. Pathol., 82, 655-659.

68a. ALPERS, C.E. and BECKSTEAD, J.H. (1985). Enzyme histochemistry in plastic-
     embedded sections of normal and diseased kidneys. Am. J. Clin. Pathol., 83,
     605-612.

69. TROYER, H. and NUSBICKEL, F.R. (1975). Enzyme histochemistry of

undecalcified bone and cartilage embedded in glycol methacrylate. Acta Histochem., 53, 198-202.

70. RICHIE, J.P. and SKINNER, D.G. (1981). Renal neoplasia. In The Kidney, 2nd Edition, Vol 2. [Eds. B.M. Brenner and F.C. Rector (Jnr)]. W.B. Saunders, Philadelphia, 2109-2136.

71. JASMIN, G. and RIOPELLE, J.L. (1968). Renal adenomas induced by dimethyl-nitrosamine. Enzyme histochemistry in the rat. Arch. Pathol., 85, 298-305.

72. OHMORI, T., HIASA, Y., MURATA, Y. and WILLIAM G.M. (1982). Gamma-glutamyltraspeptidase activity in carcinogen-induced epithelial lesions of rat kidney. Gann, 73, 543-548.

73. TSUDA, H., MOORE, M.A., ASAMOTO, M., SATOH, K., TSUCHIDA, S., SATO, K., ICHIHAWA, A. and ITO, N. (1985). Comparison of the various forms of glutathione S-transferase with glucose-6-phosphate dehydrogenase and gamma-glutamyltranspeptidase as markers of preneoplastic and neoplastic lesions in rat kidney induced by N-ethyl-N-hydroxyethylnitrosamine. Gann, 76, 919-929.

74. ALBERT, Z., RZUCIDLO, Z. and STARZYK, H. (1970). Comparative biochemical and histochemical studies on the activity of gamma-glutamyltranspeptidase in the organs of fetuses, newborns and adult rats. Acta Histochem., 37, 34-39.

75. ALBERT, Z., RZUCIDLO, Z. and STARZYK, H. (1970). Biochemical and histochemi-cal investigations of the gamma-glutamyltranspeptidase in the embryonic and adult organs of man. Acta Histochem., 37, 74-79.

76. KUNZE, E., SCHAUER, A. and KRUSSMAN, G. (1973). Focal loss of alkaline phos-phatase and increase of proliferation in preneoplastic areas of the rat urothelium after administration of N-butyl-N(4-hyroxybutyl)-nitrosamine and N-4-(5-nitro-2-furyl)-2-thiazolyl formamide. Z. Krebsforch., 84, 143-160.

77. KUNZE, E., SCHAUER, A. and CALVÖR, R. (1969). Sur histochemie von hamblasen papillomen der ratte, induziert durch dibutylnitrosamin. Naturwissenschaf-ten, 56, 639.

78. KUNZE, E. and SCHAUER, A. (1971). Enzymhistochemische und autoradiographische Untersuchungen an dibutyl nitrosamin-induzierten harnlasenpapillomen der ratte. Z. Krebsforsch, 74, 146-160.

79. KUNZE, E. (1979). Development of urinary bladder cancer in the rat. Curr. Top. Pathol., 67, 145-232.

80. STILLER, D. and RAUSCHER, H. (1971). Irreversible preneoplastic defect in alkaline phosphatases in cancer initiation of transitional epithelium. Exp. Pathol., 5, 255-258.

81. ITO, N., MATAYOSHI, K., ARAI, M., YOSHIOTIA, Y., KAMAMOTO, Y., MAKIURA, S. and SUGIHARA, S. (1973). Effect of various factors on induction of urinary bladder tumours in animals by N-butyl-N-(4-hydroxybutyl)nitrosamine. Gann, 64, 151-159.

82. OZONO, S., HOMMA, Y. and OYASU, R. (1985). Gamma-glutamyl-transpeptidase ac-tivity in rat urothelium treated with bladder carcinogens. Cancer Lett., 29, 49-57.

83. DAWSON, J., SMITH, D., BOAK, J. and PETERS, T.J. (1979). Gamma-glutamyltransferase in human and mouse breast tumours. Clin. Chim. Acta, 96, 37-42.

84. DE YOUNG, L., RICHARDS, W., BONZELET, W., TSAI, L. and BOUTWELL, R. (1978). Localization and significance of gamma-glutamyltranspeptidase in normal and neoplastic mouse skin. Cancer Res., 38, 3697-3701.

85. FIALA, S. and TROUT, E (1979). Histochemical detection of high gamma-glutamyltransferase activity in human epithelial tumours. J. Cell Biol., 83, (Abst Z2928).

86. FIALA, S., TROUT, E., PRAGANI, B. and FIALA, E. (1979). Increased gamma-glutamyltransferase activity in human colon cancer. Lancet, 1, 1145.

71

87.   DEMPO, K., ELLIOT, K.A., DESMOND, W. and FISHMAN, W.H. (1981). Demonstration
        of gamma-glutamyltranspeptidase, alkaline phosphatase, CEA, and HGG in human
        lung cancer. Oncodev. Biol. Med., 2, 21-37.

88.   MORIYAMA, S., KAWAOI, A. and HIROTA, N. (1983). Gamma-glutamyltranspeptid-
        ase in putative precancerous thyroid lesions of rats treated with
        diisopropanolnitrosamine. Br. J. Cancer, 47, 299-307.

89.   HANIGAN, M.H. and PITOT, H.C. (1985). Gamma-glutamyltranspeptidase - its
        role in hepatocarcinogenesis. Carcinogenesis, 6, 165-172.

90.   VANDERLAAN, M., FANG, S. and KING, E.B. (1982). Histochemistry of NADPH
        diaphorase and gamma-glutamyltranspeptidase in rat bladder tumours. Carcino-
        genesis, 3, 397-402.

91.   VARMA, R.S. and VARMA, R. (eds) (1982). Glycoaminoglycans and Proteoglycans
        in Physiological and Pathological Processes of Body Systems. S. Karger,
        Basel.

92.   CULLING, C.F.A. (1974). Handbook of Histopathological and Histochemical
        Techniques. Butterworth, London.

93.   CHAYEN, J., BITENSKY, L. and BUTCHER, R.G. (1973). Practical Histochemistry.
        Wiley-Interscience, London.

94.   HOROBIN, R.W. (1982). Histochemistry. An Explanatory Outline of Histo-
        chemistry and Biophysical Staining, Chapter 3. Gustav Fischer, Stuttgart.

95.   FURUSATO, M. (1977). Ultrastructure and histochemistry of the medullary in-
        terstitial matrix of rat kidney. Acta Pathol. Jpn., 27, 331-344.

96.   SCOTT, D.E. and DORLING, J. (1965). Differential staining of acid
        glycosaminoglycans (mucopolysaccharides) by Alcian blue in salt solutions.
        Histochemie, 5, 221-233.

97.   YAMADA, K. (1973). The effect of digestion with Streptomyces hyaluronidase
        upon certain histochemical reactions of hyaluronic acid-containing tissues.
        J. Histochem. Cytochem., 21, 794-803.

98.   YAMADA, K. (1974). The effect of digestion with chondroitinases upon certain
        histochemical reactions of mucosaccharide-containing tissues. J. Histochem.
        Cytochem., 22, 266-275.

99.   LONGLEY, J.B., BURTNER, H.J. and MONIS, B.(1963). Mucous substances of ex-
        cretory organs: a comparative study. Ann. N.Y. Acad. Sci., 106, 493-501.

100.   KASHGARIAN, M. (1985). Mesangium and glomerular disease. Lab. Invest., 52,
        569-571.

101.   BERTANI, T., DOGGI, A., DOZZONI, R., DELAINI, F., SACCHI, G., THOUA, Y.,
        MECCA, G., REMUZZI, G. and DONATI, M.B. (1982). Adriamycin-induced nephrotic
        syndrome in rats - sequence of pathologic events. Lab. Invest., 46, 16-23.

102.   McAULIFFE, W.G. (1980). Histochemistry and ultrastructure of the inter-
        stitium of the renal papilla in rats with hereditary diabetes insipidus. Am.
        J. Anat., 157, 17-26.

103.   McAULIFFE, W.G. and OLESEN, O.V. (1983). Effects of lithium on the structure
        of the rat kidney. Nephron, 34, 114-124.

104.   GLOOR, F.J. (1978). Changing concept in the pathogenesis and morphology of
        analgesic nephropathy as seen in Europe. Kidney Int., 13, 27-33.

105.   BURRY, A. (1978). Pathology of analgesic nephropathy: Australian experience.
        Kidney Int., 13, 34-40.

106.   MOLLAND, E.A. (1978). Experimental renal papillary necrosis. Kidney Int.,
        13, 5-14.

107.   BACH, P.H., GRASSO, P., MOLLAND, E.A. and BRIDGES, J.W. (1983). Changes in
        the medullary glycosaminoglycan histochemistry and microvascular filling
        during the development of 2-bromoethanamine hydrobromide-induced renal
        papillary necrosis. Toxicol. Appl. Pharmacol., 69, 333-344.

108.   GREGG, N., COURTAULD, E.A. and BACH, P.H. (1987). High resolution light

morphological and microvascular changes in acutely-induced renal papillary necrosis. Br. J. Exp. Pathol. (submitted).

109. BACH, P.H. and BRIDGES, J.W. (1985). Chemically induced renal papillary necrosis and upper urothelial carcinoma. CRC Crit. Rev. Toxicol., 15, 217-439.

110. TUCKER, E., LUPTON, C.H. and McMANUS, J.F.A. (1959). A new inclusion of the visceral epithelium of the renal pelvis: The presence of these inclusions in a papillary carcinoma of the kidney and its metastases. Cancer, 12, 1052-1057.

111. ALROY, J., PAULI, B.U. and HAYDEN, J.E. (1979). Intracytoplasmic lumina in bladder carcinomas. Human Pathol., 10, 549-555.

112. HUKILL, P.B. and VIDONE, R.A. (1965). Histochemistry of mucus and other polysaccarides in tumours. I. Carcinoma of the bladder. Lab. Invest., 14, 1624-1635.

113. GREGG, N., IJOMAH, P., COURTAULD, E.A., and BACH, P.H. (1987). Two-stage experimentally induced upper urothelial dysplasia following initiation with N-butyl-N-(4-hydroxybutyl)-nitrosamine and an acutely induced renal papillary necrosis. (submitted for publication).

114. IOZZO, R. (1985). Biology of disease. Proteoglycans: Structure, function and role in neoplasia. Lab. Invest., 53, 373-396.

115. SMETS, L.A. and VAN BEEK, W.P. (1984). Carbohydrates of the tumour cell surface. Biochim. Biophys. Acta, 738, 237-249.

116. ROTH, J. (1978). The Lectins, Molecular Probes in Cell Biology and Membrane Research, Exp. Pathol., Suppl. 3, Gustav Fischer Verlag, Jena.

117. LE HIR, M. and DUBACH, U.C. (1982). The cellular specificity of lectin binding in the kidney. I. A light microscopical study in the rat. Histochemistry, 74, 521-530.

118. LE HIR, M. and DUBACH, U.C. (1982). The cellular specificity of lectin binding in the kidney. II. A light microscopic study in the rabbit. Histochemistry, 74, 531-540.

119. LE HIR, M., KAISSLING, B., KOEPPEN, B.M. and WADE, J.B. (1982). Binding of peanut lectin to specific epithelial cell types in kidney. Am. J. Physiol., 242, C117-C120.

120. HOLTHÖFER, H. (1983). Lectin binding sites in kidney. A comparative study of 14 animal species. J. Histochem. Cytochem., 31, 531-537.

121. HOLTHÖFER, H., VIRTANEN, I., PETTERSSON, E., TOERNROTH, T., ALFTHAN, O., LINDER, E. and MIETTINEN, A. (1981). Lectins as fluorescence microscopic markers for saccharides in the human kidney. Lab. Invest., 45, 391-399.

122. HOLTHÖFER, H., MIETTINEN, A., PAASIVUO, R., LEHT, V.P., LINDER, E., ALFTHAN, O. and VIRTANEN, I. (1983). Cellular origin and differentiation of renal carcinomas. A fluorescence microscopic study with kidney specific antibodies, anti-intermediate filament antibodies, and lectins. Lab. Invest., 49, 317-326.

123. ROTH, J. (1983). Application of immunocolloids in light microscopy. II. Demonstration of lectin binding sites in paraffin sections by the use of lectin-gold or glycoprotein-gold complexes. J. Histochem. Cytochem., 31, 547-552.

124. STOWARD, P.J., SPICER, S.S. and MILLER, R.L. (1980). Histochemical reactivity of peanut lectin. Horse radish peroxidase conjugation. J. Histochem. Cytochem., 28, 979-990

125. WATANABE, M., MURAMATS, T., SHIRANE, T. and UGAI, K. (1981). Discrete distribution of binding sites for Dolichos bioflorus agglutinin (DBA) and for peanut agglutinin (PNA) in mouse organ tissues. J. Histochem. Cytochem., 29, 779-790.

126. MURESAN, V., IWANIJ, V., SMITH, Z.D.J. and JAMIESON, J.D. (1982). Purification and use of Limulin. A sialic acid-specific lectin. J. Histochem. Cytochem., 30, 938-946.

127. FARAGGIANA, T., MALCHIODI, F., PRADO, A. and CHURG, J. (1982). Lectin-peroxidase conjugate reactivity in normal human kidney. J. Histochem. Cytochem., 30, 451-458.

128. LUCOCQ, J.M. and ROTH, J. (1984). Applications of immunocolloids in light microscopy. III. Demonstration of antigenic and lectin-binding sites in semithin resin sections. J. Histochem. Cytochem., 32, 1075-1083.

129. BACH, P.H. and GREGG, N.J. (1986). Unpublished data.

130. FALKENBERG, F.W., MÜLLER, E., RIFFELMANN, H.-D., BEHRENDT, B. and WAKS, T. (1981). The production of monoclonal antibodies against glomerular and other antigens of the human nephron. Renal Physiol., 4, 150-156.

131. FALKENBERG, F.W., GANTENBERG, W., JURGENLIEMK, I., MAYER, M., PIERARD, D., RIFFELMANN, H.-D., BEHRENDT, B. and WAKS, T. (1983). Development aspects of immunologically characterized proteins. Clin. Biochem., 16, 10-16.

132. LEDOUX, S., GUTKOWSKA, J., GARCIA, R., THIBAULT, G., CANTIN, M. and GENEST, J. (1982). Immunohistochemical localization of tonin in rat salivary glands and kidney. Histochemistry, 76, 329-340.

133. SCHENK, E.A., SCHWARTZ, R.H. and LEWIS, R.A. (1971). Tamm-Horsfall mucoprotein. 1. Localisation in the kidney. Lab. Invest., 25, 92-95.

134. WACHSMUTH, E.D. and TORHORST, A. (1974). Possible precursors of aminopeptidase and alkaline phosphatase in the proximal tubules of kidney and the crypts of small intestine of mice. Histochemistry, 38, 43-56.

135. WACHSMUTH, E.D. (1980). Assessment of immunocytochemical techniques with particular reference to the mixed aggregation immuno-cytochemical technique. In Trends in Enzyme Histochemistry and Cytochemistry. Ciba Found. Symp. 73. Excerpta Medica, Amsterdam, 135-160.

136. TAUGNER, R., HACKENTHAL, E., INAGAMI, T., NOBILING, R. and POULSEN, K. (1982). Vascular and tubular renin in the kidneys of mice. Histochemistry, 75, 473-484.

137. MIETTINEN, A. and LINDER, E. (1976). Membrane antigens shared by renal proximal tubules and other epithelia associated with absorption and excretion. Clin. Exp. Immunol., 23, 568-577.

138. MENDRICK, D.L., RENNKE, H.G., COTRAN, R.S., SPRINGER, T.A. and ABBAS, A.K. (1983). Monoclonal antibodies against rat glomerular antigen production and specificity. Lab. Invest., 49, 107-117.

139. WACHSMUTH, E.D. and STOYE, J.P. (1976). Differentiation of epithelial cells in human jejunum - localisation and quantification of aminopeptidase, alkaline phosphatase and aldolase isozymes in tissue sections. Histochemie, 48, 101-109.

140. NATHRATH, W.B.J., HEIDENKUMMER, P., BJÖRKLUND, V. and BJÖRKLUND, (1985). Distribution of tissue polypeptide antigen (TPA) in normal human tissues. J. Histochem. Cytochem., 33, 99-109.

141. CARNEGIE, J.A., McCULLY, M.E. and ROBERTSON, H.A. (1980). Embedment in glycol methacrylate at low temperature allows immunofluorescent localization of a labile tissue protein. J. Histochem. Cytochem., 28, 308-310.

142. TSURUTA, J., YAMAMOTO, T., KOZONO, K. and KAMBARA, T. (1985). Application of a new method of antibody-enzyme conjugation with maleimide derivative for immunohistochemistry: Hepatocellular production, interstitial tissue distribution and renal cell reabsorption of plasma albumin in the guinea pig. J. Histochem. Cytochem., 33, 767-777.

143. FUKASAWA, K.M., FUKASAWA, K., SAHARA, N., HARADA, M., KONDO, Y. and NAGATSU, I. (1981). Immunohistochemical localization of dipeptidyl aminopeptidase IV

in rat kidney, liver and salivary glands. J. Histochem. Cytochem., 29, 337-343.

144. SIEGEL, G.J., HOLM, C., SCHREIBER, J.H., DESMOND, T. and ERNST, S.A. (1984). Purification of mouse brain (Na^+, K^+)-ATPase catalytic unit, characterisation of antiserum, and immunocytochemical localised in cerebellum, choroid and kidney. J. Histochem. Cytochem., 32, 1309-1318.

145. McKENZIE, J.C., TANAKA, I., MISONO, K.S. and INAGAMI, T. (1985). Immunocytochemical localisation of atrial natriuretic factor in the kidney, adrenal medulla, pituitary and atrium of rat. J. Histochem. Cytochem., 33, 828-832.

146. SPICER, S.S., STOWARD, P.J. and TASHIAN, R.E. (1979). The immunohistolocalisation of carbonic anhydrase in rodent tissue. J. Histochem. Cytochem., 27, 820-831.

147. YOKOTA, S., TSUJI, H. and KATO, K. (1985). Immunocytochemical localisation of cathepsin D in lysosomes of cortical collecting tubule cells of the rat kidney. J. Histochem. Cytochem., 33, 191-200.

148. LIN, C.-T., GARBERN, J. and WU, J.-Y. (1982). Light and electron microscopic immunocytochemical localization of clathrin in rat cerebellum and kidney. J. Histochem. Cytochem., 30, 853-863.

149. BENDAYAN, M., REDDY, M.K., HASHIMOTO, T. and REDDY, J.K. (1985). Immunocytochemical localization of fatty acid metabolizing heat-stable and heat-labile enoyl-coenzyme A (CoA) hydratases in liver and renal cortex. J. Histochem. Cytochem., 31, 509-516.

150. GHAZARIAN, J.G. and GARANCIS, J.C. (1979). Immunofluorescent localization of 25-hydroxyvitamin-D_3-1α-hydroxylase ferredoxin in the renal tissue of chick. J. Histochem. Cytochem., 27, 1041-1045.

151. NISHINAKA, H., MINAMIURA, N., MATOBA, K., FURUSAWA, M. and YAMAMOTO, T. (1982). On the origin of alpha-glucosidase in human urine. J. Histochem. Cytochem., 11, 1186-1189.

152. ØRSTAVIK, T.B., NUSTAD, K., BRANDTZAEG, P. and PIERCE, J.V. (1976). Cellular origin of urinary kallikreins. J. Histochem. Cytochem., 24, 1037-1039.

153. SIMSON, J.A.V., SPICER, S.S., CHAO, J., GRIMM, L. and MARGOLIUS, H.S. (1979). Kallikrein localisation in rodent salivary glands and kidney with the immunoglobulin-enzyme bridge technique. J. Histochem. Cytochem., 27, 1567-1576.

154. DANIELSON, K.G., SEIGO, O. and HUANG, P.C. (1982). Immunochemical localisation of metallothionein in rat liver and kidney. J. Histochem. Cytochem., 30, 1033-1039.

155. LACASSE, J., BALLAK, M., MERCURE, C., GUTKOWSKA, J., CHAPEAU, C., FOOTE, S., MÉNARD, J., CORVOL, P., CANTIN, M. and GENEST, J. (1985). Immunocytochemical localization of renin in juxtaglomerular cells. J. Histochem. Cytochem., 33, 323-332.

156. HOFFMAN, N.A. and HARTROFT, P.M. (1971). Application of peroxidase-labelled antibodies to the localization of renin. J. Histochem. Cytochem., 19, 811-813.

157. IWAO, H., NAKAMURA, N., IKEMOTO, F. and YAMAMOTO, K. (1983). Whole body autoradiographic distribution of exogenously administered renin in mice. J. Histochem. Cytochem., 31, 776-782.

158. FARAGGIANA, T., GRESIK, E., TANAKA, T., INAGAMI, T. and LUPO, A. (1982). Immunohistochemical localization of renin in the human kidney. J. Histochem. Cytochem., 30, 459-465.

159. CAMILLERI, J.-P., PHAT, V.N., BARIETY, J., CORVOL, P. and MENARD, J. (1980). Use of a specific antiserum for renin detection in human kidney. J. Histochem. Cytochem., 28, 1343-1346.

160.   THAETE, L.G., CROUCH, R.K. and SPICER, S.S. (1985). Immunolocalisation of copper-zinc superoxide dismutase. II. Rat. J. Histochem. Cytochem., 33, 803-808.

161.   THAETE, L.G., CROUCH, R.K., SCHULTE, B.A. and SPICER, S.S. (1983). The immunolocalisation of copper-zinc superoxide dismutase in canine tissues. J. Histochem. Cytochem., 31, 1399-1406.

162.   NAKANO, M. (1982). Localisation of renal and intestinal trehalase with immunofluorescence- and enzyme-labelled antibody techniques. J. Histochem. Cytochem., 30, 1243-1248.

163.   COURTOY, P.J., TIMPL, R. and FARQUHAR, M.G. (1982). Comparative distribution of laminin, type IV collagen and fibronectin in the rat glomerulus. J. Histochem. Cytochem., 30, 874-886.

164.   MARTINEZ-HERNANDEZ, A. and CHUNG, A.E. (1984). The ultrastructural localisation of two basement membrane components Enactin and Laminin in rat tissue. J. Histochem. Cytochem., 32, 289-298.

165.   OBERLEY, T.D., CHUNG, A.E., MURPHY-ULLRICH, J.E. and MOSHER, D.F. (1981). Studies on the localisation of the glycoprotein GP-2 within the renal glomerulus in vivo and in cultured kidney cell strains in vitro. J. Histochem. Cytochem., 29, 1237-1242.

166.   HARA, M., MASE, D., INABA, S., HIGUCHI, A., TANIZAWA, T., YAMANAKA, N., SUGISAKI, Y., SADO, Y. and OKADA, T. (1986). Immunochemical localisation of glomerular basement membrane antigens in various renal diseases. Virchows Arch. Pathol. Anat., 408, 403-419.

167.   LINDER, E., MIETTINEN, A. and TÖRNROTH, T. (1980). Fibronectin as a marker for the glomerular mesangium in immunohistology of kidney biopsies. Lab. Invest., 42, 70-75.

168.   CASANOVA, S., DONINI, U., ZINI, N., MORELLI, R. and ZUCCHELLI, P. (1983). Immunohistochemical staining of hydroxyethyl-methacrylate-embedded tissues. J. Histochem. Cytochem., 31, 1000-1004.

169.   SHINDO, N., KOBAYASHI, E. and OKADA, M. (1984). Immunoelectron microscopic (IEM) studies on glutaraldehyde-fixed renal specimen. J. Histochem. Cytochem., 32, 501-509.

170.   ANDERS, M.W. (1980). Metabolism of drugs by the kidney. Kidney Int., 18, 636-647.

171.   RUSH, G., SMITH, J.H., NEWTON, J.F. and HOOK, J.B. (1984). Chemically induced nephrotoxicity: role of metabolic activation. CRC Crit. Rev. Toxicol., 13, 99-160.

172.   DEES, J.H., PARKHILL, L.K., OKITA, R.T., YASUKOCHI, Y. and MASTERS, B.S. (1982). Localization of NADPH-cytochrome P-450 reductase and cytochrome P-450 in animal kidneys. In Nephrotoxicity, Assessment and Pathogenesis. [Eds. P.H. Bach, F.W. Bonner, J.W. Bridges and E.A. Lock]. Wiley, Chichester, 246-249.

173.   DEES, J.H., MASTERS, B.S.S., MULLER-EBERHARD, U. and JOHNSON, E.F. (1982). Effect of 2,3,7,8-terachlorodibenzo-p-dioxin and phenobarbital on the occurrence and distribution of four cytochrome P-450 isozymes in rabbit kidney. Cancer Res., 42, 1423-1432.

174.   FLEISCHNER, G., ROBBINS, J. and ARIAS., I.M. (1972). Immunological studies of Y-protein. A major cytoplasmic organic anion-binding protein in rat liver. J. Clin. Invest., 57, 677-684.

175.   KIRSCH, R., FLEISCHNER, G., FEINFELD, D., GOLDSTEL, E., KAMISAKA, K. and ARIS, I.M. (1975). Renal ligandin - structure, function and role in diagnosis. Clin. Res., 23, A431.

176.   FLEISCHNER, G.M., ROBBINS, J.B. and ARIAS, I.M. (1977). Cellular localisation of ligandin in rat, hamster and man. Biochem. Biophys. Res. Commun.,

74, 992-1000.

177.   CAMPBELL, J.A.H., BASS, N.M. and KIRSCH, R.E. (1980). Immunohistological localization of ligandin. Cancer, 45, 503-510.

178.   GEE, N.S. and KENNY, A.J. (1985). Proteins of the kidney microvillar membrane. Biochem. J., 230, 753-764.

179.   KENNY, A.J. and MAROUX, S. (1982). Topology of microvillar membrane hydrolases of the kidney and intestine. Physiol. Rev., 62, 91-128.

180.   SCHWARTZ, R.H., LEWIS, R.A. and SCHENK, E.A. (1972). Tamm-Horsfall mucoprotein. 3. Potassium dichromate-induced renal tubular damage. Lab. Invest., 27, 214-217

181.   BACH, P.H., WIRDNAM, P.K., DAWNAY, A.B. ST. J. and LU, Q.H. (1984). Unpublished data.

182.   SABATINI, S., ALLA, V., WILSON, A., CRUZ-SOTO, M., DE WHITE, A., KURTZMAN, N.A. and ARRUDA, J.A.L. (1982). The effects of chronic papillary necrosis on acid excretion. Pfluegers Arch., 393, 262-268.

183.   PICH, A., BUSSOLATI, G. and CARBONARA, A. (1976). Immunocytochemical detection of casein and casein-like proteins in human tissues. J. Histochem. Cytochem., 24, 940-947.

184.   MOLIN, S.-O., ROSENGREN, L., BAUDIER, J., HAMBERGER, A. and HAGLID, K. (1985). S-100 Alpha-like immunoreactivity in tubules of rat kidney. A clue to the function of a "brain-specific" protein. J. Histochem. Cytochem., 33, 367-374.

185.   CORRADINO, R.A. and TAYLOR, A.N. (1983). 1,25-Dihydroxyvitamin D_3-induced calcium-binding protein: Localization in organ-cultured embryonic chick duodenum. J. Histochem. Cytochem., 33, 477-479.

185a.   TAYLOR, A.N., McINTOSH, J.E. and BOURDEAU, J.E. (1982). Immunocytochemical localisation of vitamin D-dependent calcium-binding protein in renal tubules of rabbit, rat and chick. Kidney Int., 21, 765-773.

186.   ØRSTAVIK, T.B. (1980). The kallikrein-kinin system in exocrine organs. J. Histochem. Cytochem., 28, 881-889.

187.   LINDOP, G.B.M. and LEVER, A.F. (1986). Anatomy of the renin-angiotensin system in the normal and pathological kidney. Histopathology, 10, 335-362.

188.   ØRSTAVIK, T.B. and INAGAMI, T. (1982). Localisation of kallikrein in the rat kidney and its anatomical relationship to renin. J. Histochem. Cytochem., 30, 385-390.

189.   MEHLMAN, M.A. (Ed.) (1984). Renal Effects of Petroleum Hydrocarbons, Princeton Scientific, Princeton.

190.   ALDEN, C.L., RIDDER, G., STONE, L. and KANERVA, (1985). Pathology of petrochemical fuels in male rats. Acute toxicity. In Renal Heterogeneity and Target Cell Toxicity. [Eds. P.H. Bach and E.A. Lock]. Wiley, Chichester, 416-472.

191.   ROY, A.K. and RABER, D.L. (1972). Immunofluorescent localisation of alpha-2u-globulin in the hepatic and renal tissues of rat. J. Histochem. Cytochem., 20, 89-96.

192.   SIMPSON, M.G., FOSTER, J.R., MILLARD, J., PHILLIPS, P., ISAACS, K., STONARD, M.D. and LOCK, E.A. (1985). Histochemical observations on the relationship between chemically induced hyaline droplet accumulation in the rat kidney and alpha-2u-globulin. Proc. Royal Microsc. Soc., 20(5), TOX 11.

193.   ANTAKLY, T., LAPERCHE, Y. and FEIGELSON, P. (1982). Synthesis and immunocytochemical localization of alpha-2u-globulin in the duct cells of the rat submaxillary gland. J. Histochem. Cytochem., 30, 1293-1296.

194.   CORDON-CARDO, C., BANDER, N.H., FRADET, Y., FINSTAD, C.L., WHITMORE, W.F., LLOYD, K.O., OETTEGEN, H.F., MELAMED, M.R. and OLD, L.J. (1984). Immunoanatomic dissection of the human urinary tract by monoclonal antibodies.

J. Histochem. Cytochem., 32, 1035-1040.

195. ACHTSTATTER, T., MOLL, R., MOORE, B. and FRANKE, W.W. (1985). Cytokeratin polypeptide patterns of different epithelia of the human male urogenital tract: Immunofluorescence and gel electrophoretic studies. J. Histochem. Cytochem., 33, 415-426.

196. WANG, E. and KRUEGER, J.G. (1985). Application of a unique monoclonal antibody as a marker for non-proliferating subpopulations of cells of some tissue. J. Histochem. Cytochem., 33, 587-594.

197. CHAPMAN, C.M., ALLHOFF, E.P., PROPPE, K.H. and PROUT, G.R. (1983). Use of monoclonal antibodies for the localization of tissue isoantigens A and B in transitional cell carcinoma of the upper urinary tract. J. Histochem. Cytochem., 31, 557-561.

198. WALDHERR, R. and SCHWECHHEIMER, K. (1985). Co-expression of cytokeratin and vimentin intermediate sized filament in renal cell carcinomas. Comparative study of the intermediate sized filament distribution in renal cell carcinomas and normal human kidney. Virchows Arch. A, 408, 15-27.

199. CLYNE, D.H., NORRIS, S.H., MODESTO, R.R., PESCE, A.J. and POLLACK, V.E. (1973). Antibody enzyme conjugates. The preparation of intermolecular conjugates of horseradish peroxidase and antibody and their use in immunohistology of renal cortex. J. Histochem. Cytochem., 21, 233-246.

200. HEMMING, F.J., MESGUICH, P., MOREL, G. and DUBOIS, P.M. (1983). Cryoultramicrotomy versus plastic embedding: Comparative immunocytochemistry of rat anterior pituitary cells. J. Microscopy, 131, 25-34.

201. WELLS, B. (1985). Low temperature box and tissue handling device for embedding biological tissue for immunostaining in electron microscopy. Micron Miscrosc. Acta, 16, 49-53.

202. ROTH, J., BENDAYAN, M., CARLEMALM, E., VILLIGER, W. and GARAVIRTRO, M. (1981). Enhancement of structural preservation and immunocytochemical staining in low temperature embedded pancreatic tissue. J. Histochem. Cytochem., 29, 663-671.

203. CARLEMALM, E., GARAVITRO, R.M. and VILLIGER, W. (1982). Recent development for electron microscopy and an analysis of embedding at low temperature. J. Microsc., 126, 123-143.

204. NAKANE, P.K. (1971). Application of peroxidase labelled antibodies to the intracellular localization of hormones. Acta Endocrinol. (Suppl.), 153, 190-204.

205. HOPFEL-KREINER, I. and VON MAYERSBACK, H. (1978). The influence of glycol methacrylate (GMA) and paraffin embedding on freeze substituted and fixed tissues for enzyme histochemistry. Acta Histochem., 63, 224-234.

206. FRANKLIN, R.M. (1984). Immunohistochemistry on semithin sections of hydroxypropyl methacrylate embedded tissues. J. Immunol. Methods, 68, 61-72.

207. VALENTINO, K.L., CRUMRINE, D.A. and REICHARDT, L.F. (1985). Lowicryl K4M embedding of brain tissue for immunogold electron microscopy. J. Histochem. Cytochem., 33, 969-973.

208. COONS, A.H., LEDUC, E.H. and CONNOLLY, J.M. (1955). Studies on antibody production. I. A method for the histochemical demonstration of specific antibody and its application to a study of the hyperimmune rabbit. J. Exp. Med., 102, 49-60.

209. TAKAMIYA, H., BATSFORD, S.R., TOKUNAGA, J. and VOGT, A. (1979). Immunohistological staining of antigens on semithin sections of sections embedded in plastic (GMA-Quetol 523). J. Immuno. Methods, 30, 277-288.

210. TAKAMIYA, H., BATSFORD, S.R. and VOGT, A. (1980). An approach to postembedding staining of protein (immunoglobulin) antigen in plastics: prerequisites and limitations. J. Histochem. Cytochem., 28, 1041-1049.

211. MOZDZEN, J.J. and KEREN, D.F. (1982). Detection of immunoglobulin A by immunofluorescence in glycol methacrylate-embedded human colon. J. Histochem. Cytochem., 30, 532-535.

212. CLAYTON, B.P. (1959). The action of fixatives on the unmasking of lipid. Quart. J. Microsc. Soc., 100, 269-274.

213. BAKER, J.R.J. (1946). Histochemical recognition of lipine. Quart. J. Microsc. Sci., 87, 441-470.

214. ELFTMAN, H. (1958). Effects of fixation in lipid histochemistry. J. Cytochem. Histochem., 6, 317-321.

215. BAKER, J.R. (1957). Lipid globules in cells. Nature, 180, 947-949.

216. BERG, N.O. (1951). A histological study of masked lipids. Acta Pathol. Microbiol. Scand., Suppl XC, 1-192.

217. WOLMAN, M. (1959). The use of chemical agents in the histochemical demonstration of lipids. Acta Histochem., Suppl. 2, 140-154.

218. HIGH, O.B. (1984). Lipid Histochemistry. Oxford University Press, Oxford.

219. BACH, P.H. and SCHOLEY, D.J. (1984). Unpublished data.

220. BOJESEN, I. (1974). Quantitative and qualitative analyses of isolated lipid droplets from interstitial cells in renal papillae from various species. Lipids, 9, 835-843.

221. BURRY, A., CROSS, R. and AXELSEN, R. (1977). Analgesic nephropathy and the renal concentrating mechanism. Pathol. Annu., 12, 1-31.

222. MOLLAND, E.A. (1976). Aspirin damage in the rat kidney in the intact animal and after unilateral nephrectomy. J. Pathol., 120, 43-48

223. MOLLAND, E.A. (1982). Renal papillary necrosis produced by long-term fat-free diet. In Nephrotoxicity, Assessment and Pathogenesis. [Eds. P.H. Bach, F.W. Bonner, J.W. Bridges and E.A. Lock]. Wiley, Chichester, 200-205.

224. MITATSCH, M.J., HOFER, H.O., GUDAT, F., KNUSLI. C., TORHORST, J. and ZOLLINGER, U. (1984). Capillary sclerosis of the lower urinary tract and analgesic nephropathy. Clin. Nephrol., 20, 285-301.

225. BACH, P.H., LU, Q.H. and DUFFY, M.J. (1986). Unpublished data.

226. APFFEL, C.A. and BAKER, J.R. (1964). Lipid droplets in the cytoplasm of malignant cells. Cancer, 17, 176-184.

227. MASIN, F. and MASIN, M. (1976). Sudanophilia in exfoliated urothelial cells. Acta Cytol., 20, 573-576.

228. KALOYANIDES, G.J. and FELDMAN, S. (1981). Gentamicin induces a phospholipidosis in the rat. In Nephrotoxicity [Ed. J.-P. Fillastre]. INSERM, Rouen, 131-139.

229. KUMAR, A. and RANA, S.V.S. (1982). Lipid accumulation in chromium poisoned rats. Int. J. Tissue React., 4, 291-295.

230. WONG, L.C. and DI STEFANO, V. (1966). Rapid accumulation of renal fat in cats after single inhalation of carbon tetrachloride. Toxicol. Appl. Pharmacol., 9, 485-494.

231. STEINER, G., BRADFORD, W. and CRAIG, J.M. (1985). Tetracycline-induced abortion in the rat. Lab. Invest., 14, 1456-1463.

232. MADHAVAN, T.V., TULPULE, P.G. and GOPALAN, C. (1965). Aflatoxin-induced hepatic fibrosis in rhesus monkeys. Arch. Pathol., 79, 466-469.

233. MADHAVAN, T.V. and SURYANARAYANA RAO, K. (1967). Tubular epithelial reflux in the kidney in aflatoxin poisoning. J. Pathol. Bacteriol., 93, 329-331.

234. GROND, J., WEENING, J.J. and ELEMA, J.D. (1984). Glomerular sclerosis in nephrotic rats. Comparison of the longterm effects of adriamycin and aminonucleoside. Lab. Invest., 51, 277-285.

235. ARCHIBALD R.W.R. and ORTON, C.C. (1970). Specific identification of free and esterified fatty acids in tissue sections. Histochem. J., 2, 411-417.

236. TRIFILLIS, A.L., REGEC, A.L., HALL-CRAGGS, M. and TRUMP, B.F. (1985).

Effects of cyclosporine on cultured human renal tubular cells. In Renal Heterogeneity and Target Cell Toxicity. [Eds. P.H. Bach and E.A. Lock]. Wiley, Chichester, 545-548.

237. LÜLLMAN, H., LÜLLMAN-RAUCH, R. and WASSERMANN, O. (1975). Drug induced phospholipidosis. II. Tissue distribution of the amphilic drug chlorphentermine. CRC Crit. Rev. Toxicol., 4, 185-218.

238. DIXON, K.C. (1968). Fatty deposition: a disorder of the cell. Quart. J. Exp. Physiol., 43, 139-159.

239. DUNN, M.J. and HOOD, V.L. (1977). Prostaglandins and the kidney. Am. J. Physiol., 233, F169-F184.

240. DUNN, M.J. and ZAMBRASKI, E.J. (1980). Renal effects of drugs that inhibit prostaglandin synthesis. Kidney Int., 18, 609-622.

241. WRIGHT, J.T. and CORDER, C.N. (1979). NAD^+-15-Hydroxyprostaglandin dehydrogenase distribution in rat kidney. J. Histochem. Cytochem., 27, 657-664.

242. SMITH, W.L. and WILKIN, G.P. (1977). Distribution of prostaglandin-forming cyclooxygenase in rat, rabbit and guinea pig kidney as determined by immunofluorescence. Fed. Proc., 36, 309.

242a. SMITH, W.L. and WILKIN, G.P. (1977). Immunochemistry of prostaglandin endoperoxide-forming cyclo-oxygenases: The detection of the cyclooxygenases in rat, rabbit and guinea pig kidneys by immunofluorescence. Prostaglandins, 13, 873-900.

243. SMITH, W.L. and BELL, T.G. (1978). Immunohistochemical localisation of the prostaglandin-forming cyclooxygenase in renal cortex. Am. J. Physiol., 235, F451-F457.

244. MORI, Y. and MINE, M. (1981). The localisation of prostaglandins in the rabbit kidney demonstrated with indirect immunofluorescence. Biomed. Res., 2, 281-284.

245. PEREZ, G. and McGUCKIN, J. (1972). Cellular localisation of prostaglandin A_2 in the rat kidney. Prostaglandins, 2, 393-398.

246. JANSZEN, F.H.A. and NUGTEREN, D.H. (1971). Histochemical localisation of prostaglandin synthetase. Histochemie, 27, 159-164.

247. JANSZEN, F.H.A. and NUGTEREN, D.H. (1973). A histochemical study of the prostaglandin biosynthesis in the urinary system of rabbit, guinea pig, golden hamster and rat. Adv. Bio. Sci., 9, 287-292.

248. LITWIN, J.A. (1977). Does diaminobenzidine demonstrate prostaglandin synthetase? A study on polyunsaturated fatty acid-induced DAB oxidation in sheep vesicular glands and rabbit kidney medulla. Histochemistry, 53, 301-315.

249. LITWIN, J.A. (1979). Histochemistry and cytochemistry of 3,3'-diaminobenzidine. A review. Folia Histochem. Cytochem., 17, 3-28.

250. AL-ANI, L.M. and FOURMAN, J. (1979). Histochemical study of prostaglandin synthetase in the mouse kidney. IRCS Med. Sci. 7, 379.

250a. BACH, P.H. and BRIDGES, J.W. (1984). The role of prostaglandin synthase mediated metabolic activation of analgesics and non-steroidal anti-inflammatory drugs in the development of renal papillary necrosis and upper urothelial carcinoma. Prostagland. Leukotri. Med., 15, 251-274.

251. SMITH, W.L., BELL, T.G. and NEEDLEMAN, P. (1979). Increased renal tubular synthesis of prostaglandins in the rabbit kidney in response to ureteral obstruction. Prostaglandins, 18, 269-277.

252. TANNENBAUM, J., PURKERSON, M.L and KLAHR, S. (1983). Effects of unilateral ureteral obstruction on metabolism of renal lipids in the rat. Am. J. Physiol., 245, F254-F262.

253. MORRISON, A.R., NISHIKAWA, K. and NEEDLEMAN, P. (1978). Thromboxane A_2

biosynthesis in the ureter obstructed isolated perfused kidney of the rabbit. J. Pharmacol. Exp. Ther., 205, 1-18.

254.   ALTMAN, F.P., MOORE, D.S. and CHAYEN, J. (1975). The direct measurement of cytochrome P450 in unfixed tissue sections. Histochemistry, 41, 227-232.

255.   NOVIKOFF, A.B. and GOLDFISCHER, S. (1969). Visualisation of peroxisomes (microsomes) and mitochondria with diaminobenzidine. J. Histochem. Cytochem., 17, 675-680.

256.   GOLDFISCHER, S. (1969). Further observations on the peroxidatic activities of microbodies (peroxisomes). J. Histochem. Cytochem., 17, 681-685.

257.   ESSNER, E. (1970). Observations on hepatic and renal peroxisomes (microbodies) in the developing chick. J. Histochem. Cytochem., 18, 80-91.

258.   GOECKERMANN, J.A. and VIGH, E.I. (1975). Peroxisome development in the metanephric kidney of mouse. J. Histochem. Cytochem., 23, 957-973.

259.   REDDY, J.K., RAO, M.S., MOODY, D.E. and QURESHI, S.A. (1976). Peroxisome development in the regenerating pars recta (P_3 segment) of proximal tubules of the rat kidney. J. Histochem. Cytochem., 24, 1239-1248.

260.   BEARD, M.E., BAKER, R., CONOMOS, P., PUGATCH, D. and HOLTZMAN, E. (1985). Oxidation of oxalate and polyamines by rat peroxisome. J. Histochem. Cytochem., 33, 460-464.

261.   GILLOTEAUX, J. and STEGGLES, A.W. (1983). Histoenzymatic alterations in kidney catalase activity following hormonal treatment of Syrian hamsters. Cell Biol. Int. Rep., 7, 31-33.

262.   ASGHAR, K., REDDY, B.G. and KRISHNA, G. (1975). Histochemical localization of glutathione in tissues. J. Histochem. Cytochem., 23, 774-779.

263.   CHIECO, P. and BOOR, P.J. (1983). Use of low temperatures for glutathione histochemical stain. J. Histochem. Cytochem., 31, 975-976.

263a.   SMITH, M.T., LOVERIDGE, N., WILLS, E.D. and CHAYEN, J. (1979). The distribution of glutathione in the rat liver lobule. Biochem. J., 182, 103-108.

264.   BACH, P.H. (1981). Unpublished data.

265.   DOLEZEL, S. (1967). Monoaminergic innervation of kidney aorticorenal ganglion - a sympathetic ganglion supply renal vessels. Experientia, 23, 109-111.

266.   FALCK, B., HILLARP, B.F., THIEME, G. and TORP, A. (1961). Fluorescence of catecholamines and related compounds condensed with formaldehyde. J. Histochem. Cytochem., 10, 348-354.

267.   DINERSTEIN, R.J., VANNICE, J., HENDERSON, R.C., ROTH, L.J., GOLDBERG, L.I. and HOFFMANN, P.C. (1979). Histofluorescence techniques provide evidence for dopamine-containing neuronal elements in canine kidney. Science, 205, 497-499.

268.   DANSCHER, G. and MØLLER-MADSEN, B. (1985). Silver amplification of mercury sulfide and selenide: A histochemical method for light and electron microscopic localization of mercury in tissue. J. Histochem. Cytochem., 33, 219-228.

269.   SUMI, Y., MURAKI, T. and SUZUKI, T. (1980). Histochemical staining in cadmium with benzothiazolylazophenol derivatives. Histochemistry, 68, 231-236.

270.   MORSELT, A.F.W., BROEKAERT, D., JONGSTRA-SPAAPEN, E.J., COPIUS-PEEREBOOM-STEGEMAN, J.H.J. (1984). Histochemical changes in protein disulphide bonds in rat liver and kidney after chronic cadmium administration, and the possible relation to metallothionein. Arch. Toxicol., 55, 155-160.

271.   MORSELT, A.F.W., VAN DE HAMER, C.J.A., PRINSEN, L., JONGSTRA-SPAAPEN, E.J., COPIUS PEEREBOOM-STEGEMAN, J.H.J. and BOSCH, K.S. (1985). Large increase in disulphide bonds containing cytosol proteins after chronic cadmium

administration, estimated in isolated rat liver cells. Histochemistry, 83, 227-229.

272. BENARD, P., BURGAT, V. and RICO, A.G. (1985). Applications of whole-body autoradiography in toxicology. CRC Crit. Rev. Toxicol., 15, 181-216.

272a. HOUSLEY, T.L. and FISHER, D.B. (1976). The efficiency of ^{14}C detection in autoradiographics of semithin plastic sections. J. Histochem. Cytochem., 23, 678-680.

273. ROGERS, A.W. (1979). Techniques of Autoradiography, 3rd edition. Elsevier/North-Holland Biomedical Press, Amsterdam.

274. WILLIAMS, M.A. (1977). Autoradiography and Immuncytochemistry. Practical Methods in Electron Microscopy, Vol. 6. [Series Ed. A.M. Glauert]. North-Holland, Amsterdam.

275. BERGERON, J.J.M., RACHUBINSKI, R., SEARLE, N., BORTS, D., SIKSTROM, R. and POSNER, B.I. (1980). Polypeptide hormone receptors in vivo: Demonstration of insulin binding to adrenal gland and gastrointestinal epithelium by quantitative radioautography. J. Histochem. Cytochem., 28, 824-835.

276. MIYAZAKI, H., MATSUNAGA, Y. and HASHIMOTO, M. (1978). Distribution of [^{14}C]labelled purines in the mouse. A whole body autoradiographic assessment of purine metabolism in mammals. J. Histochem. Cytochem., 26, 661-676.

277. SCHULTZE, B., MAURER, W. and HAGENBUSCH, H. (1976). A two emulsion autoradiographic technique and the discrimination of the three different types of labelling after double labelling with ^{3}H- and ^{14}C-thymidine. Cell Tissue Kinet., 9, 245-255.

278. MURAKAMI, M. and HIROSAWA, K. (1977). Electron microscope autoradiography of mouse kidney after administration of ^{109}Cd. J. Electron. Microsc., 26, 275.

278a. MURAKAMI, M., TOHYAMA, C., SANO, K., KAWAMURA, R. and KUBOTA, K. (1983). Autoradiography studies on the localisation of metallothionein in proximal tubular cells of the rat kidney. Arch. Toxicol., 53, 185-192.

279. HELLMAN, B., ARGY, R. and ULLBERG, S. (1984). The in vivo uptake of tritiated thymidine as a potential short-term test of toxic effects of polycyclic aromatic hydrocarbons in different organs. Toxicology, 29, 183-194.

280. TOBACK, F.G., DODD, R.C., MAIER, E.R. and HAVENER, L.J. (1983). Amino acid administration enhances renal protein metabolism after acute tubular necrosis. Nephron, 33, 238-243.

281. BALAZS, T. (1974). Development of tissue resistance to toxic effects of chemicals. Toxicology, 2, 247-255.

282. LAURENT, G., MALDAGUE, P., CARLIER, M.B. and TULKENS, P.M. (1983). Increased renal DNA synthesis in vivo after administration of low doses of gentamicin to rats. Antimicrob. Agents Chemother., 24, 586-593.

283. REITER, R.J. (1965). Cellular proliferation and deoxyribonucleic acid synthesis in compensating kidneys of mice and the effect of food and water. Lab. Invest., 14, 1636-1643.

284. GREGG, N., IJOMAH, P., MATTINGLEY, G., COURTAULD, E.A. and BACH, P.H. (1986). The hyperplastic response of the renal pelvis and ureter epithelial cell layer to an acutely-induced renal papillary necrosis. (submitted for publication).

285. AUKLAND, K. (1980). Methods for measuring renal blood flow; total flow and regional distribution. Annu. Rev. Physiol., 42, 543-555.

286. SOLEZ, K., MILLER, M., QUARLES, P.A., FINER, P.M. and HEPSTINSTALL, R.H. (1974). Experimental papillary necrosis of the kidney. IV. Medullary plasma flow. Am. J. Pathol., 76, 521-528.

287. SOLEZ, K., PONCHAK, S., BUONO, R.A., VERNON, N., FINER, P.M., MILLER, M. and HEPSTINSTALL, R.H. (1974). Inner medulla plasma flow in the kidney with

ureteral obstruction. Am. J. Physiol., 231, 1315-1321.

288. DAVIES, D.J. and TANGE, J.D. (1982). Factors influencing the severity and progress of ethyleneimine-induced papillary necrosis. J. Pathol., 137, 305-319.

289. MOLLAND, E.A. (1976). Unpublished data.

290. VERNON-BOOTH, B. (1972). The Macrophage. Cambridge University Press, Cambridge, 94.

291. JORIS, I., DE GIROLAMI, U., WORTHAM, K. and MAJNO, G. (1982). Vascular labelling with Monastral Blue B. Stain Technol., 57, 177-183.

292. ZIMMERHACKL, B., PAREKH, N., BRINKHUS, H. and SPEINHAUSEN, M. (1983). The use of fluorescent labeled erythrocytes for intravital investigation of flow and local hematocrit in glomerular capillaries in the rat. Int. J. Microcirc. Clin. Exp., 2, 119-129.

293. DOLCINI, H.A., ZAIDMAN, I., LICHTENBERG, F. and GRAY, S.J. (1960). Effects of serotonin on circulation in the rat kidney. Am. J. Physiol., 199, 1153-1156.

294. SIPPEL, T.O. (1973). The histochemistry of thiols and disulphides. I. The use of N-(4-aminophenyl)maleimide for demonstrating thiol groups. Histochem. J., 5, 413-423.

295. HANSSEN, O.E. (1958). A histochemical method for evaluation of excreted sodium ferrocyanide in isolated tubules of the mouse kidney. Acta Pathol. Microbiol. Scand., 44, 363-371.

296. BAINES, A.D., BAINES, C.J. and DE ROUFFIGNAC, C. (1969). Functional heterogeneity of nephrons. I. Intraluminal flow velocities. Pflugers Arch., 308, 244-259.

297. HANSSEN, O.E. (1961). The relationship between glomerular filtration and length of the proximal convoluted tubule in mice. Acta Pathol. Microbiol. Scand., 53, 265-79.

298. DE ROUFFIGNAC, C. and BONVALET, J.P. (1972). Use of sodium ferrocyanide as glomerular indicator to study the functional heterogeneity of nephrons. J. Biol. Med., 45, 243-253.

299. BACH, P.H. and BRIDGES, J.W. (1982). Chemical associated renal papillary necrosis. In Nephrotoxicity: Assessment and Pathogenesis. [Eds. P.H. Bach, F.W. Bonner, J.W. Bridges and E.A. Lock]. Wiley, Chichester, 437-459.

300. KLEEMAN, C.R. and EPSTEIN, F.H. (1956). Fate and distribution of ^{59}Fe labelled ferrocyanide in humans and dogs. Proc. Soc. Exp. Biol. Med., 92, 228-233.

301. GRAHAM, R.C. and KARNOVSKY, M.J. (1966). Glomerular permeability: Ultrastructural cytochemical studies using peroxidases as protein traces. J. Exp. Med., 124, 1123-1133.

302. GRAHAM, R.C. and KARNOVSKY, M.J. (1966). The early stages of absorption of injected horseradish peroxidase in the proximal tubules of mouse kidney: Ultrastructural cytochemistry by a new technique. J. Histochem. Cytochem., 14, 291-302.

303. ANDERSON, W.A. (1972). The use of exogenous myoglobin as an ultrastructural tracer. Reabsorption and translocation of protein by the renal tubule. J. Histochem. Cytochem., 20, 672-684.

304. STRAUS, W. (1975). Altered reabsorption of protein by the renal cortex in rats treated with hypertonic saline or mannitol. J. Histochem. Cytochem., 23, 707-721.

305. STRAUS, W. (1977). Altered renal cortical reabsorption of protein and urinary excretion of sodium in relation to vascular leakage induced by horseradish peroxidase. J. Histochem. Cytochem., 25, 215-225.

306. SJAASTAD, Ø., BLOM, A.K. and HAYE, R. (1984). Hypotensive effects in cats

caused by horseradish peroxidase mediated by metabolites of arachidonic acid. J. Histochem. Cytochem., 32, 1328-1330.

307.   BAREGGI, R., NARDUCCI, P., GRILL, V., MALLARDI, F., ZWEYER, M. and FUSAROLI, P. (1986). Localization of an aminoglycoside (streptomycin) in the inner ear after its systemic administration. Histochemistry, 84, 237-240.

308.   EGORIN, M.J., HILDEBRAND, R.C., CIMINO, E.F. and BACHUR, N.R. (1974). Cytofluorescence localization of adriamycin and daunorubicin. Cancer Res., 34, 2243-2245.

3

CRYOMICROTOMY OF RENAL TISSUE, AND THE USE OF X-RAY MICROANALYSIS AND AUTORADIOGRAPHY AT THE LIGHT AND ELECTRON MICROSCOPIC LEVELS

J.R.J. BAKER

INTRODUCTION

The topics covered by the title of this chapter are in a sense disparate and yet are interrelated in the context of renal study in that they are aspects of the discipline which we know as cytochemistry.

Although the three areas share certain common features it will be most convenient for the reader if they are treated as separate technical entities pointing out overlap where appropriate. Clearly, it will be deemed desirable by readers of this series to examine the role of cryomicrotomy, X-ray microanalysis and autoradiography in existing studies of renal function and malfunction. Nevertheless we should also be concerned with the future exploitation of these techniques in kidney investigation. Hence it will from time to time be advantageous to illustrate certain methods by reference to non-renal examples in the absence of evidence in the kidney itself.

I. CRYOMICROTOMY

There are various reasons why the investigator might choose to study sections of frozen (i.e. "cryo-fixed") kidney. The complex physiology of the nephron often precludes the use of chemical fixatives or any other aqueous treatment in the preparation of sections for microscopy with the result that the aqueous phase must be changed and/or lost with minimal disturbance of tissue solutes. This almost inevitably means that the tissue has to be frozen and possibly dried, avoiding any fluid phase.

A detailed description of the physical chemistry of the freezing process in biological systems is beyond the scope of this chapter and the reader is advised to consult one of the many excellent reviews of this subject[1]. If cryotechniques are to be used success-fully, the user must be aware of the consequences of the freezing, sectioning and drying processes. These will be considered during the course of the chapter.

A.   Cryomicrotomy for the light microscope

Here we shall deal with methods and applications other than those used in autoradiography. The histopathologist more often than not relies upon the speed with which cryosections can be produced, fixed and stained[2]. Moreover, the cytochemist may have no alterna-tive if he is to visualize his reaction products with any anatomical fidelity.

Chayen and colleagues have used cryosections in the region of 10 μm to develop cytochemical assays of polypeptide hormones[3,4]. Segments of guinea pig kidney were incubated with bovine parathyroid hormone, frozen and sectioned in a cryostat. The sections were reacted for marker enzymes such as glucose-6-phosphate dehydrogenase, NADPH-diaphorase, alkaline phosphatase and carbonic anhydrase. The reaction products were quantified using a Vickers M85 scanning and integrating microdensitometer and compared with the initial hormone concentration. There was a characteristic pattern of enzyme response (activation) depending upon the nephron region examined. In doubt, however, must be the authors' assertion that "chilling" rapidly to -70 °C allowed the tissue to remain supercooled, in other words, free of ice (see below).

It has been possible to retain and localize certain enzymes after chemical fixation prior to cryosectioning. Ericsson fixed rat renal cortex in 4% formaldehyde for 24 h at 0-4 °C before prepar-ing frozen sections for histochemical demonstration of acid phos-phatase in proximal convoluted tubules[5].

A fundamental problem when sampling renal tissue for microscopy is loss of kidney volume, i.e. nephron patency[6]. Karunanayake et al.[7] have used in situ freezing of kidneys of the rat to minimize this artifact.

B.   Cryomicrotomy for the electron microscope (cryoultra-microtomy)

Since the first published description of ultrathin cryosection preparation[8], there have been a large number of reports on their use for purposes of improved ultrastructural preservation, enzyme cytochemistry, immunocytochemistry, X-ray microanalysis and, oc-casionally, autoradiography. For present purposes an ultrathin cryosection may be considered always to be less than 0.5 μm thick and usually between 50 and 150 nm in the hydrated state.

It is the purpose of this account to give an overview of the technical aspects of cryo-ultramicrotomy so that the reader is aware of the options available to him and of the problems he might expect to encounter.

1.   Specimen preparation prior to freezing

    1a. Chemical fixation. It is generally accepted that chemical
fixation prior to freezing and sectioning makes the sectioning
process much easier to perform, but under what circumstances is
this justifiable or desirable? Bernhard and collaborators developed
a technique for renal and other tissues whereby immersion fixation
in glutaraldehyde or formaldehyde was followed by impregnation
with thiolated gelatin with or without dimethyl sulphoxide
(DMSO)[9,11]. Freezing, usually in liquid nitrogen, was followed by
ultrathin section preparation using a cryostat-mounted MT-1
Porter-Blum microtome with a knife trough filled with DMSO. Such
sections when negatively stained could be used for both ultrastructural study and cytochemistry such as for brush-border alkaline
phosphatase localization in the proximal tubule.
    1b. Cryoprotection. One of the problems of cooling biologi-
cal and therefore aqueous specimens is the formation of ice crystals
which can distort microanatomy and displace solutes. Cryoprotectants can inhibit or reduce the formation of crystalline ice when
freezing biological specimens. Indeed Echlin et al.[12] have reported
success in the use of hydroxyethyl starch (HES) and polyvinyl
pyrolidone (PVP) when a 25% (w/w) solution of either proved useful as both support medium and cryoprotectant in an X-ray
analytical study.
    If the purpose of a study is to localize or measure highly
soluble substances in their in vivo state then it is for the individual to decide whether he can afford to risk contact with a
fluid phase, however viscous this is and however brief contact
might be. If the risk is taken, then the burden of justification lies
with the investigator.

2.   Freezing

When biological samples are cooled to sub-zero temperatures they
do not immediately "freeze" in the sense of forming ice crystals
but, depending upon the cell type and rate of temperature reduction, become supercooled[1], a term which has latterly been replaced
by the unfortunate word "sub-cooled". Below -15 °C most tissues
begin to form crystalline ice. Paradoxically, the conditions of cooling which are of greatest use to the microscopist are those which
destroy viability by causing homogenous nucleation of ice. This
means that large numbers of small ice crystals are formed intracellularly and extracellularly when relatively rapid rates of cooling
are employed. Clearly, from a morphological point of view this is
preferable to heterogeneous nucleation where gradual cooling of the
specimen causes relatively few large ice crystals to form which,
while minimizing membrane damage, cause gross structural deform-
ity.
    Perhaps the most convenient approach to freezing a biological
specimen for ultrastructural study is to mount small pieces on to
metal specimen supports with or without the aid of a mounting
medium (e.g. methyl cellulose) prior to immersion in a cryogen at
its melting point. Baker and Appleton used liquid nitrogen slush

87

(-210 °C) to freeze pieces of mouse kidney cortex (<1 mm³) mounted at the apex of conical brass specimen holders[13]. A similar method has been described by Seveus in which small silver "pins" were used for sample mounting[14,15].

The important point about direct immersion in liquid cryogens, whether nitrogen, Freon or isopropane, is that these should always be used at their melting and not boiling points otherwise the gas bubbles which form around the specimen during boiling exert an insulating effect. This then seriously reduces the rate of specimen cooling. Some workers have sought to overcome this problem by avoiding contact between the fresh specimen and liquid cryogen. Christensen achieved this by bringing his specimens, mounted on suitable chucks, into contact with a polished copper surface standing in liquid nitrogen at -196 °C[16]. Sitte et al.[17,18] have adopted a similar though more sophisticated approach.

No matter which technique is used for specimen preparation it is virtually impossible to achieve vitrification of ice in the absence of cryoprotectants. This is especially true of substantial tissue samples such as might be obtained from kidneys. Even the fastest cooling rates achievable, i.e. 10,000-20,000 degrees C per second, usually leave a peripheral zone in the specimen which is free of ice crystal damage of only 10-15 μm[19]. Frederik and Busing demonstrated that cortex samples from rat kidneys frozen in Freon 22 at its melting point have a peripheral zone free of measurable ice crystals of barely more than 10 μm[20,21]. These observations were made in both carefully dried ultrathin cryosections and freeze-fracture replicas (Figure 1).

Van Venrooij et al.[22] have drawn some fascinating conclusions from their measurements and calculations of cooling rates in model systems made from silver cylinders filled with dilute glycerol (a cryoprotectant)[22]. These investigators ascertained that the cooling rates at the periphery and centre of the cylinders when plunged into Freon 22 were faster than in the intermediate zones. In support of these data, freeze-fracture studies showed that ice crystals were small at the centre as well as the periphery while they were much larger in the slower-cooling intermediate zone. Unfortunately no data have yet been published which show this phenomenon in biological specimens.

3.   Storage of frozen specimens

In most instances it is convenient and economic to freeze more specimens than can be immediately sectioned. Hence the specimens must be stored in an environment which maintains their physical state at the completion of cooling. A temperature at which the vapour pressure of water in the presence of ice is virtually zero is thus required. The most common means of fulfilling this condition is to hold specimens in liquid nitrogen (-196 °C) which is relatively cheap and simple to store.

4.   Preparation of ultrathin cryosections

4a.   Instrumentation.   A brief consideration only can be given to the cryo-ultramicrotomes available. In recent years these have become sophisticated and purpose-designed since the manufacturers have recognized the viable market which now exists.

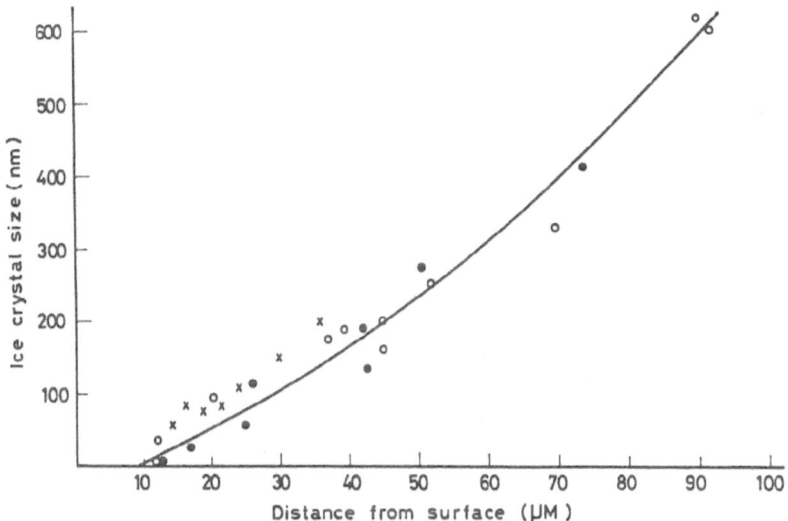

Figure 1 Relationship between ice crystal size and distance from the tissue surface. Unfixed, unglycerinated rat kidney frozen in Freon 22 and cryosectioned (X), freeze-fractured (O) or freeze-dried and embedded in Epon (●). From Frederik and Busing, 1981[20], J. Microsc., 121, 191. By permission of the Journal of Microscopy.

Basically, the requirements of a suitable instrument are that ultrathin cryosections may be produced in an atmosphere that can be cooled to -80 °C and less; that knife, specimen and storage area temperatures can be independently monitored and controlled; and that condensation of water vapour on to vital surfaces can be avoided or reduced to a minimum. So far, these conditions have been sought in two principal ways, namely, cryostat ultramicrotomes or cryo-attachments for ultramicrotomes.

The cryostat approach was reported in detail by Appleton, who used one of a limited edition of three specially constructed machines incorporating a modified LKB Ultratone III installed in a refrigerated cryostat designed by Slee Medical Equipment Ltd (London)[23]. The commercial derivative of this was the Slee TUL cryostat cryo-ultramicrotome, in which the ultratome used was a motorized Porter-Blum MT-1 with a modified MT-2 stage (Figure 2).

The alternative cryo-attachment systems have become more popular over recent years because the major ultratome manufacturers supply attachments and tools which allow their ultratomes to be modified as cryo-ultramicrotomes.

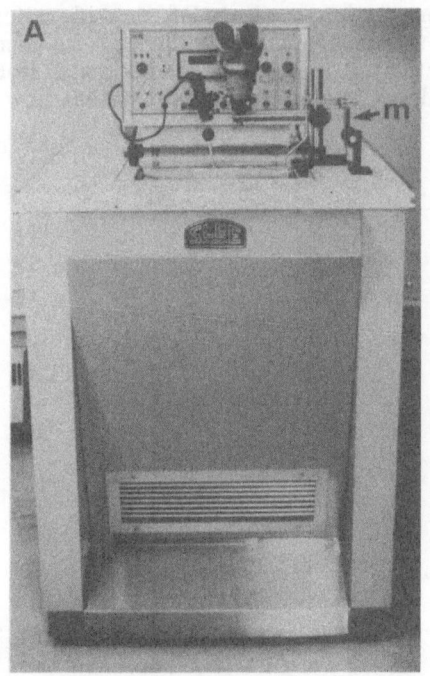

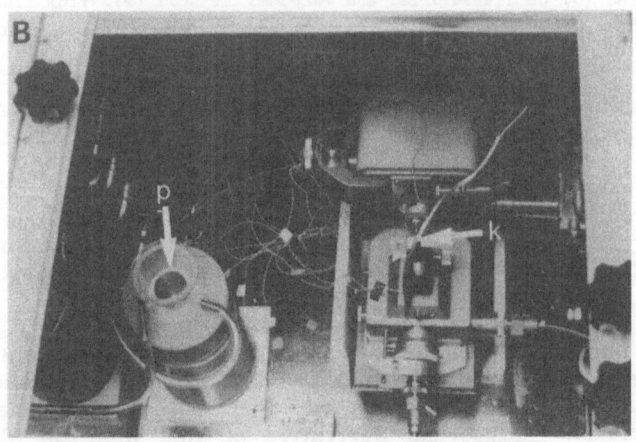

Figure 2 A. External view of the Slee TUL cryostat cryo-ultramicrotome, m - micromanipulator for vacuum line used for section recovery. B. Internal view of the cryostat chamber showing the ultramicrotome, k - glass knife, p - temperature-controlled platform for freeze-drying of sections.

The Dupont-Sorvall FS-100 has been designed to be used with the Sorvall MT-5000 ultramicrotome and was developed along the lines of the system used by Christensen, in which liquid nitrogen was fed into a polystyrene chamber which housed both knife and specimen[24,25] (see also Biddlecombe et al.[26]). In this system the specimen is connected to the ultratome arm via a "bridge" which passes over the side of the cryochamber. This is in contrast with the LKB Cryokit 14800. This employs a low conductivity specimen arm which enters the cryochamber via a hole sealed by a flexible plastic collar which inevitably becomes less flexible as the temperature is lowered. The bridge concept was retained by Reichert-Jung for their FC-4 which is designed for users with the Reichert OmU4 Ultracut ultramicrotome (Figure 3). Here, cooling of the aluminium side walls is achieved by liquid nitrogen filling of adjacent tanks plus nitrogen gas flushing of the chamber itself. Cryosorption (frosting) is minimised by incorporation of heaters in the specimen holder, knife holder, preparation plate and chamber walls (in the latter case for use when the machine is brought to ambient temperature).

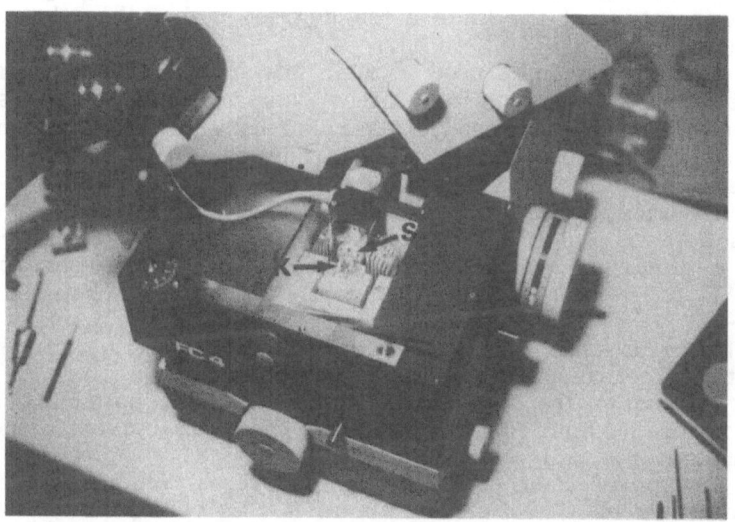

Figure 3 View of the chamber of the FC4 cryochamber fixed to a Reichert OmU4 Ultracut ultramicrotome, k - knife-holder containing two glass knives for sectioning between which lies an elliptical steel trimming knife; s - specimen holder.

4b. The sectioning process. The specimen, frozen on to its holder and most probably having been stored in liquid nitrogen, is transferred rapidly to the specimen chuck of the ultratome whose temperature and that of the surrounding atmosphere should be no higher than -70 to -80 °C in order to avoid rapid ice crystal growth (see below). Time should always be allowed for specimens to equilibrate to chuck temperature before sectioning commences. The decision whether or not to trim the frozen specimen will depend upon the preferred method of recovery. If ribbons of sections are required then trimming becomes desirable (although not absolutely necessary). Appleton has described trimming to a more or less square face[27]. This has the disadvantage that some if not all of the least ice-damaged zone is lost on all sides of the specimen face. A better compromise is to trim the leading and trailing edges (i.e. those parallel to the knife edge) but to leave the sides untrimmed, thereby retaining the maximum possible zone of best preserved tissue.

It is not possible to generalize about the precise conditions governing the cutting procedure since these will depend to some extent upon the equipment used and the tissue itself. Baker and Appleton produced sections of mouse renal cortex (nominal thickness 100 nm) in an ultramicrotome cryostat whose chamber temperature was between -80 and -90 °C[13]. Similarly, Frederik and Busing used a chamber temperature of -80 °C in an LKB Cryokit to obtain sections of rat kidney cortex[20]. Many workers have found that cutting and collecting sections is made easier by arranging to have the temperature of the knife a few degrees higher than that of the specimen[15].

The type of knife used is much less critical than for conventional resin ultramicrotomy. Although special steel and diamond knives are sometimes used, glass knives are most common. It should be remembered that glass at or below -80 °C is a much harder substance than at room temperature.

Recommended cutting speeds are slow and usually range between 0.5 and 2.0 mm per second[23,28]. In recent years there has been a tendency to recommend cutting temperatures as low as -140 °C (specimen) and knife and air temperatures between -100 and -120 °C[15,29]. An important issue raised by the work of Kirk and Dobbs is that the lower range of cutting temperatures may result in fractioning rather than true sectioning, as could be seen from replicas of the "cut" block surface[30]. This possibility seems to have been forgotten or ignored by those who advocate the use of temperatures well below -100 °C.

One phenomenon of the sectioning process which has received the attention of a number of authors is that of a potential melting zone arising from the energy input of the advancing knife. This raises the possibility of redistribution of soluble substances and could negate the entire rationale of the procedure. An overall conclusion which may be drawn is that such a melting zone is either negligible or so restrictied as to impose no real limitation on the technique[21,23,31,32].

4c. Section retrieval. There can be little doubt that this procedure can be the most frustrating and difficult of all the manipulations involved in cryo-ultramicrotomy. The use of an organic trough fluid such as DMSO can give pleasing results and simplify section handling[11], but DMSO has been found to extract certain elements from sections[33]. The safe rule therefore is that for any studies involving the localization of diffusible substances, sections must be collected "dry", i.e. without contact with external fluids.

There are many variants to retrieval of dry sections but these may be categorized in two principal ways. Most workers have chosen to manipulate sections singly or in ribbons on to support film-bearing grids using a "hair-probe"[28], or mounted needle[26], and then to press the sections on to the grid with a variety of devices such as the end of a polished copper or Teflon rod[25]. The main alternative to this is the vacuum collecting system introduced by Appleton (Figure 2)[23]. In this method a flattened syringe needle connected to a vacuum line and held in a micromanipulator is used to pull the leading edge of a ribbon of sections from a trimmed block face away from the knife edge. When the ribbon is of sufficient length it is lowered on to a support film-carrying grid placed below the knife edge. When the vacuum is switched off, the "needle" can be withdrawn and the ribbon pressed down with a polished copper rod. The latter method has the advantage that it helps reduce both the tendency of the sections to roll and the compression inherent in dry cut ultrathin cryosections.

4d.   Preparation of ultrathin cryosections for electron microscopy. The final choice facing the cryo-ultramicrotomist is to decide the physical state in which sections should be transferred and examined in the EM.

There is some evidence that sections which have been allowed to melt prior to drying have a pleasing ultrastructural appearance[25], and bear no signs of ice-crystal damage[20]. It is likely that soluble electrolytes will be redistributed under these circumstances[33]. When dried sections were allowed to rehydrate in laboratory air, previously compartmentalized sodium has been shown by X-ray microanalysis to redistribute evenly within sections[23].

A common means of examination of ultrathin cryosections when serious attempts are to be made at solute study is to freeze-dry prior to transfer to the electron microscope. After mounting sections on to grids, these are conveniently stored within the cryo-ultramicrotome at a "holding" temperature at which freeze-drying cannot take place, e.g. -130 °C or less[23]. When sufficient grids with sections have been collected they can be freeze-dried.

Successful freeze-drying of ultrathin cryosections requires an awareness of the process known as "recrystallization". This entails the growth of some ice crystals at the expense of others when the temperature of frozen specimens is raised, and if permitted in sections destined for EM examination, will lead to distortion of microstructure usually beyond recognition. In practice, the temperature at which recrystallization begins to occur rapidly in biological specimens is around -60 °C[23]. It follows then that if freeze-drying is to take place at atmospheric pressure it must be carried out at a temperature at which an adequate rate of ice sublimation can be achieved (i.e. > -130 °C) but at which rapid ice crystal growth is not possible (i.e. < 60 °C). Under atmospheric pressure, freeze-drying temperatures of -70 °C[23], or -90 °C have been used[13,26] freeze-drying being safely completed within 3 hours and probably within 1 hour. It is essential that no water remains in the specimen when its temperature is raised, and equally important that heat "sinks" and/or desiccators are used to prevent rehydration of the sections prior to transfer to the electron microscope. Naturally, freeze-drying can be accelerated and the hazards of a moist atmosphere reduced by use of mild evacuation[20]. Further precautions against rehydration of these hygroscopic sections may be taken. The most common of these is evaporation of a carbon layer on to the sections[13,26,34].

It has been claimed that a major drawback of freeze-drying ultrathin cryosections is that this leads to gross distribution of electrolytes in tissue compartments lacking an organic matrix[35]. The most obvious way to avoid this problem is to allow the sections to remain hydrated up to and during examination and analysis. In addition, low-temperature examination of sections, especially in the scanning transmission (STEM) mode, should help to minimize beam damage[36]. Essentially, the requirement is that sections, once mounted, are retained at a temperature at which they cannot dry even within the vacuum of an electron microscope column, and the most useful agent for achieving this condition is inevitably liquid nitrogen.

Various systems have been reported which allow safe transfer of sections from ultratome to microscope cold stage, ranging from self-assembled systems to commercially developed ones for specific electron microscopes[29,37]. It has become apparent, however, that there are some major drawbacks concerning the use of fully hydrated sections. For example, energy dispersive X-ray microanalysis of these results in inferior peak to background ratios at energies below around 3 keV when compared with spectra obtained from the same sections after freeze-drying in the microscope column[29,37]. A further problem is that full hydration reveals much less structural detail in a section that can be observed upon complete freeze-drying[36].

The foregoing account of cryomicrotomy, primarily at the ultrathin level, is by no means a comprehensive or exhaustive review of the topic - for such a review see Robards and Sletyr[38]. Rather, it is an attempt to present to the newcomer a feel for the complexity of the technology and to dissuade the uncommitted from embarking upon this field. On the positive side, it is hoped that the following sections will include data and arguments which illustrate the goals which can be achieved by diligent and dedicated use of ultracryomicrotomy.

II. X-RAY MICROANALYSIS

When an electron beam interacts with a specimen many events ensue, all of which may be put to some form of analytical use (Figure 4). To the transmission electron microscopist most important of all are the electrons which penetrate the specimen and form the image. These may be unscattered or undergo a change of direction maintaining their initial energy (elastically scattered) or lose a portion of it (inelastically scattered). Some electrons from the primary beam are so attenuated that their energy is totally absorbed within the specimen, being transformed into heat or light. The latter gives rise to the phenomenon of cathodoluminescence. Events above the specimen are of more concern to the scanning electron microscopist. Interactions of the incident beam with atoms at or below the surface of the specimen produce secondary electrons of low energy, and it is these that can be collected by a secondary detector using a positive bias voltage and thus form an image of surface detail. Electrons which are backscattered from the upper side of the specimen and which lose negligible energy may, by the use of a suitable directional detector, provide information on surface contrast, especially where elements of high and differing atomic numbers are present.

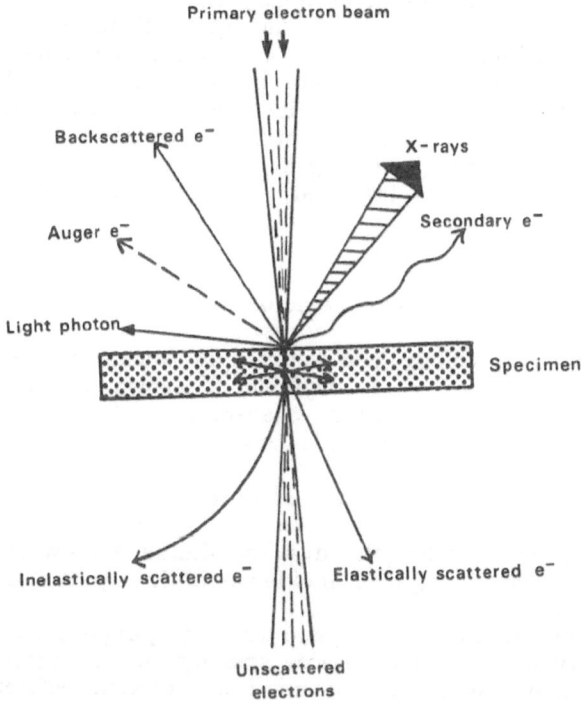

Figure 4 Diagrammatic representation of the interaction of an electron beam with a relatively thin specimen.

Of particular importance for the discussion of the next few pages is that orbital "shell" electrons can be excited by the primary electron beam such that an incident electron with sufficient energy removes an electron from the atom altogether, a process we know as "ionization". For the atom to retain energetic stability the vacant shell is filled by an electron from an outer shell with obvious possible "knock-on" effects. The outer electrons must lose energy in order to fill inner orbits which are at lower energy levels, and this is achieved by emission of X-rays, characteristic in number, energy and wavelength for a given element. It follows then that in ionizing a specimen with an electron beam we have a means to perform elemental analysis on the volume of specimen under irradiation.

Another category of X-rays is formed as a result of the slow-ing (or braking) effect of positive atomic nuclei on beam electrons. These X-rays are variously termed "bremsstrahlung", "background", "white" or "continuum" radiation and contribute to the overall spectrum of X-ray energies.

A. Collection and recording of X-ray information

The design and disposition of X-ray detectors are constrained by many factors, perhaps the most important of which is the need to optimize the efficiency of X-ray collection. To achieve this it is necessary to collect an adequate solid angle of the X-ray emiss-ions, and this entails bringing the detector as close as possible to the specimen without interfering with the electron beam.

There are three basic types of X-ray detector and the follow-ing brief description is intended to outline the principles involved for each.

1. Wavelength dispersive detector

The principles involved are essentially those of X-ray crystal-lography "in reverse", i.e. crystals of known lattice spacings are used to diffract and thus characterize X-rays of unknown wavelength according to Bragg's Law:

$$n\lambda = 2d \sin\theta$$

where = X-ray wavelength; d = the distance between the crystal lattice planes; Θ = angle of incidence of X-ray and crystal and n is an integer.

The spectrometers designed for this purpose contain a range of crystal types of various lattice spacings whose diffracting angles can be "tuned" so as to optimize the radiation reflected into the detector. The latter is an electronic gas flow counter producing pulses proportional to the energy of the X-rays entering it. The pulses, once amplified, are "gated" through a preset narrow volt-age range (in a pulse height analyser) which results in the predominant recording of selected X-rays and generally provides a good signal to noise ratio.

2. Gas flow proportional counter

This device, as well as being used to detect X-ray energies in crystal spectrometers, can be used directly as a detector. It is also known as a "non-dispersive" detector because, unlike its use in the spectrometer in which only one X-ray wavelength can be detected at a time, it can be made to receive all the X-ray wavelengths coming from the specimen. Thus a range of X-ray energies, inversely proportional to wavelength, will produce an ar-ray of pulses representing all elements present but with poor resolution. These can be displayed using a cathode ray oscillo-scope. Gas-flow proportional counters are further used in conjunction with wavelength dispersive microanalysis to measure continuum radiation which is necessary for some forms of quantification (see below).

3.   Energy dispersive detector

The advantage of this type of detector is that it permits analysis of all elements within a specimen simultaneously. The principle behind this device (Figure 5) is that the semiconductor silicon can be used to transduce X-rays into electrical signals which can be discriminated, quantified and displayed. The body of the detector is a silicon crystal wafer between 2.5 and 5 mm in thickness which, as a result of incoming X-rays, undergoes ionizations creating a cascade of "electron-hole" pairs. The "holes" act as free positive charges and migrate to the front of the detector where a negative voltage is maintained at a thin layer of gold. The opposite side of the crystal, also metal-coated, is held at a positive bias. This is connected to a field effect transistor (FET) and receives the electrons. The total charge is then amplified and passed into a multichannel analyser (MCA).

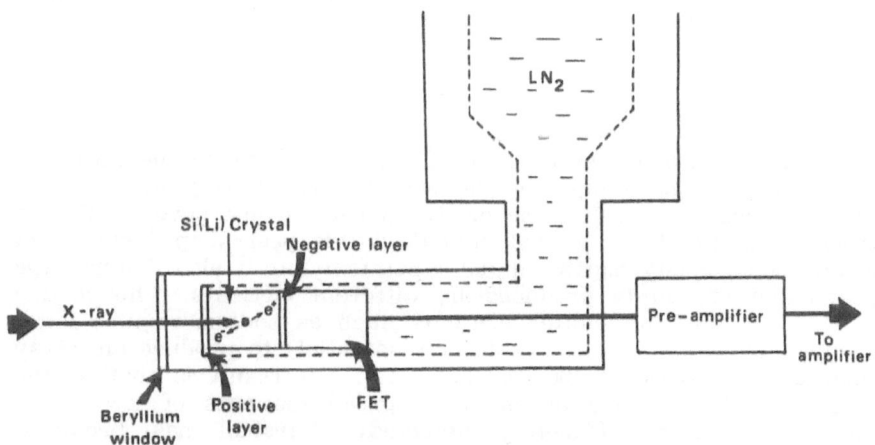

Figure 5   Schematic drawing of an energy-dispersive X-ray detector, FET - field effect transistor.

An important feature of modern energy dispersive detectors is that their resistivity is increased by diffusing lithium ions into the silicon crystal, thereby neutralizing electron-accepting impurities which are present in crystals of even the highest specification. The detector and FET are held at liquid nitrogen temperature to reduce electronic noise. A thin beryllium window isolates the detector from the exterior and effectively prevents entry of low energy "organic" X-rays. Quantification of the charge produced relies upon the fact that it takes 3.8 eV (electron volts) of energy to produce one electron-hole pair such that:

$$C_t = \frac{Ex}{3.8}$$

where C_t = total charge; Ex = X-ray energy.

The multichannel analyser stores the output voltages corresponding to these charge differences in terms of pulse amplitude and final display of the energy spectrum can be via a monitor or some form of "hard copy".

B.   Specimen size and spatial resolution

The area of specimen surface irradiated by the primary electron beam is usually less than that from which X-rays emanate due to diffusion and spread of electrons within the specimen. The extent to which this phenomenon occurs in practice depends upon specimen thickness, density, composition (i.e. atomic number) and energy of incident electrons (accelerating voltage). Thus it is not justified to assume that because the diameter of the incident beam is known this represents the area (and thus volume) from which X-rays are being collected by the detector.

1.   Bulk specimens

Specimens of 0.5 μm or more in thickness tend to be the norm for examination in scanning electron microscopes (SEMs) and, as can be seen from Figure 6, some electrons can diffuse several microns from the point of entry. Not only does this pear-shaped spread of electrons seriously impair spatial resolution but it also distorts the proportion of counts produced by different elements. This is due to the fact that the lighter elements such as sodium require lower electron energies (critical excitation potential) to produce an X-ray than heavier elements like calcium. The net result is that at the extremity of the zone of electron spread elements of low atomic number are most efficiently detected. Marshall has produced measurements showing that a 7 kV beam can penetrate to a depth of at least 15 μm to reveal radiation from a Si substrate below dried biological tissues, in contrast to a previous estimate[39] which gave a figure of 4.4 μm. Despite these problems count rates from bulk specimens are generally good, and produce useful elemental peaks.

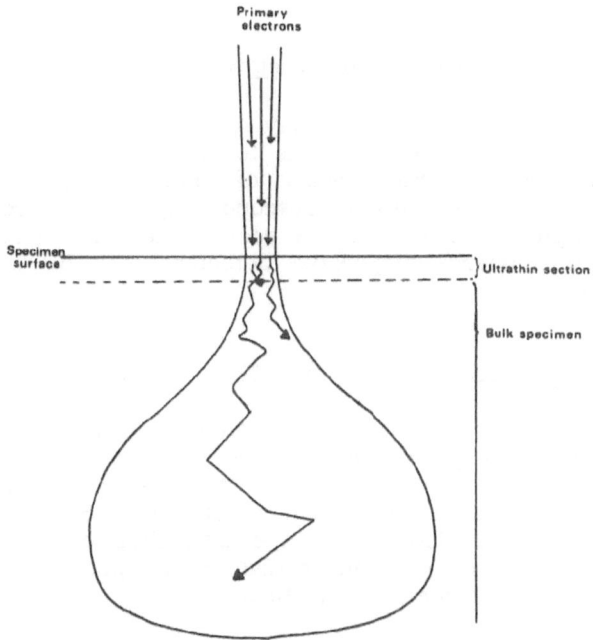

Figure 6 Schematic drawing of the penetration of the primary electron beam in a bulk specimen. The pear-shaped volume of excitation means that spatial resolution of X-ray detection is much less than that which would be obtained from the probe diameter in an ultrathin section.

2.   Ultrathin sections

For the transmission electron microscopist the problems of beam spread in sections of 200 nm or less are negligible for most practical purposes. There are data which show that lateral beam spread is considerably lower in freeze-dried sections than in sections of embedded tissue[40].

Although spatial resolution in ultrathin sections usually approximates to the incident beam diameter, and can be considered good, it must be remembered that a very small volume of tissue is irradiated, which means that when the massive organic matrix is taken into account, characteristic peak to background ratios of elements of interest can be modest. Hence there is little merit in obtaining the ultimate in spatial resolution when low count rates produce statistically unsatisfactory results.

C.   Electron optical instrumentation for X-ray microanalysis

Although X-ray microanalysis has become a widespread technique through its introduction to electron microscopists over the past 15 years it can be attributed to Castaing, who described the first purpose-built microprobe analyser in 1951[41].

1.   Electron-probe microanalyser (EPMA)

This instrument contains a relatively simple electron optical column usually incorporating scanning coils to provide an electron-derived image. However, the main means of specimen visualization and manipulation is via a light microscope. Specimens are generally thick, although sections of a few microns can be analysed. Both wavelength and energy-dispersive detectors may be used in the microanalyser.

2.   Scanning electron microscope (SEM)

This instrument provides and relies upon a much more sophisticated electron imaging system than the microanalyser. The secondary electron image is used to view the specimen (usually bulk) and very fine probe diameters can be obtained. Scanning electron microscopes generally have large specimen chambers allowing convenient interfacing of wavelength-dispersive spectrometers and/or solid-state energy-dispersive detectors.

3.   Transmission electron microscope (TEM)

Most modern transmission electron microscopes are designed with spare ports around the specimen stage which allow attachment of X-ray detectors (usually energy-dispersive). As already mentioned, when ultrathin sections are irradiated by the electron beam the volume of excited atoms producing X-rays for analysis is very small. It follows therefore that particular attention must be paid to detector-specimen geometry in order to allow the best possible solid angle of collection to be achieved (Figure 7). It is equally important to minimize unwanted peaks from the metallic elements of the specimen environment. Consequently it is necessary to choose grid materials carefully so that no spurious X-ray peaks are produced close to those of interest in the energy spectrum. In addition, non-standard specimen holders are required with low atomic number inserts such as graphite or beryllium.

4.   Scanning transmission electron microscope (STEM)

Despite the high spatial resolution obtainable in the TEM there is some operational inconvenience associated with analysis in this mode. The formation of the analytical probe is not compatible with simultaneous viewing of the transmitted image and alignment errors can lead to analysis of the wrong areas. Moreover, constant irradiation of the specimen during imaging may do much unseen damage, especially in volatilizing some lighter elements. These problems can be overcome or reduced by imaging thin specimens in the STEM mode using either an expensive dedicated STEM instrument or a STEM attachment for a conventional TEM. In this way the specimen, during imaging, receives a lower dose of electrons since the beam is scanned across it rather than remaining static. Additionally, the use of slowly decaying phosphors in the cathode ray monitor permits precise positioning of the analysing probe over the scanning image before this fades. In some scanning attachments the position of the probe can be defined by X-Y control of a dot or of line intersections superimposed on the TV image.

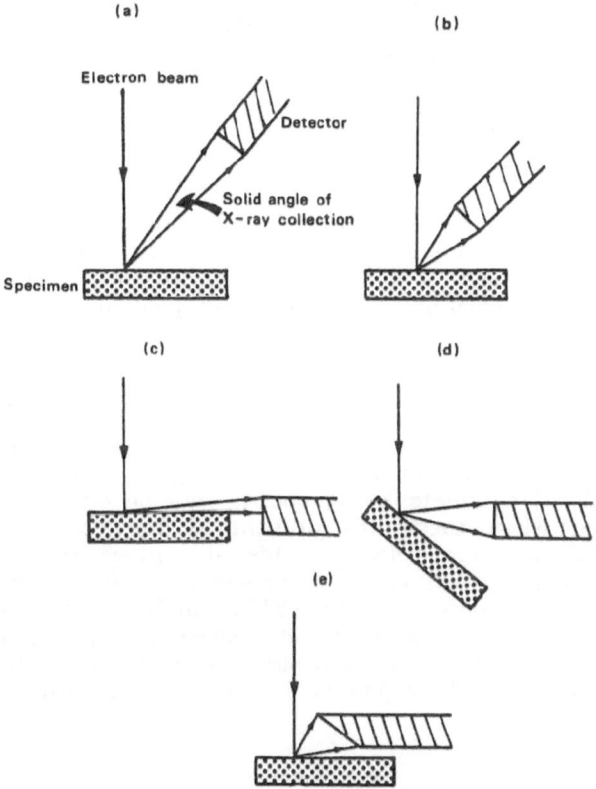

Figure 7 Diagrams to illustrate factors which influence the solid angle of X-ray collection. (a) A standard detector at a high take-off angle to a horizontal specimen results in a moderate solid angle of collection; (b) if the detector is moved closer to the specimen the solid angle increases further; (c) a horizontal standard detector acquires a low take-off angle from a horizontal specimen; (d) if the specimen is tilted toward the detector the solid angle increases; (e) if both specimen and detector are horizontal but the detector is of the high "take-off" angle type, the solid angle of collection will be large.

D. Choice of analytical mode

1. X-ray mapping

If the analyser is instructed to select one or more characteristic X-ray lines from a single element, this can become the output signal which is displayed on the cathode ray monitor of a SEM or STEM. The resultant image is a "map" of the distribution of the element within a given area of specimen and appears as a density distribution of bright spots which can be photographed. This type of "analysis" is feasible only when elemental concentrations are high. This means that in biological specimens its usefulness is usually confined to examinations of mineralized tissues, those with pathological or toxicological build-up of metal deposits or some enzyme-cytochemical preparations.

2. Line scanning

An alternative to the above approach is to scan the electron probe across a particular line on the specimen. By use of a suitable ratemeter, this permits a quantitative representation of the given elemental X-rays according to the height of peak in the trace.

3. Static probe analysis

By focusing the stationary electron beam to a very small diameter of as little as 20 nm and by use of long counting times (100 seconds or more) adequate X-ray counts may be obtained for many elements even when these are present at low concentrations in ultrathin sections. Quite clearly, this also gives the optimum in spatial resolution. Nevertheless, emphasis on spatial resolution increases the risk of poor sampling. This can be reduced by use of larger spot sizes or, in scanning instruments, by replacement of the static probe by scanning of a small selected area which on the basis of morphological homogeneity is judged to be within a single structure.

E. Specimen preparation

The methods available for preparation of biological specimens for X-ray microanalysis are numerous. The choice depends upon the physico-chemical nature of the elements under investigation and to a lesser extent upon the sample size and degree of quantitative sophistication required.

For comprehensive treatment of the problems of preparation of biological specimens in general the reader is referred to other reviews of the subject[42,43]. Many of the requirements for specimen preparation for detection and analysis of soluble elements in TEM and STEM modes were dealt with in the section on ultracryotomy. The following account is a very brief consideration of preparative possibilities which might apply to renal analysis. Since it is improbable that precise information can be gained from analysis of bulk kidney samples it will be assumed that thin or ultrathin sections are normally required.

The elements of interest in renal study fall into two broad categories. The first includes metals which produce toxic effects in kidney cells as a result of their role as pollutants or their side-effects when administered as therapeutic agents. In general, these occur as intracellular deposits which are so stable that they present no real problems of specimen preparation and can be adequately retained by conventional methods involving chemical fixation, dehydration and embedding. Examples will be given in the section below on applications of X-ray microanalysis in renal research.

The other category of elements includes soluble electrolytes and elements of partial solubility whose distribution and concentration can be modified by toxic events. For faithful retention these require methods which either avoid chemical fixation or involve modification of conventional techniques as in freeze substitution and precipitation plus embedding.

1.   Freeze substitution

Freeze substitution involves rapid freezing whereupon ice is replaced by immersion in an organic solvent such as acetone or ether at low temperature. This substitution is followed by replacement of the solvent in turn by an embedding medium for light or transmission electron microscopy. On many occasions chemical fixatives have been added to the solvents to enhance structural preservation[44]. Many investigators have recognized the need to section dry, i.e. in the absence of an ultratome trough fluid[45].

Claims for the extent of elemental retention possible with freeze substitution are often impressive[43,46]. Freeze substitution of rat kidney using diethyl ether at -80 °C has been shown to retain 99% of ^{68}Ge (from germanic acid) by the final embedding stage in Spurr resin[47]. Nevertheless many questions remain unanswered. For ultimate fidelity in solute micro-retention, it is unlikely that freeze substitution is as safe as ultracryotomy in spite of the ultrastructural shortcomings of the latter.

2.   Precipitation and embedding

Cations may be arrested within tissues by techniques other than those based on freezing. A controversial but commonly used approach has been the use of precipitating anions followed by "conventional" preparative techniques. The overwhelming majority of such applications have been performed with potassium pyroantimonate ($K[Sb(OH)_6]$) which was initially introduced for localizing sodium ions[48]. Nevertheless, it has become apparent that pyroantimonate, especially when added to osmium tetroxide as the primary fixative, has a superior affinity for calcium ions[49]. Due to overlap of Sb L_α and Ca K_α lines, however, there is a requirement to "strip" away a proportion of the counts attributable to antimony when using energy-dispersive analysis. Fortunately most modern analyser software packages include a routine to handle this type of problem.

An alternative to dehydration and embedding with epoxy or acrylic resins is to fix in the presence of a precipitating agent and to embed in situ by means of a glutaraldehyde/urea mixture. Yarom et al.[50] used this method for the retention and analysis of sodium and chloride in skeletal and cardiac muscle, silver acetate being used to precipitate chloride ions.

It should be remembered that the very act of creating visible deposits of precipitate in tissues must involve migration of ions to the "nucleus" of precipitation. Hence, pin-point resolution is essentially unattainable either by visual or analytical means, and the most realistic mode of analysis is to use a selected area raster scan rather than a static probe.

F.   Applications of X-ray microanalysis in renal research

1.   Physiology

X-ray microanalysis has often been used to study the composition of renal tubular filtrates and urine ex vivo, thereby avoiding any special requirements for specimen preparation except that of ensuring that the analyte remains stable in the electron beam.

One of the earliest investigations of the potential of electron microprobe analysis on biological fluids used a synthetic test specimen of known K^+ and Cl^- composition[51]. In this study a microprobe analyser incorporating a wavelength-dispersive spectrometer was used to establish the feasibility of measuring these ions with acceptable accuracy and reproducibility. Although nanolitre samples could be analysed, K concentrations of 1 mEq/litre or less resulted in large standard deviations. Comparable instrumentation was used by Morel et al.[52] to analyse 0.4 nl micropuncture samples collected from proximal distal convolutions of kidney tubules of rats undergoing different levels of salt diuresis. Tubular fluid to plasma concentration ratios (TF/P) of Na, K, Cl, P, Ca, Mg and Fe (from $Fe(CN)_6$ as a filtration marker) were determined using calibration curves of K_α, counts per unit time versus concentration of standard solutions. Good agreement was obtained with values from other forms of measurement with especially high correlations for flame photometric determinations of Na and K. The same group of investigators used a very similar system to measure identical elements in non-diuretic rat kidneys[53]. The results indicated that 20% of filtered Mg was absorbed along the proximal tubule whereas 64% was resorbed by the loop of Henle. In addition P, purportedly all in the form of phosphate, was shown to be actively resorbed, notably in the proximal tubule but also in the late distal or collecting tubules.

Acute plasma loading with $MgCl_2$ revealed that late proximal tubular TF/P of Mg/In ([^{3}H]inulin was used to monitor filtration rate) remained proportional to the filtered load[54]. An active and saturable mechanism for Mg resorption appeared to be present in the loop of Henle. Furthermore, early distal Mg filtrate/plasma ratios were below urine/plasma values. This can be interpreted as indicating a net Mg tubular excretion by the terminal nephron segments or a medullary Mg ion pool resulting from the loading process.

This ambiguity emphasizes the limitation of studying only extracellular fluids and the need to analyse intracellular electrolyte compartments to help explain the processes responsible for measured filtrate and urine composition.

Freeze-dried ultrathin cryosections of unfixed rat kidney have been used to assess the results of ion pump inhibition in proximal tubule cells following 24 h incubation in hypoxic medium at 0-4 °C[55]. In this study an electron probe microanalyser with transmission electron and energy-dispersive X-ray detectors measured "intracellular" Na, Cl and K before and after the incubation period. Quantification of results prior to standard curve calibration was undertaken initially by net peak to background ratio according to the following formula:

$$\frac{P-B}{B}$$

where P = peak + background counts (i.e. total counts within a defined "window" above the energy axis); B = background (i.e. counts remaining after substration of net peak count).

An alternative formula for quantification of results was:

$$\frac{P-B}{B_2}$$

where B_2 represents "background" or "continuum" counts measured within a window which does not contain characteristic elemental peaks.

This method, originally devised by Hall, works on the principle that dividing the net peak counts for a given element by a constant continuum value will provide correction for variations in thickness of the specimen[56]. This is because the X-ray emission is proportional to the mass of tissue being irradiated assuming the electron beam current is constant, a condition which effectively remains true as long as the net peak and continuum values are obtained from the same energy spectrum. The value given by the second formula is often termed "relative mass fraction" and will be referred to later. Trump et al.[55] compared absolute Na, Cl and K concentrations obtained with both formulae and showed that values derived from the second are in better agreement with those obtained by chemical analysis.

Saubermann et al.[57] and Bulger et al.[58] have analysed 0.5 μm cryosections of fresh rat renal papillae at a temperature of -175 °C in an SEM operated in the STEM mode. However, since

105

these sections were cut at between -40 and -50 °C and structure was easily discerned, it is probable that these sections were only partially hydrated. Collecting duct cytoplasm was shown to be lower than interstitial space in Na, Cl and S, similar in K and higher in P. When sections were fully dried by warming inside the instrument, mass fractions increased proportionally in all compartments, indicating that the differences observed were not the result of differences in water content.

The study described by Bulger et al.[58] showed that papillary interstitial cells contained Na at 898 ± 194 mmol/kg wet weight. They suggest that if the Na is unbound it is these cells which make an important contribution to papillary adaptation to the hypertonic environment. This study used the continuum method[56], but included an important correction not previously mentioned, i.e. that of subtracting from the total continuum count a continuum value obtained for analysis of the grid support film alone. This corrects not only for the support film component but also for counts attributable to the metallic environment of the specimen.

As mentioned previously, bulk specimens of kidney are limited in the degree of precision of elemental concentrations which may be derived from their analysis. In spite of this, Lechene et al.[59] have performed some interesting experiments on hemisected frozen kidneys from antidiuretic (urine 2828-3130 mOsM) and diuretic (urine 95 mOsM) rats. Wavelength dispersive line scans from outer cortex to papilla tip were performed with spectrometers set for Na, K, Cl and P. In the antidiuretic (water-deprived) rat, Na and Cl were markedly increased in the inner medulla from its boundary with the outer medulla. In the diuretic rat the highest Na and Cl counts were at this boundary and fell away in the medulla. Figures 8 and 9 show the sodium profile for both conditions. This result supports the view that the inner medulla plays an important role in the mechanism of salt concentration in the kidney.

In recent years detailed results on intracellular electrolyte composition have come from the laboratory of Dörge and Rick (Beck et al.[60]). This group analysed 1 μm freeze-dried cryosections of rat kidney which had been frozen with an outer layer of albumin containing known concentrations of Na, K and Cl to serve as an in situ standard. Energy-dispersive analysis in a SEM operated in the STEM mode was carried out on raster-scanned selected areas of 1 μm^2. Proximal and distal tubule profiles were examined from only the superficial layers of cortex, since this region was best preserved and was adjacent to the in situ standard. Quantification was achieved by a derivation of the "ratio" method of Russ[61], according to the following equation:

$$Cu = Iu \, (Ck/Ik)$$

where Cu = mass of unknown element/unit volume; Iu = X-ray intensity of unknown element; Ck = mass of known (i.e. standard) element/unit volume; Ik = X-ray intensity of known (standard element).

The final elemental values were expressed as mmol/kg wet

weight and are summarized in Figure 10. The concentrations of Na and Cl were significantly lower in distal tubular nuclei than those of proximal tubules. Measurements performed in the centrally located cytoplasm of proximal and distal tubule cells next to nuclei showed similar Na and K concentrations to those in nuclei. Wherever the scanned areas included extracellular space, there was a fall in P and K and an increase in Na and Cl.

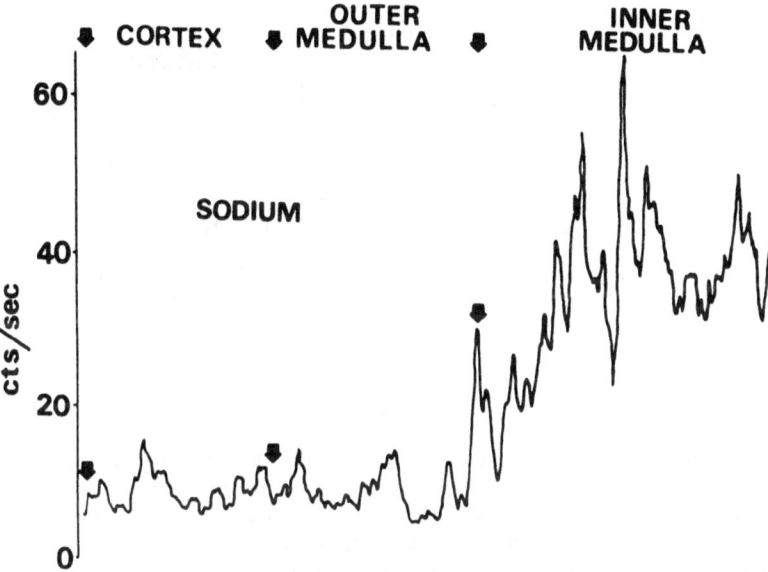

Figure 8 X-ray intensity profile of sodium along the corticomedullary axis of a kidney taken from a water-deprived rat producing a urine of 3130 mOsm. The kidney was quench-frozen in isopentane, hemisected with a circular saw in liquid nitrogen and analysed frozen-hydrated at -156 °C. Note the marked increase in sodium signal near the boundary between outer and inner medulla. The irradiating beam was focused and its accelerating voltage was 2 kV. The tracing represents a continuous recording of characteristic X-ray intensity as the specimen was moved along the corticomedullary axis beneath the beam. From Lechene et al., 1979[59]. Reproduced by permission of Academic Press, Orlando, Florida.

The same group has used similar techniques to assess the effect of model ischaemia on intracellular electrolyte composition[62]. Ischaemia was caused by hilar ligation of the renal artery and proceeded in an aerobic or nitrogen-filled atmosphere, and in some instances was followed by reperfusion. When a kidney was maintained in air during ischaemia the elemental composition of cells to a depth of 50 μm differed little from controls. An atmosphere of nitrogen, however, caused all cells to undergo electrolyte changes, namely increases in Na and Cl and decreases in K and P. This state of affairs took longer to establish in distal than in proximal tubules. Sodium and potassium changes were attributed to disturbances of the Na/K pump while Cl and P alterations resulted from fluid influx into cells. Reperfusion rapidly reversed all electrolyte disturbances but there was evidence of a return of elemental imbalances in some proximal tubule cells 18 hours after restoration of blood flow.

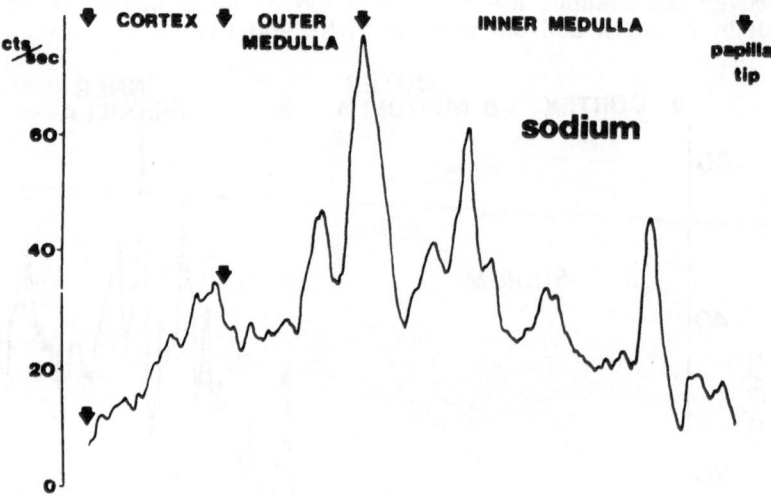

Figure 9 X-ray intensity profile of sodium along the corticomedullary axis of a kidney taken from a water-diuretic rat producing a urine of 95 mOsm. Preparation as for Figure 8. Sodium characteristic X-ray line signal decreases from outer-inner medullary border to papilla tip. Beam accelerating voltage 10 kV. The beam was continuously scanned over an area of 50 μm². From Lechene et al., 1979[59]. Reproduced by permission of Academic Press, Orlando, Florida.

2.   Metal toxicity

Heavy metals can accumulate in the kidney as a result of environmental pollution or therapeutic side-effects. Very often the resulting deposits are easily imaged in the electron microscope and may be analysed with little need for precautions in specimen preparation. Because toxicological and pathological events progress in a highly variable way, much less emphasis has generally been placed upon accurate quantification than in physiological studies.

Rheumatoid arthritis has often been treated with gold salts which may sometimes lead to harmful side-effects. This has prompted microanalytical studies of both experimentally and clinically affected kidneys. Stuve and Galle have studied gold deposits which appeared in proximal tubule organelles of rats dosed acutely or chronically with subcutaneous aurothiopropanol sulphonate[63]. Primary fixation with osmium tetroxide and Epon embedding followed by wavelength-dispersive analysis permitted identification of the inclusions as gold. Affected organelles were extruded into the tubule lumen and tubule damage regressed following cessation of gold salt injections. The organelles containing the gold inclusions were originally described as mitochondria. However, the authors have subsequently concluded that these structures correspond to lysosomes or phagolysosomes (personal communication).

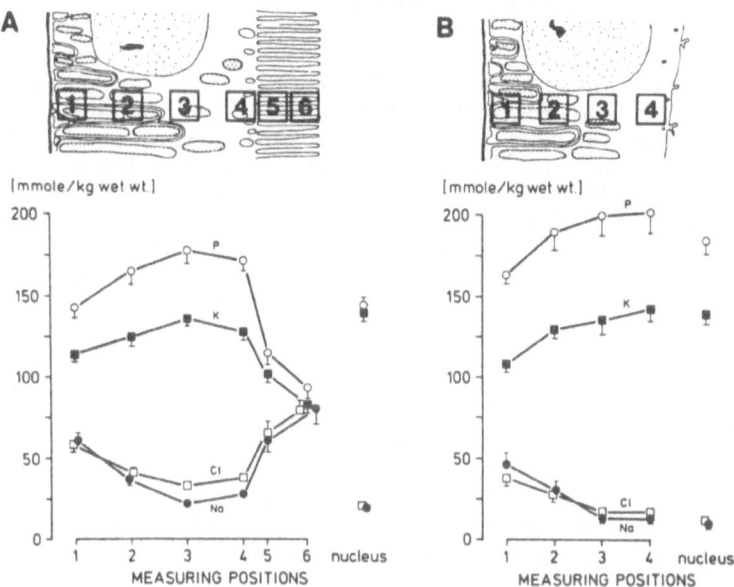

Figure 10 Concentrations of phosphorus, potassium, chloride and sodium given as mean ± SEM, obtained in the different regions of 15 proximal (A) and eight distal (B) tubular cells, which are indicated in the accompanying sketches. Reproduced from Beck et al., 1980[60]. By permission of Springer-Verlag, Heidelberg.

Yarom et al.[64] were also able to detect gold in energy-dispersive analysis of damaged proximal tubule mitochondria of biopsy from a rheumatoid patient who had received gold sodium thiomalate and who had developed massive albuminuria. Once again osmium fixation and Epon embedding were sufficient to preserve the dense deposits of gold. Another patient who had been treated with gold sodium thiomalate, and who had developed the nephrotic syndrome, was studied by Ainsworth et al.[65] using energy-dispersive analysis of glutaraldehyde-fixed biopsy material. Proximal tubule cells not only contained Au and S positive "aurosomes" in the cytoplasm but the nuclei also possessed Au positive inclusions.

Platinum in the form of cisplatin has been used as an anti-tumour agent but its long-term toxicity in many organs including kidney has limited its therapeutic use. Chronic (8 month) i.p. administration of cisplatin to rats resulted in the appearance of platinum in proximal tubular lysosomes as revealed by Berry et al.[66] using wavelength-dispersive analysis in a microprobe analyser.

X-ray microanalysis has revealed some fascinating differences with respect to renal mercury poisoning depending upon whether exposure is acute or chronic and single or in combination with other intoxicating elements. Nabarra et al.[67] found that single dosing of rats with $HgCl_2$ produced mitochondrial alterations which were especially marked in proximal tubule S_3 cells. Those mitochondria with spicule-like crystals contained low concentrations of Hg.

Separate and combined chronic administration to rats of mercuric chloride and sodium selenate (Na_2SeO_4) has been monitored by Carmichael and Fowler[68]. $HgCl_2$ alone produced renal tubular necrosis while Na_2SeO_4 resulted in a more severe retardation of growth but no obvious pathological changes in the kidney. Simultaneous administration resulted in protection against weight loss and histopathological effects except for electron dense nuclear inclusions in proximal tubule cells. Energy-dispersive analysis showed these inclusions to contain both Hg and Se always in a ratio of 1 to 2, suggesting that the elements may be present in chemical combination with concomitant reduction of their toxic effect. The nuclei of rat proximal tubule cells were also found to be sites of dense body formation following bismuth subnitrate treatment for 2-6 days[69]. These bodies were positive for Bi upon subjecting ultrathin Epon sections to energy-dispersive analysis.

Other metals such as chromium have been found in lysosomes. Chronic intraperitoneal dosing of rats with potassium dichromate showed Cr X-ray peaks in proximal tubule organelles identified as lysososomes by the Gomori method for acid phosphatase[70].

Cadmium metallothionein administered i.v. to rabbits as a single dose induced formation of lysosomes dose-dependent[71]. These possessed significant Cd which was absent from surrounding cytoplasm of perfusion-fixed kidneys. This study revealed much necrosis of S_1 and S_2 proximal tubule segments while S_3 cells appeared more resistant to damage.

A fully quantitative investigation of physiological and toxicological consequences of cadmium dosing in mouse kidney has been reported by Kendall et al.[72] Freeze-dried ultrathin frozen sections of unfixed cortex were examined by energy-dispersive analysis. The results were expressed as mg/kg dry weight using a commercially available software package which depends upon the use of standards and is based upon the continuum method of Hall[56,73]. The test animals received two subcutaneous nephrotoxic doses of $CdCl_2$ (0.7 μmol each). The most significant result of the induced nephrotoxicity was an increase in cytoplasmic and mitochondrial S in distal tubules. Also evident was a loss of Mg, P, Cl, K and especially Na from mitochondria. It was suggested that the sulphur increase arose from induction of metallothionein, one third of whose amino acids are cysteine. This peptide can bind several metals including cadmium, as already mentioned.

3.   Pathology

When pathological events result in deposition of highly stable elemental complexes the latter are usually amenable to X-ray microanalytical study. Such was the case at autopsy of a patient who had Wegener's granulomatosis[74]. Crystalline deposits were found in glomerular basement membrane (renal failure had set in before death). Energy-dispersive analysis showed marked Ca and P presence in these deposits which were absent from almost all other basement membranes.

4. Enzyme histochemistry

When X-ray microanalysis became familiar to the majority of electron microscopists, many believed that it would extend the use of light microscopic cytochemical methods to the electron microscope by making electron transparent inorganic reaction products detectable. In reality this "revolution" never came about, but some work along these lines has been carried out with promising results. Rosen and Beeuwkes mapped the distribution of Na/K dependent ATPase in 10 μm cryosections of kidney samples from human, rabbit and rat[75]. The reaction medium, at pH 9, contained KCl, $MgCl_2$ p-nitrophenyl phosphate and DMSO. Reaction product could be made visible by $(NH_4)_2S$ to precipitate CoS. Wavelength-dispersive analysis in a microprobe analyser was used to create X-ray maps of thick ascending limbs of the loop of Henle (Figure 11). Plotting counting rates for P against reaction time showed that reaction product formation was linear for the first 10 minutes.

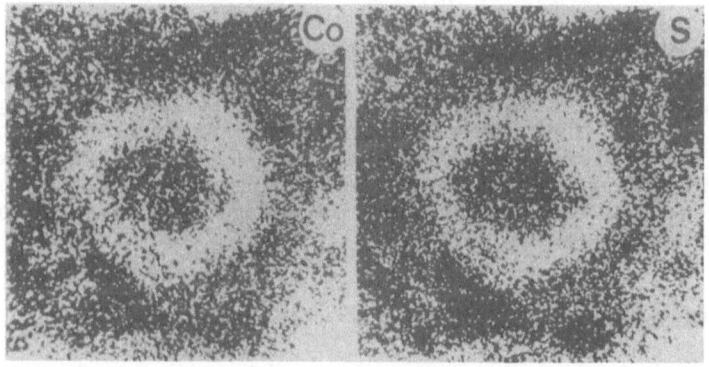

Figure 11 X-ray elemental maps (15,000 counts/element). Sections were incubated to demonstrate potassium-dependent ouabain-sensitive transport ATPase, subsequently treated with $CoCl_2$, then exposed to $(NH_4)_2S$ and dehydrated. The final reaction product, CoS, delineates this thick ascending Henle's limb. Reproduced from Rosen and Beeuwkes, 1979[75]. By permission of Academic Press, Orlando, Florida.

111

G. Comparison of X-ray microanalysis with other analytical techniques

Some of the aforementioned examples of X-ray microanalytical renal study have compared analysis results with those from other techniques such as atomic absorption spectroscopy and flame photometry, with impressive agreement. However, comparison with conventional physiological methods (e.g. ion-selective microelectrodes) must be made bearing in mind that X-ray microanalysis records total elemental fraction irrespective of ionic state and physiological availability[76]. Thus, X-ray microanalysis must ultimately be considered as a complementary technique. It has nevertheless a unique advantage in its potential to measure elemental composition in biological specimens at the organellar level[77], and will continue to make a valuable contribution in the study of renal physiology, pathology and toxicology.

III. AUTORADIOGRAPHY

X-ray microanalysis offers an opportunity to study endogenous substances (elements) be they physiological or pathologically or toxicologically acquired. Autoradiography can be considered a complementary technique (or set of techniques) in that it also permits the investigation of substances in situ with a high level of structural correlation. The fundamental difference is that in autoradiography the substances investigated are introduced into the organism or organ albeit they can be chemically identical to the non-radiolabelled endogenous substances.

Although radioisotopes of many elements are suitable for autoradiography[78,79], tritium and carbon-14 are most frequently used due to their versatility in the radiosynthesis of organic molecules[80]. Autoradiography can permit location of radiochemicals from the whole organism to the sub-organellar level, and has played a significant role in renal physiology, pathology, toxicology and pharmacology.

A. Whole-body autoradiography

Although it is the primary purpose of this section to describe light and electron microscopic contributions of autoradiography to renal study, an important starting point is the consideration of macro- or whole-body autoradiography. In respect of animal work the major pioneer of the technique was Ullberg[81,82]. Animals, dosed with radiolabelled compounds, were rapidly frozen to immobilize both bound and soluble label, and sections were cut using a sledge-type microtome in a sub-zero chamber (cryostat). The sections, supported on adhesive tape, were allowed to freeze-dry and were firmly apposed to X-ray film. After exposure, the sections were removed from the film which was developed leaving an image usually of high anatomical detail and providing an instant impression of organs in which radiolabel was most concentrated.

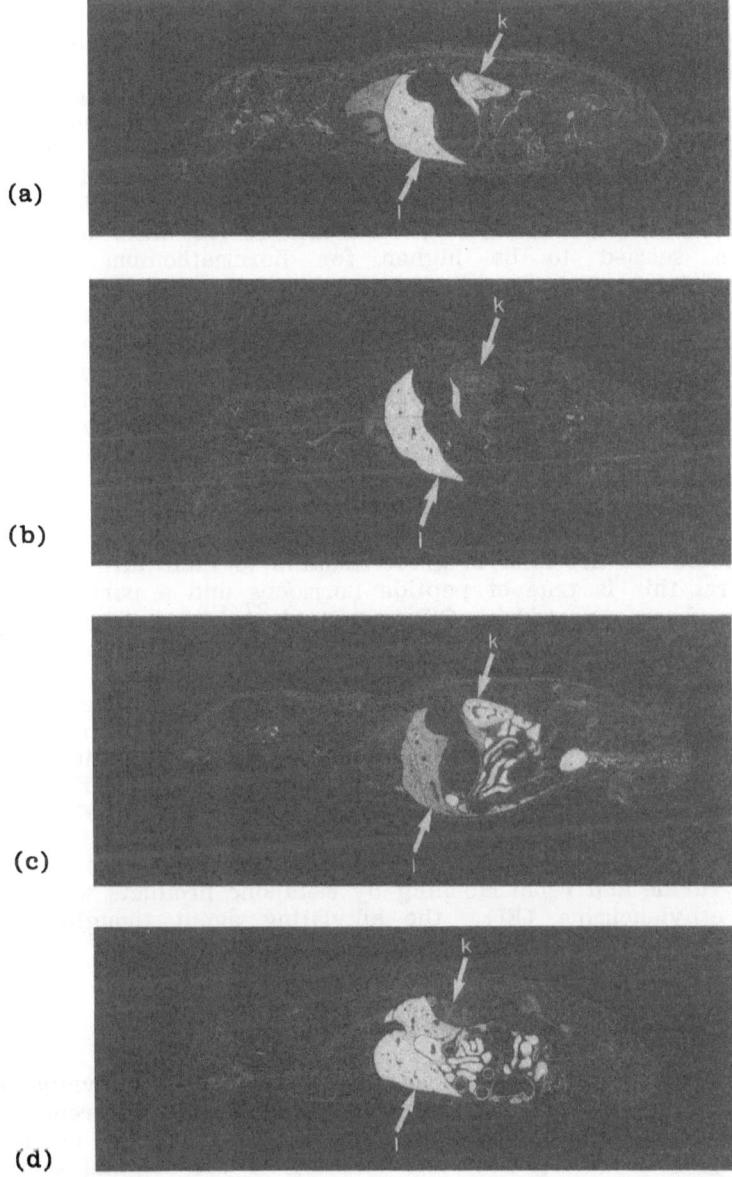

Figure 12 Whole-body autoradiographs showing the differing pattern of metabolism in the rat of two synthetic analogues of somatostatin. When $[4\text{-}^3H\text{-}Phe^7]\text{-}[des\text{-}AA^{1,2,3,4,13,14}\text{-}D\text{-}Trp^8, Gaba^{12}]$somatostatin was injected intravenously the metabolism at 3 min (a) or 40 min (c) could be seen to be shared between the kidneys (k) and liver (l). When however $[4\text{-}^3H\text{-}Phe^6]\text{-}[des\text{-}AA^{1,2,3,4,13,14}, D\text{-}Trp^8, \beta\text{-}(\alpha\text{-}naphthyl) Gaba^{12}]$somatostatin was identically administered the metabolism at 3 (b) or 40 (d) min was almost exclusively hepatic.

113

Whole-body autoradiography has become a widespread and standard technique in the evaluation of the distribution of radiopharmaceuticals. Using this method it has become possible to determine with relative ease which of a series of analogues are most readily metabolized in the kidney (Figure 12)[83].

The relative importance of kidney as an organ of metabolism also changes within an homologous series. Wasserman showed that the kidneys of mice injected with the bis-quaternary ammonium compound [^{3}H]hexamethonium became more heavily labelled than the liver[84]. Moreover, when mice were labelled with [^{14}C]hexamethonium and [^{14}C]decamethonium the rate of urinary excretion seemed to be higher for hexamethonium than for decamethonium[85].

The extent of renal metabolism varies not only with respect to chemical modification but also to species. This was elegantly illustrated in the whole-body distribution of L-tyrosine-O-[^{35}S]sulphate[86]. When the ester was injected i.p. into rats it rapidly accumulated in renal inner cortex where it is metabolized, whereas in the mouse the label was not metabolized and therefore concentrated in the renal pelvis.

On many occasions whole-body autoradiography has vividly illustrated that physiological and pharmacological mediators which are highly potent do not bind in great amounts to their target organs. In general this is true of peptide hormones and a particular example has been reported by O'Byrne et al.[87] Intravenous labelling of mice with [^{125}I]Tyr^3-relaxin failed to show an affinity of the hormone for its target organs, i.e. pubic symphysis, uterus or cervix. Radiolabel was most concentrated in renal cortex but in parallel experiments was shown to represent degradation products.

As well as serving a useful function in pharmacokinetic and metabolic investigations, whole-body autoradiography can provide valuable information on renal toxicology. Intraperitoneal administration of the renal papillary necrosis-inducing agent 2-bromo-[1-^{14}C]ethan-1-amine (BEA) upon whole-body investigation, revealed primarily urine and renal labelling by metabolic products which may contain ethyleneimine (EI), the alkylating agent thought to be responsible for the papillary lesions[88].

1.   Whole-organ macroautoradiography

It is possible to apply the whole-body procedure to individual organs such as kidneys. In this way histological differences in radiochemical distribution may be revealed and especially enhanced by photographic enlargement and staining of the original section. Baynton and Mercer adopted this modification when studying the disposition of [^{14}C]urea in rat kidneys in terms of its contribution to total osmotic pressure[89]. Figure 13 shows a particular build-up of radiolabel in the inner medulla and papillary tip region. An identical distribution of ^{22}Na was demonstrated by Dartigues et al.[90] who compared the actions of diuretics. These authors were able to show that treatment with hydrochlorothiazide did not alter the control pattern of distribution for ^{22}Na whereas furosemide, a so-called "loop" (of Henle) diuretic abolished the medullary label.

114

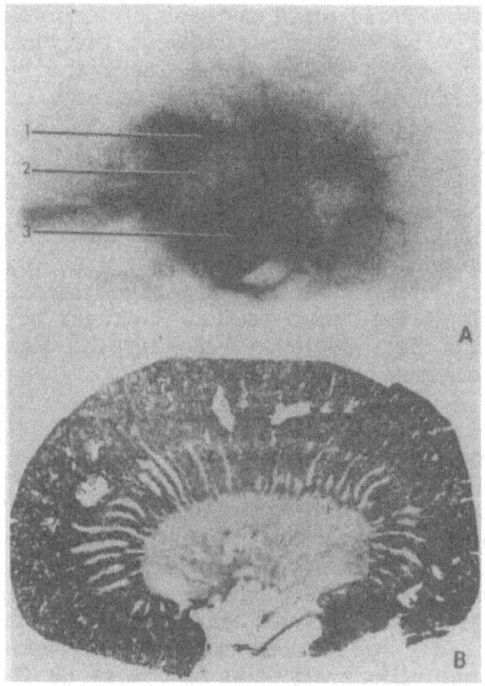

Figure 13 A. Autoradiograph of a kidney from a rat given a constant infusion of [^{14}C]urea. Arrow 1 indicates the increased deposition of [^{14}C]urea in the outer medulla. Arrow 2 shows the lower deposition of radiolabel in the outer zone of the inner medulla. Arrow 3 points to the increasing deposition in the medulla and papillary tip. B. Section adjacent to that in A stained with haematoxylin and eosin. Reproduced from Baynton and Mercer, 1968[68]. By permission of the National Research Council of Canada.

2. Quantification of whole-body autoradiography

Whole-body autoradiography is generally regarded as a qualitative or at best semi-quantitative technique. Berlin and Ullberg created a standard scale from fixed X-ray film dipped into solutions of radiolabel[91]. Squares were cut from sheets which had been treated with a range of radiolabel concentrations and made into a scale which was attached to X-ray film and exposed simultaneously with freeze-dried animal sections. After development, visual comparison of the scale and tissue label densities permitted semi-quantitative comparisons to be made. Cross et al.[92] extended this principle using microdensitometric comparisons of tissue and scale radiolabels in an attempt to make measurements more quantitative. Longshaw and Fowler used "beta-radiography" to evaluate the extent of quenching of beta particles in sections used for autoradiography[93]. This involved a thin sheet of $[^{14}C]$polymethyl methacrylate used as a radiation source. Freeze-dried sections of unlabelled rat ranging from 10 to 60 μm were sandwiched between the plastic source and X-ray film. After exposure and development the percentage light transmission recorded revealed the range of beta particle attenuation which might be expected as a result of variation in tissue density. The results suggested that sections which were 10 or 15 μm thick underwent uniform beta quenching in soft tissues (between 44 and 48%) whilst bone absorbed up to 57% of light. At higher section thickness, beta (i.e. light) absorption was greater and more variable with very high values in bone (up to 89%). The problem of beta particle quenching in tissues labelled with tritium is of course much reduced, and section thickness is of little importance since all the beta particles reaching the film emanate from the top few micrometres only.

B. Light microscopic autoradiography

A major factor in any autoradiographic work is whether the handling or nature of the radioisotope within the tissue will enable it to be retained by conventional "wet" chemical preparation and, if not, how this problem can best be overcome. Thus, autoradiography is subdivided in terms of "fixable" and "soluble" (or "diffusible") substances and renal applications can be conveniently treated in terms of these subdivisions. It must of course be remembered that there are many substances which fall into a "grey area" of qualified fixability or diffusibility. Ultimately the responsibility lies with the investigator to define the class of substance he is handling.

1. Autoradiography of chemically fixable substances

The most commonly encountered "fixable" radiochemicals are those which act as precursors in macromolecular synthesis, or which in some other way form covalent bonds with some fixable tissue constituent or with chemical fixatives.

<u>1a. Nucleoside uptake, nucleic acid synthesis and cellular turnover in the kidney.</u> Nucleoside incorporation measured both radiometrically and autoradiographically can provide an index of cellular regeneration in kidneys following exposure to toxic agents. The aminoglycoside gentamicin, which can cause proximal tubular necrosis, has been found after low-level dosing in rats to stimulate incorporation of $[^{3}H]$thymidine in the cortex[94]. Microautoradiography showed the labelling of many nuclei in both proximal tubule epithelia and interstitial cells.

The anti-depressive agent lithium is known to produce polyuria in some patients even at therapeutic doses. Rats succumb similarly and have been studied by enzyme histochemistry and $[^{3}H]$thymidine autoradiography following daily dosing with Li for up to 21 days[95]. Between 7 and 21 days, collecting ducts exhibited hyperplasia, increase in mitochondrial oxidative enzyme activity and increase in DNA synthesis. The authors concluded that these compensatory modifications occur in response to cellular changes in the distal tubule.

Oestrogen transplants can produce tumours in hamster kidneys which, following administration of [^{3}H]thymidine or [^{3}H]uridine, exhibit enhanced nuclear autoradiographic labelling of proximal tubule cells[96]. The increased RNA synthesis observed may reflect increased protein biosynthesis of intracellular oestrogen receptors since autoradiography also revealed enhanced uptake of [^{3}H]oestradiol.

Other tumour types such as the mesenchymal and corticol epithelial neoplasms have been related to their respective originating cell types by autoradiography of perfusion-fixed kidneys from rats[27]. These animals were treated with the carcinogen dimethyl nitrosamine and received daily i.v. injections of [^{3}H]thymidine for 3 to 10 days after treatment. Autoradiographic analysis of the proliferative activity of renal cell sub-populations was carried out (Figure 14). The main proliferation was in cortex for epithelial cells and in cortex and outer stripe, outer medulla for interstitial (mesenchymal) cells. The results indicated that a correlation exists between the ability of a carcinogen to cause toxic injury to target cells, to stimulate a pulse of early proliferation in the same populations and to induce tumours of a histological type consistent with the cell types involved in the early phase of injury.

1b. Study of renal function. The major site of metabolism of many proteins and peptides is the kidney, and examples of this process will be described below in the section on EM autoradiography.

Sottiurai traced the major site of resorption and metabolism of [^{131}I]insulin in the rat to the renal proximal convoluted tubule epithelium[98]. A further conclusion was that inhibition of glomerular filtration permitted reduced but significant uptake (33%) from peritubular capillaries. It must be questioned, however, on the basis of the inappropriate choice of isotope (^{125}I would be better resolved) and the many basal invaginations of the tubular cell membranes, whether the autoradiographic silver grains truly represented intracellular radiolabel.

The octapeptide [^{3}H]angiotensin II when administered intra-arterially to rats has been found to bind specifically to mesangial cells[99]. Specificity was claimed in the light of the fact that labelling was inhibited by pretreatment with 8-Ileu-angiotensin II. The claim was made that mesangial cells may be a target for the hormone. In spite of this, it does generally seem to be the case that peptide hormones are highly potent and therefore do not concentrate at their respective target organs. In fact, concentration of radiolabel derived from these molecules can indicate metabolism[83].

Autoradiography has also contributed to investigation of anabolic kidney function. For example Pegg et al.[100] have studied the renal distribution of ornithine decarboxylase in androgen-treated mice using the covalent inhibitor α[5-^{14}C]difluoro-methylornithine. Silver grains were located predominantly in

117

proximal tubule cells (Figure 15). Such incorporation was markedly reduced by prior treatment with cycloheximide.

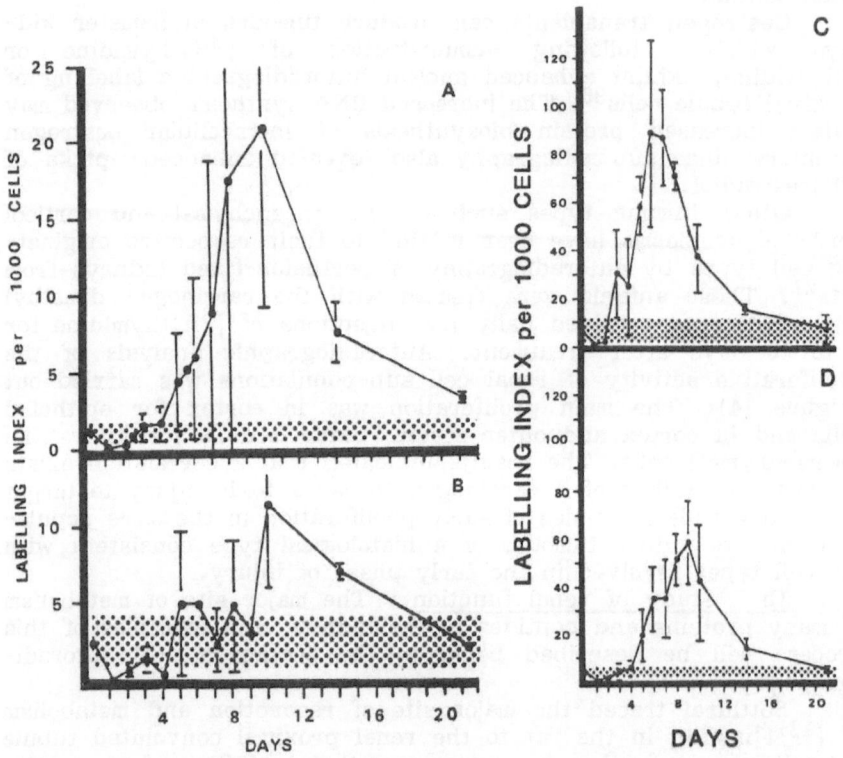

Figure 14 Effect of 60 mg/kg dimethyl nitrosamine on the uptake of [^{3}H]thymidine by proximal tubule epithelium (A & B) and in the free interstitial cells (C & D) of the various kidney zones. (A & C), convolutions of proximal tubules, distal convoluted tubules, some collecting tubules and glomeruli, (B & D) pars recta of proximal tubules, straight portions of distal tubules and collecting tubules. The stippled band represents ± standard deviation from the mean of 10 control values. Each test point is the mean value determined from at least three rats ± S.D. Redrawn from Hard, 1975[97]. By permission of Cancer Research, Inc.

1c. Study of renal toxicity. Whereas X-ray microanalysis has the advantage of permitting the localization of exogenous elements such as renal xenobiotics, autoradiography allows organic molecules to be localized. The furan derivative 4-ipomeanol is particularly nephrotoxic in mice[101]. Radiolabelling of the compound with ^{14}C or ^{3}H and subsequent autoradiography showed covalent binding of the 4-ipomeanol in proximal tubules which corresponded with tubular necrosis. Pretreatment with piperonal butoxide prevented formation of tubular lesions and markedly reduced radiolabelling.

118

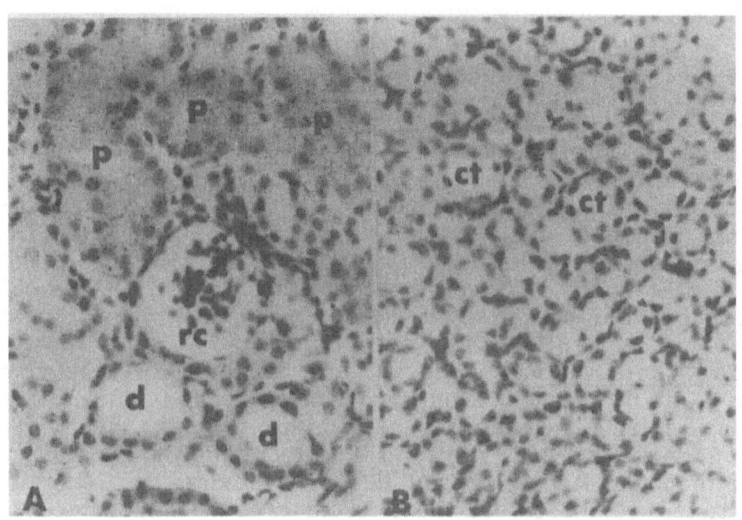

Figure 15 Microautoradiographs from androgen-induced kidney of mice treated with [^{14}C]difluoromethylornithine. Tissues were perfused with 10% neutral buffered formalin, embedded in polyester wax and sectioned at 10 μm. Sections were exposed for 6 weeks at 4 °C in Kodak NTB-2 emulsion. A. Section of cortex showing extensive labelling of the proximal convoluted tubules (p) and much less activity over the glomeruli (rc) and distal convoluted tubules (d). B. A section of medulla with only sparse labelling over the collecting tubules (ct). From Pegg, A.F., Science, 217, 68-70, 1982. Copyright 1982 by the American Association for the Advancement of Science.

2.   Autoradiography of diffusible substances

The primary requirement for successful autoradiographic localization of diffusible compounds is that the handling of specimens prevents redistribution or loss of radiolabel up to the moment of photographic development. The most straightforward way to achieve this is yet again to freeze the specimen after labelling and to allow no further contact with fluids until exposure is complete. From this principle two major approaches have been developed.

The method of Appleton uses cryostat sections of frozen tissue which, under safelighting[102], are mounted without thawing on to slides or coverslips at sub-zero temperatures bearing a preformed emulsion layer. Exposure proceeds at cryostat temperatures (e.g. -15 to -30 °C) during which freeze-drying takes place. At the end of exposure the sections are chemically fixed, developed and stained. Appleton has shown[103] that the "resolution" (image spread) obtainable with this technique is satisfactory even for the energetic positron emitter sodium-22.

The major alternative is the method of Stumpf and Roth[104].

This involves freeze-drying of cryosections under vacuum before mounting on to a preformed emulsion layer at room temperature. The atmospheric humidity must therefore be low and not more than 25%.

Each of these methods has its particular advantages and Rogers has found the results from both, in his hands, to be of comparable quality[105].

Some investigators have not been satisfied with the histological appearance of cryosections whose stainability is undoubtedly impaired after freeze-drying. Stirling et al.[106] traced the trans-intestinal transport of tritiated glucose and galactose by freeze-drying and resin embedding the labelled tissue[106]. Silicone oil was added to the resin prior to polymerization. This "waterproofing" inhibited but did not eliminate loss of radiolabel when 1 or 2 μm sections were cut on to water.

2a. Localization of physiological markers. Frozen sections for the light microscopic level and fixed embedded material for the electron microscopic level have been used to study the glomerular filtration markers [^{14}C]inulin and [^{14}C]polyvinylpyrolidone[107]. Although the bulk of the material in both instances was excreted, a small amount (0.3-0.4%) of the injected dose was endocytosed into the proximal tubules. Preloading did not affect renal storage of these compounds, which was modest. This indicates that the uptake of the markers is passive and related to tubular fluid absorption by the epithelium.

Soluble compound autoradiography has advanced our understanding of modifications to tubular epithelial transport when experiments have been performed in vitro. For example, the glycoside phlorizin, a transepithelial transport inhibitor, selectively binds in vivo to proximal tubule brush border membranes where it competes for carriers. Weeden and Vyas used rat kidney cortex slices to show that phlorizin inhibited secretion of [^{3}H]p-aminohippuric acid (PAH) from cell to lumen in proximal tubules[108]. It was concluded that increased [^{3}H]PAH uptake and the delayed washout induced by phlorizin might be attributable to increased efflux inhibition at the antiluminal membrane.

2b. Localization of compounds with fixable and soluble metabolites. Clearly, when radiochemicals undergo metabolism the final autoradiographic image derived from them will depend upon the position of the radioisotope within the molecule. Furthermore, the requirements of tissue preparation will depend upon the need to image either bound metabolites or total radiolabel. Such considerations were paramount in a study of the diabetogenic drug streptozotocin by Karunanayake et al.[7,109]. Streptozotocin, ^{14}C-labelled in three specific positions (Figure 16) was administered to rats from which autoradiographs were prepared using both frozen and fixed tissues to investigate binding to "target" (pancreatic islet) versus metabolic tissues (liver and kidney). Quantitative assessment of autoradiographs from fixed tissues showed modest grain densities except where the radiolabel was in the methyl group of the side-chain. In this case the pancreatic islets were quickly labelled whereas renal cortex, liver and pancreatic exocrine tissue became labelled much later. It thus appears that streptozotocin acts by alkylation, possibly of nucleic acid, and that the

120

glucopyranose moiety facilitates distribution and cell uptake of the molecule or terminal methyl group.

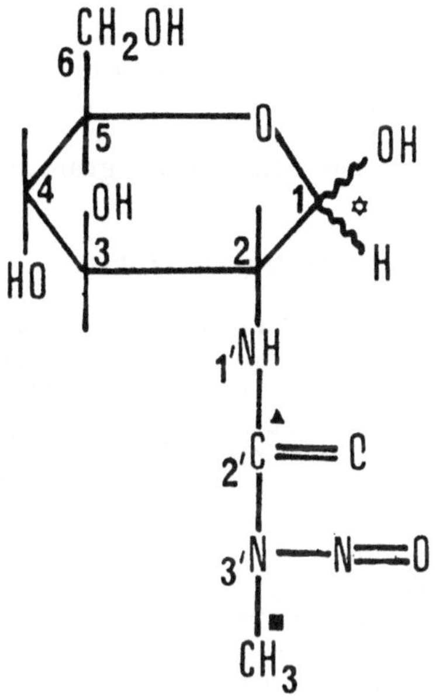

Figure 16 Streptozotocin (2-deoxy-2(3'-methyl-3'-nitrosoureido)-D-glucopyranose) labelled in one of three positions with ^{14}C; * - [1-^{14}C]streptozotocin, ▲ - [2'-^{14}C]streptozotocin, ■ - [3'-methyl-^{14}C]streptozotocin. From Karunanayke et al., 1976[7]. Reproduced by permission of Springer-Verlag, Heidelberg.

2c. **Localization of soluble pharmaceuticals.** Since pharmaceuticals may be subdivided into several classes with respect to their solubility and histological retention there is a range of preparative regimes which can give usable results when autoradiographs are prepared.

Gusterson et al.[110] used a modification of the Appleton technique to assess the relative density of opiate binding sites in the Syrian hamster following intraperitoneal injection of [^{3}H]diprenorphine. The highest grain density was in the amygdala of the brain (136 grains/500 μm^2) while renal cortex and medulla were almost identical at around 15 grains/500 μm^2.

Odlind and Dencker used a somewhat less cautious method in their microautoradiographic study of the diuretic [^{35}S]furosemide in hens[111]. These investigators prepared their autoradiographs from sections of freeze-dried kidney pieces which had been paraffin embedded in vacuo. One minute after drug administration via the portal circulation proximal tubule cells were shown to be most heavily labelled. By 4 minutes the pattern was dramatically altered, most silver grains appearing in the lumen of the collecting ducts.

A recently developed method was specifically introduced to permit receptor binding of ligands such as opiates which do not readily cross the blood-brain barrier[112]. Essentially this approach

121

involves in vitro labelling of fresh or lightly formaldehyde-fixed cryosections prior to apposition of a preformed emulsion layer. Summers and Kuhar have extended this method to localize β-adrenoceptors in rat kidney using $[^{125}I]$cyanopindolol (CYP)[113]. This study indicated that in the rat kidney, high concentrations of β-adrenoceptors are associated with glomeruli, distal tubules and cortical collecting ducts. In this case, specificity of binding was confirmed by preincubation with the competitor (-)-isoprenaline which eliminated all but low non-specific grain density.

C.   Electron microscopic autoradiography

Autoradiography is carred out at the EM level to relate distribution of radiolabel within tissue to the high spatial resolution of ultrastructure obtainable from examination of ultrathin sections in the transmission electron microscope. The value and limitations of the technique have been described elsewhere[80], but consideration of some of the major technical problems should never be absent from appraisal of renal or any other applications. The problems of limited efficiency (or sensitivity) in EM autoradiography are widely appreciated[114], although suggested remedies such as the use of scintillators are of marginal or unproven value[115]. Conversely, difficulties resulting from image (grain) spread are widely ignored while several refined methods exist for analysis of EM autoradiographs. These will be described in outline later.

1.   EM autoradiography of fixable substances

1a.   Toxic substances.   The toxicity of cadmium in the kidney is well known. It has recently been shown in rats that dosage form strongly influences the zone of the nephron which absorbs the cadmium and exhibits necrosis. Murakami and Webb found that subcutaneous administration of $^{109}CdCl_2$ followed by intraperitoneal L-cysteine produced marked radiolabelling in the S_3 zone of proximal tubule in the outer stripe of the outer medulla[116]. However, the same group has shown that intravenous $^{109}CdCl_2$-metallothionein produced denser radiolabelling of the convoluted zone of the proximal tubules in the cortex[117]. In both studies EM autoradiography showed that the ^{109}Cd was not concentrated in endocytotic vesicles, lysosomes or any other cellular organelle even early on after dosing, but was distributed apparently evenly throughout the epithelium. Thus even when Cd is administered and filtered as a complex with metallothionein, its liberation from the metalloprotein appears to occur very early in the resorptive process.

1b.   Protein and peptide resorption.   There is little doubt that the most productive area of renal study using EM autoradiography is the resorption and degradation of filtered or microinjected proteins and peptides. This is because the kidney is the major organ of catabolism of most proteins and polypeptides and these and many of their metabolites can be fixed and therefore retained by aldehydes.

Generally, for this type of study the most widely used radionuclide employed has been iodine-125 with rather fewer studies involving tritium. Iodine-125 has the advantage that it is relatively easily introduced into tyrosine residues which, when these become detached from the parent molecule by metabolism, are not readily reutilized for new protein synthesis[118]. The drawback of radioiodinated polypeptides is that their biological activity is compromised leading to doubts that they are handled by cells and tissues in a manner which is always identical to their unlabelled counterparts. This problem is absent from studies in which tritiated peptides are used. However, the radiolabelling of these is more complicated and since tritiated aminoacids are not recognized as "foreign", these, once detached from their parent peptide, can be reincorporated into newly synthesized proteins. The resulting autoradiographs are difficult to interpret since they contain grains produced by both anabolic and catabolic components.

A large range of molecular sizes of proteins and peptides has been studied with respect to their renal resorption and degradation using EM autoradiography. An early study used micro-injection of [125I]homologous albumin into proximal tubules of single rat nephrons to ensure sufficient radiolabel was presented to the tubular epithelium for resorption[119]. Neustein and Maunsbach injected rabbits intravenously with haemoglobin which had been synthesized in vitro by rabbit reticulocytes using [3H]DL-leucine[120].

Lysozyme, which has a molecular weight of 14,400 daltons and is readily filtered by glomeruli, has been the subject of several studies[121-125] for which it was radiolabelled with iodine-125. [125I]cytochrome C (MW 12,400) was also included in the study of Christensen and Maunsbach[123].

EM autoradiographic evaluation of renal resorption in rats or rabbits of a range of peptide hormones has been carried out during the past 12 years as follows: [125I]porcine insulin[126], synthetic tritiated adrenocorticotrophin analogues[127-128] [125I]sheep growth hormone[129], [125I]salmon calcitonin[130], and [125I]human choriogonadotrophin[131].

These examples encompass a variety of approaches to fixation of the labelled tissue. It appears that superior morphology has been achieved when kidneys were perfusion-fixed in a manner similar to that described by Maunsbach[132,133].

The overall picture emerging from these studies is that filtered proteins and peptides are rapidly absorbed from the proximal tubule lumen across the brush border by the epithelial cells within a very few minutes of administration. At this early stage, silver grains are associated with the apical region of the cells which is occupied by endocytotic vesicles and vacuoles (Figure 17). Thirty to ninety minutes after administration silver grains are usually seen in association with cytoplasmic bodies which by various criteria may be regarded as secondary lysosomes (Figure 18).

1c. Quantification and analysis of EM autoradiographs. Further consideration should not be given to the interpretation of autoradiographs from the sizeable group of studies above without an outline of the problems involved in quantification of EM autoradiographs so obviously lacking in many of these reports.

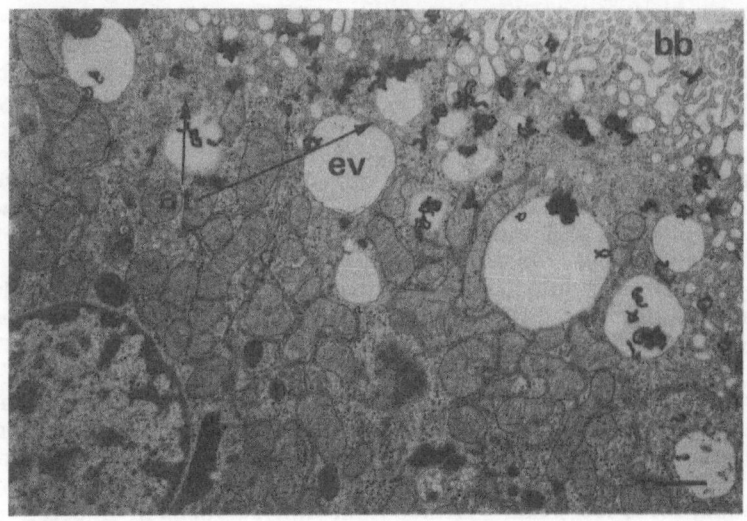

Figure 17 Electron microscopic autoradiograph of the apical region of proximal tubule cells of a rat 3 min following intravenous injection of a tritiated 1-24 ACTH analogue ([^{3}H]Tyr^2-Synacthen). Most of the silver grains appear to be in the region occupied largely by endocytotic vesicles (ev) and apical tubules (at); bb - brush border. Bar - 1 μm. From Baker et al., 1977[128]. Reproduced by permission of the Journal of Endocrinology.

It is well established that the majority of silver grains in EM autoradiographs do not directly overlie the point in the tissue section producing the isotopic decay particles (usually electrons) responsible for their formation. This can readily be demonstrated by reference to EM autoradiographs of infinitely thin line sources of radionuclides of the type illustrated in Figure 19 and first described for tritium by Salpeter et al.[134]. Several factors are responsible for this phenomenon. These include variable electron energy, section and emulsion thickness, angle of particle emission but above all, the ability of the electron microscope to resolve the discrepancy between ultrastructural detail and autoradiographic image spread. This situation therefore can lead to the formation of silver grains, some of which do not overlie the structures containing the radiolabel responsible for their formation. This process is known as "cross-fire". It follows that merely counting silver grains in relation to structures beneath them will lead to overestimates and underestimates of the distribution of radiolabel. This becomes particularly serious when the labelled structures are small.

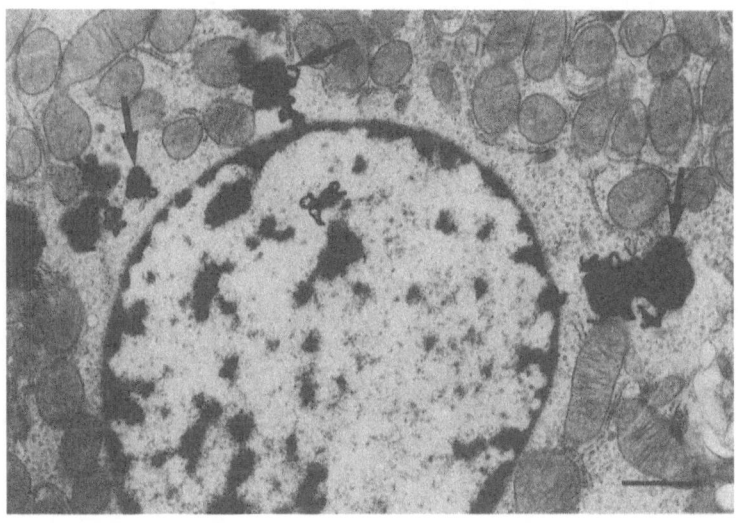

Figure 18 Electron microscopic autoradiograph of the nuclear region of a proximal tubule cell of a rat 30 min following intravenous administration of a tritiated 1-24 ACTH analogue ($[^3H]Tyr^2$-Synacthen). Most of the silver grains are associated with secondary lysosomes (arrowed). Bar - 1 μm. From Baker et al., 1977[128]. Reproduced by permission of the Journal of Endocrinology.

Salpeter and her colleagues pioneered evaluation of EM autoradiographic image spread[134]. They produced grain density distributions from line sources of the type illustrated from the author's own results in Figure 20. This introduced the concept of "half-distance" (HD), i.e. the distance from the line source within which 50% of the silver grains fall. Since, however, the majority of radiolabel in biological specimens exist as discrete points it became necessary to calculate the functions for expected grain distributions about point sources (Figure 21)[79,134-136]. Under these circumstances it is necessary to think in terms of "half-radius" (HR), which is the radius of a circle about a point of disintegration within which 50% of the grains arising from that point fall. The latter circle is often referred to as a "50% probability circle".

According to Williams[137], analysis of EM autoradiographs using image spread data falls into two basic categories: "restricted" and "unrestricted".

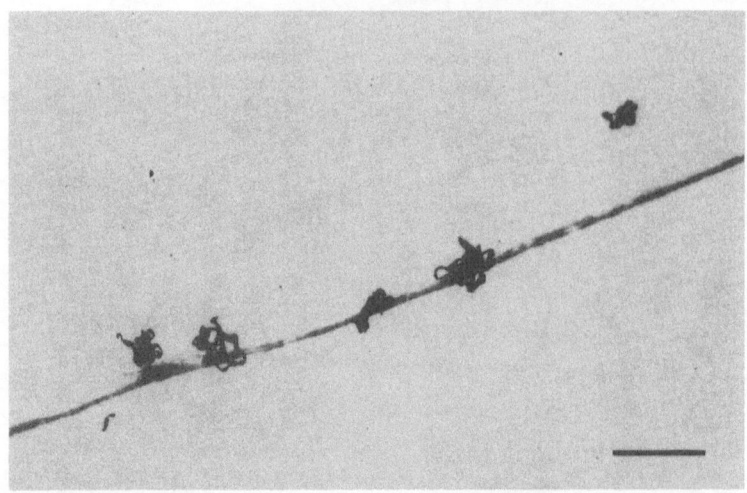

Figure 19 Electron micrograph of a thin line source of [51]Cr. Sodium [51]chromate was mixed with serum albumin and thinly painted on to a slab of polymerized epoxy resin. The layer was fixed in glutaraldehyde and dehydrated in graded ethanols prior to embedding in more epoxy resin. Section thickness, 80 nm; emulsion, Ilford L4; developer, Kodak D19. Note that not all of the silver grains lie over the source. Bar - 1 μm.

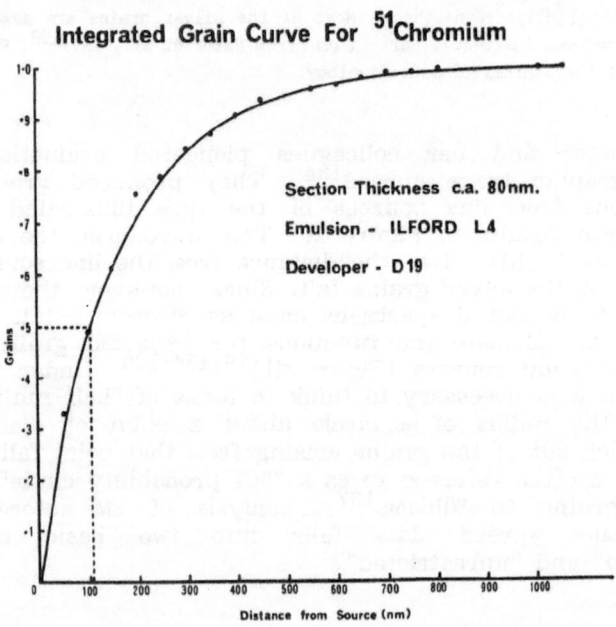

Figure 20 Cumulative range-distribution curve for a line source of ^{51}Cr under the conditions indicated. The dotted line indicates the "half-distance" (HD) which is the distance from the source within which one half of the silver grains occur - in this case 108 nm.

126

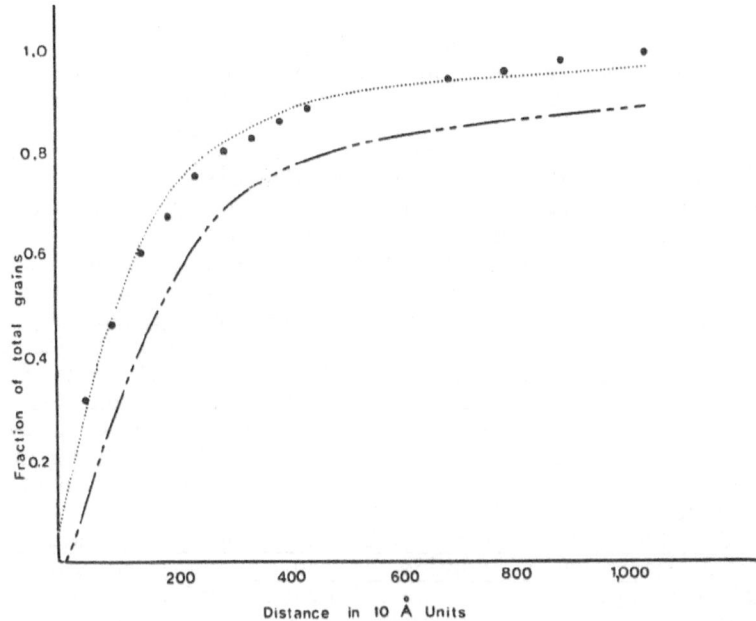

Figure 21 Cumulative range-distribution curve for a line source of ^{55}Fe ($\cdots\bullet\cdots\bullet\cdots\bullet\cdots\bullet\cdot$) and the calculated curve for a point source ($——\text{ }--\text{ }——\text{ }--$). After D.M. Parry and N.M. Blackett. Reproduced from the Journal of Cell Biology, 1973, 57, 16-26, by copyright permission of the Rockefeller University Press.

"Restricted" analysis permits prediction and testing of radiolabel distribution about sources of regular geometry (bands, discs, etc.) as described by Salpeter et al.[134,138] The method described by Salpeter and her colleagues required the analysed structures to be not only of similar shape but also of similar size. Recently, Downs and Williams have introduced a mathematical refinement which allows a range of structure sizes to be included within a single analysis[136].

"Unrestricted" methods attempt to derive estimates of activity for all structures within the cells and tissues under investigation. Williams introduced a simple but quite useful method in which regular or random sampling of subcellular structures ("items") gave effective area measurements against which grain distributions could be compared and assessed for randomness using the chi-squared test[139,140]. 50% probability circles were used for both morphometric and grain sampling. Moreover, dividing the number of grains by morphometric circles for defined groups of items gave estimates of relative specific radioactivity for those items.

The first unrestricted analytical method which took into account all the cross-fire possible in the system was the "hypothetical grain" method introduced by Blackett and Parry[135,141]. In this method a computer program is used to compare hypothetical grain distributions with the real grain distribution. Depending upon the hypothesis being tested, hypothetical sources of radiolabel are established by applying to the autoradiographs a transparent overlay screen. This contains computer-predicted source-to-site (of silver grain) distances which generate the hypothetical silver grains "emanating" from these sources. The directions of the hypothetical decays are, of course, random. The distances are derived from the range distribution curves for point sources previously mentioned[134]. Hence a rectangular matrix of cross-fire is created, there being invariably more sites than sources. Estimates of radiolabel in the various sources derive from systematic modification of the hypothetical source values by a minimizing subroutine until the hypothetical and real grain distributions fit optimally for the designated sites as assessed by the chi-squared test. On one occasion it has been possible to confirm predictions from the hypothetical grain method by biochemical means[142]. Subsequent published methodologies have been very similar to the hypothetical grain method[143], or based on the same principles of cross-fire measurement while offering an alternative to the use of a minimizing subroutine by solution of sets of simultaneous equations[144,145].

    1d. The use of EM autoradiographic analysis in studies of the renal resorption of peptide hormones. In some studies of radiolabelled peptide uptake into rat proximal tubule cells the silver grains have been characterized and quantified by use of a circle whose diameter is similar to the longest axis of the grains[119,129,130]. By merely counting grains in this way, not only is much of the cross-fire ignored but also no account is taken of the frequency of the subcellular organelles.

    Baker et al.[128] used the "circle method" of Williams to analyse their EM autoradiographs of tritiated adrenocorticotrophin analogues[139,140], in which the position of the labelled residues was varied, as was the time of fixation following i.v. administration. Figure 22 shows that this method of analysis is able to reveal approximate relative tritium specific activities in various proximal tubule organelles at times between 3 and 60 minutes. Furthermore, it appears that intracellularly, the carboxy-terminus of the 24 residue compound labelled in the tyrosine of position 23 was more rapidly hydrolysed by the lysosomes than the amino-terminus which in a separate experiment was tritiated in the tyrosine of position 2.

    However, it was necessary to use the hypothetical grain method of the Blackett and Parry to implicate the very small apical tubules in the process of transfer of radiolabel from the pinocytotic apical vesicles to secondary lysosomes (Table 1).

2. EM autoradiography of diffusible substances

It has become clear that the only safe approach to the EM autoradiographic localization of highly diffusible substances must be via the use of freeze-dried ultrathin sections of unfixed frozen tissue as described earlier. Only a few investigators have explored this technology[13,146-150]. The most logical way to apply nuclear emulsions to the hygroscopic freeze-dried sections has been to protect the latter with an evaporated carbon layer before application of the emulsion in loop form. Baker and Appleton have shown that this procedure probably does not result in measurable loss or diffusion of electrolyte using X-ray microanalysis[13]. The previously unpublished data in Table 2 show that microanalysis of mouse erythrocyte cryosections before and after application of a simulated nuclear emulsion (minus silver halide to permit analysis and visualization) could detect no elemental loss as a result of emulsion application.

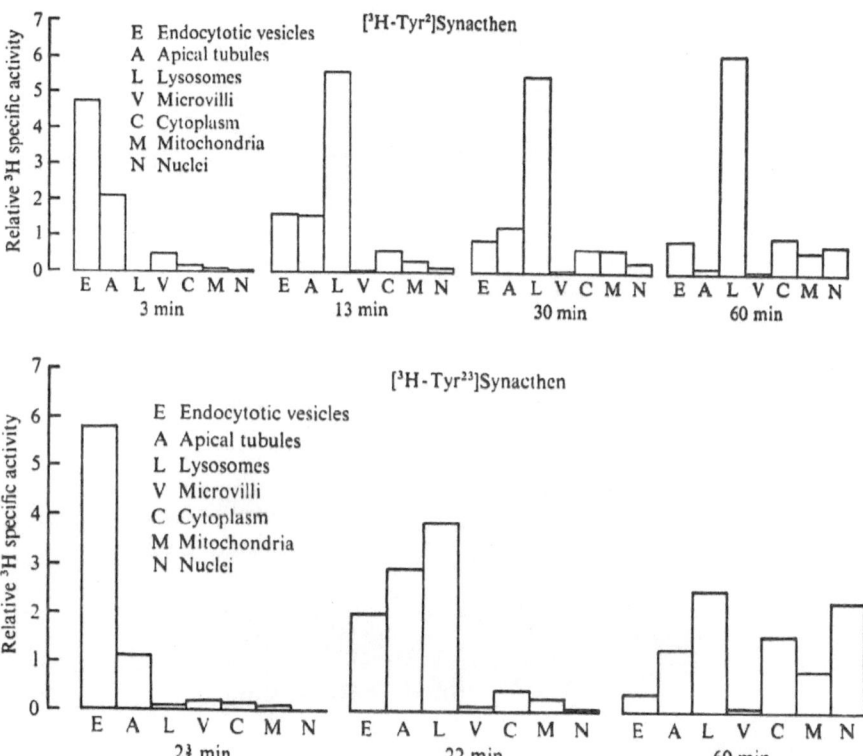

Figure 22 An example of the use of the "circle method" of Williams to analyse EM autoradiographs of rat kidney proximal tubule cells at the time intervals shown following intravenous injection of tritiated Synacthen. (a) When the radiolabel is in the tyrosine of position 2 (amino-terminus) there is some resistance to lysosomal hydrolysis of this terminus even at 60 min; (b) when the radiolabel is in the tyrosine of position 23 (carboxy-terminus) there is a rapid lysosomal cleavage of the tritiated residue which is available for rapid incorporation in other organelles by protein synthesis. From Baker et al., 1977[128]. Reproduced by permission of the Journal of Endocrinology.

The main problem inherent in the method is the preservation of adequate ultrastructure. Distribution of ^{22}NaCl in mouse renal cortex was examined by Baker and Appleton (Figure 23)[13]. Although some ultrastructural detail remained it is likely that freeze-drying caused an artifactual loss of radiolabel and other solutes from extracellular spaces such that the higher extracellular sodium concentration expected as a result of Na pump activity was not reflected in the final autoradiographs.

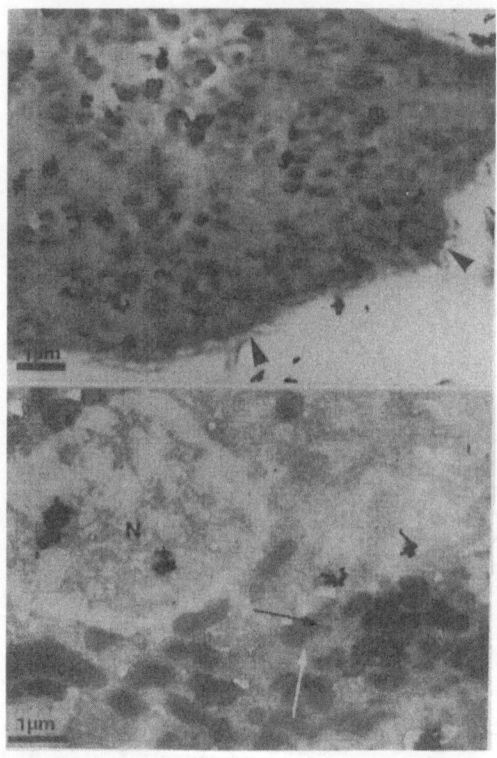

Figure 23 EM autoradiographs of mouse kidney cortex 15 min after i.p. administration of ^{22}NaCl. The autoradiographs were obtained from freeze-dried ultrathin sections of dry-sectioned unfixed material. No chemical or fluid treatments at all have been used. (a) Basal region of a proximal tubule showing basement membrane (arrows) and mitochondria (m); (b) nuclear region showing natural chromatin contrast of the nucleus (N) and some indication of mitochondrial cristae (black arrow) and invaginated basal plasma membrane (white arrow). From Baker and Appleton, 1976[13]. J. Microsc., 108, 307. By permission of the Journal of Microscopy.

Clearly much remains to be done before it can be claimed that an established technique exists for the EM autoradiography of

soluble   substances.   While   the   widespread   use   of   X-ray
microanalysis will obviate the need for autoradiography of soluble
elements at the EM level it is difficult to envisage an alternative
which could be acceptable for ultrastructural localization of soluble
organic molecules.

Table 1 Hypothetical grain analysis for [^{3}H-Tyr^2]C41795 Ba (an octadecapeptide analogue of adrenocorticotrophic hormone) 7 minutes after injection and [^{3}H-Tyr^{23}]Synacthen 22 minutes after injection. (From J.R.J. Baker et al.[128])

Organelle	Activity (mean ± SEM)	Relative area	Relative specific activity
[^{3}H-Tyr^2]C41795-Ba			
Endocytotic vesicle	51.8 ± 5.5	80	0.648
Apical tubule	36.6 ± 6.0	47	0.779
Lysosome	11.7 ± 1.6	44	0.266
[^{3}H-Tyr^{23}]Synacthen			
Endocytotic vesicle	1.5 ± 6.7	80	0.019
Apical tubule	55.7 ± 6.8	47	1.185
Lysosome	42.8 ± 2.7	44	0.973

Table 2 Integrated peak counts from energy-dispersive X-ray analytical spectrum of mouse spleen red blood cells before and after application of simulated Ilford L4 emulsion. (J.R.J. Baker and T.C. Appleton, unpublished)

Element	Before application	After application
P	149 ± 48	145 ± 32
S	777 ± 56	870 ± 228
Cl	1160 ± 27	1157 ± 95
K	424 ± 27	526 ± 84
Ca	126 ± 29	152 ± 69
Cu	170 ± 56	83 ± 43
Zn	370 ± 48	428 ± 51

REFERENCES

1.   Mazur, P., Cryobiology: The freezing of biological systems, Science, 168, 939, 1970.

2.   Pearse, A.G.E., Histochemistry Vol.1, J. & A. Churchill Ltd., London, 1968, 13.

3.   Chayen, J., Daly, J.R., Loveridge, N. and Bitensky, L., The cytochemical bioassay of hormones, Rec. Prog. Horm. Res., 32, 33, 1976.

4.   Chambers, D.J., Schaefer, H., Laughorn, J.A. Jnr., Johnstone, J., Zanelli, J.M., Parsons, J.A., Bitensky, L. and Chayen, J., Dose-related activation by PTH of specific enzymes in various regions of the kidney, in Endocrinology of Calcium Metabolism, Copp, D.H. and Talmage, R.V., Eds., Excerpta Medica, Amsterdam - Oxford, 216, 1978.

5.   Ericsson, J.L.E., Transport and digestion of hemoglobin in the proximal tubule, Lab. Invest., 14, 1, 1965.

6.   Griffith, L.E., Bugler, R.E. and Trump, B.F., The ultrastructure of the functioning kidney. Lab. Invest., 16, 220, 1967.

7.   Karunanayake, E.H., Baker, J.R.J., Christian, R.A., Hearse, D.J. and Mellows, G., Autoradiographic study of the distribution and cellular uptake of (^{14}C)-streptozotocin in the rat, Diabetologia, 12, 123, 1976.

8.   Fernández-Morán, H., Application of the ultrathin freezing-sectioning technique to the study of cell structures with the electron microscope, Ark. Fys., 4, 471, 1952.

9.   Bernhard, W. and Leduc, E.H., Ultrathin frozen sections I. Methods and ultrastructural preservation, J. Cell. Biol., 34, 757, 1967.

10. Leduc, E.H., Bernhard, W., Holt, S.J. and Tranzer, J.P., Ultrathin frozen sections II. Demonstration of enzymic activity, J. Cell. Biol., 34, 773, 1967.

11. Bernhard, W. and Viron, A., Improved techniques for the preparation of ultrathin frozen sections, J. Cell. Biol., 49, 731, 1971.

12. Echlin, P., Lai, C.E. and Hayes, T.L., Low temperature X-ray microanalysis of the differentiating vascular tissue in root tips of Lemna minor, J. Microsc., 126, 285, 1982.

13. Baker, J.R.J. and Appleton, T.C., A technique for electron microscope autoradiography (and X-ray microanalysis) of diffusible substances using freeze-dried fresh frozen sections, J. Microsc., 108, 307, 1976.

14. Sevéus, L., The subcellular distribution of electrolytes. A methodological study using cryoultramicrotomy and X-ray microanalysis, Thesis, University of Stockholm, Sweden, 1979.

15. Sevéus, L. Cryoultramicrotomy as a preparation method for X-ray microanalysis, Scanning Electron Microscopy, 4, 161, 1980.

16. Christensen, A.K., A way to prepare frozen thin sections of fresh tissue for electron microscopy, in Autoradiography of Diffusible Substances, Roth, L.J. and Stumpf, W.E., Eds., Academic Press Inc., New York, 1969, 349.

17. Sitte, H., Neumann, K., Haessig, H., Kleber, H. and Kappl, G., FC4-cryochamber for the Reichert-ultramicrotome OmU4-Ultracut, Arzneim. Forsch., 29, 1809, 1979.

18. Sitte, H., Neumann, K., Haessig, H., Kleber, H. and Kappl, G., FC4-cryochamber for Reichert-OmU4-ultramicrotome Ultracut, Proc. 7th Eur. Reg. Conf. Electron Microscopy, The Hague, 1, 540, 1980.

19. Elder, H.Y., Gray, C.C., Jardine, A.G., Chapman, J.N. and Biddlecombe, W.H., Optimum conditions for cryoquenching of small tissue blocks in liquid coolants, J. Microsc., 126, 45, 1981.

20. Frederick, P.M. and Busing, W.M., Ice crystal damage in frozen thin sections

- freezing effects and their restoration, J. Microsc., 121, 191, 1981.

21. Frederick, P.M. and Busing, W.M., Strong evidence against section thawing whilst cutting on the cryo-ultratome, J. Microsc., 122, 217, 1981.

22. Van Venrooij, G.E.P.M., Aertsen, A.M.H.J. and Hax, W.M.A., Freeze-etching: freezing velocity and crystal size at different locations in samples, Cryobiology, 12, 46, 1975.

23. Appleton, T.C., A cryostat approach to ultrathin "dry" frozen sections for electron microscopy: a morphological and X-ray analytical study, J. Microsc., 100, 49, 1974.

24. Christensen, A.K., A simple way to cut frozen thin sections of tissue at liquid nitrogen temperatures, Anat. Rec., 157, 227, 1967.

25. Christensen, A.K., Frozen thin sections of fresh tissue for electron micros-copy with description of pancreas and liver, J. Cell. Biol., 51, 772, 1971.

26. Biddlecombe, W.H., McEwan Jenkinson, D., McWilliams, S.A., Nicholson, W.A.P., Elder, H.Y. and Dempster, D.W., Preparation of cryosections with a modified Sorvall MT2B ultramicrotome and cryoattachment, J. Microsc., 126, 63, 1982.

27. Appleton, T.C., The contribution of cryoultramicrotomy to X-ray analysis in biology, in Electron Probe Microanalysis in Biology, Erasmus, D.A., Ed., Chapman and Hall, London, 148, 1978

28. Frederick, P.M., Busing, W.M. and Persson, A., Concerning the nature of the cryosectioning process, J. Microsc., 125, 167, 1982.

29. Ross, A., Sumner, A.T. and Ross, A.R., Preparation and assessment of frozen-hydrated sections of mammalian tissue for electron microscopy and X-ray microprobe analysis, J. Microsc., 121, 261, 1981.

30. Kirk, R.G. and Dobbs, G.H., Freeze-fracturing with a modified cryoultratome to prepare large intact replicas and samples for X-ray microanalysis, Sci. Tools, 21, 2, 1975.

31. Hodson, S. and Marshall, J., Evidence against through-section thawing whilst cutting on the ultramicrotome, J. Microsc., 95, 459, 1972.

32. Karp, R.D., Silcox, J.C. and Somlyo, A.V., Cryoultramicrotomy: evidence against melting and the use of a low temperature cement for specimen orien-tation, J. Microsc., 126, 157, 1982.

33. Sjöström, M. and Thornell, L-E., Preparing sections of skeletal muscle for transmission electron analytical microscopy (TEAM) of diffusible elements, J. Microsc., 103, 101, 1975.

34. Barnard, T. and Sevéus, L., Preparation of biological material for X-ray microanalysis of diffusible elements II. Comparison of different methods of drying ultrathin cryosections cut without a trough liquid, J. Microsc., 112, 281, 1978.

35. Gupta, B.L. and Hall, T.A., Quantitative electron probe X-ray microanalysis of electrolyte elements within epithelial tissue compartments, Fed. Proc., 38, 144, 1979.

36. Frederik, P.M., Busing, W.M. and Hax, W.M.A., Frozen-hydrated and drying thin cryosections observed in STEM, J. Microsc., 126, RP1, 1982.

37. Hax, W.M.A. and Lichtenegger, S., Transfer, observation and analysis of frozen hydrated specimens, J. Microsc., 126, 275, 1982.

38. Robards, A.W. and Sleytr, U., Freeze-sectioning, in Low Temperature Methods in Biology, Glauert, A.M., Ed., Elsevier, Amsterdam, 201, 1985.

39. Marshall, A.T., Principles and instrumentation, in X-Ray Microanalysis in Biology, Hayat, M.A., Ed., Macmillan, London and Basingstoke, 14, 1981.

40. Russ, J.C., Resolution and sensitivity of X-ray microanalysis in biological sections by scanning and conventional transmission electron microscopy, Scanning Electron Microscopy, 73, 1972.

41. Castaing, R., Application des sondes electroniquies à une methode d'analyse ponetvelle chimique et crystallographique, Ph.D. thesis, University of Paris, Onera No. 55, 1951.

42. Chandler, J.A., X-Ray Microanalysis in the Electron Microscope, Glauert, A.M., Ed., Elsevier, Amsterdam, 1977, chap. 4.

43. Morgan, A.J., Preparation of specimens, in X-Ray Microanalysis in Biology, Hayat, M.A., Ed., Macmillan, London and Basingstoke, 1981, chap. 2.

44. Dempsey, G.P. and Bullivant, S., A copper block method for freezing non-cryoprotected tissue to produce ice-crystal-free regions for electron microscopy. I. Evaluation using freeze-substitution, J. Microsc., 106, 251, 1976.

45. Harvey, D.M.R., Hall, J.L. and Flowers, T.J., The use of freeze substitution in the preparation of plant tissue for ion localization studies, J. Microsc., 107, 189, 1976.

46. Harvey, D.M.R., Freeze-substitution, J. Microsc., 127, 209, 1982.

47. Mehard, C.W. and Volcani, B.E., Evaluation of silicon and germanium retention in rat tissues and diatoms during cell and organelle preparation for electron probe microanalysis, J. Histochem. Cytochem., 23, 348, 1975.

48. Komnick, H., Elektronenmikroscopische localisation von Na^+ und Cl^- in Zellen und Geweben, Protoplasma, 55, 414, 1962.

49. Wick, S.M. and Hepler, P.K., Selective localization of intracellular Ca^{2+} with potassium antimonate, J. Histochem. Cytochem., 30, 1190, 1982.

50. Yarom, R., Peters, P.D. and Hall, T.A., Effect of glutaraldehyde and urea embedding on intracellular ionic elements, J. Ultrastruct. Res., 49, 405, 1974.

51. Ingram, M.J. and Hogben, C.A.M., Electrolyte analysis of biological fluids with the electron microprobe, Analyt. Biochem., 18, 54, 1967.

52. Morel, F., Roinel, N. and Le Grimellec, C., Electron probe analysis of tubular fluid composition, Nephron, 6, 350, 1969.

53. Le Grimellec, C., Roinel, N. and Morel, F., Simultaneous Mg, Ca, P, K, Na and Cl analysis in rat tubular fluid I. During perfusion of either inulin or ferrocyanide. Pfluegers Arch., 340, 181, 1973.

54. Le Grimellec, C., Roinel, N. and Morel, F., Simultaneous Mg, Ca, P, K, Na and Cl analysis in rat tubular fluid II. During acute Mg plasma loading, Pfluegers Arch., 340, 197, 1973.

55. Trump, B.F., Berezesky, I.K., Chang, S.H. and Bulger, R.E., Detection of ion shifts in proximal tubule cells of the rat kidney using X-ray microanalysis, Virchows Arch. B Cell Pathol., 22, 111, 1976.

56. Hall, T.A., The microprobe assay of chemical elements, in Physical Techniques in Biochemical Research, Vol. 1A, Oster, G., Ed., Academic Press, New York, 393, 1971.

57. Saubermann, A.J., Beeuwkes III, R., Peters, P.D., Riley, W.D. and Bulger, R.E., Definition of tissue compartments in renal papilla by direct X-ray microanalysis of frozen specimens, Kidney Int., 14, 7709, 1978.

58. Bulger, R.E., Beeuwkes III, R. and Saubermann, A.J., Application of scanning electron microscopy to X-ray analysis of frozen-hydrated sections III. Elemental content of cells in the rat renal papillary tip, J. Cell Biol., 88, 274, 1981.

59. Lechene, C.P., Bonventre, J.V. and Warner, R.R., Electron probe analysis of frozen-hydrated bulk tissues, in Microbeam Analysis in Biology, Lechene, C.P. and Warner, R.R., Eds., Academic Press, New York, 409, 1979.

60. Beck, F., Bauer, R., Bauer, U., Mason, J., Dörge, A., Rick, R. and Thurau, K., Electron microprobe analysis of intracellular elements in the rat kidney, Kidney Int., 17, 756, 1980.

61. Russ, J.C., The direct element ratio model for quantitative analysis of thin sections, in Microprobe Analysis as Applied to Cells and Tissues, Hall, T., Echlin, P. and Kaufmann, R., Eds., Academic Press, London, 269, 1974.

62. Mason, J., Beck, F., Dörge, A., Rick, R. and Thurau, K., Intracellular electrolyte composition following renal ischemia, Kidney Int., 20, 61, 1981.

63. Stuve, J. and Galle, P., Role of mitochondria in the handling of gold in the kidney, J. Cell Biol., 44, 667, 1970.

64. Yarom, R., Stein, H., Peters, P.D., Slavin, S. and Hall, T.A., Nephrotoxic effect of parenteral and intraarticular gold, Arch. Pathol., 99, 36, 1975.

65. Ainsworth, S.K., Swain, R.P., Watabe, N., Brackett, N.C., Pilia, P. and Hennigar, G.R., Gold nephropathy, ultrastructural, fluorescent, and energy-dispersive X-ray microanalysis study, Arch. Pathol. Lab. Med., 105, 373, 1981.

66. Berry, J.P., Brille, P., LeRoy, A.F., Gouveia, Y., Ribaud, P., Galle, P. and Mathé, G., Experimental ultrastructural and X-ray microanalysis study of cisplatin in the rat: Intracellular localization of platinum, Cancer Trtmt. Rep., 66, 1529, 1982.

67. Nabarra, B., Galle, P., Adrianarison, I. and Lebois, E., Apport du microanalyseur à, sonde électronique dans l'étude des lésions rénales provoquées par l'intoxication aiguë mercurielle, Kidney Int., 4, 208, 1973.

68. Carmichael, N.G. and Fowler, B.A., Effects of separate and combined chronic mercuric chloride and sodium selenate administration in rats: Histological, ultrastructural, and X-ray microanalytical studies of liver and kidney, J. Environ. Pathol. Toxicol., 3, 399, 1979.

69. Fowler, B.A. and Goyer, R.A., Bismuth localization within nuclear inclusions by X-ray microanalysis, J. Histochem. Cytochem., 23, 722, 1975.

70. Berry, J-P., Hourdry, J., Galle, P. and Lagrue, G., Chromium concentration by proximal renal tubule cells: An ultrastructural, microanalytical and cytochemical study, J. Histochem. Cytochem., 26, 651, 1978.

71. Fowler, B.A. and Nordberg, G.F., The renal toxicity of cadmium metallothionein: Morphometric and X-ray microanalytical studies, Toxicol. Appl. Pharmacol., 46, 609, 1978.

72. Kendall, M.D., Warley, A., Nicholson, J.K. and Appleton, T.C., X-ray microanalysis of proximal and distal tubule cells in the mouse kidney, and the influence of cadmium on the concentration of natural intracellular elements, J. Cell Sci., 62, 319, 1983.

73. Hall, T.A. and Gupta, B.L., Quantification for the X-ray microanalysis of cryosections, J. Microsc., 126, 333, 1982.

74. Sanfilippo, F., Wisseman, C., Ingram, P. and Shelburne, J., Crystalline deposits of calcium and phosphorus: Their appearance in glomerular basement membranes in a patient with renal failure, Arch. Pathol. Lab. Med., 105, 594, 1981.

75. Rosen, S. and Beeuwkes III, R., Renal Na-K-ATPase: Quantitative X-ray microanalysis, in Microbeam Analysis in Biology, Lechene, C.P. and Warner, R.R., Eds., Academic Press, New York, 489, 1979.

76. Smith, N.K.R. and Cameron, I.L., Observations on electron probe X-ray microanalysis compared to other methods for measuring intracellular elemental concentration, Scanning Electron Microscopy, 395, 1981.

77. MacKnight, A.D.C., Comparison of analytical techniques: chemical isotopic, and microprobe analysis, Fed. Proc., 39, 2881, 1980.

78. Forberg, S., Odeblad, E., Söremark, R. and Ullberg, S., Autoradiography with isotopes emitting internal conversion electrons and Auger electrons, Acta Radiol., 2, 241, 1964.

79. Blackett, N.M., Parry, D.M. and Baker, J.R.J., Isotope decay range

distribution curves for use in the analysis of electron microscope autoradiographs, J. Histochem. Cytochem., 28, 1050, 1980.

80. Baker, J.R.J., Electron microscopic autoradiography, its value and limitations, Proc. E.M. Soc. Southern Africa, 11, 5, 1981.

81. Ullberg, S., Studies on the distribution and fate of ^{35}S-labelled benzylpenicillin in the body, Acta Radiol. (Suppl. 118), 1, 1954.

82. Ullberg, S., The technique of whole-body autoradiography: cryosectioning of large specimens, Sci. Tools, Special Issue, LKB-producter AB, Sweden, 1977.

83. Baker, J.R.J., Kemmenoe, B.H., McMartin, C. and Peters, G.E., Pharmacokinetics, distribution and elimination of a synthetic octapeptide analogue of somatostatin in the rat, Regulatory Peptides, 9, 213, 1984.

84. Wassermann, O., Studies on the pharmacokinetics of bis-quaternary ammonium compounds II. Autoradiographic studies on the distribution of ^{3}H-hexamethonium in mice, Naunyn Schmiedebergs Arch. Pharmak., 270, 419, 1971.

85. Shindo, H., Takahashi, I. and Nakajima, E., Autoradiographic studies on the distribution of quaternary ammonium compounds II. Distribution of ^{14}C-labelled decamethonium, hexamethonium and dimethonium in mice, Chem. Pharm. Bull., 19, 1876, 1971.

86. Curtis, C.G., Cross, S.A.M., McCulloch, R.J. and Powell, G.M., Whole-body Autoradiography, Academic Press, London, 51, 1981.

87. O'Byrne, E.M., Brindle, S., Quintavalla, J., Strawinski, C., Tabachnik, M. and Steinetz, B.G., Tissue distribution of injected ^{125}I-labelled porcine relaxin: Organ uptake, whole-body autoradiography, and renal concentration of radiometabolites, Annals N.Y. Acad. Sci., 380, 187, 1982.

88. Bach, P.H., Christian, R., Baker, J. and Bridges, J.W., The metabolism of 2-bromo-[1-^{14}C]ethan-1-amine (BEA): A model compound for inducing renal papillary necrosis (RPN), in Mechanisms of Toxicity and Hazard Evaluation, Holmstedt, B., Lauwerys, R., Mercier, M. and Roberfroid, M., Eds., Elsevier/North Holland Biomedical Press, Amsterdam, 533, 1980.

89. Baynton, R.D. and Mercer, P.F., The intrarenal distribution of urea-^{14}C as shown by autoradiography, Can. J. Phys. Pharm., 46, 281, 1968.

90. Dartigues, B., Laparra, J., Roquebert, J. and Blanquet, P., Autoradiographie de coupes de reins de rats au moyen du sodium 22. Application à la recherche du lieu d'action des diurétiques, C.R. Soc. Biol. (Paris), 166, 580, 1972.

91. Berlin, M. and Ullberg, S., Accumulation and retention of mercury in the mouse, Arch. Envir. Hlth., 6, 589, 1963.

92. Cross, S.A.M., Groves, A.D. and Hesselbo, T., A quantitative method for measuring radioactivity in tissues sectioned for whole-body autoradiography, Int. J. Appl. Rad. Isotopes, 25, 381, 1974.

93. Longshaw, S. and Fowler, J.S.L., A poly[methyl-^{14}C] methacrylate source for use in whole-body autoradiography and beta-radiography, Xenobiotica, 8, 289, 1978.

94. Laurent, G., Maldague, P., Carlier, M-B. and Tulkens, P.M., Increased renal DNA synthesis in vivo after administration of low doses of gentamycin to rats, Antimicrob. Ag. Chemother., 24, 586, 1983.

95. Jacobsen, N.O., Olesen, O.V., Thomsen, K., Ottosen, P.D. and Olsen, S., Early changes in renal distal convoluted tubules and collecting ducts of lithium-treated rats, Lab. Invest., 46, 298, 1982.

96. Pantic, V., Li, J. and Villee, C., Autoradiographic studies of the kidneys of hamsters bearing longterm oestrogen implants, Cytobiologie, 9, 89, 1974.

97. Hard, G.C., Autoradiographic analysis of proliferative activity in rat kidney epithelial and mesenchymal cell subpopulations following a carcinogenic dose of dimethylnitrosamine, Cancer Res., 35, 3762, 1975.

98. Sottiurai, V., The role of the convoluted segment of the proximal tubule in

the disposal of ^{131}I-insulin in the rat kidney, Am. J. Anat., 140, 181, 1974.

99. Osborne, M., Meyer, P., Droz, B. and Morel, F., Physiologie cellulaire - Localisation intrarénale de l'angiotensine tritiée dans les cellules mésangiales par radio-autographie, C.R. Acad. Sci. (Paris), 276, Série D- 2457, 1973.

100. Pegg, A.E., Seely, J. and Zagon, I.S., Autoradiographic identification of ornithine decarboxylase in mouse kidney by means of α-[5-^{14}C]difluoromethyl- ornithine, Science, 217, 68, 1982.

101. Boyd, M.R. and Dutcher, J.S., Renal toxicity due to reactive metabolites formed in situ in the kidney: Investigations with 4-ipomeanol in the mouse, J. Pharmacol. Exp. Ther., 216, 640, 1981.

102. Appleton, T.C., Autoradiography of soluble labelled compounds, J. R. Microsc. Soc., 83, 277, 1964.

103. Appleton, T.C., Resolving power, sensitivity and latent image fading of soluble-compound autoradiographs, J. Histochem. Cytochem., 14, 414, 1966.

104. Stumpf, W.E. and Roth, L.J., Vacuum freeze-drying of frozen sections for dry-mounting high-resolution autoradiography, Stain Technol., 39, 219, 1964.

105. Rogers, A.W., Techniques of Autoradiography, Elsevier/North Holland Biomedi- cal Press, Amsterdam, 174, 1979.

106. Stirling, C.E., Schneider, A.J., Wong, M-D. and Kinter, W.B., Quantitative radioautography of sugar transport of intestinal biopsies from normal humans and a patient with glucose-galactose malabsorption, J. Clin. Invest., 51, 438, 1972.

107. Schiller, A., Reb, G. and Taugner, R., Excretion and intrarenal distribution of low-molecular polyvinylpyrrolidone and inulin in rats, Arzneim. Forsch., 28, 2064, 1978.

108. Weeden, R.P. and Vyas, B.T., Phlorizin stimulation of p-aminohippurate up- take in rat kidney cortex slices, Kidney Int., 14, 158, 1978.

109. Karunanayake, E.H., Baker, J.R.J., Christian, R.A., Hearse, D.J. and Mel- lows, G., Microautoradiographic study of the distribution and uptake of (^{14}C)-streptozotocin in rat tissues, Biochem. Soc. Trans. 3, 414, 1975.

110. Gusterson, B.A., Neville, A.M., Baker, J.R.J. and Christian, R.A., Autoradiographic localization of ^{3}H-diprenorphine in the Syrian hamster, Diag. Histopath., 4, 209, 1981.

111. Odlind, B. and Dencker, L., Autoradiographic localization of 35-S-furosemide at different stages of its renal excretion, Acta Physiol. Scand., 111, 179, 1981.

112. Young, W.S. III and Kuhar, M.J., A new method for receptor autoradiography: [^{3}H]opiate receptors in rat brain, Brain Res., 179, 255, 1979.

113. Summers, R.J. and Kuhar, M.J., Autoradiographic localization of β- adrenoreceptors in rat kidney, Europ. J. Pharmacol., 91, 305, 1983.

114. Salpeter, M.M. and Szabo, M., Sensitivity in electron microscope autoradiog- raphy 1. The effect of radiation dose, J. Histochem. Cytochem., 20, 425, 1972.

115. Buchel, L.A., Delain, E. and Bouteille, M., Electron microscope fluoro- autoradiography: improvement of efficiency, J. Microsc., 112, 223, 1978.

116. Murakami, M. and Webb, M., A morphological and biochemical study of the ef- fects of L-cysteine on the renal uptake and nephrotoxicity of cadmium, Br. J. Exp. Pathol., 62, 115, 1981.

117. Murakami, M., Cain, K. and Webb, M., Cadmium-metallothionein-induced nephropathy: A morphological and autoradiographic study of cadmium distribu- tion, the development of tubular damage and subsequent cell regeneration, J. Appl. Toxicol., 3, 237, 1983.

118. Zizza, F., Campbell, T.J. and Reeve, E.B., The nature and rates of excretion of radioactive breakdown products of I^{131}-albumin in the rabbit, J. Gen. Physiol., 43, 397, 1959.

119. Maunsbach, A.B., Absorption of ^{125}I-labelled homologous albumin by rat kidney proximal tubule cells, J. Ultrastruct. Res., 15, 197, 1966.

120. Neustein, H.B. and Maunsbach, A.B., Hemoglobin absorption by proximal tubule cells of the rabbit kidney. A study by electron microscopic autoradiography, J. Ultrastruct. Res., 16, 141, 1966.

121. Christensen, E.I. and Maunsbach, A.B., Intralysosomal digestion of lysozyme in renal proximal tubule cells, Kidney Int., 6, 396, 1974.

122. Christensen, E.I. and Maunsbach, A.B., Effects of dextran on lysosomal ultrastructure and protein digestion in renal proximal tubule, Kidney Int., 16, 301, 1979.

123. Christensen, E.I. and Maunsbach, A.B., Digestion of protein in lysosomes of proximal tubule cells, in Functional Ultrastructure of the Kidney, Maunsbach, A.B., Olsen, T.S. and Christensen, E.I., Eds., Academic Press, London, 341, 1980.

124. Baumann, K., Bode, F., Ottosen, P.D., Madsen, K.M. and Maunsbach, A.B., Quantititative analysis of protein absorption in microperfused proximal tubules of the rat kidney, in Functional Ultrastructure of the Kidney, Maunsbach, A.B., Olsen, T.S. and Christensen, E.I., Eds., Academic Press, London, 291, 1980.

125. Bode, F., Ottosen, P.D., Madsen, K.M. and Maunsbach, A.B., Does transtubular transport of intact protein occur in the kidney?, in Functional Ultrastructure of the Kidney, Maunsbach, A.B., Olsen, T.S. and Christensen, E.I., Eds., Academic Press, London, 385, 1980.

126. Bourdeau, J.E., Chen, E.R.Y. and Carone, F.A., Insulin uptake in the renal proximal tubule, Am. J. Physiol., 225, 1399, 1973.

127. Baker, J.R.J., Bennett, H.P.J., Hudson, A.M., McMartin, C. and Purdon, G.E., On the metabolism of two adrenocorticotrophin analogues, Clin. Endocrinol., 5 (Suppl.), 61s, 1976.

128. Baker, J.R.J., Bennett, H.P.J., Christian, R.A. and McMartin, C., Renal uptake and metabolism of adrenocorticotrophin analogues in the rat: An autoradiographic study, J. Endocrinol., 74, 23, 1977.

129. Stacy, B.D., Wallace, A.L.C., Gemmell, R.T. and Wilson, B.W., Absorption of ^{125}I-labelled sheep growth hormone in single proximal tubules of the rat kidney, J. Endocrinol., 68, 21, 1976.

130. Warshawsky, H., Goltzman, D., Rouleau, M.F. and Bergeron, J.J.M., Direct in vivo demonstration by radioautography of special binding sites for calcitonin in skeletal and renal tissues in the rat, J. Cell. Biol., 85, 682, 1980.

131. Markkanen, S.O. and Rajeniemi, J., Lysosomal degradation of human choriogonadotrophin in the proximal tubule cells of the rat kidney, in Functional Ultrastructure of the Kidney, Maunsbach, A.B., Olsen, T.S. and Christensen, E.I., Eds., Academic Press, London, 361, 1980.

132. Maunsbach, A.B., The influence of different fixatives and fixation methods on the ultrastructure of rat kidney proximal tubule cells I. Comparison of different perfusion fixation methods and of glutaraldehyde, formaldehyde and osmium tetroxide fixatives, J. Ultrastruct. Res., 15, 242, 1966.

133. Maunsbach, A.B., The influence of different fixatives and fixation methods on the ultrastructure of rat kidney proximal tubule cells II. Effects of varying osmolality, ionic strength, buffer system and fixative concentration of glutaraldehyde solutions, J. Ultrastruct. Res., 15, 283, 1966.

134. Salpeter, M.M., Bachmann, L. and Salpeter, E.E., Resolution in electron

microscope autoradiography, J. Cell Biol., 41, 1, 1969.

135. Blackett, N.M. and Parry, D.M., A new method for analysing electron microscope autoradiographs using hypothetical grain distributions, J. Cell Biol., 57, 9, 1973.

136. Downs, A.M. and Williams, M.A., An improved approach to the analysis of autoradiographs containing isolated sources of simple shape: method, theoretical basis and reference data, J. Microsc., 136, 1, 1984.

137. Williams, M.A., Autoradiography: its methodology at the present time, J. Microsc., 128, 79, 1982.

138. Salpeter, M.M. and Salpeter, E.E., Resolution in electron microscope autoradiography II. Carbon[14], J. Cell Biol., 50, 324, 1971.

139. Williams, M.A., The assessment of electron microscope autoradiographs, Adv. Opt. Elect., Microsc., 3, 219, 1969.

140. Williams, M.A., Electron microscopic autoradiography: its application to protein biosynthesis, in Techniques in Protein Biosynthesis, Vol.3, Campbell, P.W. and Sargent, J.R., Eds., Academic Press, London, 125, 1973.

141. Blackett, N.M. and Parry, D.M., A simplified method of "hypothetical grain" analysis of electron microscope autoradiographs, J. Histochem. Cytochem., 25, 206, 1977.

142. Baker, J.R.J., Butler, K.D., Eakins, M.N., Pay, G.F. and White, A.M., Subcellular localization of ^{111}In in human and rabbit platelets, Blood, 59, 351, 1982.

143. Salpeter, M.M., McHenry, F.A. and Salpeter, E.E., Resolution in electron microscope autoradiography IV. Application to analysis of autoradiographs, J. Cell Biol., 76, 127, 1978.

144. Downs, A. and Williams, M.A., An iterative approach to the analysis of EM autoradiographs I. The method, J. Microsc., 114, 143, 1978.

145. Williams, M.A. and Downs, A., An iterative approach to the analysis of EM autoradiographs II. Estimates of sample sizes and confidence limits. J. Microsc., 114, 157, 1978.

146. Baker, J.R.J. and Appleton, T.C., Electron microscopic autoradiography of diffusible substances using ultrathin sections of unfixed frozen tissues, Acta Pharmacol. Toxicol., 41, Suppl. 1, 18, 1977.

147. Christensen, A.K. and Paavola, L.G., Frozen thin sections of fresh tissue and their possible use for autoradiography of diffusible substances, Acta Histochem. Cytochem., 5, 212, 1972.

148. Nagata, T. and Murata, F., Electron microscopic dry-mounting radioautography for diffusible compounds by means of ultracryotomy, Histochemistry, 54, 75, 1977.

149. Johnson, I.T. and Bronk, J.R., Electron microscope autoradiography of a diffusible intracellular constituent, using freeze-dried frozen sections of mammalian intestinal epithelium, J. Microsc., 115, 187, 1979.

150. Johnson, I.T. and Bronk, J.R., Distribution of actively absorbed diffusible sugars in the jejunal epithelium of the rat, J. Cell Sci., 45, 199, 1980.

4

FIXATION OF KIDNEY TISSUE FOR MORPHOMETRIC STUDY

M.A. WILLIAMS AND J.I. LOWRIE

I. THE MORPHOLOGICAL APPROACH IN THE STUDY OF KIDNEY

The classical biochemical approach to studying an organ has been to homogenize it. This technique has provided much of the present body of knowledge on intermediary metabolism, the nature of metabolites and the essential basic processes carried out in all cells. This "grind and measure" approach is especially successful in tissues and cell populations which are homogeneous. The more heterogeneous the collection of cells, the more the procedure based on destroying cell biological organization is seen to be limited in its usefulness. The kidney is heterogeneous at both a gross and a microscopic level. Cortex and medulla, though playing parts in the same overall process of urine production, are biochemically very dissimilar. Within the cortex and medulla there are numerous types of cells, each with special properties, many of which are highly directional. As a consequence the cells are polarized both along the kidney tubule length, and across its width on an axis from tubule lumen to tubule basement membrane. Methodologies that permit the study of chemical processes as they occur spatially, i.e. "anatomically based" approaches, are thus particularly pertinent to the study of the kidney and of nephrotoxicity.

A. Perspectives in the morphologically based study of kidneys

There are several ways in which the kidney anatomy can be preserved whilst functional studies (or functional inferences) are made. These include micropuncture techniques[1], single tubule isolation procedures and the cytochemical study of kidney sections. The first two of these permit or involve the voluntary observation or sampling of particular segments. The cytochemical procedure, on the other hand, involves chemical studies of "profiles" of sectioned tubules obtained from a sampling plane through the organ. In this case a segment represented in a particular profile is picked out from the assortment present, by its morphological characteristics. In addition, modern stereometric methods (morphometric methods based on stereological principles)[2,3] are available which allow data from these planes to be extrapolated rationally to a whole cell, tubule or kidney. This permits valuable studies of particular cell types in the kidney and segments of kidney tubule yielding functional insight into, for example, lysosome populations or aspects of membrane economy. In addition, cytochemical methods such as autoradiography can be backed up with, and linked to, stereometrically derived morphological data.

The methods of preparing kidneys for microscopical examination are thus of crucial importance, since they lie at the root of a large group of techniques essential to the elucidation of kidney function. The manner in which the tissue is prepared determines to a large extent the nature and quality of the images, and hence the numerical information that may be obtained.

B.   The need for tissue fixation in microscopy

Untreated tissues, and especially intact cells, are extremely labile and difficult to stain and visualize. Generally, visibility is achieved with the aid of sectioning and staining methods, but many cell components are soluble, and application and penetration of stains will imply the loss of some or all cell components including those of interest.

Fixation stabilizes the materials of interest and makes them stainable. Some procedures involve the use of controlled tissue freezing, which may be followed by chemical treatments. More generally chemical fixation methods are used.

While stabilization of particular materials is the purpose of fixation, there may be a need to preserve specific chemical groups[4] or morphology. The substance and its surroundings must be preserved in near to their original spatial relationships. This chapter describes fixation of kidney tissue in those experimental situations where the primary purpose is the preservation of morphology. Morphometric experiments in which function is being traced by quantitative estimates of structural characteristics are particularly important in the study of the glomerular filtration barrier in normal and diabetic animals[5,6], and in some studies of tubular processes, e.g. endosomal peptide degradation. Autoradiographic experiments (especially of peptides, proteins, nucleic acids and glycosaminoglycans)[4,7] are also complemented by morphometric estimates.

II.   FIXATION OF KIDNEY TISSUE FOR MORPHOMETRIC STUDIES

Some morphometric studies are still being carried out on tissue fixed in traditional chemical fixatives (e.g. neutral formalin, dichromate, mercury salts, picric acid) and embedded in paraffin wax, but these techniques are being supplanted by more discriminating methods. These methods are usually based on glutaraldehyde fixation and embedding in a resin that permits semi-thin or thin sectioning. Combined, these result in the greatly improved discrimination of detail, which is required to identify tubule segments and to study processes therein.

A. Methods of applying the fixative to the kidney

The need to preserve cells and organelles with dimensions, shapes, spacings and patterns as near as possible to those present "in life" is paramount for morphometric work. Volumetric parameters in kidney tubule lumena and glomerular cells are very markedly affected by the method of fixation, and since the tubules are patent in vivo[8,9] excision of the kidney results in collapse of the tubule cells into the lumena. Traditional methods of fixing tissues consist of excision, dicing and then immersion of fragments in the fixative. When applied to the kidney, immersion fixation results in a closed tubular configuration. Application of the fixative agent from the tubule lumena and vascular tree whilst these two systems are fluid-filled can be achieved by in vivo "perfusion" methods. Such perfusion methods result in tubules and capillaries fixed in a patent condition. It is generally felt that perfusion fixation yields a more valid picture of the functioning kidney.

B. General objectives in the preservation of tissues for morphometric analysis

When preparing tissue for morphometric study there are several objectives. The first is to retain, in the fixed specimen, the dimensions of the tissue in its fresh state - organ, cell and organelle volumes and volume-surface ratios and also its organelle (e.g. vesicle, granule) numbers. While this objective is self evident, the nature of perfusion fixation is complex and less predictable than would be desired. Every cell consists of numerous compartments each with its own shape, volume, contents, pH and tonicity. The barriers between the cells and their exterior, and between each of the "compartments" and its neighbours, are all semi-permeable and have distinct properties. The cell may have several plasmalemmal surfaces which face different extracellular environments. The fixative (a single concentration, pH, tonicity and nature of vehicle) is delivered to the cell and arrives in different concentrations and rates at each of the plasmalemmal surfaces, quickly modifying them - though they retain some selective permeability. Fixative molecules and vehicle ions enter the cell and travel towards the various compartments - disturbing internal balances of soluble substances as they go - giving rise to osmotic effects which are scarcely within the control of the experimenter. The fixative then continues by breaching the internal compartmental interfaces as it reaches them - at whatever altered concentration, tonicity and pH it now has. The primary stabilizing reactions, e.g. protein cross-linking by glutaraldehyde, proceed. Provided stabilization proceeds

143

to a point which creates a gel of most proteins without gross osmotic imbalance occurring (between cell and exterior, or organelle and its intracellular neighbour), the fixed specimen will bear a close resemblance to its pre-fixation state. However, it is possible for some organelles or whole cells to be less satisfactorily fixed than others. It is not possible to provide the ideal conditions for the preservation of all subcellular component or cell types via a single fixative treatment. The experimenter must:

1. optimize the fixation of selected organelles or cells and use a defined yardstick to evaluate his procedures; and
2. rigorously standardize the fixation protocol.

Important reference structures for fixation include: S_2 segment cells for studying peptide processing in the nephron (S_2 and S_3 cells are difficult to fix optimally in the same kidney), and the reproducibility of thickness estimates of the filtration barrier in studies on diabetic change in the glomerulus (Gundersen, personal communication). The fixation of parotid gland, where immersion fixation is necessary, was optimized by referring to the zymogen granules[10], macrophage activation studies by lysosomal preservation[11], while in lung tissue fixation careful consideration of the degree of inflation was required[12].

With the procedures at present available all components of a cell or tissue cannot be fixed optimally at the same time. Thus it is fortunate that absolute values for the structural parameters of the kidney, cells and extracellular material, are less important than reproducibility. In most experiments the particular mean value obtained for some parameter is less critical than standard error of the mean. Whilst every effort must naturally be made to reproduce the dimensions of volume and surface area present within living kidney, reproducible fixation between kidneys is the factor most likely to determine the feasibility of quantitative experiments. The experimental protocol must minimize the variance between animals that arises from technical sources, so that the real biological variation can be adequately estimated. The reproducibility with which various parameters of interest, such as the volumetric ratio of the lumen to cell; mean tubule cell volume, e.g. for proximal tubule (PT) as a whole or one particular segment, nuclear sizes in tubule cells; capillary and Bowman's space volumes in glomeruli and their ratio, is the most important test of the fixation protocol. Basement membranes of tubules are very resistant to damage, but are somewhat elastic (vide infra). The mean cross-sectional area of tubule profiles therefore provides a useful internal standard to which other data can be referred. When choosing tissue preparation protocols for morphometry it is also necessary to bear in mind the requirements of tissue sampling. All of the kidney must be treated such that in due course representative cells of a particular sort (e.g. a tubule segment) are available for study.

144

C.   Factors influencing the results of kidney perfusion with fixatives

1.   Physiological state of the kidney

The morphology of the normal kidney   in vivo   exhibits patent tubules, where the lumena probably contain very little cellular debris. This patency is generally lost, partly by cellular swelling, when the kidney is excised. This collapse is less evident in kidneys undergoing a marked water diuresis[8]. Surgical trauma necessary to expose the kidneys for perfusion fixations should therefore be carried out during a diuretic response. It is likely that quantitative data obtained from kidney fixed during heavy diuresis will differ somewhat from the "normal". It must also be realized that the interstitial environment of the renal medullary cells exhibits a gradient of tonicity,   and for   successful fixation   the fixative tonicity must be mirrored in the fixative.   Since the gradient changes with the physiological (and pathological) state of the kidney, it will be obvious that the fixation conditions will require adjustment to the tonic state that pertains at that time.

Maintenance of normal blood pressure is necessary to preserve normal architecture. Loss of blood pressure results in macroscopic changes in the kidney - loss of turgidity and deepening colour,   and kidney tissue can then be fixed satisfactorily within the next few seconds only[8]. In experiments where the fixation follows the administration of a drug or precursor, and some predetermined lapse of time, lowering of blood pressure can occur gradually due to deepening anaesthesia. The perfusion pressure (discussed below) must provide an adequate substitute for, and a smooth transition from, the normal blood pressure.

Ether anaesthesia causes local vasoconstriction in the renal medulla[13] and drug-induced vasoconstriction can also compromise perfusion fixation. Generally, fixation solutions must be at body temperature,   otherwise   the   entry   of   cool   fixative   causes vasoconstriction which affects the distribution of the fixative. Early perfusion experiments were done with osmium tetroxide fixatives[8,14,15],   which strongly contracts blood vessels, but which if the concentration gradient is steep works well, because the vessels are fixed before they can contract. When glutaraldehyde is used[16],   1% $NaNO_2$ is often added to prevent vasoconstriction. It must be realized that as fixation proceeds both the ability to contract and the elasticity of the blood vessels become modified. Thus even if the hydrostatic pressure with which the fixative is delivered mimics normal blood pressure, the flow rate and the viscosity of fixative in the vessels is unlikely to be similar to that of blood.

2.   Fixative tonicity

The tonicity of the fixative must "match" that of the cell type of interest. In practice this generally means that the tonicity of the fixative and any prior washing solution should match that of the local environment of the cell   in vivo. It is not surprising, therefore, that a fixative tonicity of 350 mosmol/kg was deemed appropriate for proximal tubule S_1 and S_2 segments of the rat, whilst Bohman[13] concluded that 1000 and 1300 mosmol/kg were satisfactory for outer and middle medulla respectively and 1800 mosmol/kg for papillary cells. Generally, it is more successful to approach the most appropriate osmolality by experiment (rather than theory) although published data[17] are a good guide.

3.   Fixative colloid osmotic potential

Fixatives destroy cellular respiratory activity (and hence the cation pump necessary for fluid transport)[42,43], and thus if the cells remain at the same time osmotically active, fixation could result in cell swelling. Colloids are therefore often added to fixatives, but it is not clear to what extent the addition of dextran (the most frequently used) is beneficial. Some authors have suggested that the addition of colloids is more justifiable as a means of adjusting fixative viscosity.

4.   Fixative viscosity

In vitro the viscosity of whole blood at 37 °C is 3-4 cp, the precise value being dependent upon the method of measurement and the haematocrit, but the viscosity in vivo is apparently lower, 2.5 cp[18]. Low-concentration glutaraldehyde fixatives for perfusion fixation show much lower viscosities than blood, circa 1 cp at 37 °C. This means that for the maintenance of a "physiological" pressure gradient in blood vessels the fixative would be flowing about three times as fast as blood. Several groups of workers have sought to adjust the viscosity of their fixatives by adding macromolecular plasma substitutes, usually dextran. The addition of a plasma substitute appears to be very reasonable in experiments where the vascular system is an important part of the structures being subjected to morphometry. (For extensive discussion see Thorball and Tranum-Jensen[19].) In studies on rats with experimental diabetes[5,20] glutaraldehyde fixative containing 2.25% w/v dextran T40, (total osmolality 330-357 mosmol/l) was used.

The addition of dextran seems advantageous in glomerular studies since the glomerulus has a large vascular component, but it is less clear that any advantage accrues in studies of tubule cells. In our studies of proximal tubule cells, where assessment of fixative regimes was made by estimating the mean and "between-animal" variance for PT cell volume, the addition of dextran T40 seemed mostly detrimental (see below).

Many of the observations necessary for evaluating fixative protocols can be made using the light microscope. Tissue fixed in aldehyde then osmium tetroxide solutions (see Glauert[32] for review) and embedded in Araldite, Epon or Vestopal, gives excellent light microscopy images from sections of 0.5-2.0 μm thickness (see Figures 1-4). Such preparations easily permit the evaluation of lumen patency and of the degree of "between-cell" swelling.

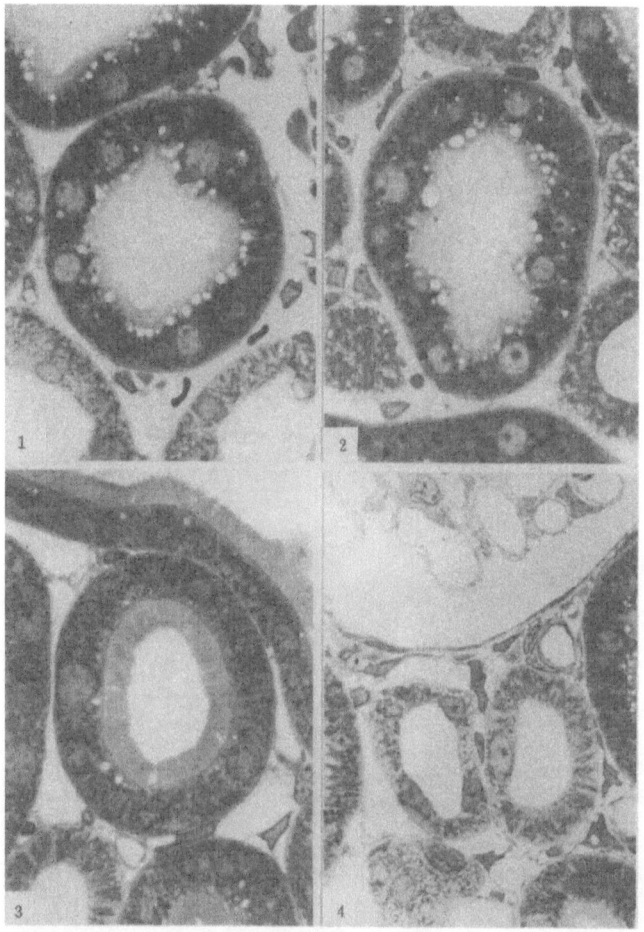

Figure 1 Rat kidney perfusion-fixed using 1% glutaraldehyde in modified Tyrode solution delivered at a pressure of 120 mmHg. Profile of S_1 segment of proximal tubule. Araldite embedding, 0.5 μm section stained with toluidine blue (x450).

Figure 2 Rat kidney perfusion-fixed using 1% glutaraldehyde in modified Tyrode solution delivered at a pressure of 120 mmHg. Profile of S_2 segment of proximal tubule. Araldite embedding, 0.5 μm section stained with toluidine blue (x450).

Figure 3 Rat kidney perfusion-fixed using 1% glutaraldehyde in modified Tyrode solution delivered at a pressure of 120 mmHg. Profile of S_3 segment of proximal tubule. Araldite embedding, 0.5 μm section stained with toluidine blue (x450).

Figure 4 Rat kidney perfusion-fixed using 1% glutaraldehyde in modified Tyrode solution delivered at a pressure of 120 mmHg. Profiles of distal tubules. Araldite embedding, 0.5 μm section stained with toluidine blue (x450).

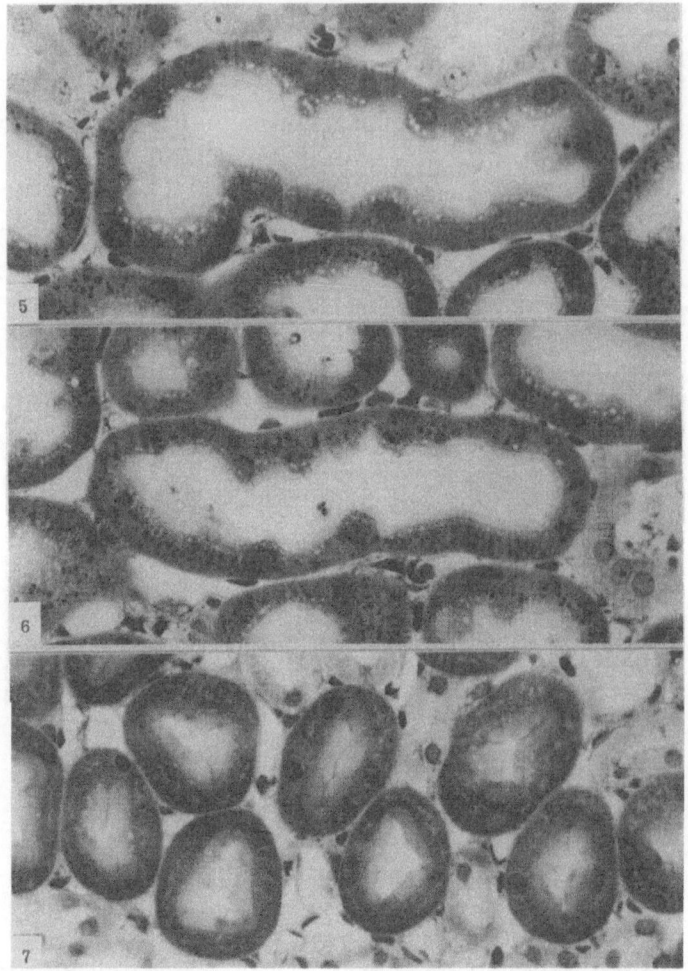

Figure 5 Rat kidney perfusion-fixed using 1% glutaraldehyde in modified Tyrode solution at 120 mmHg. Profile of S_1 segment. Tissue embedded in JB4 resin, 2 μm section, toluidine blue stain (x380).

Figure 6 Rat kidney perfusion-fixed using 1% glutaraldehyde in modified Tyrode solution at 120 mmHg. Profile of S_2 segment. Tissue embedded in JB4 resin, 2 μm section, toluidine blue stain (x380).

Figure 7 Rat kidney perfusion-fixed using 1% glutaraldehyde in modified Tyrode solution at 120 mmHg. Profiles of S_3 segments. Tissue embedded in JB4 resin, 2 μm section, toluidine blue stain (x380).

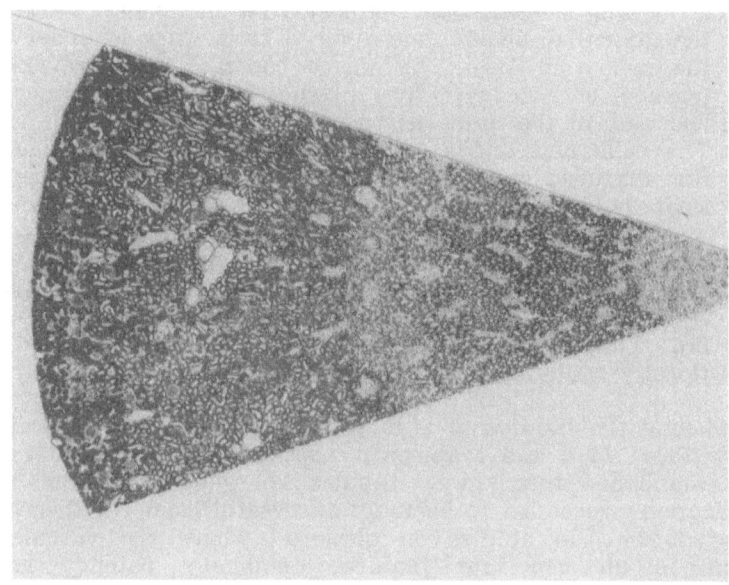

Figure 8 Low-power view of a rat kidney well-fixed by the perfusion approach. Note the patent tubule profiles throughout the organ. JB4 embedding, 2 μm section, toluidine blue staining (x16).

Even morphometric assessments by point counting (for methods see Williams[2]; Aherne and Dunnill[21]; Baak and Oort[22]) are possible for lumen versus cell; tubule versus extracellular space, and nucleus versus cytoplasm. The EM has of course to be employed for studies at the organelle level. Embedding in glycolmethacrylate resin (see Figures 5-7) permits the cutting of sections of whole kidney of species such as the rat. This resin does not yield as fine detail of cells as Araldite or Epon, but it is a valuable approach for evaluating the perfusion of the whole kidney (Figure 8).

III.   CRITERIA FOR THE JUDGEMENT OF GOOD FIXATION

Over the years in which biological transmission electron microscopy was almost exclusively evaluated qualitatively, and reported by verbal descriptions of morphological appearances, a set of general criteria grew up for what was to be regarded as "good" fixation for normal tissues. A consensus was achieved on the following:

1.   There should be membrane continuity, i.e. no sharp ends or obvious breaks.
2.   No empty spaces should be present within the cells.
3.   Large intercellular spaces should be absent.
4.   There should be no obvious signs of distortion,   such as

stretching compression, explosion or shrinkage. Particularly, the structure should not diverge from what is observable in the cells in vivo by phase contrast or Nomarski inter- ference microscopy. The tissue should look intact, and "normal" in the light microscope.

5. The cells and tissue as imaged should appear well-ordered, fine-textured and distinct. Much of the human perception of what is to be counted beautiful is attributable to order, balance and harmony. It has thus been widely accepted as a guiding principle in electron microscopy that, given a selec- tion of images of the same material, the more aesthetically satisfying one is the one most likely to represent the state in life. This assertion that "beauty is truth" has proved opera- tionally sound in practice.

Considering the fixation of kidney in particular, the applications of the criteria, 1, 2 and 3 above are self-evident. In addition, since it is established that kidney tubules are generally patent in life, the fixation procedure to be truly successful must fix them with an "open" lumen. In studies on glomeruli where the vascular com- ponent is an important feature, capillary patency must be achieved. Johnston et al.[23] observed that endothelial and mesan- gial cell swelling were sensitive indices of poor perfusion fixation. It is important to appreciate that in morphometric studies reproducibility of fixation is vital. A few superbly fixed kidneys are not adequate. Thus when morphometry is contemplated, the variance between kidneys must be estimated. Achieving good fixa- tion must in part consist of minimizing the "between-animal" variance.

A.   Choosing a tissue preparation protocol

It is generally true that a fixative protocol yielding optimal results for one part of a complex organ is unlikely to yield optimal results for other portions of the same organ. Indeed, the same argument can be made about the fixation of organelles within a cell (vide supra). It is necessary therefore to choose which portions of the organ are most important to the study and then to decide how their quality of fixation should be assessed. Clearly, the vital cells or components must be conserved. Conservation being achieved, then two further things must be aimed at:

1. physiological "normality" of conformation (in practice this is likely to mean lack of demonstrable physiological anomaly); and
2. minimization of "between-animal" variance for some pertinent parameter(s), e.g. V_V tubule lumen, V_{cell}, thickness of filtration barrier etc. The minimization may be approached by a factorially designed experiment[33] on "treatments" of the parameter of interest. Treatments which may be tested could include fixative delivery pressure, viscosity, pH and tonicity.

B. A case study: fixation of S_1 and S_2 for charting the economy of membranes during peptide endocytosis

Using a 2 x 2 factorial design, a test was made of the effects of increasing perfusion pressure (90 versus 120 mmHg), and fixative viscosity (presence and absence of the dextran T40) on the various parameters that may be used to describe S_2 segment fixation in the rat kidney. The anatomical parameters evaluated with this design included V_V lumen, V_V PT cells in tubule, $V_{cell(PT)}$, V_V PT tubules in whole kidney: and V_V values for nuclei, mitochondria, lysosomes, ER and ground cytoplasm in PT cells. Some of the results are summarized in Table 1. The addition of dextran T40 to the perfusate decreased the mean cross-sectional area of the PT at low and high perfusion pressure. However, the data indicate that the decrease in cortical volume occupied by PT, although associated with the diminution of tubule diameter, is also due to a small increase in extracellular volume. Increasing the hydrostatic pressure of perfusion also decreased tubule diameter if dextran was not present. The basal lamina is evidently elastic, extending in area by up to 40%.

Table 1 Stereometric data for proximal tubule cells (S_1 + S_2) of the rat kidney, perfusion fixed in four manners, six kidneys per treatment.

Structural parameter	Perfusion pressure			
	90 mmHg	90 mmHg + Dextran	120 mmHg	120 mmHg + Dextran
C.S.A. PT (μm^2)	2959 ± 14	2117 ± 11	2570 ± 21	2208 ± 19
V_V (PT in cortex)	0.130 ± 0.017	0.077 ± 0.010	0.152 ± 0.020	0.092 ± 0.038
V_V (Lumen in PT)	0.180 ± 0.020	0.105 ± 0.022	0.221 ± 0.019	0.128 ± 0.013
Mean cell PT volume (μm^3)	1608 ± 370	1980 ± 275	1180 ± 198	1364 ± 395
V_V (nuclei in PT cells)	0.089 ± 0.002	0.086 ± 0.003	0.106 ± 0.003	0.095 ± 0.004

Notes: All kidneys were sampled by an unbiased procedure (Figures 17 and 18). SEM values are quoted for "between-animal" means. Between-animal variances were >90% of total variance in all cases. Cell volumes were estimated as described in ref. 31.

Inside the tubules, increasing pressure increased lumenal volume, and mean PT cell volume fell. Increased pressure was perhaps therefore applied to the PT cells from both lumenal and basal directions. When the cell volume (using this particular mode of estimation) went over 2000 μm^3 the lumen was essentially occluded. Increased perfusion pressure decreased mean PT cell volume. It seems likely that the lower cell volumes seen were the ones nearest to the state in vivo, and the higher values therefore represent cell swelling. The appearances of cells fixed at 120 mmHg pressure with no added dextran are shown in Figures 9-12. This treatment also yielded the lowest "between-animal" variance for PT cell volume - the parameter that appeared to be the most appropriate one for choosing a fixation routine for this study.

Morphometric studies indicate that when the PT cells swell the process is largely cytoplasmic, the organelles swelling and shrinking largely in parallel. Thus whilst the tubules can be considered to be a compartment separate from the extratubular material, inside the tubules the cytoplasm, nuclei and tubule lumena can also be considered distinct compartments. In a study of rat S_3 cells Goncalves and Sobrinho-Simoes[24] found that most cell parameters including mean cell volume were similar in immersion and perfusion fixed kidneys.

C. Examples of perfusion fixation methods applied to the kidneys of various species

Perfusion fixation techniques have been applied to the kidneys of several species including mice, rats[5], rabbits[34], pigs[25], and humans. In smaller species it is sometimes possible to effect perfusion by introducing fixative into the functioning blood circulation of the live animal. Generally, however, perfusion fixation is effected by pumping fixative through an isolated part of the vasculature or even through an excised kidney. Figures 13-16 illustrate the surgical arrangement for passage of fixative via the beating heart (mouse) or via the aorta (rat). In the mouse the heart will keep beating for many minutes after fixative is introduced to the left ventricle, effecting circulation to the kidney and other viscera.

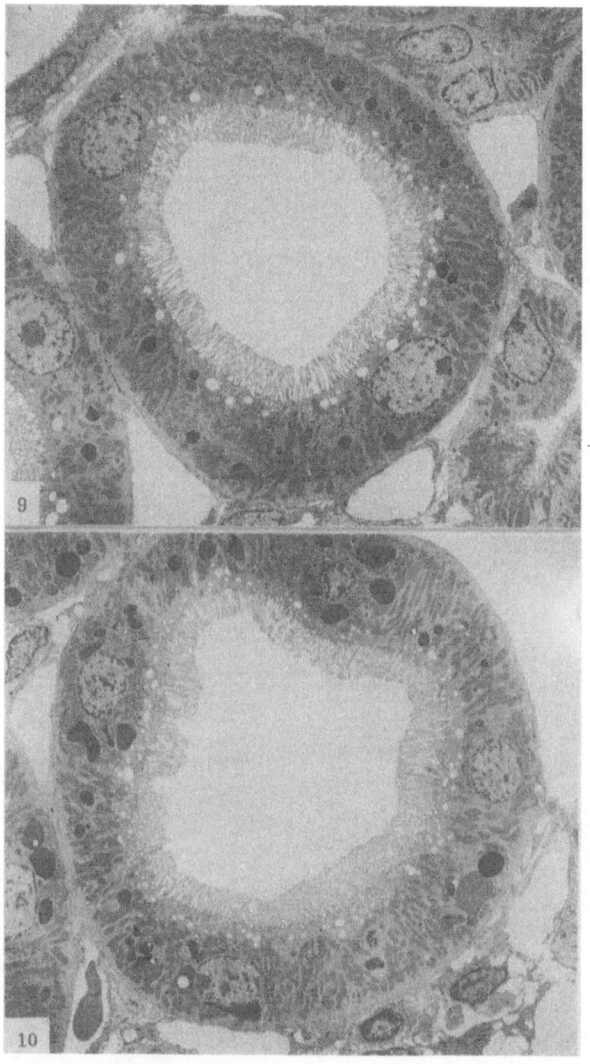

Figure 9 Electron micrograph of an S_1 profile. Tissue fixed as described in Figures 1-4. Reynolds lead citrate stain (x715).
Figure 10 Electron micrograph of an S_2 profile. Tissue fixed as described in Figures 1-4. Reynolds lead citrate stain (x715).

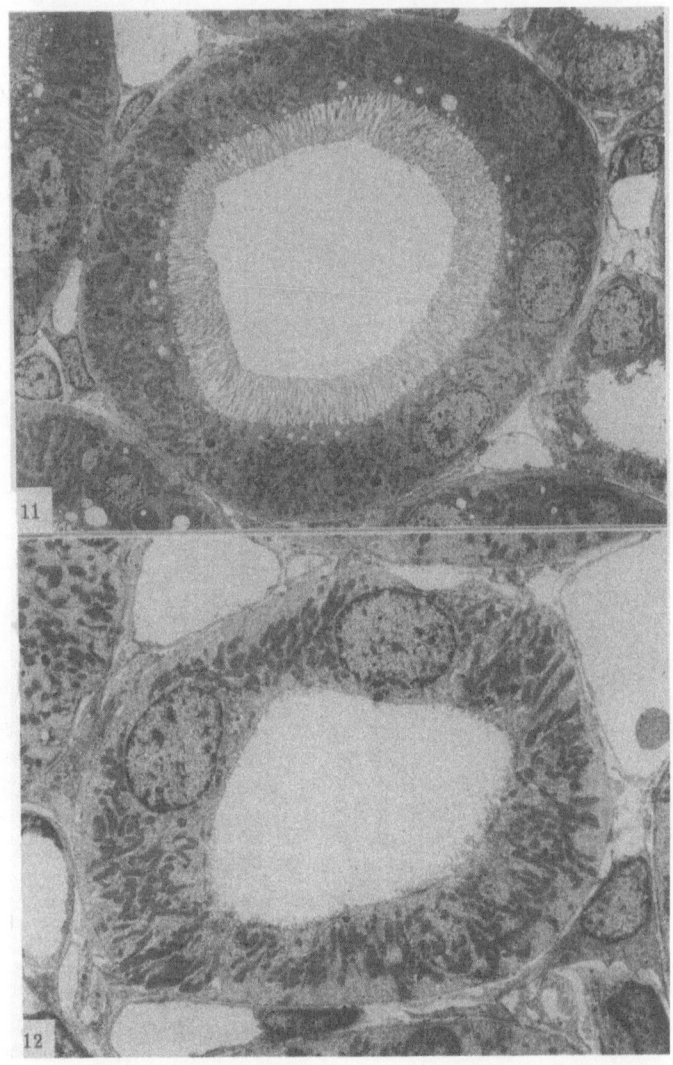

Figure 11 Electron micrograph of an S_3 profile. Tissue fixed as described in Figures 1-4. Reynolds lead citrate stain (x715).
Figure 12 Electron micrograph of a distal tubule profile. Tissue fixed as described in Figures 1-4. Reynolds lead citrate stain (x1100).

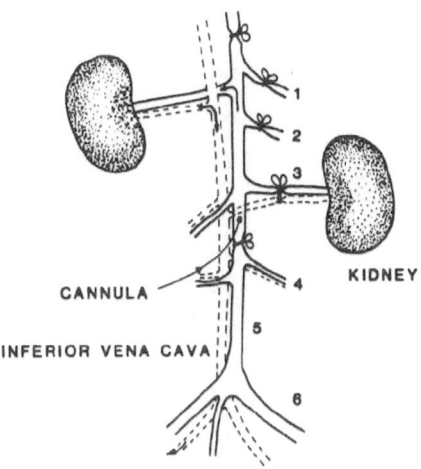

Figure 13 Surgical layout for perfusion fixation of rat kidney.

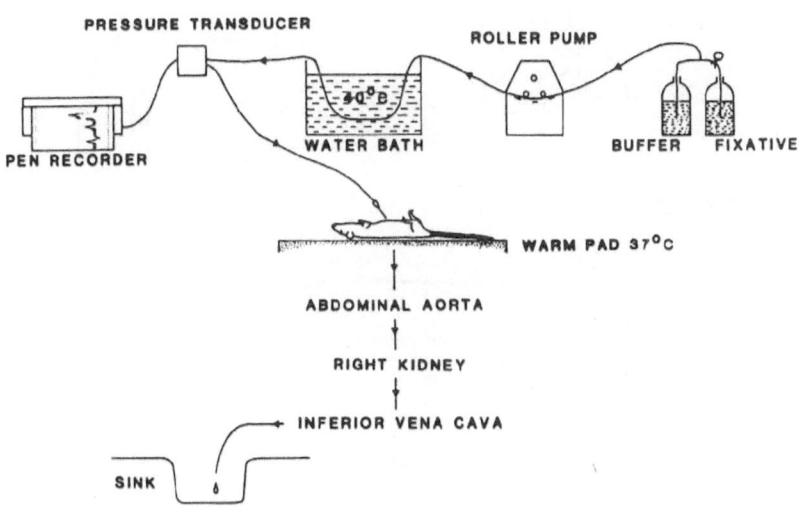

Figure 14 Rig for perfusion fixation of rat kidney.

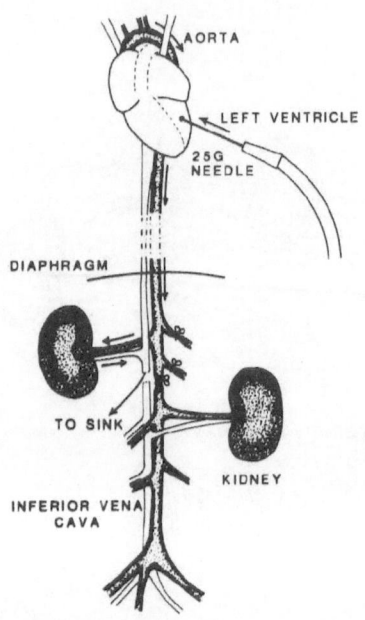

Figure 15 Surgical layout for perfusion fixation of mouse organs via the left ventricle.

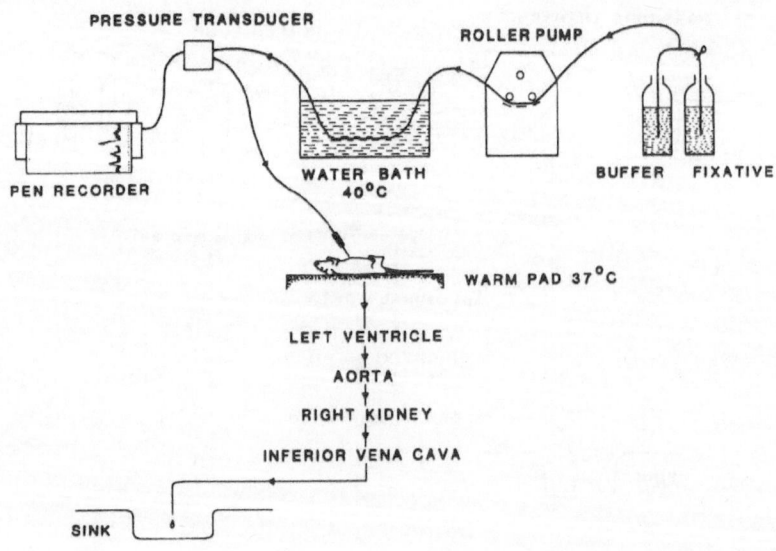

Figure 16 Rig for perfusion fixation of the mouse via the heart.

156

IV. SAMPLING THE PERFUSION-FIXED KIDNEY

A useful consequence of perfusion fixation is that it produces an organ rigid enough to be easily sliced. For valid morphometric studies to be possible, sampling must be unbiased. All parts of the kidney must have an equal chance of appearing in the sample taken. To achieve this the kidney must be sliced at positions determined relative to an external point. The most satisfactory procedure is to create a slicing device which, for EM work, cuts thin slices at spaced intervals. The thicker intervening slices can be used for LM work if desired (see Figure 17). This procedure is essentially that proposed by Pfaller[26].

For high power LM, or for EM studies of any particular segment of the nephron (or zone of the cortex or medulla), it is necessary to excise one or more strips from each slice. The strips must be generous in length and include more than the full depth of the zone under study (e.g. if the cortex is to be studied, then the strips must penetrate right down into the medulla). Thin sections, if they are to be taken, must give equal chance to all parts of the strip. Micrographs should be positioned by reference to an external point by a standard method, e.g. one or two per grid square always at the same corners (for discussion of this procedure see refs. 3 and 21).

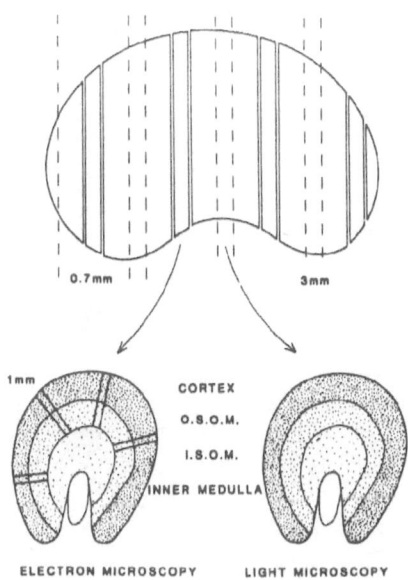

Figure 17 Slicing of the perfused kidney to achieve unbiased sampling.

The aim must always be to construct a hierarchical sampling tree in each kidney which gives rise to a defined number of blocks (each from a separate slice) and each block to several micrographs (Figures 18 and 19).

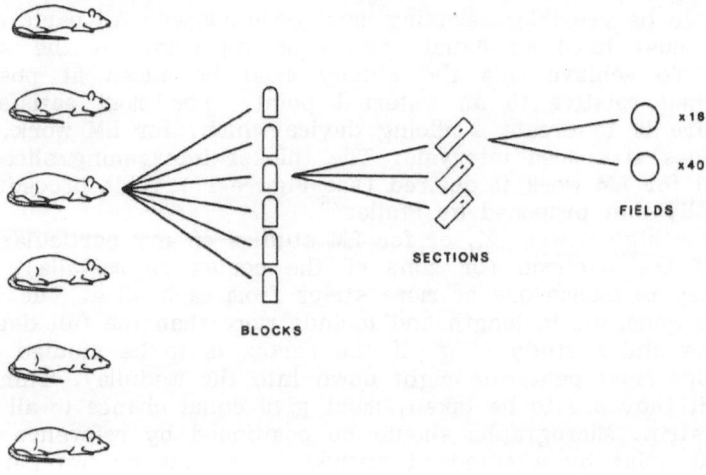

Figure 18 Sampling tree used by the authors in morphometric evaluation of perfusion fixation routines.

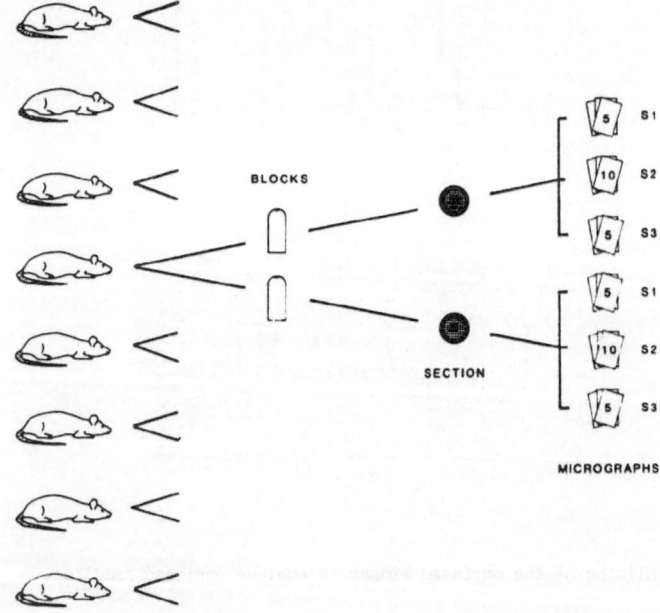

Figure 19 An example of a sampling tree for ultrastructural morphometry of the rat kidney proximal tubule.

If the tree is well constructed the total variance between replicate animals will consist largely of "between-animal" variance, and only a minor component will originate in "between-micrograph" variance. Usually "between-block" variance is extremely small[27-29]. It is perhaps worth noting that variance between animals is less if kidneys from the same side are used. An example of a sampling tree used to study S_1, S_2 and S_3 cells of the rat kidney is given in Figure 19. Further examples of sampling regimes for morphometric study of the kidney have been described by Wehner[30].

A.   Immersion fixation methods in kidney morphometry

Despite the very considerable advantages of the perfusion fixation approach in kidney studies, there are circumstances in which immersion-fixed tissue such as biopsies and surgical wedge biopsies are used as a source for morphometric data[35,36]. In addition, post mortem material is often fixed by immersion[37]. Such specimens are widely used in diagnostic nephropathology (see ref. 30 for review) and in which area morphometry yields a more precise description of changes present than does subjective assessment[35].

Although steps can be taken to ensure that any biopsy which is taken is thoroughly sampled in an unbiased fashion, needle biopsies are not generally highly representative of the whole kidney. This is because certain parts of the kidney have almost zero chance of being sampled. Even when the cortex alone is considered (the intended site of most biopsies) the most superficial and deeper parts are usually less likely to be taken by the needle than the cortical midzone. In addition some nephropathologies are focal. In glomerular studies there may be anxiety that an insufficient number of glomeruli might be found in a biopsy. In many clinical pathology laboratories a minimum of six glomeruli is regarded as the target for diagnostic work. Wehner[30] based his biopsy-derived morphometric observations on ten glomeruli, whereas Gundersen and Osterby[27] have shown that three glomeruli per kidney may be sufficient in experimental work.

V.   MAGNIFICATION OF IMAGES TO BE EMPLOYED FOR MORPHOMETRY

Studies of membranes and organelles naturally require the use of electron microscope images. Generally these will be most useful when the prints (or final projected images) are at 15,000-30,000 x magnification. Such images must be of accurately calibrated magnification, perhaps using a replica of a "crossed" grating (see ref. 2 for details). Often grosser morphometric estimates are necessary as well as (or instead of) these higher magnification ones. In this case low magnification EM or LM (100 x oil immersion lens) images must be employed. Many useful studies have also been done at this magnification, but LM images must be calibrated by photographing a stage micrometer along with the fields of tissue section. Useful work can be undertaken with images prepared with a LM fitted with high-quality x 40 and x 100 planapochromat objectives, the highly planar semi-thin resin sections, when carefully stained, providing almost ideal objects for photomicrography (see Figures 1-4).

A.   Reference volumes

Most morphometric data are based on ratio estimates and yield "density" values (Table 3). For example: endoplasmic reticulum - 600 μm^2 membrane/1000 μm^3 of cytoplasm. Such data are most useful if they can be related to a reference volume. The reference volume might be the whole kidney, whole cortex or glomerulus, whole tubule or perhaps the whole cell. When this is done ratio estimates become translated into estimates of absolute values of volume, area, length or number, which is naturally more informative. Thus if in the above example the cell volume, i.e. the reference, equals 2500 μm^3 the endoplasm reticulum area estimate becomes converted to 1500 μm^2/cell. A further reason for referring data to reference volumes is that, as a result of experimental treatment, developmental change or a pathological process, the reference can change. The kidney could be greater in volume, perhaps, or the glomeruli enlarged. The volume of the whole kidney may be determined by the immersion methods[2], and estimations of mean cell volume in various ways[2,31]. One useful type of calculation for estimating mean cell volume is shown below in the brief synopsis of morphometric computations.

B.   Morphometric procedures and principles

It is not appropriate here to give a detailed exposition on morphometric procedures and principles, but a very brief summary may be in order. Using morphometric methods volumes, areas, lengths and numbers of components (in cells or tissues or organs) can be estimated with reference to a chosen reference dimension (such as volume, surface), to give volume per unit volume, surface per unit surface, length per unit volume, etc. The major possibilities and the symbols for them are summarized in Tables 2 and 3. Note that each quantity is attributable to one or more reference, to give a number that can be referred to volume or surface, the reference being attached to the quantity as a subscript, thus creating and denoting the various ratio estimates. The ratio estimates can all be calibrated by using a reference volume, see above.

160

Table 2 Some common morphometric symbols

V_V	volume density	$\mu m^3/\mu m^3$
S_V	surface density	$\mu m^2/\mu m^3$
N_V	numerical density	$N/\mu m^3$
L_V	length density	$\mu m/\mu m^3$
N_S	number per unit surface	$N/\mu m^2$
S_S	surface/unit surface	$\mu m^2/\mu m^2$
v (e.g. v_{cell}, v_{kidney})		μm^3
S/V	surface/volume ratio	$\mu m^2/\mu m^3$
t	section thickness	μm
N_A	number profiles or particles per unit area section	$N/\mu m^2$
H	diameter of a particle (caliper diameter)	μm
$\bar{H}$	mean particle diameter (caliper diameter)	μm
D	diameter of a sphere	μm
$\bar{D}$	mean sphere diameter	μm
d	profile diameter	μm
$\bar{d}$	mean profile diameter	μm
A_A	area fraction of a component	$\mu m^2/\mu m^2$
P_P	fraction of points over a feature	

Table 3 Listing of tissue component densities and their dimensions

Component	Reference			
	Volume, V (μm^3)	Surface, S (μm^2)	Length, L (μm)	Number, N (μm^o)
Volume V (μm^3)	V_V μm^o			
Surface S (μm^2)	S_V μm^{-1}	S_S μm^o		
Length L (μm)	L_V μm^{-2}	L_S μm^{-1}	L_L μm	
Number (μm^o)	N_V μm^{-3}	N_S μm^{-2}	N_L μm^{-1}	N_N μm^o

See also Table 2 for explanation of symbols

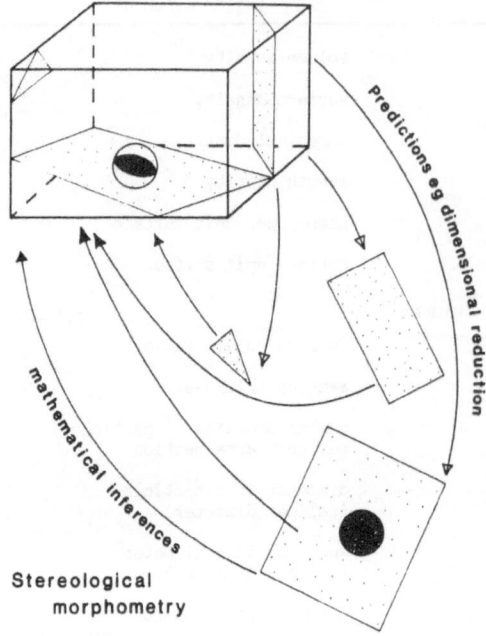

Stereological
morphometry

Figure 20 Diagram illustrating the two limbs of the process of stereological morphometry.

The basic estimates

Classical methods

<u>Estimation of V_V</u>, e.g. V_V lumen - fraction of kidney cortex occupied by tubule lumen. V_V estimation depends on the principle of Delesse[41] (see also Sorby[38]). Thus it is mathematically proven that, irrespective of the component form, the area of component per unit area of reference in the measuring fields on the sections (referred to as A_A) equals V_V.

A_A can be measured conveniently, by <u>point counting</u> (to obtain the ratio, P_P) using perhaps a square array of points laid over the micrographs or LM fields. For details of point counting methods see the introductory account by Williams[2]. It can also be measured by line intercept length estimate, L_L or by a tracing technique to give A_A directly.

$$V_V \text{ thus equals } A_A = P_P = L_L$$

Surface density, S_V

$$m = \frac{I \times \pi}{2L}$$

$$S_V = \frac{4M}{\pi}$$

where I = intersection number, L = line length applied,
e.g. surface area of microvillous plasmalemma per PT cell.

Length density, L_V

L_V = 2QA (see Weibel[3], p.109)
e.g. length of PT per unit volume of kidney cortex.

Numerical density, N_V

$$N_V = \frac{NA}{\overline{H} + t}$$

after Dehoff and Rhines[39] where t = section thickness;
$\overline{H}$ = particle diameter (mean)
e.g. number of DT nuclei per kidney.

Reference volumes

Whole kidney volumes can be estimated by fluid displacement (for
account see Williams[2], pp.71-2).
    Estimates of mean cell volumes can be obtained, e.g. for
kidney cells from:

$$\text{mean cell volume} = \frac{4/3\pi(\overline{D}/2)^2}{V_V \text{ nucleus in cell}}$$

(see Cope and Williams[31] for examples), or

$$\overline{V}_{cell} = \frac{V_V}{N_V}$$

In this case, N_V must be estimated from the N_A value for the
nuclei of the cell type concerned.

Example:

N_A (S_1 nuclei in cortex) $= 604/253973$ N/μm^2 = 2.38 x 10^{-3}

V_V (nuclei S_1 in cortex) $= 0.086$

*N_V (S_1 nuclei in cortex) $= 3.19$ x 10^{-4}/μm^3

v (S_1 nucleus) $= 269.7$ μm^3

Thus: cell volume $= 3.13$ x 10^3 μm^3

* From the formula explained in ref.44, i.e.:

$$N_V = K/\beta \times (N_A)^{3/2}/(V_V)^{\frac{1}{2}}$$

The brief list given above covers merely the quantities commonly estimated. An increasing number of more refined parameters can also be determined including estimates of surface curvature, connectivity of particles, thickness of layers and width of projections. The last two find a place in kidney research in the study of the thickness of the filtration barrier and the width of foot processes[20]. Accounts of many of the refined estimates can be found in Weibel[2], and a useful discussion and summary of nomenclature can be found in the article by Underwood[40].

As well as the above classical formulations appropriate for data collection from unbiased sections, certain other methods are available in which data are collected from sections in selected planes or from pairs of planes. Worthy of mention here are estimations of N_V by the disector approach[45], e.g. of cells in a glomerulus; estimation of V_V from systematic sections[46], useful for example for cortex : medulla ratios; and the use simply of vertical cell sections, which allows the exclusive use of cell profiles in which the tubule segment may be unambiguously identified[47].

REFERENCES

1.   Walker, A.M. and Oliver, J., Methods for the collection of fluid from single glomeruli and tubules of the mammalian kidney, Am. J. Physiol., 134, 562, 1941.

2.   Williams, M.A., Quantitative methods in biology, in Practical Methods in Electron Microscopy, Glauert, A.M., ed., North Holland Press, Amsterdam, 6, 1977.

3.   Weibel, E.R., Stereological methods, Vol. 1, Practical methods in biological morphometry, Academic Press, London, 1979.

4.   Williams, M.A., Autoradiography and immunocytochemistry, in Practical methods in Electron Microscopy, Glauert, A.M., ed., North Holland Press, Amsterdam, 6, 1977.

5.   Sayer-Hansen, K., Hansen, J. and Gunderson, H.J.G., Renal hypertrophy in experimental diabetes. A morphometric study, Diabetologia, 18, 501, 1980.

6.   Osterby, R. and Gundersen, H.J.G., Fast accumulation of basement membrane material and the rate of morphological changes in acute experimental

diabetic glomerular hypertrophy, Diabetologia, 18, 493, 1980.

7. Williams, M.A., Electron microscopic autoradiography: its application to protein biosynthesis, in Techniques in Protein Biosynthesis, Campbell, P.N. and Sargent, J.R., eds., Academic Press, London and New York, 3, 125, 1973.

8. Griffith, L.D., Bulger, R.E. and Trump, B.F., The ultra-structure of the functioning kidney, Lab. Invest., 16, 220, 1967.

9. Longley, J.B. and Burstone, M.S., Intraluminal nuclei and other inclusions as agonal artifacts of the renal proximal tubules, Am. J. Pathol., 42, 643, 1963.

10. Cope, G.H. and Williams, M.A., Improved preservation of parotid tissue for electron microscopy. A method permitting collection of valid stereological data, J. Cell. Biol., 60, 292, 1974.

11. Mayhew, T.M. and Williams, M.A., A quantitative morphological analysis of macrophage stimulation. II. Changes in granule number, size and size distributions. Cell Tissue Res., 150, 529, 1974.

12. Weibel, E.R., Morphometry of the human lung: the state of the art after two decades. Extrait du bulletin european de physiopathologie respiratoire, 15, 999, 1979.

13. Bohman, S.O., The ultrastructure of rat renal medulla as observed after improved fixation methods, J. Ultrastruct. Res., 47, 329, 1974.

14. Palay, S.L., McGee-Russell, S.M., Gordon, S. and Grillo, M.A., Fixation of neural tissues for electron microscopy by perfusion with solutions of osmium tetroxide, J. Cell Biol., 12, 385, 1962.

15. Pease, D.C., Histological techniques for electron microscopy, New York, Academic Press, 1960.

16. Maunsbach, A.B., The influence of different fixatives and fixation methods on the ultrastructure of rat kidney proximal tubule cells, J. Ultrastruct. Res., 15, 242, 1966.

17. Gottschalk, C.W. and Mylle, M., Micropuncture study of pressures in proximal and distal tubules and peritubular capillaries of the rat kidney during osmotic diuresis, Am. J. Physiol., 189, 323, 1957.

18. Folkow, B. and Neil, E., Circulation, Oxford University Press, New York, 33, 1971.

19. Thorball, N. and Tranum-Jensen, J., Vascular reactions to perfusion fixation, J. Microsc., (Oxford), 129, 123, 1983.

20. Seefeldt, T., Gundersen, H.J.G. and Osterby, R., Stereological determination of the true width and distribution of glomerular epithelial foot processes and its application in experimental nephrosis, Stereol. Jugosl., 3, Suppl. 1, 443, 1981.

21. Aherne, W.A. and Dunnill, M.S., Morphometry, Arnold, London, 205, 1982.

22. Baak, J.P.A. and Oort, J., A manual of morphometry in diagnostic pathology, Springer-Verlag, Heidelberg and New York, 205, 1983.

23. Johnston, W.H., Latta, H. and Ostvaldo, L., Variations on glomerular ultrastructure in rat kidneys fixed by perfusion, J. Ultrastruct. Res., 45, 149, 1973.

24. Goncalves, V. and Sobrinho-Simoes, M.A., Comparative morphometric studies of the cells of the third proximal segment of the rat kidney under different conditions of fixation, Experientia, (Basel), 33, 761, 1977.

25. Elling, F., Hasselager, E. and Fruus, C., Perfusion fixation of kidneys in adult pigs for electron microscopy, Acta Anatomica, 98, 340, 1977.

26. Pfaller, W., Structure-function correlation on rat kidney - quantitative correlation of structure and function - a review, Adv. Anat. Embryol., 70, 1, 1982.

27. Gundersen, H.J.G. and Osterby, R., Optimizing sampling efficiency of

stereological studies in biology or "Do more less well", J. Microsc., 121, 65, 1981.

28. Shay, J., Economy of effort in electron microscope morphometry, Am. J. Pathol., 81, 503, 1975.

29. Gupta, M., Mayhew, T.M., Bedi, K.S., Sharma, A.K. and White, E.H., Inter-animal variation and its influence on the overall precision of morphometric estimates based on nested sampling designs, J. Microsc., 131, 147, 1983.

30. Wehner, H., Morphometry in nephro-pathology, Stereol. Jugosl., 3, Suppl. 1, 449, 1981.

31. Cope, G.H. and Williams, M.A., Restitution of granule stores in the rabbit parotid gland after isoprenaline-induced secretion: stereological analysis of volume parameters, Cell Tissue Res., 209, 315, 1980.

32. Glauert, A.M., Fixation, dehydration and embedding of biological specimens, North Holland Press, Amsterdam, 209, 1975.

33. Bailey, N.T.J., Statistical methods in biology, English Universities Press, London, 1972.

34. Kaisling, B. and Kriz, W., Structural analysis of the rabbit kidney, Adv. Anat. Embryol. Cell Biol., 56, 1, 1979.

35. Romppanen, T. and Collan, Y., Morphometrical method for analysis of kidney biopsies in diagnostic histopathology, Stereol. Jugosl., 3, Suppl. 1, 435, 1981.

36. Wehner, H., Quantitative pathomorphologie des glomerulum der menschlichen niere, Fisher Verlag, Stuttgart, 1974.

37. Hanberg-Sorensen, F., Quantitative studies of the renal corpuscles. III. The influence of post mortem delay before taking renal tissue samples and of the duration of tissue fixation. Acta Pathol. Microbiol. Scand., Section A, 83, 251, 1975.

38. Sorby, H.C., On slaty cleavage as exhibited in the Devonian limestones of Devonshire, Phil. Mag., 11, 20, 1856.

39. Dehoff, R.T. and Rhines, F.N., Determination of number of particles per unit volume from measurements made on random plane sections: the general cylinder and the ellipsoid, Trans AIME, 221, 975, 1961.

40. Underwood, E.E., A standardised system of notation for stereologists, Stereol. Jugosl., 3, Suppl. 1, 715, 1981.

41. Delesse, A., Procède mechanique pour determines la composition des roches (extrait), CR Acad. Sci., (Paris), 25, 544, 1847.

42. Grantham, J.D., Ganote, C.E., Burg, M.B. and Orloff, J., Paths of transtubular water flow in isolated renal collecting tubules, J. Cell. Biol., 41, 562-576, 1969.

43. Linshaw, M.A., Effects of metabolic inhibitors on renal tubule cell volume, Am. J. Physiol., 239, F 562-579, 1980.

44. Weibel, E.R. and Gomez, D.M., A Principle for counting tissue structures on random sections, J. Appl. Physiol., 17, 343, 1962.

45. Sterio, D.C., Unbiased estimation of arbitrary particles, J. Microsc., (Oxford), 134, 127, 1984.

46. Cruz-Orive, L.M. and Myking, A.D., Stereological estimation of volume ratios by systematic sections, J. Microsc., (Oxford), 122, 143, 1981.

47. Baddeley, A.J., Gundersen, H.J.G. and Cruz-Orive, L.M., Estimation of surface area from vertical sections, Proc. 4th European Symposium on Stereology, Goteburg, Paper 11, 1985.

CORRELATING STRUCTURAL AND FUNCTIONAL CHANGES IN NEPHROTOXIC RENAL INJURY

D.C. DOBYAN, G. EKNOYAN AND R.E. BULGER

INTRODUCTION

The mammalian kidney is particularly susceptible to a variety of toxic agents. The fact that the kidneys receive approximately 20-25% of the cardiac output and yet make up only about 1% of the total body weight probably accounts for this susceptibility. As such, the structural integrity of the renal tubule is frequently compromised in response to ischaemic and toxic insults. Probably the most common lesion seen in experimental models of acute renal injury is necrosis of the proximal tubular epithelium. Prolonged renal ischaemia or direct exposure to a wide variety of toxins are the usual causes of acute tubular injury. The term acute renal failure has often been equated with acute tubular necrosis. While the interchangeable use of these two terms is reasonable for most experimental models where renal dysfunction is associated with a definitive lesion, the presence of underlying extensive tubular injury in clinical forms of acute renal failure is not prominent. Hence, the question of whether morphological injury precedes or contributes to the development of renal dysfunction remains controversial, at least in the clinical setting.

Over the past several years, a number of investigators have been rigorous in their attempts to correlate the structural changes seen in experimental renal disease with concomitant physiological observations. A better understanding of the relationship between structure and function might help elucidate the mechanisms which contribute to the development of kidney dysfunction. In this respect there are a number of important principles which need to be applied when structural-functional correlations are desired in experimental models of nephrotoxicity. First of all, it is imperative to establish the physiological state of the animal at the time of study. Secondly, it is important to utilize varied morphological approaches to provide the most complete assessment of the degree of structural change in any particular model. Finally, the employment of extensive morphometric analysis is essential in order to avoid unintentional bias and to permit the statistical analysis of the morphological changes that occur.

APPROACHES FOR QUANTITATING RENAL TUBULAR AND GLOMERULAR INJURIES

There are a number of important factors that must be considered in any attempt to quantitate the morphological changes in the kidney. To begin with, a system which assesses separately the severity of injury and the extent of injury must be employed other than the more frequently used and simple but imprecise grading system in which only one rating is provided (rating lesions from 0 to 4+). A second and very important component of any morphometric study must be the randomization of samples analysed. It is also imperative for the individual making judgments concerning the severity and extent of injury to be completely unaware of the treatment regimen given the animal under investigation. Additionally, the criteria to be used in any multiple grading of degrees of injury must be clearly defined prior to the initiation of counting procedures. Finally, the mode of visualization for quantitative study must be carefully considered. The use of light microscopy of paraffin sections is generally the method of choice for morphometric study of renal injury because it allows for the sampling of areas of tissue containing large numbers of cells. This is particularly important in organs like the kidney that are characterized by discrete anatomical zones and heterogeneous segments. It should be pointed out, however, that in certain types of studies, for example, evaluation of organelle lesions, transmission and scanning electron microscopy must be used. However, the use of electron micrographs requires more time-consuming and exact technical procedures on small pieces of tissue and therefore limits significantly the number of cells which can be examined.

A. Fixation

Certainly one of the most important aspects of any morphological study is the optimization of tissue preservation at the time of study. This is particularly relevant to those studies which attempt to correlate subtle changes in structure with physiological measurements made in the same animal. There is probably general agreement among morphologists that the most suitable method of tissue fixation for routine morphometric analysis entails the vascular perfusion of fixative solutions, preferably in vivo, prior to removal of the organs. This approach maximizes structural details and significantly minimizes the otherwise numerous artifacts associated with immersion fixation (Figures 1 and 2). Vascular perfusion is particularly important for the study of well-vascularized organs like the kidney in which tubular lumen and vessel patency is dependent on the maintenance of normal blood pressures. There have been several methods described for both in vivo and in vitro vascular perfusion in animals and these should be consulted for more detailed accounts[1-6]. We have previously employed both the in vivo method using a variety of experimental animal species

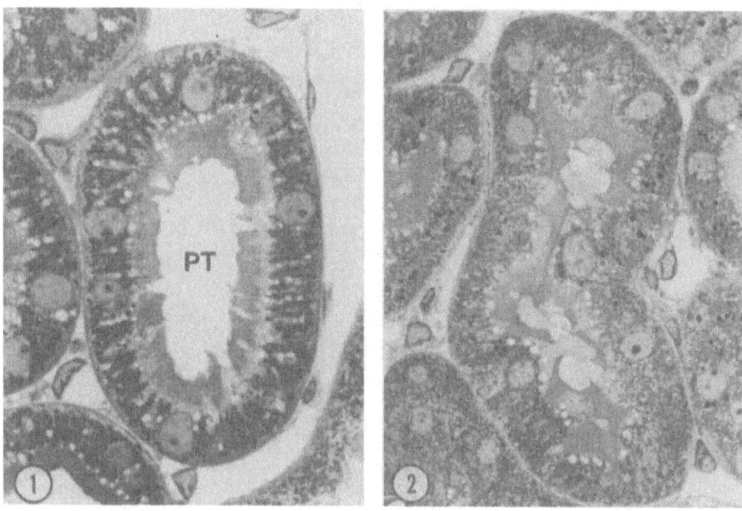

Figure 1 Light micrograph showing a well-perfused control rat kidney (plastic embedded section). Note the lumen of the proximal tubule (PT) is patent (toluidine blue, x740). **Figure 2** Light micrograph showing a poorly fixed control rat kidney (plastic embedded section). Note how the lumen of the proximal tubule has collapsed (toluidine blue, x580).

including rats, mice, rabbits, dogs, and primates and the in vitro method for studying human kidneys which were harvested for transplantation but for various reasons were unusable. In these procedures the fixative, usually a combination of buffered glutaraldehyde and formaldehyde, is introduced into the abdominal aorta at physiological pressures in the anaesthetized animal in vivo or directly into the renal artery in the in vitro approach[6].

B. Nephron heterogeneity

One of the more difficult aspects of investigations designed to evaluate structural alterations in the kidney is the heterogeneity of its nephrons. The mammalian kidney contains numerous heterogeneous segments, each with distinct physiological and morphological characteristics (Figure 3). It has become readily apparent that the large numbers of nephrotoxins currently utilized in experimental models of acute renal failure are quite specific with respect to the site along the nephron where they exert their major damaging effects. For example, heavy metals such as mercuric

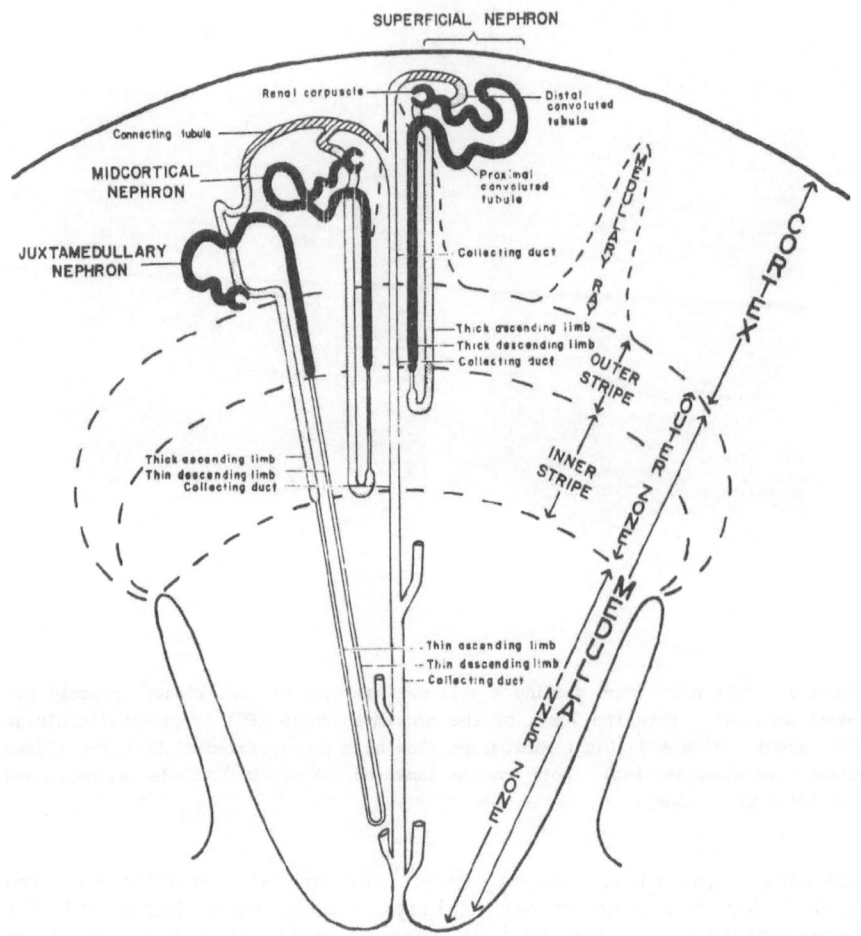

Figure 3 Schematic diagram showing superficial, midcortical, and juxtamedullary nephrons showing the relationship of the segments of the urinary tubule to the different zones of the kidney.

chloride, cis-platinum, and uranyl nitrate cause predominantly selective necrosis of the S_3 segment of the proximal tubule located in the outer stripe of the medulla[7-12] (Figure 4). Other agents including the aminoglycoside antibiotic, gentamicin, cephaloridine, and the putative redox compound, 6-hydroxy-3,4-dihydroxyphenyl-alanine, cause necrosis of the proximal S_2 segment[13-15] (Figure 5). Damage to the ascending thick segment of the distal tubule has been reported after the administration of isopropylhydrazine and folic acid[16]. The prolonged ingestion of analgesics such as aspirin and phenacetin has been shown to damage the thin limbs of the loop of Henle, vasa recta, collecting ducts, and interstitial cells

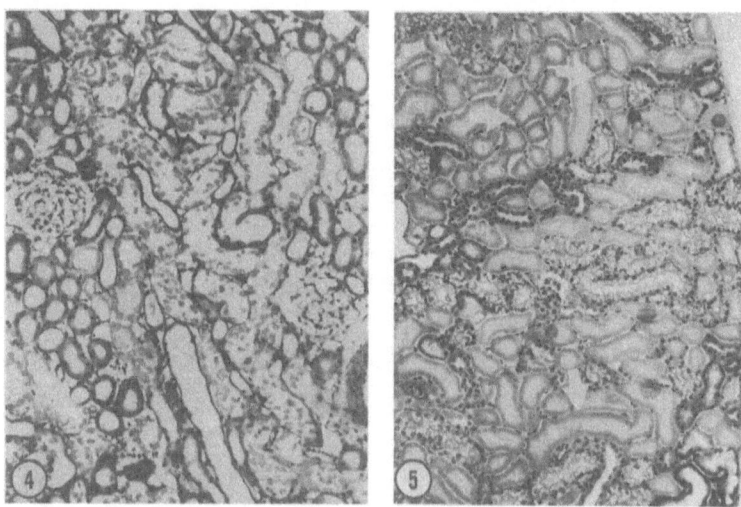

Figure 4 Light micrograph showing the outer stripe of the medulla of the rat kidney 24 hours after the administration of mercuric chloride. Note the selective necrosis involving the S_3 segment of the proximal tubules located in this region (haematoxylin and eosin, x88). **Figure 5** Light micrograph showing the outer cortex of the mouse kidney 24 hours after the administration of the putative redox compound, 6-OH-DOPA. Note the selective lesion involving only the S_2 segments (arrows) of the proximal tubule (haematoxylin and eosin, x88).

in the inner medulla and papilla[17].

These differential toxicities may be a consequence of regional blood flow within the kidney, drug concentration within a specific zone or nephron segment, binding or uptake of the toxin by different regions, or metabolic activation of the agent into more toxic compounds. In any case, these observations underlie the importance of extensive morphological quantitation for the accurate documentation of the specific site of injury along the nephron. Thoroughly comparing the segmental damage induced by known toxins with established functional characteristics of a particular region of the nephron, allows for the better elucidation of mechanisms of cellular injury.

1.   Methods for quantitating renal tubular injury -
       correlation with functional parameters

The kidneys should be fixed by vascular perfusion at the conclusion of assessment[6] of renal function. In our laboratory, this is generally after either inulin or endogenous creatinine clearances

171

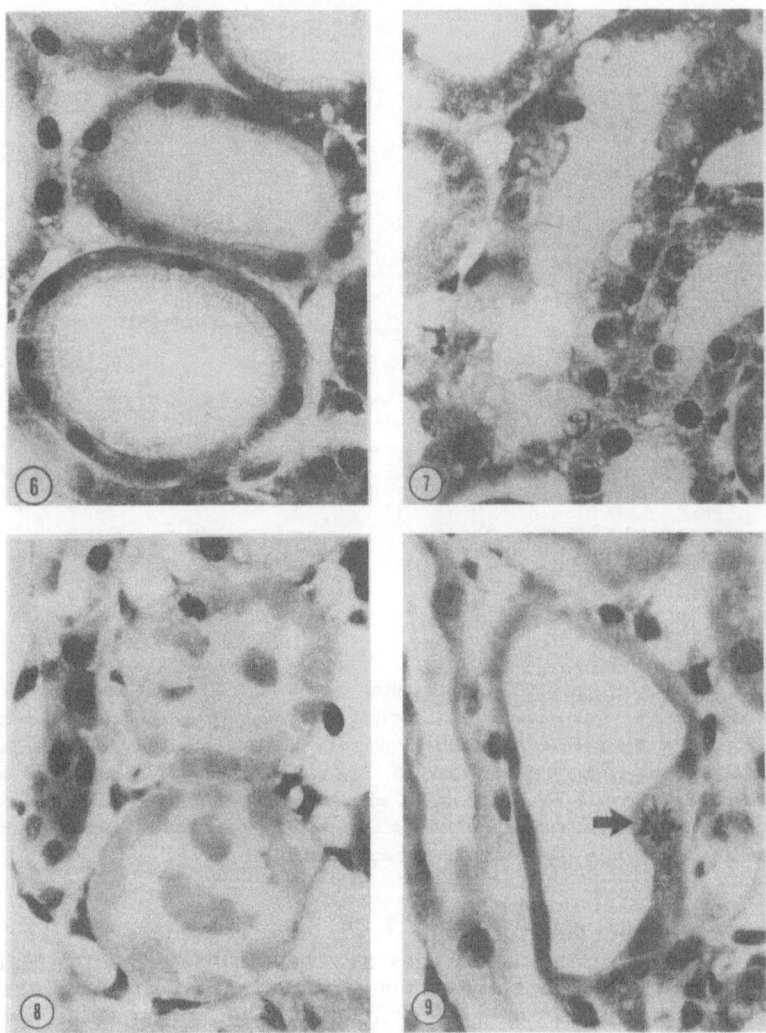

Figure 6 Light micrograph showing the appearance of proximal tubule cells categorized as normal (haematoxylin and eosin, x580). **Figure 7** Light micrograph showing proximal tubule cells categorized as injured. There is a focal loss of brush border from proximal tubule cells and an increase in apical vesicles and vacuoles (haematoxylin and eosin, x545). **Figure 8** Light micrograph showing proximal tubule cells categorized as necrotic. Cell membrane integrity and nuclear staining is lost. Some cells have detached from the basement membrane and lie within the tubule's lumen (haematoxylin and eosin, x590). **Figure 9** Light micrograph showing the appearance of proximal tubule cells categorized as regenerating. Epithelial cells lining these tubules are low in height and a brush border is lacking. A mitotic figure is apparent (arrow) (haematoxylin and eosin, x680).

(metabolic cage studies). The fixative which we normally use contains 2.5% glutaraldehyde and 2% formaldehyde buffered with either 0.04 M potassium phosphate or sodium cacodylate at a pH of 7.4. The kidneys are subsequently excised and are cut in a manner which allows sampling of the entire cortex through inner medulla and papilla. Additional samples are also taken and processed for transmission and scanning electron microscopy.

Paraffin sections are routinely used for the quantitative assessment of renal tubular injury. The number of specific regions to be evaluated is predetermined and depends to a large extent on the distribution of lesions within the kidney (see section on Nephron heterogeneity) and on the particular species under investigation. In general, five areas of each of the following regions are analysed: the pars convoluta of the proximal tubule in the inner and outer cortex, the pars recta of the proximal tubule in the inner and outer cortical medullary rays, and the pars recta (S_3 region) of the proximal tubule. This type of quantitation is preferred because the proximal tubule represents the most frequent site of injury in nephrotoxic models. An area is first centred at low magnification in a random fashion and then the high power objective is positioned for viewing the field at random, without moving the specimen stage to bias the chosen area. Using a Leitz-Wetzlar overhead projector microscope, the image is projected upon a screen onto which 144 points have been inscribed. The structure lying under or nearest each point is classified by one observer without prior knowledge of the source of the specimen being examined. Each of the proximal tubule cells counted are assigned to one of the following categories: (1) normal when indistinguishable from controls, (2) injured when the cell reveals no evidence of necrosis but the cell shape is altered to a low cuboidal or simple squamous type or reveals extensive apical vacuolization in addition to loss of brush border, (3) necrotic when the cell shows irreversible damage such as a loss of membrane integrity or loss of nuclear staining, and (4) regenerating when lining cells are low in height and are markedly basophilic and frequently show mitotic figures (Figures 6-9). The data for each specific region are then combined to yield a single value per region per animal. In this manner, comparisons can be made between different segments and regions of the kidney, as well as between animal groups receiving different treatment regimens. Values are routinely expressed per animal group as means ± SEM. Parametric tests like the Student's t-test and non-parametric tests such as the Mann-Whitney rank sum test are used to evaluate differences between experimental and control groups.

Table 1 illustrates a representative morphometric assessment of proximal tubular injury in rats subjected to mercuric chloride ($HgCl_2$) toxicity with and without pharmacological intervention. Mercuric chloride administration to laboratory animals produces a model of acute renal failure characterized by a reduction in glomerular filtration rate, an increase in fractional sodium excretion, and acute tubular necrosis of the S_3 segment of the proximal tubule[9]. In this study, Group I rats represent the sham injected controls. Group II rats received a sham injection of saline followed by $HgCl_2$ administration.

Table 1 Morphological changes in the proximal tubules in the outer stripe region of the outer medulla 24 hours after saline or mercuric chloride administration in rats pretreated with either chlorpromazine (CPZ) or saline

	Group I (n = 7) (CPZ + saline)	Group II (n = 5) (saline + HgCl$_2$)	Group III (n = 8) (CPZ + HgCl$_2$)
Normal(%)	99.7±0.2	5.0±2.5$^{a\pi}$	32.8±10.3$^{ab\pi}$
Injured(%)	0.3±0.2	6.3±2.9	40.8± 6.7* *
Necrosis(%)	0.0±0.0	88.1±3.6$^{\pi}$	26.5± 8.9$^{+\pi}$

Values are means ± SEM in percentage of proximal tubule cells that appeared normal, injured or necrotic. Some of these results have been previously reported, Laboratory Investigation, 50, 578, 1984.

[a] Groups II and III compared to Group I.
[b] Group III compared to Group II.
+ = P<0.05; * = P<0.005; π = P<0.001

Group III rats received an injection of the anaesthetic amine, chlorpromazine (CPZ), a putative protective agent, followed by HgCl$_2$ administration. Renal clearances were performed 24 hours after the sham injection of either saline or mercuric chloride. Both of the groups which received HgCl$_2$ exhibited significant renal tubular injury which was confined to the S$_3$ segment of the proximal tubule when compared to controls. Using the morphometric techniques described, the degree of injury in the CPZ-pretreated rats was significantly less than animals receiving HgCl$_2$ alone. These morphological observations suggest that CPZ affords partial protection against HgCl$_2$-induced acute tubular necrosis[18]. This method of quantitation allows for the quantitative assessment of both the degree as well as the site of injury, thereby providing a more accurate estimate of the beneficial effects of this or any other protective agents.

In these same groups, renal dysfunction was also significantly less impaired in the CPZ-treated animals. An analysis was performed relating the percentage of proximal tubular necrosis to glomerular filtration rate or to fractional sodium excretion. A significant correlation was noted between the structural injury observed and both the glomerular filtration rate (r = 0.81; P<0.01; Figure 10) and the urinary excretion of sodium (r = 0.65; P<0.01; Figure 11). Although these observations fail to establish a cause and effect relationship, they nevertheless illustrate one type of quantitative correlation between morphological and functional changes in nephrotoxic models of acute renal injury.

There have been increasing numbers of studies appearing in the literature which have shown correlations between renal structural changes and various parameters of renal function in ischaemic and nephrotoxic models of acute renal failure[9,19-24].

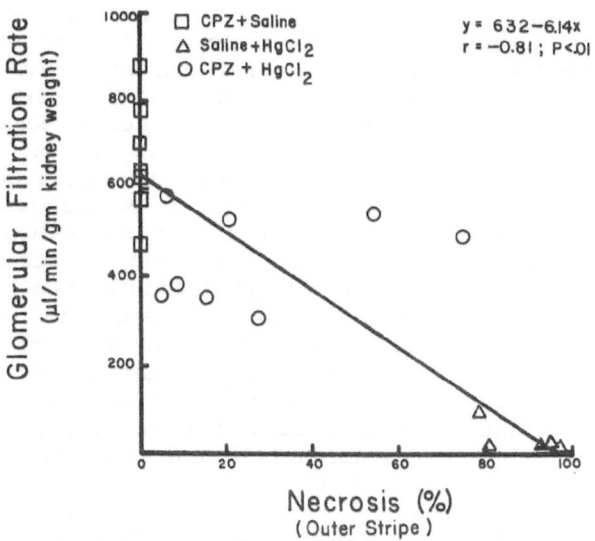

Figure 10 Relationship between the glomerular filtration rate and the percentage of necrotic cells in the pars recta of the proximal tubule in the inner cortical region. Values were obtained 24 hours after sham injection of either saline or mercuric chloride with and without pretreatment with chlorpromazine (CPZ). A significant correlation is demonstrated (y = 632 - 6.14x; r = 0.81; P < 0.01).

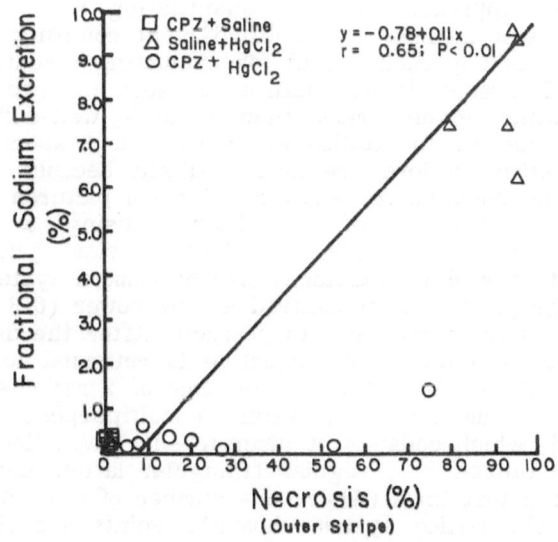

Figure 11 Relationship between the fractional sodium excretion and the percentage of necrotic cells in the pars recta of the proximal tubule in the inner cortical region. Values are obtained 24 hours after sham injection of either saline or mercuric chloride with and without pretreatment with CPZ. A significant correlation exists between these two parameters (y = 0.78 + 0.11x; r = 0.65; P < 0.01).

Eknoyan and co-workers[9] evaluated the effects of the centrally active sympathomimetic agent, clonidine, in a nephrotoxic model induced by the injection of mercuric chloride. They showed a good correlation between the degree of inner and outer stripe necrosis involving the proximal tubule and both the glomerular filtration rate and fractional sodium excretion. In a model of ischaemic renal injury induced by clamping the renal pedicle in rabbits for 1 hour, Solez and colleagues[20] showed a significant correlation between the serum creatinine and that of the number of cortical casts and of the severity of vasa recta lesions. Similar correlations between serum creatinine and the presence of casts, accumulations of leukocytes in the vasa recta, interstitial inflammation, tubular necrosis, and tubular dilatation have also been noted in glycerol and gentamicin-induced models of acute renal failure[21,22]. Quantitative assessment of structural changes can also be related to biochemical parameters. For example, Dobyan and colleagues[25] demonstrated a significant correlation between tubular injury and renal cortical sodium and potassium content in gentamicin-induced acute renal failure in dogs. Finally, it is interesting to note that recent reports by Solez and co-workers[21,24] provided evidence suggesting correlations may exist between structure and function in human acute renal failure. They analysed biopsies from 50 patients who had acute renal failure at the time of study and from seven patients who had recovered from the renal impairment. They noted that the extent of necrosis and loss of tubular epithelial cells were significantly greater in patients with established acute renal failure at the time of biopsy compared to patients whose renal failure had resolved.

Another approach used for quantitating renal morphological data utilizes test lattices and modified point counting methods. We have found this approach useful for evaluating structural changes which are of a more diffuse nature, as seen in chronic renal injury, and which involve more than a single well-defined tubular segment and lesion. In studies where there is a spectrum of renal lesions, paraffin sections are again utilized because of the large area of tissue available for analysis. Random pictures are obtained from different regions of the kidney using a conventional photomicroscope. We utilize a Leitz-Wetzlar photomicroscope equipped with a Wild Photoautomat MPS 55 camera system. The area to be photographed is first centred at low power (6.3 x) and then the 16 x objective is rotated into position. After the area has been photographed, the low-power objective is returned to the original position and the field is moved a distance of 2 mm (using an optical reticle) for the next photograph. A multipurpose test system[26] is then used, which consists of discrete short test lines whose end points are arranged in a regular triangular lattice using an array of n rows of n test lines (where n = number of rows and lines and varies with the lattice system chosen). Points are classified into various categories such as normal and abnormal proximal tubules, normal and abnormal distal tubules, tubules with casts, normal and abnormal glomeruli (sclerotic and hypercellular), interstitium, areas of inflammation, and tubules which are not identifiable. A typical micrograph with overlying lattice is shown in Figure 12.

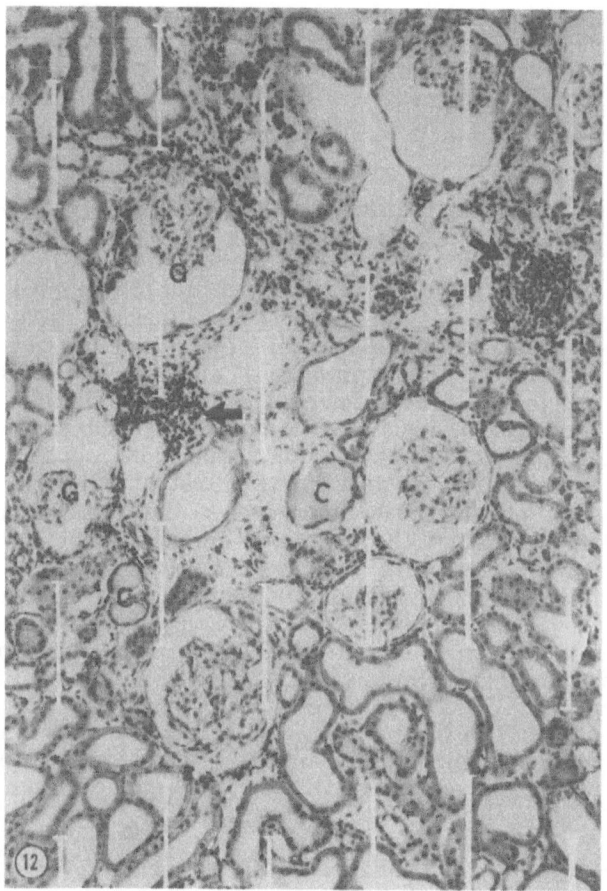

Figure 12 Light micrograph showing a paraffin section of the inner cortical region of the kidney of a rat 15 months after a single injection of cis-platinum. A transparent overlay illustrates the method of point counting. Note the abnormal glomeruli (G), areas of chronic inflammation (arrows), and tubules filled with casts (C) (haematoxylin and eosin, x120).

This figure illustrates the chronic nature of renal injury taken from a rat injected with the antineoplastic agent, cis-platinum, and then examined 15 months after injection. In this study, morphometric evaluation of renal injury revealed that cis-platinum-treated rats had a significantly greater number of abnormal proximal tubules, sclerotic glomeruli, areas of chronic inflammation and interstitial fibrosis, and dilated tubules filled with hyaline casts when compared to age-matched control rats. In close agreement with these observations was a significant impairment in renal function. In these same animals the glomerular filtration rate and urinary osmolality (520±59 μl/min per g kidney weight and 871±194 mOsm/kg H_2O) were significantly reduced compared to respective values in the control group[27] (799±100 μl/min per g kidney weight and 1471±162 mOsm/kg H_2O; P<0.01).

D. Methods for quantitating glomerular injury - correlation with functional parameters

Most studies which have examined the effects of nephrotoxic agents on the structure of the kidney have been directed at the pathological changes that occur in the renal tubules. Several groups have recently investigated how changes in the structure of the renal corpuscle might influence or relate to normal glomerular function. Such assessments seem warranted considering that one of the earliest functional disturbances seen in nephrotoxic renal failure is a reduction in glomerular filtration rate. Furthermore, the ability of physiologists to measure the glomerular capillary ultrafiltration coefficient (K_f), defined as the product of the effective hydraulic permeability and the capillary surface area, has prompted investigators to seek correlating morphological changes involving the renal corpuscle. For example, a decrease in K_f has been reported in uranyl nitrate-induced acute renal failure[28], after aminoglycoside administration[29,30], after angiotensin infusion[28], and in ischaemic acute renal failure[31]. The current literature regarding the presence or absence of a discrete glomerular lesion, however, remains controversial and additional careful morphometric analyses are necessary to resolve this important question.

1. Changes in visceral epithelial cells (glomerular podocytes)

The visceral epithelial cell of the renal corpuscle, frequently referred to as the glomerular podocyte, represents one of the most complex cell types found within the kidney. The main cell body of the podocyte is somewhat removed from the glomerular capillary wall and is separated from the underlying glomerular basement membrane by a layer of numerous cytoplasmic projections. Primary processes or trabeculae emanating from the main cell body radiate and branch into secondary and tertiary processes which eventually terminate in small club-shaped foot processes called pedicels (Figure 13). These pedicels interdigitate extensively with pedicels from adjacent podocytes to form an elaborate system of slits that are part of the glomerular filtration barrier. Because of this elaborate three-dimensional architecture, the method of choice for assessing changes in glomerular podocyte morphology has been scanning electron microscopy. Using this technique, some investigators have reported alterations in podocyte morphology in experimental acute renal failure[32-38] while other investigators, using

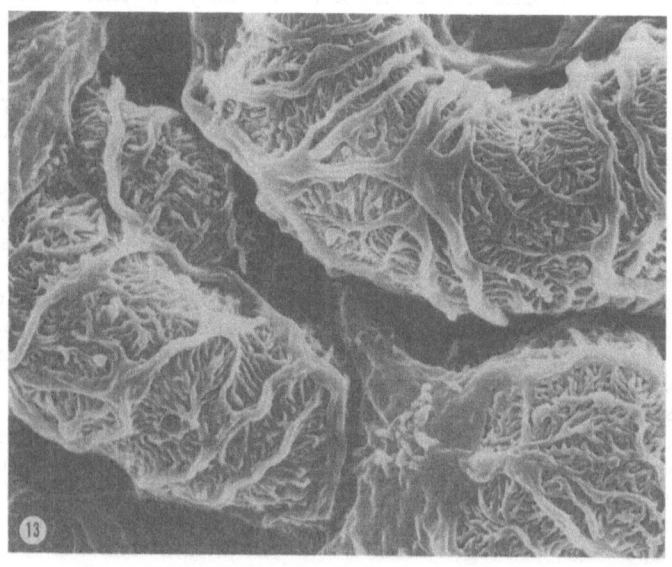

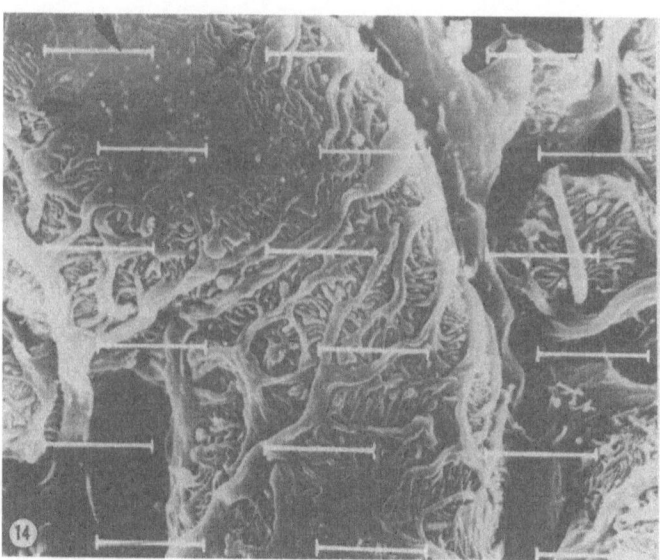

Figure 13 Scanning electron micrograph with overlay showing a normal glomerulus from a rat kidney. Note the elaborate appearance of the visceral epithelial cells (podocytes) and the fine pedicels or foot processes which form an elaborate series of channels (x3,480). **Figure 14** Scanning electron micrograph with overlay showing a glomerulus with alterations in normal glomerular podocyte structure. The abnormal area is marked by arrows (x3,540).

similar as well as different models, have failed to show changes[29,39-43]. One major problem in many of these studies was the lack of morphometric quantitation. Also, several of these investigations were performed during different phases of the renal impairment (initiation versus maintenance). Correlating structural changes observed at later time periods with functional impairment measured shortly after injury is a major problem of some studies.

As previously discussed, the kidneys of animals to be studied should be fixed by vascular perfusion at the conclusion of physiological determinations and the tissue processed for scanning electron microscopy using conventional methods[44]. The major advantages of using scanning techniques are the relative ease of sample preparation and the ability to view pieces of tissue containing all regions of the kidney. In razor-blade sliced tissue sections, the visceral epithelial cells investing the glomerular capillaries are easily visualized because Bowman's capsule is usually removed during sample preparation.

In our laboratory[45], we routinely take an equal number of low-power scanning electron micrographs from glomeruli situated in the outer, mid, and inner cortical regions of the kidney at a final magnification of 3000 x. The micrographs of experimental and control groups are photographed in a blind and random manner to avoid bias. The simplest approach is to quantitate the areas of the

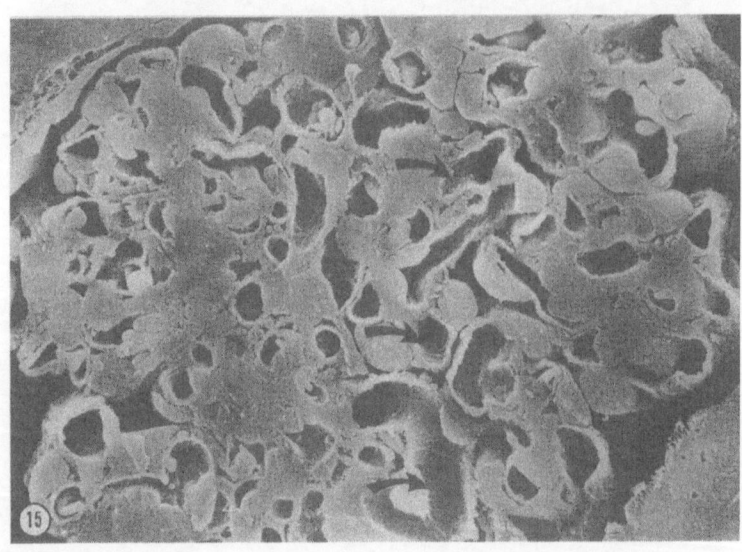

Figure 15 Low-power scanning electron micrograph showing a freeze-cracked glomerulus from a control rat kidney. For quantitating the glomerular epithelium we chose areas where the capillary loops are cracked parallel to their long axis and those with widely patent lumens (arrows) (x1,055).

glomerular capillary surface which appear either normal or abnormal. Areas which are considered abnormal are first circumscribed and then, using test lattices and point counting methods (previously described), the percentage of each selected area can be determined (Figure 14). In this manner, the changes in podocyte structure can be correlated with various parameters of glomerular function.

Racusen and Solez[38] have used a similar approach to evaluate podocyte changes in human renal biopsies obtained 1 hour post-transplant. They compared podocyte morphology of kidneys with normal renal function in the early post-transplant period with podocytes from kidneys that developed post-ischaemic acute renal failure. In this study, they determined the area of glomerular surface area covered by podocyte foot processes and fine epithelial cell processes (less than 1 mm in diameter on the micrograph) and compared these observations with areas covered by epithelial cell bodies and major processes greater or equal to 1 mm in diameter. Their results showed altered glomerular podocyte cell bodies over much of the capillary surface, reducing the area covered by fine pedicels from 60% in controls to 38% in those with acute renal failure. They also observed a significant positive correlation between the percentage of capillary surface area covered by only fine processes and the serum creatinine levels on the third post-transplant day.

Another aspect of glomerular morphology which has generated significant interest concerns possible structural alterations in glomerular capillary endothelium. The cells which line the glomerular capillary are perforated with numerous fenestrae or pores, which probably accounts for the increased hydraulic permeability of this specialized capillary. In this respect, investigators have been focusing on the potential role which changes in endothelial pore size and density may play in experimental models of renal toxicity. More specifically, they have been searching for correlations between endothelial alterations and decreases in parameters such as glomerular filtration rate and ultrafiltration coefficient. In the past, a thorough quantitative study of the glomerular capillary surface was difficult because the standard preparative procedures for scanning electron microscopic observation exposed only a small percentage of the total endothelial surface area. The introduction of freeze-cracking techniques by Tanaka[46] has provided a simple method for exposing large areas of the endothelium for study. In this method, fixed tissue is dehydrated in ethanol, cracked by immersion into liquid nitrogen, and then processed for scanning electron microscopy using conventional methods[6,46].

To quantitate endothelial morphology, we select at random four to six cortical and four to six juxtamedullary glomeruli at random from mounted tissue specimens. The glomeruli to be studied are photographed at a low magnification (24 x) and the positive print is used to map areas with exposed endothelial surfaces (Figure 15). The regions selected to be photographed are those areas of the capillary loops which have been cracked parallel to their long axis and those with widely patent lumens. Pictures of the selected areas are taken at a final magnification of 24,000 x.

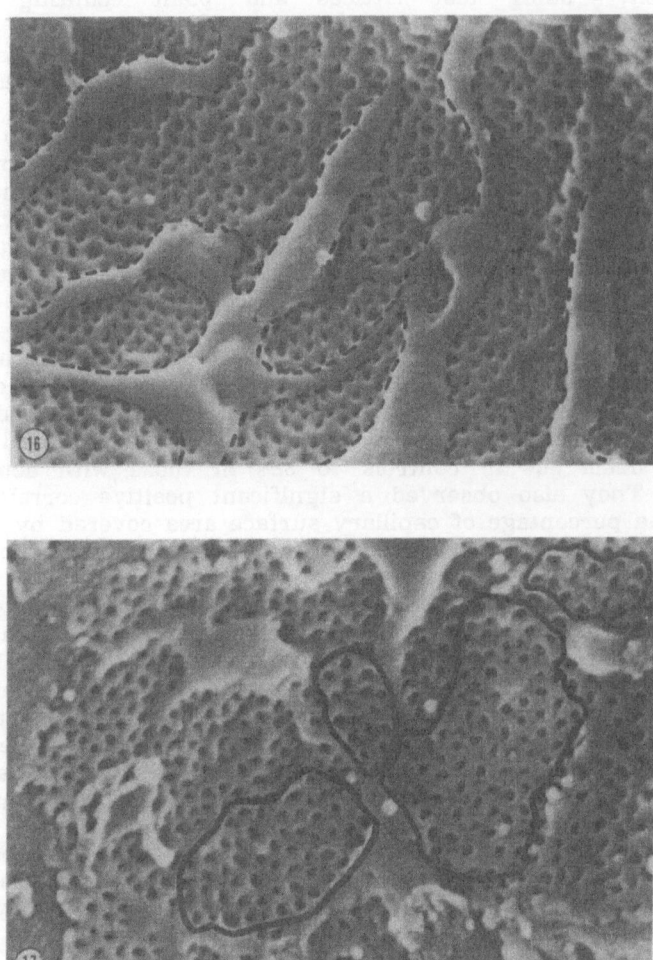

Figure 16 Scanning electron micrograph showing the endothelial surface of the glomerular capillary from a control rat kidney. The cytoplasmic ridges of the endothelial cells are outlined with dashed lines, while the fenestrated regions occupy the remaining areas. The percentages of capillary surface area occupied by ridges or fenestrae are determined from such micrographs (x24,800). **Figure 17** Scanning electron micrograph showing the glomerular capillary endothelium from a normal rat kidney. For estimates of pore area and pore density, flat areas of the capillary surface parallel to the plane of the photograph showing attenuated endothelium with pores are encircled. Individual pore areas within a circled region, as well as the total area of the circled region, are measured using a digitizer (x25,300).

Great care must be taken to ensure the accuracy of recorded magnifications. This is accomplished through daily calibration of the scanning electron microscope. Of the total prints taken per animal, we select twelve at random for subsequent quantitative analysis.

In our laboratory, two different quantitative methods are performed sequentially. We initially determine and define endothelial surface morphology in normal animals. Xerox copies of randomly selected micrographs are made for each animal under investigation. The following structures are circumscribed on each copy: (1) cytoplasmic ridges; (2) attenuated areas with endothelial pores; (3) non-fenestrated areas (assumed to overlie the nucleus); and (4) areas not pertaining to the endothelium (Figure 16). The regions corresponding to the first three categories of endothelial surface are cut out and weighed on an analytical balance. The percentage component of each type of surface structure is determined and these percentages are averaged for each group at the completion of study. For example, we have quantitated the percentage composition of normal surface morphology of the rat capillary endothelium[47]. In this study, 53.6±2.7% of the surface was made up of fenestrated areas, 31.2±1.5% by areas with cytoplasmic ridges, and 15.5±4.0% non-fenestrated regions. This type of quantitative evaluation is essential to avoid errors committed in the past, whereby pathological changes described in the endothelium have since been shown to be normal components of the capillary surface structures. Similar measurements can be easily performed using any of the standard digitizers currently available.

The second approach which we use to quantitate endothelial surface characteristics involves determination of the effective pore area and density. The fenestrae of the glomerular endothelium exhibit a wide diversity in shape and size. Several studies which have reported changes in endothelial pore size in models of experimental acute renal failure have relied on measurements of diameters of endothelial pores as a representative expression of pore size. This assumes that endothelial pores represent perfect circles which upon inspection of Figures 16 and 17 is clearly not the case.

In our laboratory, after assessing endothelial surface morphology, the micrographs are printed at a final magnification of 72,000 x. Flat areas of the capillary surface parallel to the plane of the micrograph, and which exhibit attenuated endothelium with pores, are circumscribed (Figure 17). A Laboratory Computer Systems, Micro-plan II Image Analysis System (Digital Planimeter) equipped with an alpha numerical printer is used to measure individual pore areas within the outlined area of each photograph. Pore density (expressed as number of pores per μm^2) is calculated by determining the number of pores per unit area measured. Individual values for each micrograph are then combined to yield a single value for each parameter measured for each animal studied. This type of quantitation permits an estimate of the total area occupied by endothelial fenestrae and emphasizes the considerable variation in "normal" pore size. For example, Dobyan and colleagues[6] reported pore areas ranging in size from 1130 to 2608 nm^2 for the human glomerular capillary endothelium, and Bulger and associates reported pore areas of 1494±75 nm^2 in control rats[47].

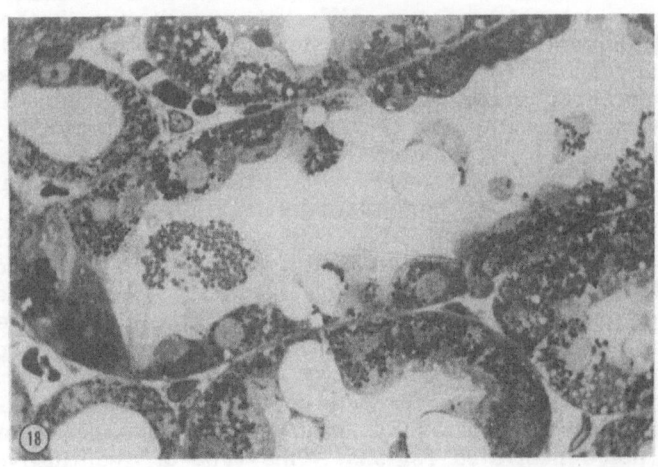

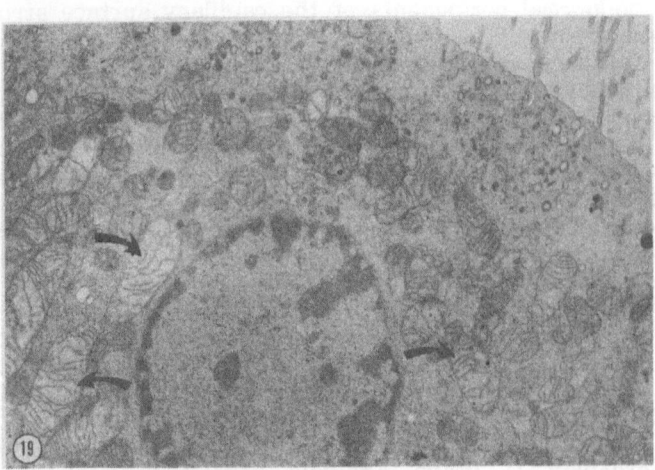

Figure 18 Light micrograph showing a plastic embedded section of a mouse kidney after the injection of the putative redox compound, 6-OH-DOPA. Notice the numerous structural changes which can be identified in these semi-thin plastic sections. There is a focal loss of brush border, the cells have rounded it, and the mitochondria are markedly abnormal (toluidine blue, x600). **Figure 19** Transmission electron micrograph showing a proximal tubule cell exhibiting numerous ultrastructural changes consistent with various stages of cellular injury. There is a focal loss of brush border and the mitochondria exhibit high amplitude swelling (arrows) (x7200).

184

Most of the information which has been described in this present report has centred on either light microscopic or scanning electron microscopic observations of structural damage and concomitant physiological correlations. Additional important information can be gleaned from studies which utilize either semi-thin (0.5-1.0 μm) plastic embedded sections or transmission electron microscopy. While the use of these techniques requires more tedious methodology and limits the sampling size, the improved resolution allows for a more accurate assessment of renal injury at the cellular and subcellular levels. Using plastic embedded sections, more subtle and discrete changes can be identified by light microscopy (Figure 18). Transmission electron microscopy allows for the examination of changes in organellar structure which is important for documenting sublethal and lethal cellular injury (Figure 19). In this respect we have been attempting to correlate the progression of organellar changes with specific mechanisms of toxicity. We have recently observed that the sequential alterations in proximal tubule cells seen after the administration of the redox compound, 6-OH-DOPA, are quite different from those induced either by ischaemia or by alkylating agents. This suggests that differences may exist in the mechanisms initiating the cell injury among these models, and emphasizes the potential importance of quantitating injury at the ultrastructural level.

In summary, there are increasing numbers of reports in the literature which emphasize the apparent close correlation between structural changes and various parameters of renal function in toxic models of renal injury. These observations support the viewpoint that structure and function are inextricably related. The continuous rigorous application of morphometric techniques to evaluate structural changes and its blending with functional and biochemical approaches will undoubtedly increase our knowledge and understanding of the mechanisms which underlie the development, maintenance, and resolvement of cellular injury in the kidney.

REFERENCES

1. Ericsson, J.L.E., Glutaraldehyde perfusion of the kidney for preservation of proximal tubules with patent lumens, J. Microsc., 5, 97, 1966.

2. Maunsbach, A.B., The influence of different fixatives and fixation methods on the ultrastructure of the rat kidney proximal tubule cells. I. Comparison of different perfusion fixation methods of the glutaraldehyde, formaldehyde and osmium tetroxide fixative, J. Ultrastruct. Res., 15, 242, 1966.

3. Griffith, L.D., Bulger, R.E. and Trump, B.F., The ultrastructure of the functioning kidney, Lab. Invest., 16, 220, 1967.

4. Hall-Craggs, M., Little, J.R., Sadler, J.H. and Trump, B.F., Structural changes following hypothermic preservation of human cadaveric kidneys, Human Pathol., 11, 23, 1980.

5. Moller, J.C., Skriver, E., Olson, S. and Maunsbach, A., Perfusion fixation of human kidneys for ultrastructural analysis, J. Ultrastruct. Res., 3, 375, 1982.

6. Dobyan, D.C., Eknoyan, G., Magill, L.S., Sarrafian, M. and Bulger, R.E., A

quantitative evaluation of the glomerular capillary endothelium in rat and human kidneys: Utilization of vascular perfusion, freeze-cracking of tissue, and scanning electron microscopy, J. Electron Microsc. Tech., 1, 185, 1984.

7.   Siegel, F.L. and Bulger, R.E., Scanning and transmission electron microscopy of mercuric chloride-induced acute tubular necrosis in rat kidney, Virchows Arch. (Cell Pathol.), 18, 243, 1975.

8.   Dobyan, D.C., Levi, J., Jacobs, C., Kosek, J. and Weiner, M.W., Mechanism of cis-platinum nephrotoxicity: II. Morphological observations, J. Pharmacol. Exp. Ther., 235, 551, 1980.

9.   Eknoyan, G., Bulger, R.E. and Dobyan, D.C., Mercuric chloride-induced acute renal failure in the rat. I. Correlation of functional and morphological changes and their modification by clonidine, Lab. Invest., 46, 613, 1982.

10. Haley, D.P., Bulger, R.E. and Dobyan, D.C., The long-term effects of uranyl nitrate on the structure and function of the rat kidney, Virchows Arch. B. Cell Pathol. Molec. Pathol., 41, 181, 1982.

11. Choie, D.D., Longnecker, D.S. and delCampo, A.A., Acute and chronic cisplatin nephrotoxicity in rats, Lab. Invest., 44, 397, 1981.

12. Chopra, S., Kaufman, J.S., Jones, T.W., Hong, W.K., Gehr, M.K., Hamburger, R.J., Flamenbaum, W. and Trump, B.F., Cis-diamminedichloro-platinum-induced acute renal failure in the rat, Kidney Int., 21, 54, 1982.

13. Kosek, J.C., Mazze, R.I. and Cousins, M.J., Nephrotoxicity of gentamicin, Lab. Invest., 30, 48, 1974.

14. Porter, G.A. and Bennett, W.M., Nephrotoxic acute renal failure due to common drugs, Am. J. Physiol., 241, F1, 1981.

15. Dobyan, D.C., Smith, C.V., Mitchell, J.R. and Bulger, R.E., Heterogeneous proximal tubule (PT) injury produced by 6-OH-DOPA, in Renal Heterogeneity and Target Cell Toxicity, Bach, P. and Lock, E.A., Eds., John Wiley and Sons, Chichester, 1985, 43

16. Byrnes, K.A., Ghidoni, J.J. and Mayfield, E.D., Response of the rat kidney to folic acid administration. II. Morphologic studies, Lab. Invest., 26, 184, 1972.

17. Gloor, F.J., Changing concepts in pathogenesis and morphology of analgesic nephropathy as seen in Europe, Kidney Int., 13, 27, 1978.

18. Dobyan, D.C. and Bulger, R.E., Partial protection by chlorpromazine in mercuric chloride-induced acute renal failure in rats, Lab. Invest., 50, 578, 1984.

19. Eknoyan, G., Senekjian, H.O., Bulger, R.E. and Dobyan, D.C., Functional and morphological correlates of protection from gentamicin (G) nephrotoxicity by oral clonidine in the rat, Kidney Int., 23, 203, 1983.

20. Solez, K., D'Agostini, R.J., Stowowy, L., Freedman, M.T., Scott, W.W., Jr., Siegelman, S.S. and Heptinstall, R.H., Beneficial effect of propranolol in a histologically appropriate model of post-ischemic acute renal failure, Am. J. Pathol., 88, 163, 1977.

21. Solez, K., Morel-Maroger, L. and Sraer, J.D., The morphology of "acute tubular necrosis" in man: Analysis of 57 renal biopsies and a comparison with the glycerol model, Medicine, 58, 362, 1979.

22. Kourilsky, O., Solez, K., Morel-Maroger, L., Whelton, A., Duhoux, P. and Sraer, J.D., The pathology of acute renal failure due to interstitial nephritis in man with comments on the role of interstitial inflammation and sex in gentamicin nephrotoxicity, Medicine, 61, 258, 1982.

23. Richards, C.J. and DiBona, G.F., Acute renal failure: Structural-functional correlation, Proc. Soc. Exp. Biol. Med., 146, 880, 1974.

24. Solez, K. and Finckh, E.S., Is there a correlation between morphologic and functional changes in human acute renal failure? in Acute Renal Failure.

Correlations Between Morphology and Function, Solez, K., and Whelton, A., Eds., Marcel Dekker, New York, 1984, 3.

25. Dobyan, D.C., Cronin, R.E. and Bulger, R.E., Effect of potassium depletion on tubular morphology in gentamicin-induced acute renal failure in dogs, Lab. Invest., 47, 586, 1982.

26. Weibel, E.R., Kistler, G.S. and Scherle, W.R., Practical stereological methods for morphometric cytology, J. Cell Biol., 30, 23, 1966.

27. Dobyan, D.C., Long term consequences of cis-platinum-induced renal injury: A structural and functional study, Anat Rec., 212, 239, 1985.

28. Blantz, R.C., The mechanism of acute renal failure after uranyl nitrate, J. Clin. Invest., 55, 621, 1975.

29. Baylis, C., Rennke, H.R. and Brenner, B.M., Mechanisms of the defect in glomerular ultrafiltration associated with gentamicin administration, Kidney Int., 1, 344, 1977.

30. Schor, N., Ichikawa, I., Rennke, H.G., Troy, J.L. and Brenner, B.M., Pathophysiology of altered glomerular function in aminoglycoside-treated rats, Kidney Int., 1, 344, 1981.

31. Williams, R.H., Thomas, C.E., Navar, L.G. and Evan, A.P., Hemodynamic and single nephron function during the maintenance phase of ischemic acute renal failure in the dog, Kidney Int., 19, 503, 1981.

32. Cox, J.W., Baehler, R.W., Sharma, H., O'Dousio, T., Osgood, R.W., Stein, J.H. and Ferris, T.F., Studies on the mechanism of oliguria in a model of unilateral acute renal failure, J. Clin. Invest., 53, 1564, 1974.

33. Stein, J.H., Gottschall, J., Osgood, R.W. and Ferris, T.F., Pathophysiology of a nephrotoxic model of acute renal failure, Kidney Int., 8, 27, 1975.

34. Flamenbaum, W., Hamburger, R.J., Huddleston, M.L., Kaufman, J., McNeil, J.S., Schwartz, J.H. and Nagle, R., The initiation phase of experimental acute renal failure: An evaluation of uranyl-nitrate-induced acute renal failure in the rat, Kidney Int., 10, S115, 1976.

35. Barnes, J.L., Osgood, R.W., Reineck, H.J. and Stein, J.H., Glomerular alterations in an ischemic model of acute renal failure, Lab. Invest., 45, 378, 1981.

36. Solez, K., Ideura, T., Silvia, C.B., Hamilton, B. and Saito, H., Clonidine after renal ischemia to lessen acute renal failure and microvascular damage, Kidney Int., 18, 309, 1980.

37. Racusen, L.C., Prozialeck, D.H. and Solez, K., Glomerular epithelial cell changes after ischemia or dehydration. Possible role of angiotensin II. Am. J. Pathol., 114, 157, 1984.

38. Racusen, L.C. and Solez, K., Podocyte changes in post-ischemic ARF, in Acute Renal Failure. Correlations Between Morphology and Function, Solez, K., and Whelton, A., Eds., Marcel Dekker, 1984, 134.

39. Myers, W.D., Langlinais, P. and Merrill, R.H., Glomerular alterations by scanning electron microscopy in acute renal insufficiency in man, Kidney Int., 12, 531A, 1977.

40. Dobyan, D.C., Nagle, R.B. and Bulger, R.E., Acute tubular necrosis in the rat kidney following sustained hypotension. Physiologic and morphologic observations, Lab. Invest., 37, 411, 1977.

41. Cronin, R.E., DeTorrente, A., Miller, P.D., Bulger, R.E., Burke, T.J. and Schrier, R.W., Pathogenic mechanisms in early norepinephrine-induced acute renal failure: Functional and histological correlates of protection, Kidney Int., 14, 115, 1978.

42. Baehler, R.W., Kotchen, T.A., Burke, J.A., Galla, J.H. and Bhathena, D., Considerations of the pathophysiology of mercuric chloride-induced acute renal failure, J. Lab. Clin. Med., 90, 330, 1977.

43.   Zager, R.A., Baltes, L.A., Sharma, H.M. and Couser, W.G., Glomerulopathy does not increase renal susceptibility to acute ischemic injury, Am. J. Physiol., 246, F272, 1984.

44.   Bulger, R.E. and Dobyan, D.C., Morphological techniques for the study of the kidney, in Methods in Pharmacology, Vol. 4B, Martinez-Maldonado, M., Ed. Plenum Press, New York, 1978, 1.

45.   Bulger, R.E., Cronin, R.E. and Dobyan, D.C., Glomerular architectural changes after a two-hour infusion of norepinephrine, Am. J. Anat., 159, 379, 1980.

46.   Tanaka, K., Freezed resin cracking method for scanning electron microscopy of biological materials, Naturwissenschaften, 2, 77, 1972.

47.   Bulger, R.E., Eknoyan, G., Purcell, D. and Dobyan, D.C., Endothelial characteristics of glomerular capillaries in normal, mercuric chloride-induced and gentamicin-induced acute renal failure in the rat, J. Clin. Invest., 72, 128, 1983.

6
NATURALLY OCCURRING RENAL DISEASE IN NON-HUMAN PRIMATES

P.N. SKELTON-STROUD AND J.R. GLAISTER

INTRODUCTION

Non-human primates have a long established place in biomedical research and have contributed much valuable and useful data for comparison with that derived from man. The popularity of non-human primates for research has been based upon them being members of the same order as man, with many similarities in anatomy, physiology and metabolism, psychological and reproductive behaviour, immunology and also their susceptibility to a wide range of human diseases[1-8].

The kidney is of particular interest in non-human primates used as animal models for spontaneous disease syndromes in man, and also for predictive toxicology. The models of disease include pyelonephritis, nephrocalcinosis, immune complex glomerulonephritis, congenital malformations, hypospadia, hydronephrosis of pregnancy, leptospirosis, psychogenic polyuria/polydipsia, vesicoureteral reflux, malaria and schistosomiasis[7,9-11]. To this comprehensive list must now be added those of kidney transplant surgery with its associated procedures[12,13].

In toxicology the primary concern is with the identification of the substances which exert a detrimental effect upon the normal physiological function of the kidneys. In such nephrotoxicity studies in non-human primates it is necessary to know the range, incidence and severity of macroscopic and histological lesions that may be encountered, and which may confound the interpretation of chemically induced lesions. This is particularly important in view of the low numbers of primates used when compared to other species of laboratory animals such as the rat.

There has been little comprehensive information published which has dealt specifically with non-human primate kidney pathology[14]. Only a few incidental comments had been made on early zoological cases before Fox reported on non-human primate material as part of a more general survey on mammalian kidney pathology. He observed not only an incidence of 20% kidney disease at necropsies of apes, but that monkeys with uraemia showed signs similar to those seen in man[15,16]. Several more recent reports on monkey kidney pathology have each dealt with a diversity of species and ages. Although some described a high incidence of pathological findings, significant kidney disease was found only in some surveys, and in particular species. In toxicology the majority of animals, whether wild-caught or laboratory bred, are usually immature or young adults, and background pathology is relatively minor in most instances. However, more substantial lesions are occasionally encountered and these are included in this review.

ANATOMY

The anatomical position of the kidneys can vary between species. In Old World monkeys (Papio, Macaque, Erythrocebus and Cercopithecus spp.) the right kidney is situated more cranially than the left one[5,17]. In the marmoset a variety of positions - either cranially, level or caudally - may be found. Individual variations exist among anthropoid apes. In man the right kidney is commonly situated caudal to the left kidney. The paired adrenal glands are positioned in close proximity to the kidneys and can be found either in contact with the cranial pole or sometimes slightly towards the medial side[17]. This arrangement can be involved in adrenorenal ectopism which has been seen in Old World monkeys[18-20].

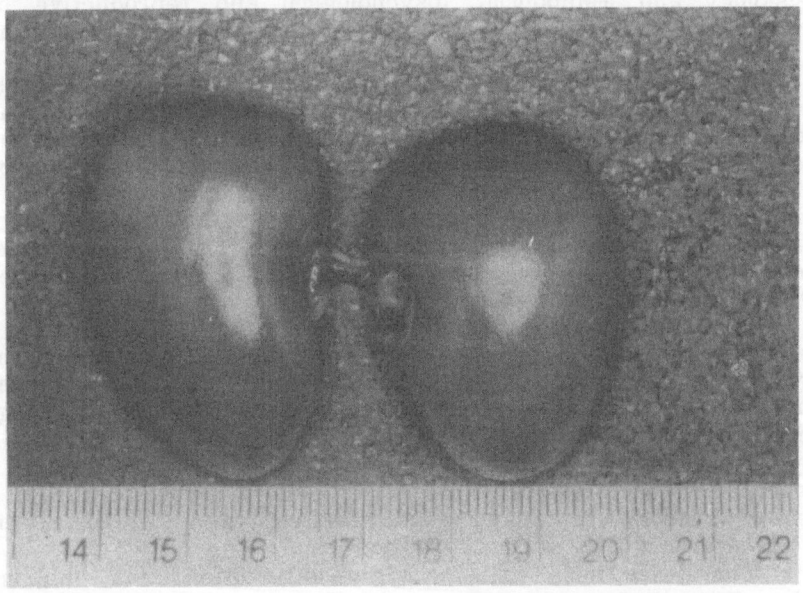

Figure 1 Kidneys from an immature baboon. The outline and surfaces (capsules removed) are smooth and show no evidence of lobulation (x0.7)

190

In their external appearance the kidneys of man are singular among primates in showing definite external lobulation at the fetal stage and also at birth[17]. In other species the kidneys are smooth (Figure 1). This is certainly so in adult baboons (Papio spp.) rhesus (Macaca mulatta) and cynomolgus (Macaca fascicularis) monkeys, and also in marmosets (Callithrix jacchus). The presence of lobulation, however limited, gives no indication of specific internal structures in any primate, and is entirely superficial[21]. This is in contrast to the deeply lobulated kidneys of other mammals such as the cow, bear, elephant, otter and rhinoceros. The most important feature in any comparison of human and monkey kidneys is that of internal structure. Only man and the spider monkey (Ateles spp.) possess multipyramidal kidneys and have a true renal pelvis that is divided into proper calyxes[22]. In man several papillae are commonly present. In spider monkeys only two or three may be found. The formation of primary pyramids is also more clearly defined in man. All other non-human primates are unipyramidal, like the dog and the rat. There is further variation in the form of the single pyramid in monkeys and apes. Some show a papilla and others have divisions into papillary ridges[17].

Little information is available on the relative areas of the cortex and medulla in different primate species. In man the cortex is relatively thin. In baboons the ratio of cortex to the medulla is approximately equal[21]. More glomeruli are found in the outer cortex in man, with the largest glomeruli in the inner cortex adjoining the medulla. This is similar in almost all non-human primate species irrespective of age[17]. Reductions in the number of glomeruli with increasing age occur in both man and monkeys[23,24].

CONGENITAL ABNORMALITIES

These are generally uncommon in non-human primates and only a few different types have been reported[25]. These include unilateral hypoplasia or aplasia, double ureters, cystic conditions, ectopic adrenal foci within kidney tissue, and a single case of renal fusion with ectopy and aberrant blood vessels[26-35].

Aplasia or hypoplasia has been reported at a very low incidence, usually single examples, among a wide range of species. Some were accompanied by other minor morphological alterations which generally affected the ureter. Compensatory hypertrophy and hyperplasia of the remaining kidney was normally observed in both rhesus monkeys and baboons but not in a single incidence in an adult female langur nor in baboons following unilateral nephrectomy[1,28]. No examples of bilateral hypoplasia, however slight, have been reported. The unusual case of renal fusion and ectopy in a squirrel monkey (Saimiri sciurea) showed the mass located at the bifurcation of the abdominal aorta and supplied by a single large artery[29]. Double ureters were found on one kidney of an otherwise normal rhesus monkey, but without hydronephrosis[36]. Unilateral hydronephrosis and ureter distension were seen, however, together with contralateral hypertrophy in an adult male Cercopithecus[28].

Single cysts have been found in many different monkey

191

species[17,20-26,35-39]. Again the reported incidence is low when considering the numbers of non-human primates used in biomedical research. Cysts in juvenile or older animals may be seen macroscopically at necropsy as transparent, pale or dark subcapsular lesions containing pale or dark fluid[20,36]. They usually vary in size from 2 to 10 mm and can be solitary or multiple, although large single cysts 26 mm by 35 mm replaced the entire kidney in two separate individual cases in lemurs[25,26]. Microscopically the smaller cysts contain a pale granular eosinophilic fluid, are lined by flattened and attenuated epithelium and compress adjacent tissue (Figure 2). Significant inflammatory infiltrates are not usual[36]. Cysts are generally unilocular and are of no consequence in toxicology. A familial cause due to inbreeding was suggested by a high incidence of small cortical cysts in a batch of chacma baboons (Papio ursinus) caught from the wild in a particular area of South Africa[38]. Such a cause was again suggested by an incidence of cysts in five yellow baboons (Papio cynocephalus) from a group of 68 animals[35].

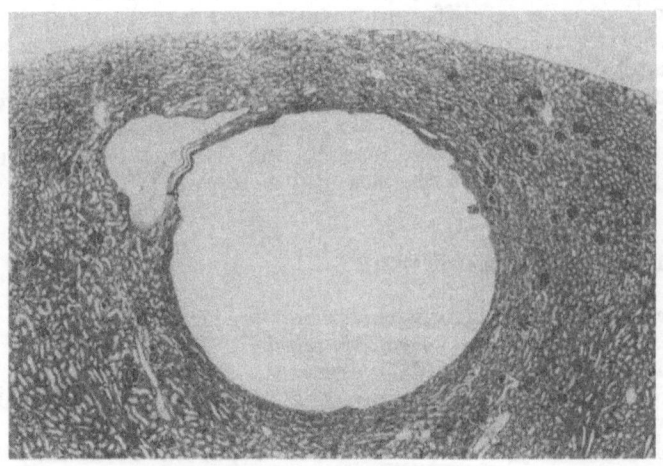

Figure 2 Cysts in the outer cortex were seen at necropsy as small dark fluid-filled foci. Some compression of adjacent tissue is present (x5).

A more severe infantile polycystic disease, similar to that seen as both hereditary and congenital in man, has been reported in an infant rhesus monkey which died shortly after birth[40]. Kidney pathology was characterized by bilateral enlargement, abnormal shape and multiple small cysts throughout the parenchyma. A polycystic condition was also described in a pregnant adult pigtailed macaque (Macaca nemestrina), in which the unequally enlarged and irregular kidneys showed cysts in both cortex and medulla. The fluid-filled cysts were multilocular, varied in size from 1 mm to 2 cm and occupied 50% of the parenchyma[29]. A further instance of adult polycystic change occurred in a 16 year old male rhesus, where the combination of clinical signs and pathological changes closely resembled a specific type of polycystic disease seen in man[41].

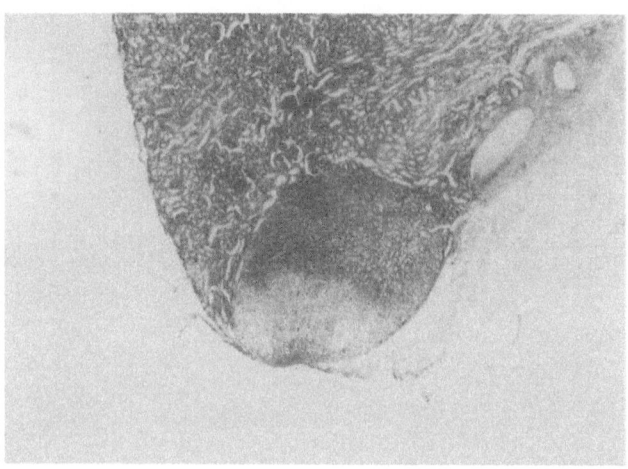

Figure 3 Ectopic adrenal cortical tissue in a kidney from an immature baboon (x5).

The adrenal glands develop in close proximity to the kidneys and ectopic adrenal tissue may be found closely adjacent to the outer kidney capsule or beneath it in the parenchyma (Figure 3)[18-20]. Such ectopic adrenal rests have been reported at an incidence of 1 in 600 (0.16%) in rhesus monkeys[19]. A single focus also in a rhesus monkey contained cells from the three zones of the adrenal cortex and reacted like the adrenal gland proper following treatment with an antimalarial drug[18]. In baboons an incidence of 2 in 504 (0.4%) has been found[20]. Such foci are often visible at necropsy as pale circular flat or slightly raised nodular areas from 1 mm to 5 mm in size. Microscopically they can contain cells from any of the three zones of adrenal cortical tissue. No cells from the adrenal medulla have been found. Foci are usually solitary, but a few separate foci in the same kidney may be seen occasionally.

VASCULAR LESIONS

As in man, these are usually found in older animals and are generally infrequent in the younger non-human primates used in toxicological studies. However, a proliferative arteriopathy found in the kidneys of a few macaque monkeys during such an investigation was a good example of the way in which a background lesion with a sporadic incidence can confound the interpretation of particular toxicity studies[42],[43]. The arteriopathy was characterized by eccentric nodular thickening in disorientated proliferating cells (Figure 4).

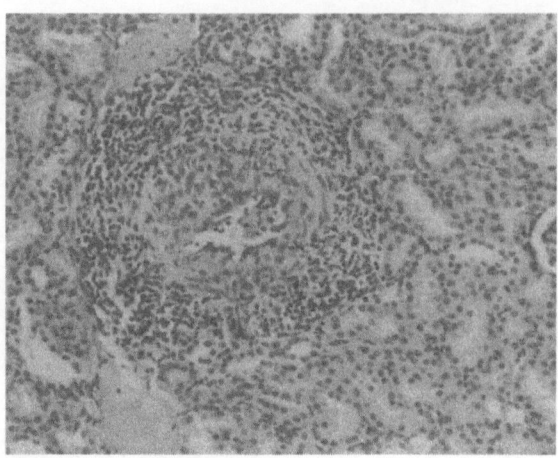

Figure 4 Proliferative arteriopathy with surrounding mononuclear cell infiltrates occurs spontaneously in macaque monkeys (x27). (Material kindly provided by J. E. Beach).

Such cells were seen to extend through the thickness of the vessel wall from the endothelium to the tunica adventitia, and the latter often contained a generally mononuclear cell infiltrate. In a few cases the lesions were not restricted to the kidneys. Confirmation that this was a background lesion was given by identification of the same arterial change in untreated control monkeys. They had been used in a series of studies related to this particular test substance. It was also found in macaque monkeys from several different locations used in entirely unrelated studies, and also in some untreated stock animals. The incidence rates of 19 in 161 (11.8%) in treated animals and 5 in 103 (4.8%) in control animals in the particular studies and of 14 in 2000 (0.7%) in unrelated monkeys demonstrated the sporadic nature of the lesion. Yet further evidence that this type of lesion was restricted to macaque monkeys occurred more recently. A chronic renal proliferative arteriopathy with similar histological changes was seen in three wild-born and two colony-born pigtailed macaques, an incidence of 0.7%. Lesions were generally segmental, but in one instance they were diffuse, and were also present in both splenic and cardiac arteries in addition to the kidneys. No relationship with altered haemodynamics such as ischaemia, infarction or hypertension was established, nor with any immunological alterations, veterinary medical procedures or experimental procedures. Whilst prior exposure to either toxic or infectious factors has been suggested, the precise cause still remains unknown[42,43].

Arteriosclerosis occurs naturally in non-human primates but lesions are generally rare in kidney vessels[44,45]. The arcuate vessels of two old marmosets showed arteriosclerosis in a group of six animals that died from a "wasting syndrome". The vascular changes were considered unrelated to the cause of death[46]. In a small number of old monkeys, four sacred baboons (Papio hamadryas) and one rhesus monkey, renal arterial sclerosis accompanied sclerotic changes in the abdominal aorta. The kidneys of these animals also showed pronounced nephrosclerosis[24]. A single case together with hydronephrosis was found in an unspecified species of monkey and eight out of 150 (5.3%) wild-caught rhesus monkeys (ranging from 1 to 6 years old) showed vascular changes suggestive of arteriosclerosis; but no hypertension was recorded[36,47]. A 4% incidence of renal arteriosclerosis was noted in wild-caught chacma baboons, and lesions were also found in the heart and aorta[39].

GLOMERULAR LESIONS

As with other kidney lesions glomerular pathology has been seen in many different monkey species and age ranges, and has been associated with ageing, infectious and immune phenomena. The severity of glomerular change ranged from solitary minor lesions to extensive forms of glomerulonephritis, although the latter is rare in the species commonly used in toxicity studies. In these younger animals solitary hyalinized and sclerosed glomeruli can sometimes be found randomly scattered throughout the cortex at a low incidence, for example in immature yellow baboons (Figure 5), and also in owl monkeys (Aotus trivirgatus)[35,48]. These minor lesions commonly increase in numbers and intensity with age[11,24,49].

A comparable increased severity with age has been described in pigtailed macaques. Similar glomerular and vascular changes can also be seen in man and are again closely related to ageing, and in a study on ageing in the non-human primate some 10/20 pigtailed macaques ranging from 4 to 20 years old showed evidence of glomerulonephritis[33]. It was minimal to moderate, mesangioproliferative, and was most pronounced in the oldest animal. In a retrospective study of 340 wild-born and 334 colony-born monkeys of the same species, 58 individuals showed similar glomerular lesions. In 16 of 53 adults (30%) it was considered the more advanced changes could have resulted in renal failure. Similarly in 28 out of 113 (24%) pigtailed macaques, the glomerular lesions were considered severe enough to have caused detectable kidney malfunction in five animals. The two most severe cases could have been the cause of death[49]. In one group comprising four sacred baboons and one rhesus monkey with severely wrinkled kidney surfaces, histologically pronounced glomerularsclerosis and hyalinization were accompanied by small cysts, increased connective tissue and renal arterio sclerosis. One of these animals was a 31-year-old female baboon, and it is unlikely that animals of such great age or with such severe changes would ever be encountered in routine toxicological studies.

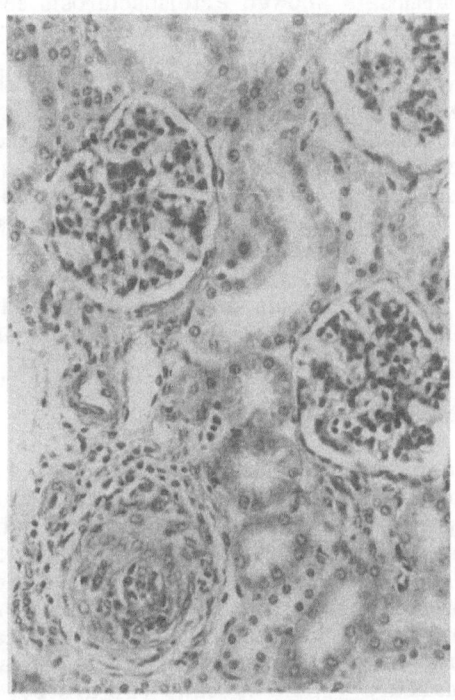

Figure 5 A solitary sclerotic glomerulus adjacent to two normal glomeruli. Baboon kidney (x43).

Glomerular changes are not, however, restricted to aged monkeys alone, and several spontaneous cases of glomerulonephritis have been found, particularly in New World species. In prosimians the most common types of glomerulonephritis were proliferative and membranoproliferative[51,52]. In the former there was hypercellularity of the tuft, crescent formation in varying sizes of tuft and adhesions. There was also tubular abnormality ranging from hydropic change to atrophy and cyst formation. In the membrano proliferative cases thickened basement membranes of tubules and glomeruli accompanied the increased mesangium in the swollen tufts[51]. Glomerulonephritis is common in owl monkeys, a New World species, where a related incidence with interstitial nephritis was established in 87 animals with haemolytic anaemia[48]. In squirrel monkeys of differing ages from both sexes 12 of 38 (31%) adult female animals showed evidence of glomerulonephritis and it was present in seven out of 36 (19%) males at the termination of a diet study[53]. Glomerular changes were considered to be secondary in several marmosets with the "wasting syndrome"[46].

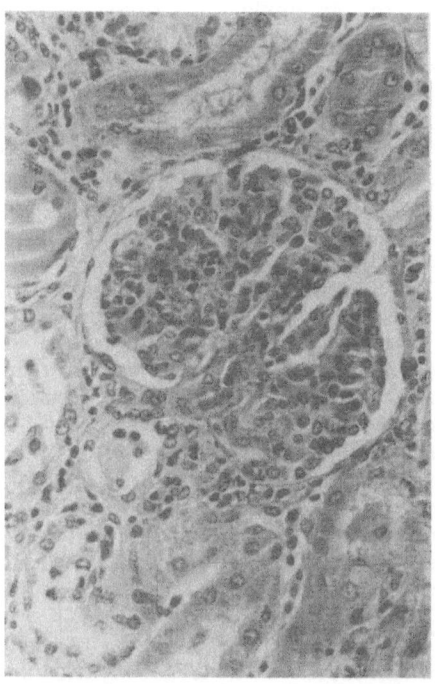

Figure 6 Proliferative glomerulonephritis in a baboon with septicaemia (x68).

Various causes have been suggested for non-human primate glomerulonephritis, such as bacterial and parasitic infections and related immune phenomena. In Old World monkeys membrano-proliferative and mesangioproliferative glomerulonephritis occurred in baboons associated with chronic infection with various bacteria following repeated or indwelling intravenous catheterization[54,55]. Staphylococcus aureus, Herellea, Streptoccoci, Klebsiella and Providencia spp. were isolated from these cases. Varying amounts of complement and immunoglobulins were identified in different in-dividuals within the capillaries and mesangium. Histological changes ranged from increased mesangial cells and matrix to crescent forma-tion, synechia, sclerosis of Bowman's capsule and generally reduced capillary patency. Tubular degeneration and atrophy some-times accompanied such glomerular lesions. A similar histological picture in a rhesus monkey suggested that it too was of bacterial origin. It displayed signs of the nephrotic syndrome and was comparable to the severe changes seen in one baboon study[54,56]. Septic embolic glomerulonephritis, again in baboons, was seen in young animals with systemic bacterial infections, and revealed complement and immunoglobulin at similar sites[49]. Another case with Salmonella septicaemia could have been similar to the varied bacterial infections identified in baboons, in which an immune-mediated response to bacteria resulted in immune complex deposition[51,54,55]. Similarly the septic emboli in baboons resulted in IgG and B_{1c} deposition, and in IgA, IgM, IgG and complement deposition in the catheterized baboons[49,54]. Septicaemia and anti-genaemia from enterocolitis or from other suppurative foci were considered as part of the pathogenesis of renal lesions in pigtailed macaques[51]. In a chimpanzee (Pan spp.) a marked diffuse bilateral case of glomerulonephritis was considered to be postinfective as is often seen in man[58]. Experimentally, muramyl dipeptide administration in baboons resulted in mesangioproliferative glomerulonephritis, in addition to lesions in other organs[59]. These closely resembled changes seen in septicaemia (Figure 6) and supported the involvement of bacterial antigenic stimulation as a prime cause of the glomerular pathology. This would agree with the mechanisms in which the "nominal" presence of immune complex present normally in the glomerulus is continually cleared, but may have stimulated the mesangium to proliferative activity[23].

Parasites are common in wild-caught monkeys, but their role as aetiological agents in glomerulonephritis is unclear. Parasitic infections, particularly those of Plasmodium brasilianum or filarial nematodes were considered to be possible causes for glomerulonephritis in owl monkeys, although a familial predisposition was also noted[53]. Malarial infections in man may result in glomerulonephritis due to immune complex deposition in severe cases. In baboons infected with Hepatocystis kochi, a common malarial parasite, no cases of glomerulonephritis have been associated with this protozoal organism[35]. Similarly, no association with Plasmodium cynomolgi and glomerular pathology has been reported in macaque monkeys. Glomerular changes consisting of immunoglobulin deposition have been found in some species irrespective of the presence of patent parasitic infections. Experimental infection of baboons with ova of Schistosoma spp. showed no significant differences in kidney pathology when compared to controls[11].

It was uncertain whether the immune complex deposition identified in pigtailed macaques was related to various combinations of infections, environmental or genetic background[33]. Immune complex deposition has also been suggested in galagos, possibly associated with infected skin wounds or intestinal protozoal parasites[52]. Autoimmune mechanisms have been suggested in owl monkeys[48,57]. Finally, in a 5-week-old galago (Galago crassicaudatus panganiensis) a congenital origin, but unknown cause, was suggested[51].

TUBULOINTERSTITIAL LESIONS

These range from minor foci of leucocyte infiltration to chronic pyelonephritis. Interstitial nephritis is the most common inflammatory renal lesion seen in many animals including non-human primates[60]. Cellular infiltrates are predominantly lymphocytic, are found mainly in the cortex and are usually of a mild degree. Such infiltrates were noted in 284 out of 456 marmosets (62%) with similar infiltrates present in other tissues, e.g. the heart and liver of the same animal[34]. Among laboratory maintained baboons incidences of 38% and 42% have been reported (Figure 7)[20,61].

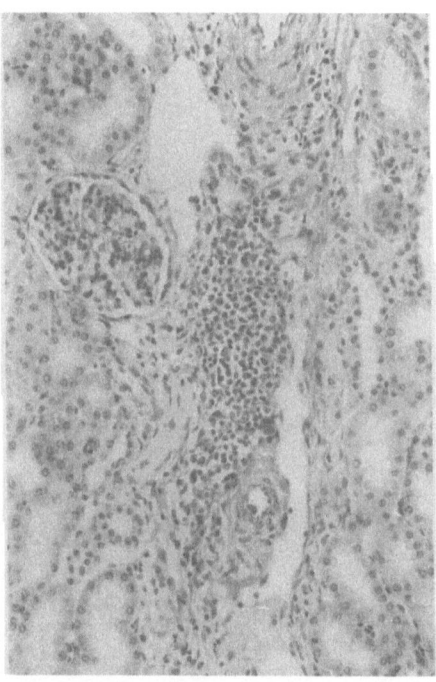

Figure 7 Minor focal lymphocytic infiltrates are common in non-human primates in the kidneys and other major organs (x27).

Trace to minimal focal lymphocytic infiltrates have also been seen at an incidence of 40 in 446 (9%) in the pelvic epithelium in immature baboons (Figure 8)[20]. It rarely progresses and has not been reported elsewhere. In other baboons, ranging in age from 1 day to over 10 years old, interstitial infiltrates occurred in 16 of 18 (89%) normal animals[49]. The infiltrates were mixed, contained plasma cells and neutrophils, and were accompanied by minor focal tubular epithelial damage. Detected only at microscopic examination they were classified as early pyelonephritis or interstitial nephritis. Interstitial infiltrates described as subacute interstitial nephritis were found around or adjacent to the arcuate arteries in adult wild-caught chacma baboons at an incidence of 24 in 100 (24%)[39].

In more animals of the same species the mainly lymphocytic infiltrates were present around Bowman's capsule and the collecting tubules, and were described as non-suppurative nephritis[62]. The incidence in the kidneys was 8.6% and in the heart and liver 6.7%. A viral cause was suggested. In four prosimian monkeys such infiltrates were diffuse and present together with tubular atrophy, cysts and some interstitial fibrosis[51]. Similar changes have been seen in a few galagos, where they coincided with glomerulonephritis[52].

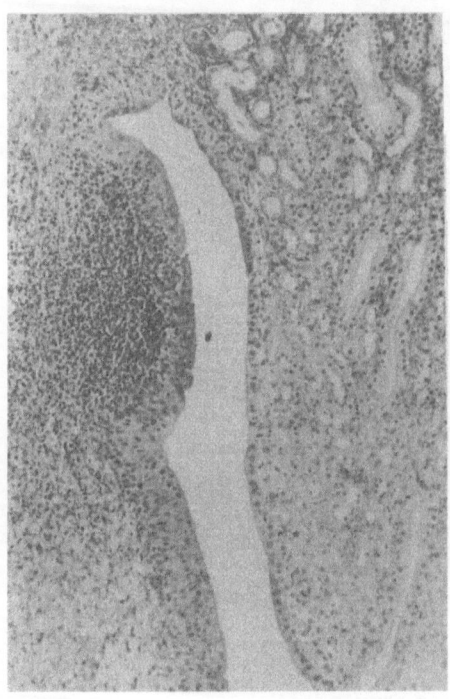

Figure 8 Minimal focal chronic pyelitis in a baboon. The inflammatory infiltrate is lymphocytic and was unilateral in this instance (x22).

An equal incidence of interstitial infiltrates and glomerulonephritis was found in owl monkeys, and a relationship suggested between haemolytic anaemia and the interstitial component[48]. Chronic tubulointerstitial disease was described in the subpelvic and corticomedullary areas in marmosets with "wasting disease"[46], but infiltrates also occurred in other animals dying from different causes which, with fibrosis and interstitial mineralization, led to nephrosclerosis. Infiltrates and mild fibrosis were common in chimpanzees[58]. In pigtailed macaques mild subacute to chronic interstitial nephritis, together with some fibrosis and tubular atrophy, were noted in 37 of 674 (5.4%) monkeys[33].

The natural incidence of pyelonephritis was investigated from a total of 590 necropsies of a wide range of both New and Old World monkeys and apes[47]. Chronic pyelonephritis occurred at a level of 0.65%, which was comparable to that found in man. It is generally an uncommon infection of non-human primates, but has been reported in several species: 7 of 674 (1.0%) macaques, over 50% of 44 squirrel monkeys where it was often accompanied by nephrocalcinosis, 1 of 22 (4.5%) prosimians, from 3 of 36 (8%) to 3 of 446 (0.6%) baboons, and 7 cases in owl monkeys[20,33,43,51,53,63,64]. The overall incidence is therefore quite low.

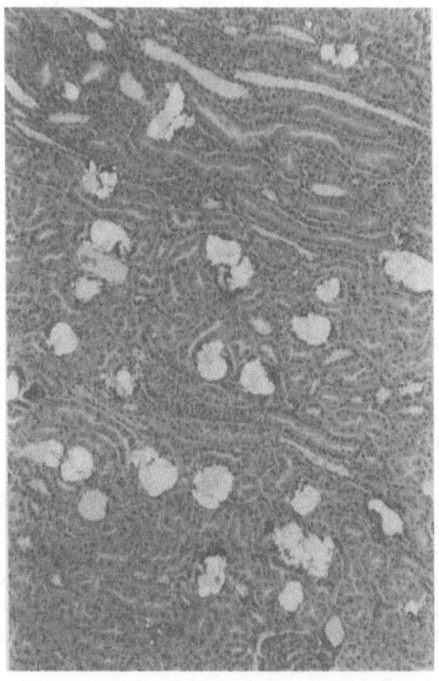

Figure 9 Intratubular oxalate crystals in a monkey were thought to be related to diet (x27).

Tuberculosis, although uncommon, is undoubtedly the most serious infection that can occur in non-human primates. Considerable preventive effort is devoted to keeping this organism out of non-human primate facilities. A recent outbreak identified Mycobacterium intracellulare (serotype 10) in two of 90 (2.2%)

rhesus monkeys. Lesions in the kidneys are generally rare, but granulomas were found in the kidneys in this instance as well as in other organs. Organisms were later isolated from the drinking water[65].

Lesions primarily involving the tubule rather than the interstitium are occasionally encountered, and may be related to therapy, stress or diet.

Antibiotic treatment for persistent diarrhoea was held responsible for nephrosis seen in 88 of 674 (13%) pigtailed macaques. It affected the proximal tubules, and concentration of the antibiotic due to dehydration was suggested as part of the pathogenesis. Non-human primates used in biomedical studies should be clinically healthy before investigations commence, and careful consideration should be given to clinical history and any previous veterinary medical treatment. Other cases of nephrosis in the same colony were ascribed to either trauma or septicaemia. In wild-caught chacma baboons examined from a field survey five of 100 (5%) showed tubular nephrosis characterized by hyaline granular casts or myoglobinuric casts. Another single example of nephrosis with myoglobin casts, again in a baboon, was comparable to the cases noted in the field survey, and the stress either of capture or of other violent procedures suggested as a causative factor[33,49]. Another individual instance in a baboon showed calcium oxalate crystals in the interstitium thought to be related to diet. Similar crystals were also seen in both tubules (Figure 9) and interstitium of the same species of baboon, together with foreign body chronic inflammatory reactions[35,38]. The same relationship to diet was suggested for 20 of 674 (3%) pigtailed macaques with oxalate crystals present within the tubules of the cortex and medulla[33].

MISCELLANEOUS LESIONS

There are several miscellaneous lesions that may be encountered. They occur only sporadically and include; mineralization, amyloidosis, lipidosis, multinucleate epithelial cells, inclusions, acquired cysts, cytomegalovirus, parasites and neoplasia.

The presence of small foci of mineralization in the interstitium of the medulla, mainly in the papilla, is common in non-human primates as in other animal species[60,66]. Such foci are found only at microscopic examination and are easily identified with routine haematoxylin and eosin staining. There are no accompanying inflammatory changes (Figure 10). These minor foci are of no routine significance, and are so common as to seldom deserve comment. From a total of 590 necropsies of different monkey species which showed 46 cases of renal disease, mineralization was found in 18 individuals (39%)[47]. Other reported incidences in baboons range from 6 in 100 (6%) to 18 in 100 (18%) and of 19 in 674 (2.8%) in pigtailed macaques[33,39,61]. Mineralization appears to be common in squirrel monkeys, a high incidence of 86% having been found in some wild-caught animals[67,68]. An equally high incidence of 144 in 169 (85%) was found in monkeys of the same species, and varied from minor focal deposits to pelvic urolithiasis[53]. Such mineraliz-

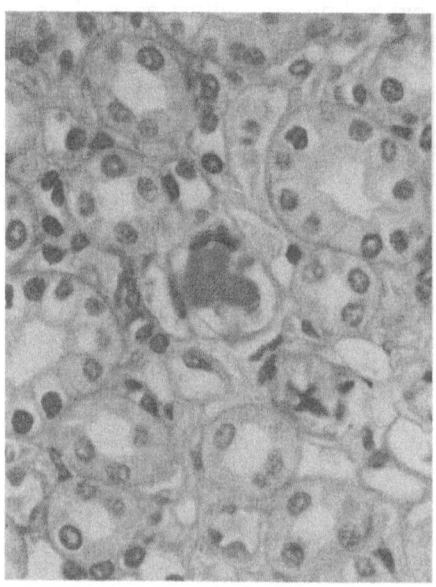

Figure 10 Interstitial focal mineralization is common in the renal medulla in many non-human primates (x54).

ation was found in wild-born, colony-born and stillborn infant squirrel monkeys. The incidence of pelvic urolithiasis in this survey was only 1%, thus confirming its earlier reported rarity[53,60]. Dystrophic mineralization is a non-specific response to tissue damage, and can occur with inflammatory states such as bacterial or parasitic infections. Nephrocalcinosis has been frequently found accompanying pyelonephritis in squirrel monkeys[42].

Non-human primates have been used as models for nephrocalcinosis by feeding diets unbalanced in magnesium and phosphorus[69]. Although the exact process of formation is not fully understood, ionic imbalance is involved. Studies of calcium metabolism in monkeys show more similarities to man than either rat or dog[70].

Amyloidosis has not been seen in immature baboons by the authors and only few cases in monkeys have been found. These have involved the kidneys in three baboons, a squirrel monkey, a single unspecified monkey, a rhesus and 13 pigtailed macaques[33,47,71-73]. This is a low total reported incidence. Tubular lipidosis possibly resulting from sudden anorexia was found in 28 of 674 (4%) pigtailed macaques; all of which were adult wild-born monkeys[33].

Multinucleated cells in the collecting ducts of immature baboons are common (Figure 11). No inclusions have been identified, and the clusters of nuclei within enlarged epithelial cells are easily identified by light microscopy. Binucleated cells are found in baboon renal pelvic epithelium as well as ureter and bladder. Although mammalian urothelium has a very low mitotic index of 0.01% comparable to man, in baboons 92% of cells were diploid[74]. There is a pronounced capacity to respond to focal or more widespread damage such as can be seen in some toxic nephropathies by greatly increased mitotic activity, as much as a 100-fold increase within 72 hours. This could be of importance in assessing histological changes at the papilla tip and in the collecting ducts in instances of nephrotoxicity.

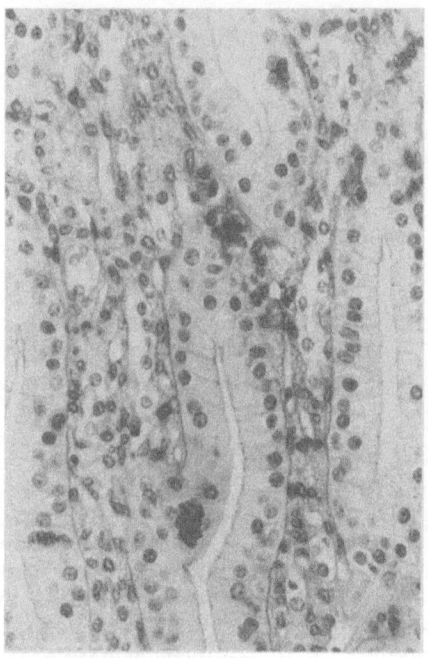

Figure 11 Multinucleate epithelial cells in the collecting ducts of both kidneys of an immature yellow baboon (x65).

In the epithelium of the pelvis, ureter and urinary bladder of both baboons and macaque monkeys, intracytoplasmic inclusions may be seen[35,39,45,75-78]. They are brightly eosinophilic and refractile, are round, oval, or comma-shaped and tend to be larger in the epithelial cells nearer the lumen (Figure 12). Their function and development are unknown. Electron microscopy and histochemistry have shown their structure is of hollow filaments in hexagonal format and composed of abnormally developed tonofilaments of keratin. Clearly they should be differentiated from any simian viruses. They are of no toxicological significance.

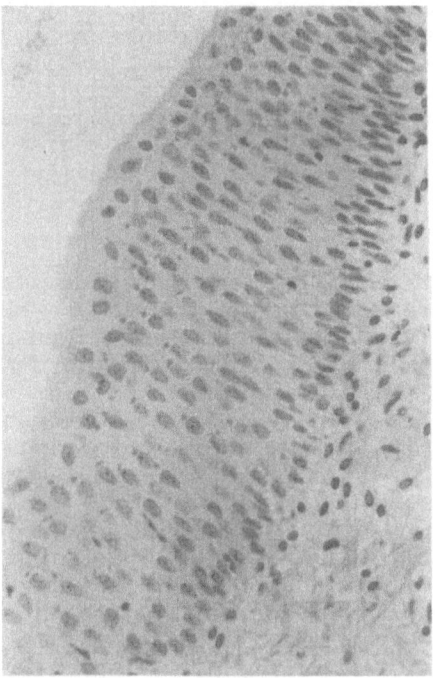

Figure 12 The intracytoplasmic inclusions in the urinary epithelium of baboons and macaques are eosinophilic and refractile (x68).

Cysts, other than those described as congenital, can also be acquired. Occasional solitary or multiple dilated tubules in either cortex or medulla can result from obstruction or inflammation, which in turn can result from infectious or ageing processes.

Cytomegalovirus has been identified in macaque kidneys[33]. Karyomegaly was seen in cortical tubules in baboons with similar change in the liver. No inclusion bodies were found[39]. Changes of a similar nature can be induced by some nephrotoxic substances.

Parasitic nephritis in non-human primates is rare, and only a few instances involving nematodes or protozoa are recorded. In rhesus monkeys aberrant nematode larvae have caused granulomatous lesions in the kidney[60]. The possible involvement of Plasmodium brasilianium in squirrel monkeys should be considered[53]. Geography of catchment areas and subsequent veterinary medical treatment is important in selecting animals for use in toxicity studies.

Only in marmosets has extramedullary haemopoiesis been found in the renal interstitium[34].

Primary renal tumours of non-human primates have been

recently reviewed[79]. A total of 47 tumours have been reported in monkeys whose ages ranged from 1 to 22 years old. The majority of tumours were in members of the macaque species, but this was probably a reflection of their popularity in biomedical research. Overall the reported incidence of primary renal tumours is low when related to the numbers of primates previously used in research, and seen in zoological collections generally. It is unlikely that a tumour would occur in routine non-human primate investigations.

CONCLUSION

Although a diversity of background kidney disease in non-human primates has been described in this chapter it is clear that certain diseases tend to occur in particular species. Both pathologists and toxicologists have to familiarize themselves with the broad patterns of kidney disease in the species they use. For example, glomerulonephritis has been reported most frequently in owl and squirrel monkeys from the New World, and macaques as a species have demonstrated a random proliferative arteriopathy which could prejudice some investigations.

However, if monkeys of good health and known clinical history are available, the reported types and incidences of background kidney disease should not prejudice their use in predictive nephrotoxicity. The background kidney lesions in monkeys used in toxicology are generally infrequent, minor and comparable with that seen in the laboratory rat or dog. It is important, however, that any significant or unusual kidney pathology in non-human primates is reported, so that pathologists have an adequate database of background pathology against which to assess lesions encountered in toxicity studies.

Acknowledgements

The authors are grateful to Mr L. A. P. Brito-Babapulle and Mr C. Sheard for photography, to Mr J. E. Beach for material depicted in Figure 4 and to Miss Christine Beckett for patient typing.

REFERENCES

1. Dicker, S. E. and Morris, C. A., Absence of compensatory hyperplasia in baboons, J. Physiol., 223, 365, 1972.
2. Ruch, T. C., Preface, in Disease of Laboratory Primates, Saunders, Philadelphia, 1959.
3. Kratochvil, C. H., Comparative evaluation of primates for medical research, Ann. N.Y. Acad. Sci., 162 (Art.1), 71, 1969.
4. Lapin, B. A., The rational use of primates in biomedical research, in Pathology of Simian primates, Part 1, T-W-Fiennes, R. N., Ed., Karger, Basel, 2, 1972.
5. Swindler, D. R. and Wood, C. D., An atlas of primate gross anatomy: baboon,

chimpanzee and man, University of Washington Press, Seattle and London, 1973.

6. Goosen, D. J., Dormehl, I. C., du Plessis, D. J. and Walters, L., Nonhuman primates as models for the study of renal physiology and disease, Int. J. Primatol., 3, 287 (0125), 1982.

7. Cornelius, C. E. and Rosenberg, D. P., Nonhuman primates with spontaneous diseases as animal models, Am. J. Med., 74(2), 169, 1983.

8. Letvin, N. L., King, N. W., Daniel, M. D., Aldrich, W. R., Blake, B. J. and Hunt, R. D., Experimental transmission of macaque AIDS by means of inoculation of macaque lymphocyte tissue, Lancet, 2, 599, 1983.

9. Voller, A., Davies, D. R. and Hutt, M. S. R., Quartan malarial infections in Aotus trivirgatus with special reference to renal pathology, Br. J. Exp. Pathol., 54(5), 457, 1973.

10. Houba, V., Experimental renal disease due to schistosomiasis, Kidney Int., 16, 30, 1979.

11. Brack, M., McPhaul, J. J., Damian, R. T. and Kalter, S. S., Glomerular lesions in "normal" and "Schistosoma mansoni-infected" baboons (Papio cynocephalu), J. Med. Prim., 1, 363, 1972.

12. Hitchcock, C. R., Kiser, J. C., Telander, R. L. and Seljeskog, E. L., Baboon renal grafts, J. Am. Med. Assoc., 189, 934, 1984.

13. Johnston, G. S., van Heerden, P. D., van Zyl, J. A., van Zyl, J. J. W., Retief, C. P. and Murphy, G. P., Renal function studies in the intact baboon, Invest. Urol., 6(2), 125, 1968.

14. Ruch, T. C., Urinary system, in Diseases of laboratory primates, Saunders, Philadelphia, 1959, 463.

15. Fox, H., Disease of captive wild mammals and birds. Incidence, description, comparison, Lippincott, Philadelphia, 1923.

16. Fox, H., Some observations on comparative constitutions in man and the lower animals, Proc. Amer. Phil. Soc., 68, 27, 1929.

17. Straus, W. L. andArcadi, J. A., Urogenitalorgane, in Primatologia, Handbuch der Primatenkunde, Hofer, H., Schultz, A. H. and Starck, D., Eds., Teil 1, Karger, Basel, 1958, 507.

18. Schmidt, I. G., An accessory adrenal cortex in the kidney of a rhesus monkey and the affects of pyrimethamine upon this tissue, Endocrinology, 59, 454, 1956.

19. Prentice, D. E. and Jorgeson, W., Ectopic adrenal tissue in the kidney of rhesus monkeys, Lab. Anim., 13, 221, 1979.

20. Skelton-Stroud, P. N., Observations on the spontaneous pathology of the baboon (Papio spp.), MVSc thesis, University of Liverpool, 1981.

21. Sperber, I., Studies on the mammalian kidney, Zool. Bidrag. Uppsala, 27, 249, 1944.

22. Straus, W. L., The structure of the primate kidney, J. Anat. Lond., 69, 93, 1934.

23. Giddens, W. E., Seifert, R. A. and Boyce, J. J., Renal disease, in Aging in Nonhuman Primates, Bowden, D. M., Ed., Van Nostrand Reinhold, New York and London, 1979, 324.

24. Lapin, B. A., Krilova, R. I., Cherkovich, G. M. and Asanov, N. S., Observations from Sukhumi (renal system), in Aging in nonhuman primates, Bowden, D. M., Ed., Van Nostrand Reinhold, New York and London, 1979, 14.

25. Osman Hill, W. C., Congenital abnormalities of the urinary tract in primates, Folia Primatol, 2, 111, 1964.

26. Scott, H., Congenital malformations of the kidney in reptiles, birds and mammals, Proc. Zool. Soc. London (Part 4), 1259, 1925.

27. Haddow, A. J., Field and laboratory studies on an African green monkey

(Cercopithecus ascanius schmidti matschie), Proc. Zool. Soc. Lond., 122 (Part II), 297, 1952.

28.   David, G. F. X. and Ramaswami, L. S., Unilateral hypoplasia of the kidney of a female langur, (Presbythis entellus entellus Dufresne), Folia Primatol., 5, 312, 1967.

29.   Maruffo, C. A. and Cramer, D. L., Congenital renal malformations in monkeys, Folia Primatol., 5, 305, 1967.

30.   Kim, C. S. and Kalter, S. S., Unilateral renal aplasia in an African baboon (Papio sp.), Folia Primatol., 17, 157, 1972.

31.   McCraw, A. P., Rotheram, K., Sim, A. K. and Warwick, M. H., Unilateral renal aplasia in the baboon, J. Med. Prim., 2, 249, 1973.

32.   Wadsworth, P. F. and Squires, P. F., Renal aplasia and hypoplasia in the rhesus monkey (Macaca mulatta), Lab. Anim., 14, 1, 1980.

33.   Giddens, W. E., Boyce, J. T., Blakley, G. A. and Morton, W. R., Renal disease in the pigtailed macaque (Macaca nemestrina), Vet. Pathol., 18 (Suppl. 6), 70, 1981.

34.   Tucker, M. J., A survey of the pathology of marmosets (Callithrix jacchus) under experiment, Lab. Anim., 18(4), 351, 1984.

35.   Skelton-Stroud, P. N., Unpublished data, 1985.

36.   Kaur, J., Chakravarti, R. N., Chugh, K. S. and Chhuttani, P. N., Spontaneously occurring renal diseases in wild rhesus monkeys, J. Pathol. Bacteriol., 95, 31, 1968.

37.   Kalter, S. S., Kuntz, R. E., Myers, B. J., Eugster, A. K., Rodriquez, A. R., Benke, M. and Kalter, G. V., The collection of biomedical specimens from baboons (Papio sp.), Kenya, 1966. Primates, 9, 123, 1968.

38.   Weber, H. W., Brede, H. D., Retief, C. P., Retief, F. P. and Melby, E. C., The baboon in medical research: Baseline studies in fourteen hundred baboons and pathological observations, in Defining the Laboratory Animal, National Academy of Sciences, Washington, DC, 1971, 529.

39.   McConnell, E. E., Basson, P. A., de Vos, V., Myers, B. J. and Kuntz, R. E., A survey of diseases among 100 free ranging baboons (Papio ursinus) from the Kruger National Park, Onderstepoort. J. Vet. Res., 41(3), 97, 1974.

40.   Baskin, G. B., Roberts, J. A. and McAfee, R. D., Infantile polycystic renal disease in a rhesus monkey (Macaca mulatta), Lab. Anim. Sci., 31(2), 181, 1981.

41.   Kessler, M. J., Roberts, J. A. and London, W. T., Adult polycystic disease in a rhesus monkey (Macaca mulatta), J. Med. Primatol., 13, 147, 1984.

42.   Beach, J. E., Blair, A. M. J. N., Pirani, C. L., Cox, C. E. and Dixon, F. J., An unusual form of proliferative arteriopathy in macaque monkeys (Macaca spp.), Exp. Molec. Pathol., 21, 322, 1974.

43.   Beach, J. E., Blair, A. M. J. N., Clarke, A. J. and Bonfield, C. T., Cromolyn sodium toxicity studies in primates, Toxicol. Appl. Pharmacol., 57, 367, 1981.

44.   McNulty, W. P. and Malinow, M. R., The cardiovascular system, in Pathology of simian primates, Part 1, T-W-Fiennes, R. N., Ed., Karger, Basel, 1972, 756.

45.   Roberts, J. A., The urinary system, in Pathology of Simian Primates, Part 1, T-W-Fiennes, R. N., Ed., Karger, Basel, 1972, 821.

46.   Brack, M. and Rothe, H., Chronic tubulointerstitial nephritis and wasting disease in marmosets (Callithrix jacchus), Vet. Pathol., 18 (Suppl. 6), 45, 1981.

47.   Roberts, J. A., Clayton, J. D. and Seibold, H. R., The natural incidence of pyelonephritis in the non-human primate, Invest. Urol., 9(4), 276, 1972.

48.   Chalifoux, L. V., Bronson, R. T., Sehgal, P., Blake, B. J. and King, N. W.,

Nephritis and haemolytic anaemia in owl monkeys (Aotus trivirgatus), Vet. Pathol., 18 (Suppl. 6), 23, 1981.

49. Brack, M., Renal pathology in captive baboons (Papio cynocephalus), Vet. Pathol., 18 (Suppl. 6.), 55, 1981.

50. Boyce, J. T., Giddens, W. E. and Seifert, R., Spontaneous mesangioproliferative glomerulonephritis in pigtailed macaques (Macaca nemestrina), Vet. Pathol., 18 (Suppl. 6), 1981.

51. Boraski, E. A., Renal disease in prosimians, Vet. Pathol., 18 (Suppl. 6), 1, 1981.

52. Burkholder, P. M., Glomerular disease in captive galagos, Vet. Pathol., 18 (Suppl. 6), 6, 1981.

53. Stills, H. R. and Bullock, B. C., Renal disease in squirrel monkeys (Saimiri sciureus), Vet. Pathol., 18 (Suppl. 6), 38, 1981.

54. Heidel, J. R., Giddens, W. E. and Boyce, J. T., Renal pathology of catheterised baboons (Papio cynocephalus), Vet. Pathol., 18 (Suppl. 6), 59, 1981.

55. Leary, S. L., Sheffield, W. D. and Strandberg, J. D., Immune complex glomerulonephritis in baboons (Papio cynocephalus) with indwelling intravenous catheters, Lab. Anim. Sci., 31(4), 416, 1981.

56. Feldman, D. B. and Bree, M. M., The nephrotic syndrome associated with glomerulonephritis in a rhesus monkey (Macaca mulatta), J. Am. Vet. Med. Assoc., 155, 1249, 1969.

57. Hunt, R. D., van Zwieten, M. J., Baggs, R. B., Sehgal, P. K., King, N. W., Roach, S. M. and Blake, B. J., Glomerulonephritis in the owl monkey (Aotus trivirgatus), Lab. Anim. Sci., 26, 1088, 1976.

58. Butler, T. M., The chimpanzee: selected topics in laboratory animal medicine, Vol XVI, U.S. Department of Commerce, Springfield, Virginia, 1973.

59. Terrell, T.G. and Haliday, S. C., Pathology of chronic treatment of cynomolgus macaques with a synthetic analog of muramyl dipeptide, Abstracts, International Symposium on Immunotoxicology, University of Surrey, 1982.

60. Casey, H. W., Ayers, K. M. and Robinson, F. R., The urinary system in Pathology of laboratory animals, Vol. I, Benirschke, K., Garner, F. M. and Jones, T. C., Eds., Springer-Verlag, New York, 1978, ch. 3.

61. Glaister, J., Principles of toxicological pathology, Taylor and Francis, London, 1986.

62. Kim, C. S., Eugster, A. K. and Kalter, S. S., Pathologic study of the African baboon (Papio sp.) in his native habitat, Primates, 9, 93, 1968.

63. Weber, H. W. and Greeff, M. J., Observations on spontaneous pathological lesions in chacma baboons (Papio ursinus), Am. J. Phys. Anthrop., 38, 407, 1973.

64. Chapman, W. L., Crowell, W. A. and Isaac, W., Spontaneous lesions seen at necropsy in 7 owl monkeys (Aotus trivirgatus), Lab. Anim. Sci., 23, 434, 1973.

65. Fleischman, R. W., du Moulin, G. C., Esber, J., Ilievski, V. and Bogden, A. E., Nontuberculous mycobacterial infection attributable to Mycobacterium intracellulare (serotype 19) in two rhesus monkeys, J. Am. Vet. Med. Assoc., 181, 1358, 1982.

66. Jubb, K. V. F. and Kennedy, P. C., Pathology of domestic animals, Academic Press, New York and London, 1970.

67. Middleton, C. C., cited by Drach and Bowen (ref. 68).

68. Drach, G. W. and Bowen, J., Nephrocalcinosis in the squirrel monkey, Surg. Forum, 17, 501, 1966.

69. du Bruyn, D. B. and Liebenberg, N.v.d.L., Histochemical and ultra structural studies of calcification in the kidneys and the adrenal glands of rats and

baboons fed a nephrocalcinogenic diet, S. Afr. Med. J., 50, 2151, 1976.

70.   Harris, R. S., Moor, J. R. and Wanner, R. L., Calcium metabolism of the normal rhesus monkey, J. Clin. Invest., 40, 1766, 1966.

71.   Gillman, J. and Gilbert, C., Primary amyloidosis in the baboon (Papio ursinus), Acta Med. Scand., 152, 141, 1955.

72.   Banks, K. L. and Bullock, B. C., Naturally occurring secondary amyloidosis of a squirrel monkey (Saimiri sciurea), J. Am. Vet. Med. Assoc., 151, 839, 1967.

73.   Casey, H. W., Kirk, J. H. and Splitter, G. A., Amyloidosis in a rhesus monkey (Macaca mulatta), J. Lab. Anim. Sci., 22, 588, 1972.

74.   Sharief, Y., Reich, C. F. and Bonar, R. A., Polyploidy in mammalian urothelial cells, Urol. Res., 8, 153, 1980.

75.   Burek, J. D., van Zwieten, M. J. and Stookey, J. L., Cytoplasmic inclusions in urinary bladder epithelium of the rhesus monkey, Vet. Pathol., 9, 220, 1972.

76.   Okada, T. and Seguchi, H., Filamentous inclusion bodies in the transitional epithelium of the urinary bladder of the crab eating monkey (Macaca iris), J. Electron. Microsc., 31(1), 87, 1982.

77.   Weckerling, A. B. and Mackenzie, W. F., Keratin inclusion bodies in the transitional epithelium of M. fascicularis monkeys, Cytobios., 12, 161, 1975.

78.   Fussell, E. N. and Roberts, V. A., Cytoplasmic inclusion bodies in the monkey ureter, Vet. Pathol., 16, 127, 1979.

79.   Jones, S. R. and Casey, H. W., Primary renal tumours in non-human primates, Vet. Pathol., 18 (Suppl. 6.), 89, 1981.

7

CHEMICALLY INDUCED EPITHELIAL TUMOURS AND CARCINOGENESIS OF THE RENAL PARENCHYMA

GORDON C. HARD

I. INTRODUCTION

The most prevalent renal neoplasm in man is renal cell carcinoma, accounting for 85% of the malignancies in this organ[27]. Although it is not amongst the leading causes of cancer-related deaths in the United States, kidney carcinoma nevertheless is an unpredictable tumour with a poor prognosis, as more than one-third of patients have obvious metastatic disease at the time of clinical diagnosis[83], and many others will develop metastases later[141]. Furthermore the neoplasm is relatively refractory to chemotherapeutics and radiation, whereas aggressive surgical management of the advanced disease results in a 5-year survival rate of only 35%[141]. It is estimated that deaths in the United States from renal malignancies will approximate 8,900 in 1985[156], and most of these will be due to renal cell carcinoma. The cancer has an even higher relative incidence in Scandinavian countries. In Iceland, for example, kidney carcinoma ranks fifth in the list of most common malignancies in males, but tenth in females[172]. As a further consideration for concern, epidemiological evidence suggests that the incidence rate for renal parenchymal tumours in man is on the increase[24,142]. Consequently, the study of experimental models of renal epithelial carcinogenesis in laboratory animals for the purpose of elucidating the possible causes, pathogenesis, and molecular mechanisms involved in cancer induction, as well as for the devising and testing of therapeutic modalities, is an important aspect of the overall cancer research effort. Although renal neoplasms can be produced in animals by viral agency or irradiation, consideration will be given here only to the induction of epithelial tumours of the renal parenchyma by chemical carcinogens.

II.   SPONTANEOUS OCCURENCE OF RENAL CELL TUMOURS

With very few exceptions the background spontaneous occurrence of renal parenchymal tumours, against which organ-specific induction by chemicals can be measured, is very low in the various types of laboratory animals. In rats, for example, the frequencies of adenoma/adenocarcinoma recorded for different strains such as the Wistar[25], Fischer 344[43,102] and Osborne-Mendel[44] are all rather similar, so that amalgamation of the figures from these separate reports suggests an average spontaneous incidence of 0.24% for males and 0.06% for females. This is higher than the spontaneous incidence of 0.01% (with no male to female variation) recorded in early studies on large numbers of feral rats[110,182] presumably reflecting an enhancement by diverse factors including the controlled breeding programmes and laboratory environment. In the laboratory mouse, a survey conducted over 60 years ago recorded a renal cell tumour frequency of 0.015%[159], while a recent report on the now commonly used B6C3F$_1$ mouse encountered 0.18% in males and 0.06% in females[177], frequencies not very different from the laboratory rat. The overall background incidence of cortical epithelial tumours in the hamster is less certain, individual surveys in relatively small samples ranging from 0%[40,134] to 2.7%[134]. In contrast to rats and mice, spontaneous renal cell tumour is extremely rare in the laboratory rabbit, there being only one report in the literature[84], whereas the entity has yet to be recorded in the guinea pig.

Renal cell tumours are also encountered in the experimental or captive non-human primate, and Jones and Casey[81] have recently tabulated these occurrences. Although the species distribution is broad, almost 50% of the cases are represented by the Rhesus monkey, Macaca mulatta.

There are two special instances in which the spontaneous occurrence of renal parenchymal tumours in laboratory mammals is very high. A Wistar variant, now known as the Eker rat, is subject to familial renal adenomas which are believed to be determined by a single dominant gene[33]. When animals heterozygous for the gene are out-crossed, approximately 50% of the F1 progeny develop renal tumours of this type. From the available evidence it could be deduced that the homozygous condition is probably lethal[34]. In mice, a substrain of BALB/c, designated BALB/cf/Cd, produced by a rigid programme of inbreeding and selection[24], is subject to a 60-70% incidence of renal parenchymal tumours[135].

III.   RENAL CARCINOGENS

Sempronj and Morelli[151] first showed in 1939 that kidney tumours could be produced "at a distance" in laboratory rats by a parenterally adminstered chemical, namely β-anthraquinoline, over 100 chemical compounds of diverse structure have been recorded as inducing kidney tumours in this species. Like the kidney tumours produced by subcutaneous β-anthraquinoline[151], many of the compounds are associated with the induction of cortical epithelial tumours; some are listed in Table 1.

Table 1 Some chemicals associated with renal cortical epithelial tumour induction in experimental animals

---

Metals
  Lead acetate, phosphate
  Nickel sulphides, arsenides
  Methylmercury chloride
Aromatic and heterocyclic amines and amides
  2-acetylaminofluorene (AAF)
  O-anisidine
  4'-fluoro-4-aminobiphenyl
  N-(4'-fluoro-4-biphenylyl)acetamide (FBPA)
Furyl compounds
  Formic acid 2-[4-(5-nitro-2-furyl)-2-thiazolyl]hydrazine (FNT)
  3-hydroxymethyl-1{[3-(5-nitro-2-furyl)allydidene]amino}hydantoin
Nitroso and related compounds
  Dimethylnitrosamine (DMN)
  Diethylnitrosamine (DEN)
  N-ethyl-N-hydroxyethylnitrosamine (EHEN)
  N-nitrosomorpholine
  N-methylnitrosourea
  N-butylnitrosourea
  Streptozotocin
  B-D-glucosyloxyazoxymethane (cycasin)
  Methylazoxymethanol
Mycotoxins
  Aflatoxin B_1, G_1
  Citrinin
  Ochratoxin A
Iatrogenic compounds
  Bleomycin
  Daunomycin
  Niridazole
  (Streptozotocin)
Organohalides
  Chloroform
  Chlorothalonil
  1,2-dibromo-3-chloropropane
  Dichloroacetylene
  Hexachloro-1:3-butadiene (HCBD)
  Pentachloroethane
  Trichloroethylene
  Tetrachloroethylene
  Tris(2,3-dibromopropyl)phosphate
  Vinylidene chloride
Miscellaneous compounds
  Diethylstilboestrol
  Nitrilotriacetate
  Potassium bromate

Of the inorganic metals, the potent renal cancer inducing ability of lead salts in the rat has been known for some time[186]. The compounds are also weakly carcinogenic for the mouse and hamster kidney[176]. Lead salts are unique amongst renal carcinogens in that prolonged exposure results in the formation of intranuclear inclusions consisting of the metal complexed with an acidic non-histone protein[46]. It has been suggested that the complexing protein may function to sequester the lead in order to protect cellular organelles, but whether this reservoir plays a role in tumour induction is unknown. Lead is also unique in being the only chemical recorded as a likely environmental renal carcinogen for wild rodents. In 1962, Kilham and colleagues[86] surveyed adult feral rats inhabiting refuse dumps in New Hampshire, and found carcinomas of the renal cortex in about 5% of those examined. Assays of the wild rat tissues for lead revealed high concentrations in the kidneys, while histologically these same organs were characterized by intranuclear inclusion bodies typical of chronic lead poisoning. With respect to other metallic compounds, certain nickel sulphides and arsenides[79,164] have been shown to be carcinogenic for renal parenchyma when administered to rats by the intrarenal route. The heavy metal, mercury, in an organic form as methylmercury chloride, has also induced a high incidence of adenomas/adenocarcinomas in ICR mice[118].

The heterocyclic amines and amides contain two related compounds, 4-fluoro-4-aminobiphenyl[109] and N-(4'-fluoro-4-biphenylyl)acetamide (FBPA)[74] which, when administered in the diet for a long term, induce high incidences of renal cell tumours. In particular, FBPA represents a useful model for the study of renal carcinogenesis.

Nitrosocompounds are versatile carcinogens with specificity for a wide range of organs. They are also ubiquitous compounds, being found in the environment associated with polluted air, foods, cosmetics and tobacco products, as well as in a number of occupational settings[14]. The representatives which have induced renal parenchymal tumours are too numerous to list here, and just a few are presented in Table 1. Dimethylnitrosamine (DMN) has induced these neoplasms in the rat[55,121], mouse[170], hamster[119] and in the amphibian, Xenopus borealis[85]. In rats, DMN is carcinogenic for the kidney following single high doses, producing mainly renal mesenchymal (connective tissue) tumours in the young, but predominantly adenomas and adenocarcinomas in mature animals[53]. Like DMN, diethylnitrosamine (DEN) is a potent renal carcinogen after only one dose in the rat, but induces exclusively the epithelial neoplasm[120]. With respect to species diversity, DEN is one of the most versatile of carcinogens and has produced renal cell tumours not only in the rat, but also in the pig[148], cat and chicken[147]. N-ethyl-N-hydroxyethylnitrosamine (EHEN) has recently become popular, particularly in Japan, as a model for these tumours in rats[68]. In contrast to DMN and DEN, a 2-week regimen is required for inducing a high frequency of neoplasms with this compound. In Germany, N-nitrosomorpholine by chronic administration has been well studied in the rat, and is associated with the induction of oncocytomas as well as the more conventional types of cortical epithelial tumours[10-12]. Streptozotocin is a further example of an effective single-dose renal cell carcinogen in rats[137]. In mice no high-frequency system for renal cell tumour induction existed until recently, when streptozotocin was recorded as producing a near 100% incidence following a single intravenous injection[56]. Cycasin and its aglycone, methylazoxymethanol, are metabolically related to nitrosamines and display similar renal carcinogenic activity to DMN[93]. Both of these toxic substances are found naturally in the Cycad palms of tropical and subtropical regions of the world. Methylazoxymethanol is the only chemical to date which, in trials conducted by the National Cancer Institute, has induced renal carcinoma in non-human primates, namely the Rhesus monkey[1].

Organohalides are well represented as renal carcinogens in rats and mice, and as a chemical class their target specificity within the kidney is the parenchyma. A number of these compounds, such as chloroform, tri- and tetra-chloroethylene and vinylidene chloride, are industrial organic solvents, implying a possiblity for occupational exposure in man[88]. The chlorination of water can result in conversion of organic materials to trichloromethanes such as chloroform, which is a major contaminant of municipal drinking water sources. Dichloroacetylene and hexachloro-1:3-butadiene (HCBD) are common by-products of synthetic processes involving the chlorination of hydrocarbons. There is consequently significant scope for occupational access to these compounds also. Although HCBD was tested by dietary administration[89], in the case of dichloroacetylene the renal carcinogenicity in rats was demonstrated by inhalation[139], the most likely route of exposure for man. Tris(2,3-dibromopropyl) phosphate is one of the most popular flame-retardants, being utilized in children's sleepwear, home furnishings and building materials. It induces cortical epithelial tumours in both rats and mice[140].

A number of metabolic products generated by ubiquitously distributed fungi are nephrotoxins; some of these have also proved to be potent renal carcinogens in rodents when chronically administered with the diet. Of the purified aflatoxins, which are associated primarily with Aspergillus flavus, aflatoxins B_1 and G_1 are carcinogenic for rat kidney[20,36]. Ochratoxin A, found especially in A. ochraceus and Penicillium viridicatum, had induced a high incidence of cystic adenomas in mice, but a lower frequency of the solid type of renal cell tumour[82]. Citrinin, a metabolite of P. citrinin and other penicillia and aspergillia, has produced a 73% incidence of renal adenomas in Fischer 344 rats[5].

Amongst the iatrogenic compounds, bleomycin, daunomycin and streptozotocin are all antineoplastic agents, while niridazole, [1-(5-nitro-2-thiazolyl)2-imidazolidinone], is used in treating schistosomal disease.

The group comprising chemicals of miscellaneous structure includes the only hormonal system of renal epithelial tumour induction. Diethylstilboestrol (DES) is the model compound, being capable of effecting a 100% incidence of renal cell tumours in male hamsters[87], but other steroidal and stilbene oestrogens have been shown recently to have equivalent or lower carcinogenic activities[96]. The hamster appears to be the only experimental animal susceptible to hormonal renal carcinogenesis. Trisodium nitrilotriacetic acid (NTA), a polycarboxylic acid with chelating properties and used as a detergent builder in Canada, has been under consideration as a substitute for polyphosphates in household laundry detergents in the United States, raising the possibility of water supply contamination. Although able to induce renal adenomas/adenocarcinomas in rats[45] NTA is non-mutagenic, not metabolized by mammalian tissues, and like DES, currently considered an example of an epigenetic renal carcinogen[3]. Potassium bromate is an oxidant which has been widely used throughout the world as a food additive for the maturation of flour in the bread-making process, and in Japan as an additive to improve the quality of fish-paste products. It is also used as a neutralizer in hair lotions for permanent waving. This compound has produced very high frequencies of renal cell tumours in Fischer 344 rats when administered in the drinking water[92].

Consideration of the compounds above demonstrates that renal cell tumours have been induced by chemical agency in a fairly broad spectrum of experimental animal species. However, with the exception of a single "well-differentiated" kidney neoplasm encountered in a group of rabbits[94] treated chronically with DMN, the author is not aware of any unequivocal reports of the chemical induction of this renal tumour type in rabbit or guinea pig.

Table 2 Morphological classifications of cortical epithelial tumours

Tumour types	Types of histological organization	Cell types
Adenoma	Tubular	Granular
Adenocarcinoma	Lobular	Clear
Carcinoma	Solid	Eosinophilic
	Papillary	Basophilic
	Cystic	Oncocytic
	Anaplastic	Spindle cell
	Schirrhous	

IV. HISTOMORPHOLOGY OF RENAL PARENCHYMAL TUMOURS

Cortical epithelial tumours can be classified according to general type, according to the staining characteristics, texture and shape of the tumour cells, and according to histological organization within the tumour (Table 2). Regardless of type, epithelial tumours of the renal parenchyma in laboratory animals, when viewed grossly, appear as rounded, well-circumscribed lesions owing to their expansive mode of growth and, in the larger specimens, the formation of an encircling pseudocapsule (Figure 1). On section these tumours are soft and fleshy. Such characteristics serve to distinguish them from renal tumours of neoplastic connective tissue which are usually fibrous and poorly delineated from the surrounding tissue.

216

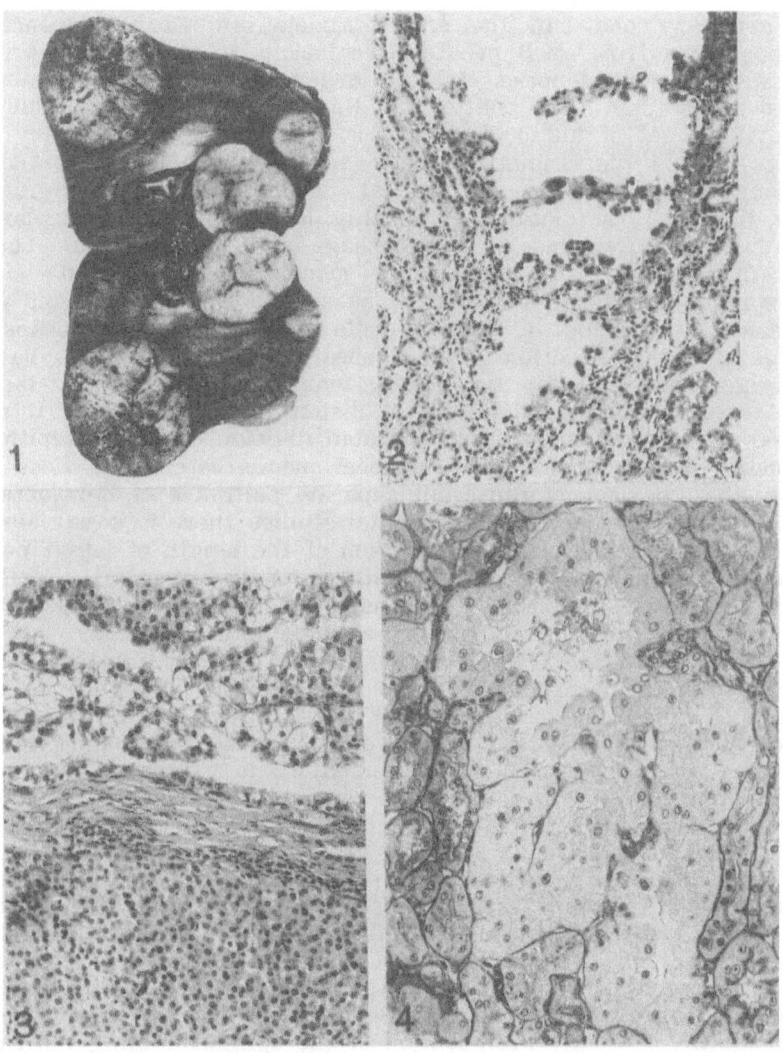

Figure 1 Gross appearance of DMN-induced cortical adenocarcinomas in rat kidney. All three tumours are rounded, expansive growths, and well circumscribed from the surrounding parenchyma. Areas of necrosis are particularly evident in the two larger neoplasms (x3). (Reproduced with permission from William Heinemann Medical Books Ltd, London.) **Figure 2** Conjoining segments of a single dilated cortical tubule with hyperplastic lining in rat kidney, 12 months after a single dose of DMN. The relationship of this end-stage cystic hyperplasia to carcinogenesis is unknown. (H & E, x112). **Figure 3** DMN-induced cortical epithelial tumour of rat shows granular cells in solid carcinomatous pattern as well as granular and clear cells in papillary organization (H & E, x225). (Reproduced with permission from Carcinogenesis[55]). **Figure 4** Oncocytic microadenoma induced in the rat by N-nitrsomorpholine. Trichrome-PAS (x245). (Reproduced with permission from Z. Krebsforsch.[11].)

217

As in man, the distinction between adenomas of the renal parenchyma and adenocarcinomas or carcinomas is, in most cases, an arbitrary one. In the animal models studied a sequence of pathogenesis from small proliferative lesions to large growths indicates that small adenomas and the larger adenocarcinomas and carcinomas are part of a continuum. Nevertheless, there is value in applying a set of histological criteria based on a discretionary size range, for discriminating between adenomas and the larger tumours. For instance, in the rat, nodular tubule proliferations less than 0.5 cm diameter invariably lack significant vascularization, or any evidence of haemorrhage and degeneration. Larger growths are well supported by a vascular network, and usually show evidence of mitotic activity, haemorrhage, necrosis, and local invasion as clumps of tumour cells beyond the pseudocapsule. Large growths compatible with adenocarcinoma or carcinoma have a malignant potential for metastasis, usually to the lungs, but in most studies the recorded rate of distant invasion is low. It must be re-emphasized that this size-related division of cortical epithelial tumours into adenomas or adenocarcinomas/carcinomas does not imply that the lesions represent separate pathways of development, but in analysing certain experimental studies there is some value in making this distinction as a reflection of the length of latent period and the associated tumorigenic potency of the chemical. Furthermore, in single-dose models of renal carcinogenesis it is clear that not all small lesions do progress inevitably to larger invasive neoplasms, and such a distinction serves to separate the latter types from adenocarcinomas/carcinomas. Similar types of decision can be applied to the renal tumours of other laboratory animals using a discretionary size range linked to the same signs of histological progression. Much further study is necessary, however, to characterize non-progressive adenoma-like lesions of the renal parenchyma and the features which distinguish them from tumours with malignant potential.

Adenomas are either solid proliferations of tubule epithelium, usually organized into small lobules, or proliferations within a cystic space, representing dilated tubule lumens, in which case they can be referred to as cystadenomas. Adenoma should not be confused with tubule hyperplasia, although the latter can progress to adenoma; the distinction again reflects lesion size and the extent of nephron involvement. Proliferation of the epithelial lining restricted to an individual tubule represents tubule hyperplasia. There may be an increase in dimensions due mainly to lumen dilatation. Frequently the change does not appear focal, that is as a single tubule cross-section, but extends along much of the length of an affected nephron (Figure 2). Where the convoluted segments of a single proximal tubule are involved, several adjacent profiles of the same tubule may give the erroneous impression of a lobular adenoma. With increase in the degree of hyperplasia, but still restricted to the luminal confines of a single tubule, the term adenomatous tubule hyperplasia has been applied by some authors[3]. As epithelial hyperplasia extends in nodular fashion beyond the limits of a single tubule, the lesion can be viewed as an adenoma. The necessity for distinction between hyperplasia and adenoma formation is not merely of academic concern. Studies with NTA have indicated that the various tubule hyperplasias induced by this compound can be reversible lesions[3]. Consequently, although renal tubule hyperplasia may represent a risk factor in renal carcinogenesis, the reversibility of the hyperplastic state must also warrant consideration in the screening of chemicals for carcinogenic potential.

The cells comprising cortical epithelial tumours may have granular cytoplasm staining in either acidophilic or basophilic fashion, or clear cytoplasm (Table 2). As in man, tumours in which clear cells predominate are referred to as clear cell carcinoma. These are quite frequent in the rat but not in mice. Terms such as hypernephroma or Grawitz tumour have been rejected in human oncology, and their use is discouraged in animals. Individual tumours may consist of an admixture of granular cells intermingled with islands of clear cells (Figure 3), either of which can display a uniformity in size or, conversely, pleomorphism. Adenomas consisting of a uniform population of large cells containing finely granular eosinophilic cytoplasm may be termed renal oncocytomas by some authors (Figure 4). They have been described in association with N-nitrosomorpholine[11] and cycasin[48] administration. Occasionally the usual epithelial contour of renal tumour cells is assumed by elongate forms in sarcoma-like pattern. Such spindle cell carcinomas are encountered particularly in the hamster[4].

The arrangement of neoplastic cells further characterizes the tumour morphologically (Table 2). Tumours in which the cells form more or less distinct tubules are designated tubular adenoma or adenocarcinoma. The integrity of these structures varies from well-formed to ill-defined tubules; the latter arrangement can be referred to as acinar. Tumours in which the cells are arranged into solid aggregates without lumens, each of which is separated by a scanty fibrous framework, are described as lobular, while those forming continuous sheets of cells without structural organization are generally designated as solid. The presence of glandular differentiation on the one hand, and solid, non-structured sheets on the other, serves to distinguish adenocarcinomas from carcinomas. Tumours in which the cells are highly pleomorphic and disorganized, and which display such invasive properties as inclusion of normal renal elements within their substance, have been termed anaplastic carcinoma. Frequently, tumour cells are arranged on either side of their fibrous tissue scaffolding to form frond-like papillary structures. Such tumours are designated papillary adenoma or adenocarcinoma. If the tumour consists of a cystic space lined by adenomatous cells it may be called a cystadenoma or, if the lining is papillated, a papillary cystadenoma. These various morphological patterns may occur in different parts of the same tumour (Figure 3) and composite terms such as tubulopapillary adenocarcinoma are frequently used. In most animal renal cell tumours the fibrous stroma is scanty and forms a ramifying network throughout the growth. Occasionally, however, the fibrous reaction is marked, widely separating the tubular or lobular structures of the neoplastic tissue and thus schirrhous in nature.

V.   ULTRASTRUCTURE

Tumours of the renal parenchyma induced in laboratory animals by chemical agents have been examined in some detail by electron-microscopy. The range of chemicals represented by these reports is broad and includes lead acetate[108], DMN[61,78], N-nitrosomorpholine[10-12], cycasin[48], FBPA[30], aflatoxin B_1[114], and DES[107]. But for the latter study in hamsters, all of the reports deal with renal tumors in the rat. It appears that there are no published ultrastructural descriptions of chemically induced cortical epithelial tumours in mice.

Regardless of the inducing chemical, the various electron-microscopic descriptions of renal cell tumours in the rat coincide in reporting neoplastic cells which, from the aspect of organelle content, bear structural conformity with epithelial cells of the renal tubules, and in particular the proximal segments. At the ultrastructural level, granular tumour cells can vary from a poorly differentiated state in which there is a general paucity of organelles but for ribosomal particles and vesicles, to darker cells which are highly differentiated and well represented by mitochondria, stacks of rough endoplasmic reticulum and Golgi apparatus. Lipid vacuoles, lysosomes, monoparticulate glycogen and cholesterol crystals can also be observed in well-differentiated tumour cells. An ultrastructural hallmark in most tumours examined is the presence of microvilli organized into brush-border profiles. This feature in particular identifies the tumour with proximal tubule. In tumours where tubular or acinar differentiation is well developed, brush-border can be oriented along the apical surfaces, although sometimes lumens are devoid of microvilli. However, in more solid or lobular tumours lacking a clear glandular pattern, attempted brush-border formation is equally evident, but at inappropriate locations, either at the boundaries between adjacent cells or especially as focal intracellular profiles (Figure 5). The latter imply deep intracytoplasmic invaginations of the cell membrane. Sometimes poorly differentiated brush-border is visualized as a haphazard tangle of transected microvilli within the cytoplasm just beneath the cell membrane (Figure 5).

Another outstanding feature which has been frequently observed in the rat renal cell tumour is an intracytoplasmic lumen or canaliculus lined by sparse, non-organized microvilli. These spaces may be solitary or multiple within individual tumour cells (Figure 6). They are not unique to kidney tumours but appear to be epithelium-specific, having been observed in a range of human adenocarcinomas arising from diverse organ sites[145]. Both the abnormal disposition of brush-border and the intracytoplasmic lumina appear to be characteristic features of neoplastic renal tubule epithelium as opposed to non-neoplastic renal tissue.

A further cytoplasmic feature which typifies the renal tumour cells are cytoplasmic vesicles. These, often found in profusion, probably represent the apical vacuoles and vesicles of normal proximal tubule cells. In addition, peroxisomes, another organelle restricted to proximal tubule, are quite frequently reported. Cell membrane interdigitations of varying complexity are described less frequently than in the normal animal where they are found

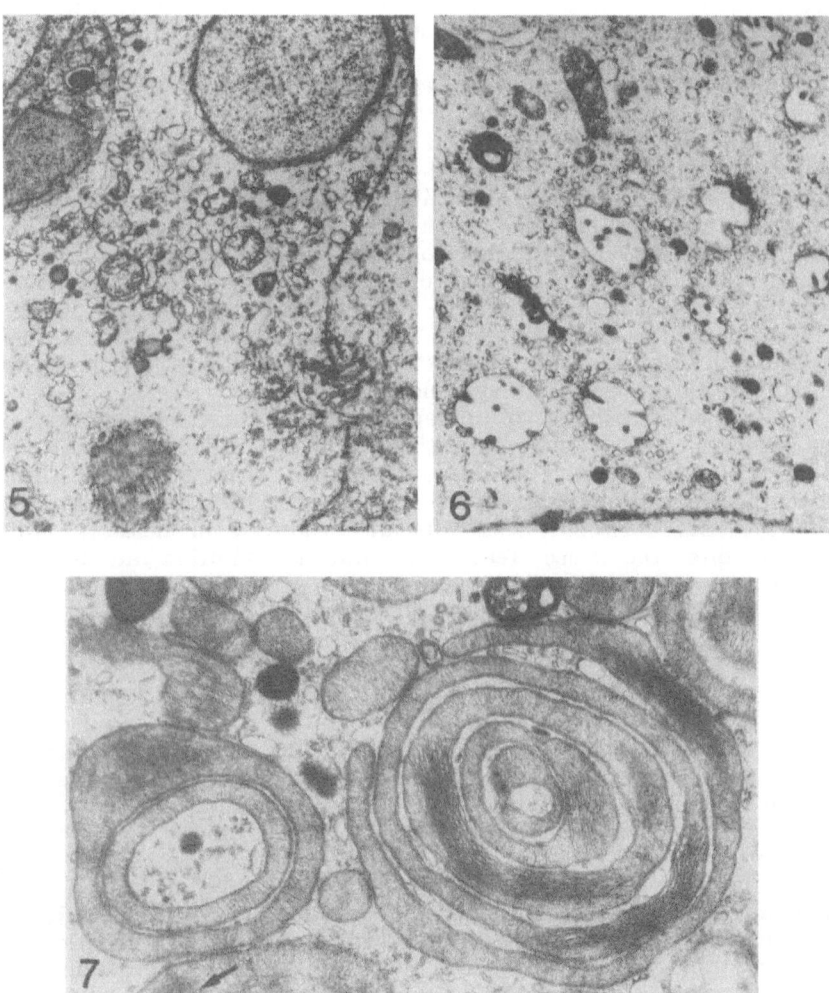

Figure 5 Electronmicrograph of DMN-induced rat renal adenocarcinoma cell shows poorly differentiated cytoplasm and a profile of internalized brush-border, presumably representing a deep surface invagination. In addition, transected microvilli can be visualized within the cytoplasm just below the cell membrane (x6,930).(Reproduced with permission from Cancer Research[61]). **Figure 6** Electronmicr ograph of DMN-induced rat renal adenocarcinoma cell with multiple microvillus-lined intracytoplasmic lumina. Vesicles similar to the apical structures in renal tubule cells are also abundant (x18,000). **Figure 7** Electronmicrographic detail of the cytoplasm of an oncocytoma induced in rat kidney by N-nitrosomorpholine. The cytoplasm is packed with mitochondrial profiles many of which are atypical, particularly appearing as concentric arrays of very elongate forms with stacks of longitudinal cristae. The arrow indicates an intramitochondrial crystalloid inclusion (x27,900). (Reproduced with permission from Z. Krebsforsch.[11].)

throughout the length of the nephron. Basement membrane is always present, invariably as a surrounding investment to the acini and lobular aggregations of tumour cells, as well as between individual cells on occasion.

As in the human counterpart, clear cell tumours of the rat are associated with excessive intracellular accumulations of monoparticulate glycogen and/or lipid bodies[10], thus contrasting with the granular cell types described above. Ultrastructurally, the oncocytomas encountered with N-nitrosomorpholine[11] and cycasin[48], display features which distinguish them from both the granular and clear cell tumours. In particular oncocytic cells are typified by excessive numbers of randomly disposed mitochondria which are frequently abnormal (Figure 7). Structural anomalies can involve striking mitochondrial elongation into linear or concentric forms, longitudinal cristae, and intramitochondrial inclusions of monoparticulate glycogen, lipid or crystalloid structures.

Electronmicroscopy of streptozotocin-induced carcinomas of mice reveals similar characteristics to the equivalent renal cell tumours of rats (G.C. Hard, unpublished observations). Thus, microvilli, vesicles and intracytoplasmic lumina have been observed. Similarly, the hormonal renal tumour produced in hamsters with DES exhibits the same features, but in addition an unusual development of highly differentiated multiple cilia, sometimes situated in deep intracellular invaginations[49,107].

VI. PATHOGENESIS

Of the many chemicals shown to be inducers of epithelial tumours of the renal parenchyma, a number have been promulgated as suitable models for in-depth study of the sequential steps involved in kidney carcinogenesis because of their potency. The most prominent of these are listed, and the essential aspects of each regime summarized, in Table 3. In particular, models based on a single administration of chemical provide an advantage for defining the sequence of precursor cell populations without perturbation by persisting toxicity which occurs with repeated or continous administrations of a carcinogen. In addition, as will be noted later, single-dose or short-term regimes permit a relatively longer survival time from the completion of carcinogenic exposure for expression of the induced tumours' malignant potential.

Regardless of the inducing chemical the latent period of induction to the stage of relatively large, palpable adenocarcinomas is long, usually requiring a term of 9 to 12 months, or sometimes more. Studies on the pathogenesis of renal cell cancer using the various models are in agreement that the sequential steps proceed via hyperplastic tubules through microscopic proliferations usually designated as adenoma, to tumours with histological features of adenocarcinoma or carcinoma. Certain cellular changes may also precede this proliferative sequence.

With most of these model chemicals, acute toxicity is induced in the target cells of renal tubules prior to the appearance of proliferative foci. In the case of DMN, early ultrastructural

Table 3 Animal models for study of renal cell tumour induction

Carcinogen	Strain	Dosage regime	Route	Incidence	Reference
Rat					
Lead	Wistar	Daily x 1% for 52 weeks	Diet	50-60%	176
FBPA	F344	Daily x 0.04% for 36-52 weeks	Diet	75-90%	74
FNT	Sprague-Dawley	Daily x 0.2% for 46 weeks	Diet	70-80%	37
DMN	Wistar	1 x 30 mg/kg	Intraperitoneal (protein deprivation)	90%	55
DEN	Sprague-Dawley	1 x 160 mg/kg	Intravenous	80%	120
EHEN	Wistar	Daily x 0.2% for 2 weeks	Diet	80%	68
Mouse					
STZ	CBA/H/T6J	1 x 250 mg/kg	Intravenous	95-100%	56
Hamster					
DES	Syrian golden	20 mg pellets for 9 months	Subcutaneous implantation	100%	87, 96

FBPA, N-(4'-fluoro-4-biphenylyl)acetamide
FNT, Formic acid 2-[4-(5-nitro-2-furyl)-2-thiazolyl]hydrazide
DMN, Dimethylnitrosamine
DEN, Diethylnitrosamine
EHEN, N-ethyl-N-hydroxyethylnitrosamine
NM, N-nitrosomorpholine
STZ, Streptozotocin
DES, Diethylstilboestrol

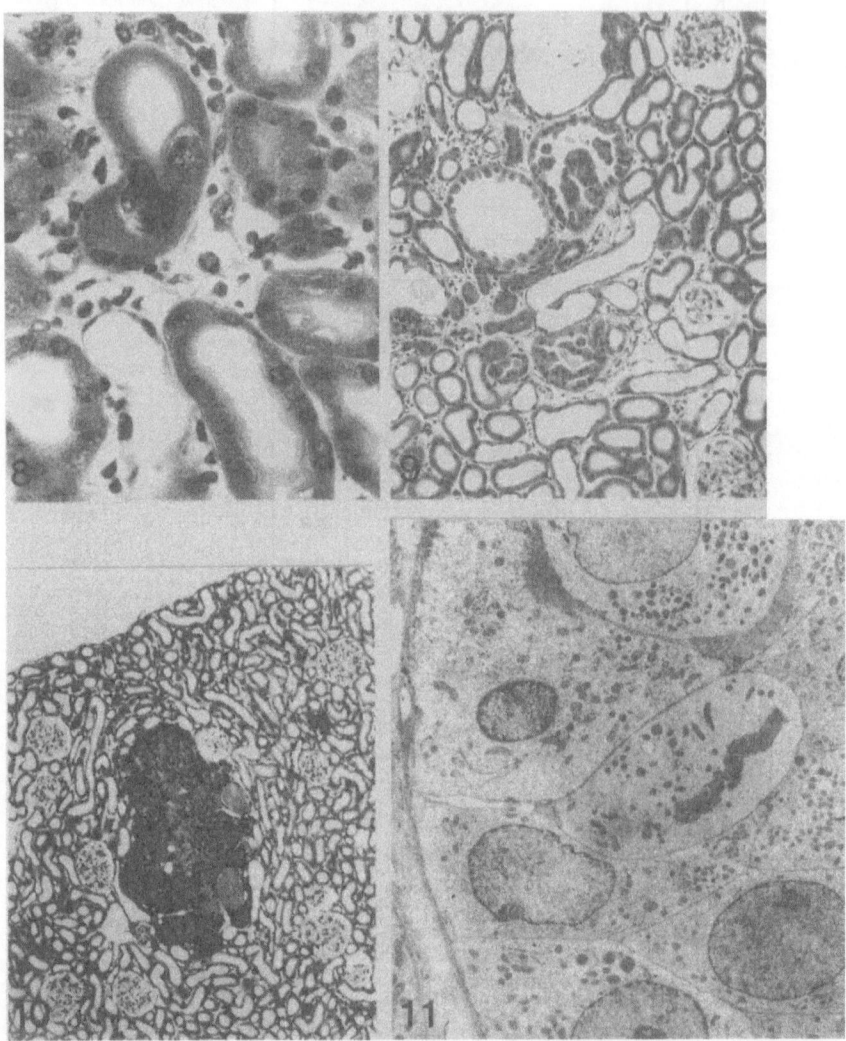

Figure 8 Karyomegaly in a proximal convoluted tubule of rat kidney 6 weeks after a carcinogenic dose of DMN (H & E, x440). **Figure 9** Atypical hyperplasia with mitosis, involving several transected profiles of a proximal convoluted tubule, in a rat 14 weeks after DMN treatment. A mild interstital reaction is associated with the lesion (H & E, x150). (Reproduced with permission from Cancer Research[60].) **Figure 10** Rat cortical adenoma induced by DMN. This lesion qualifies as a carcinoma in situ because of its rapid induction within 14 weeks of the carcinogenic treatment (H & E, x32).(Reproduced with permission from Toxicologic Pathology). **Figure 11** Electron-micrograph of a 20-week DMN-induced rat adenoma (carcinoma in situ) similar to the one illustrated in Figure 10. The solid lesion displays mitosis, poorly differentiated cells, abnormal location of brush-border, increased nucleus:cytoplasm ratio, and hypertrophied nucleoli, all features of larger adenocarcinomas (x2,880). (Reproduced with permission from Cancer Research[60].)

changes of lipid droplet accumulation and proliferation of smooth endoplasmic reticulum (SER) are seen within 24 hours of the single carcinogenic dose in proximal convoluted tubules. This is followed by scattered single-cell necrosis of cells of the S_2 tubule segment from 4 to 6 days, the same specific site where SER proliferation is observed[62]. In the ensuing period of regeneration, peaks of DNA synthesis and mitotic activity occur in the cortical (both proximal and distal) convoluted tubules[51] at day 10, while the acute phase of injury is fully resolved by 2 to 3 weeks. With the continuously administered carcinogens such as FBPA[28,29] and FNT[37], cellular injury including lipid accumulation and scattered tubule cell necrosis is observed for an extended period from the initial weeks of exposure.

A morphological aberration also preceding the development of proliferative foci with some renal carcinogens is conspicuous nuclear enlargement, termed karyomegaly or megalocytosis, affecting single cells within the renal tubules. DMN induces the alteration primarily in the proximal convoluted tubules of the cortex (Figure 8), but the location is restricted to the S_3 segment of proximal tubules with FBPA. This nuclear anomaly appears to follow as a direct result of the carcinogens' early effects on cell replication, and implies a block in G_2 of the cell cycle resulting in progressive polyploidy. The rapidity with which enlarged nuclei are induced in different organs is likely to be related to the degree of cell turnover intrinsic to the normal tissue[54]. The kidney represents a fairly permanent population with only slow cell turnover. Consequently the development of noticeable karyomegaly takes several weeks in DMN renal carcinogenesis, becoming obvious by 6 weeks after the single treatment[60]. Although this abnormality of cell division is not described as a constant kidney cell response to all renal carcinogens, it nevertheless remains feasible that, when seen, karyomegaly might be indicative of the local action of a carcinogenic compound[54]. In addition to DMN and FBPA, it has been recorded following administration of 4'-fluoro-4-aminobiphenyl[109], lead salts[186], daunomycin[162], aflatoxins B_1 and G_1[19,21] and DES[75]. Despite this association, it seems unlikely that such cytokinetically arrested cells participate in the initial formation of proliferative foci[29,60].

The time at which discrete foci of hyperplastic proliferation within cortical tubules first appear depends on the chemical system. In chronic dietary regimes such as FBPA[28] and lead[186], tubule hyperplasia is not detected for approximately 6 months after the commencement of treatment. In the single-dose DMN model, however, foci can sometimes be observed as early as 6 weeks but more frequently commencing from 12 weeks after the injection[60] (Figure 9). In rats, hyperplastic foci on the pathway to tumour formation are usually associated with some degree of cellular atypia or dysplasia[28,60,129], but beyond histological description, these very early lesions have not been well characterized. With DMN, the site for the early proliferations is within the proximal convoluted tubules of the cortex[60], although their specific origin from S_1 or S_2 segments is not yet determined. The fact that the acute cellular changes associated with DMN toxicity in the kidney are restricted to the S_2 segment of proximal tubule suggests that this might be the site of origin for DMN-induced renal cell tumours rather than S_1. In contrast, Dees and her co-workers[28,29] describe the earliest tubule proliferations with FBPA as occurring in zone 2, the outer stripe of the outer medulla, as well as in the cortical medullary rays, indicating that the straight S_3 segment of proximal tubule is the site of origin for the resultant tumours. In N-nitrosomorpholine-induced renal carcinogenesis, Bannasch considers that epithelial foci of glycogen accumulation in both proximal and distal tubules represent preneoplastic lesions for clear and eosinophilic renal cell tumours[10], while basophilic tumours are preceded by proximal tubules with unusually large basophilic or chromophobic cells[12]. Bannasch has also shown that the early stages of N-nitrosomorpholine oncocytoma formation can at times be visualized as connections to distal tubules, indicating a clear origin from this discrete part of the nephron for at least some of these lesions[11]. It is interesting to note that Eble and Hull[32] consider that human renal oncocytomas also arise from the epithelium of distal tubules.

Microscopic adenomas are presumed to develop in all systems as an increase in size of hyperplastic tubular foci. In rats this invariably involves formation of a solid proliferating nodule of epithelial cells extending well beyond the dimensions of single tubules (Figure 10). An increase in nucleus:cytoplasm ratio usually is apparent in the adenomatous cells and mitotic activity is not infrequently observed. With FBPA this stage occurs from 36 weeks onwards[28] but can sometimes be present between 12 and 20 weeks after a single dose of DMN[60]. Because such lesions appear to represent a continuum with the larger invasive tumours, they have been considered by some as carcinoma in situ[29]. Electronmicroscopic examination of these foci reveals certain features that typify the later adenocarcinomas and carcinomas (Figure 11). For instance, loss of cellular polarity, abnormal location or internalization of microvilli and brush-border, intercellular distribution of basement membrane within nodules, concentric arrangement of elongated mitochondrial profiles, and nucleolar hypertrophy and fragmentation have been described in the FBPA[29] and DMN[60] renal tumour models. Unlike the situation in liver, where preneoplastic foci are well characterized, little is known of the enzymatic activities of early kidney lesions. However, it has been determined that EHEN-induced foci have markedly reduced gamma glutamyl transpeptidase activity when compared with normal renal parenchyma[129], thus correlating with the low enzyme levels in larger kidney neoplasms[67,129].

Clinically palpable renal cell tumours can sometimes develop within 26 weeks after commencement of single-dose regime such as DMN[60], but rarely earlier than 40 weeks in systems requiring repeated administrations of carcinogen[28,37,175]. Considering tumour progression, the presence of metastatic invasion to distant organs from primary renal cell tumours is infrequent in most chemical models. Recent work with DMN in the mature rat, however, indicates that macroscopic renal cell tumours do undergo progression to malignancy providing the affected animal is able to survive for a sufficiently long period of time[55]. Statistical evaluation of tumour development has demonstrated that DMN-induced

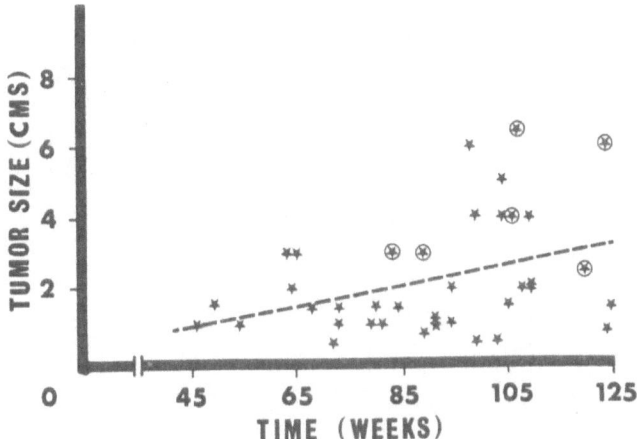

Chart I Scatter diagram plotting size of macroscopic cortical epithelial kidney tumours induced in rats by DMN (expressed as diameter in cm) against the time elaps- ing between carcinogenic treatment and death of the animal. Linear regression indi- cates an increase in size of the lesions with time and a correlation between size and age of the tumours with a tendency for metastasis (encircled points are metas- tatic tumours). (Reproduced with permission from Carcinogenesis[55].)

epithelial neoplasms of macroscopic dimensions increase in diameter by an average of 3 mm every 10 weeks, and that the parameters of time and tumour size can be correlated with a capacity for metas- tasis, mainly to the lungs. In that study (data illustrated in Chart I), almost 50% of the tumours attaining a diameter of at least 2.5 cm metastasized. This finding suggests that progression to a fully malignant stage, as supported by distant invasion, requires a cer- tain period of time for the tumour to reach a critical size. In the human disease, too, it is recognized that there is a linear relation- ship between the dimensions of renal carcinoma and the frequency of metastasis[15,150]. With feeding regimes where it is necessary to administer the carcinogen to rats for extended periods, it is con- ceivable that there may not be sufficient time available from the initial induction of the transformed state for progression to overt malignancy before the animal expires. This would explain the paucity of metastases recorded for chronic dose systems of renal carcinogenesis. The study with DMN therefore provides some reasonable justification for use of the terms "adenocarcinoma" and "carcinoma", with their connotations of malignancy, to designate chemically induced macroscopic neoplastic lesions of the renal parenchyma.

Systems of chemical renal carcinogenesis in mouse and hamster indicate a similar pattern of pathogenesis to the rat but with minor variations. The earliest proliferative lesions induced by streptozotocin in the mouse invariably are papillary extensions of the cortical tubule lining within a patent or dilated luminal space. Increase in the size of these lesions is associated with solid nodular proliferation closely resembling the macroscopic tumours

227

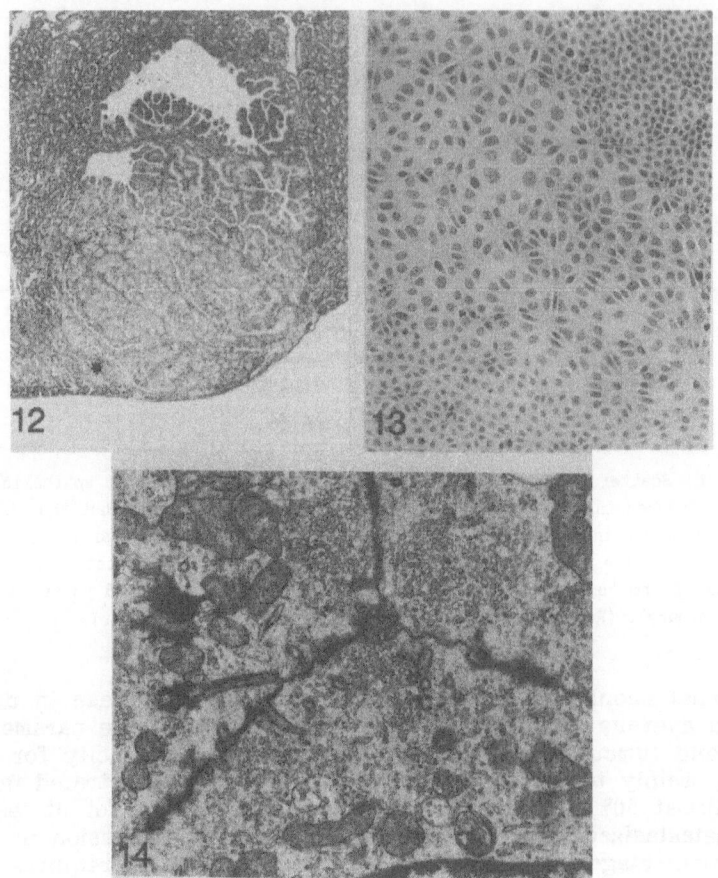

Figure 12 Medium-sized adenoma combining both papillary and solid areas, induced by a single dose of streptozotocin in the mouse. In the vicinity of the asterisk the solid portion shows local invasion by small lobules of pleomorphic cells (H & E, x47). (Reproduced with permission from Cancer Research[56].) **Figure 13** Typical mono-layer appearance of TRKE-1 shows cohesive, epithelial growth pattern, with various cell forms including large cells often arranged in rosettes, small densely crowded cells, and cells of intermediate size (H & E, x120). (Reproduced with permission from Cancer Research[63].) **Figure 14** Electronmicrograph of TRKE-1 cells grown as mul-ticellular tumour spheroids in suspension culture. There is polarization of accen-tuated junctional complexes and profuse endocytic vesicles (x14,770). (Reproduced with permission from Cancer Research[63].)

(Figure 12). In contrast to the papillary portion of the adenoma the incorporated solid areas are typified by cellular pleomorphism. In terms of neoplastic lesions the sequence of events in mice there-fore appears to be papillary or cystopapillary adenoma, mixed papillary and solid adenoma, and finally, solid carcinoma. As in the rat, the development of macroscopic tumours requires approximately 12 months. Metastasis also occurs in this system, but in animals surviving for 62 weeks or longer and bearing tumours with a maximum diameter approaching or exceeding 1.5 cm[56]. DES-induced renal cell tumours in hamsters also arise from the cortex, with the earliest foci involving convoluted tubules, particularly those in a subcapsular location, close to glomeruli, or around the arcuate vessels[75].

VII. METABOLISM AND ACTIVATION OF RENAL CARCINOGENS

Some chemical carcinogens, particularly the direct alkylating agents, are able to interact with the critical macromolecules of target cells without a prior requirement for metabolic activation. Most carcinogenic chemicals, however, do require metabolic steps to biotransform the precarcinogen to a reactive species representing the proximate or ultimate carcinogen. In the case of chemicals specific for the induction of tumours of kidney epithelium, apart from nitrosoureas such as N-ethylnitrosourea and streptozotocin, both of which induce cortical epithelial neoplasms in mice[56,98], and certain nitrosourethanes, virtually all others require metabolic conversion to reactive intermediates. However, beyond speculation, in no case is the precise identity of the ultimate carcinogen proven, nor the sequence of metabolic steps known for any cancer-causing chemical whereby the process of renal carcinogenesis is initiated. Nevertheless some information is available on the activation of certain kidney-specific, tumour-inducing chemicals with respect to the production of nephrotoxicity.

Although the liver is the body's primary organ for xenobiotic metabolism, the kidney too is well furnished with drug-metabolizing enzyme systems. Of the phase I enzymatically catalysed reactions, the cytochrome P-450-dependent mono-oxygenases appear to be exclusive to the S_2 and S_3 segments of the proximal tubules[39,47]. Morphologically, induction of renal mixed function oxidases is associated with proliferation of SER in proximal tubule cells[146]. In addition to their role in detoxification, the microsomal mono-oxygenases may be responsible for the activation of certain xenobiotics to reactive intermediates. Phase II metabolizing enzymes are predominantly associated with the cortical region also. Again such reactions may be involved in the genesis of nephrotoxicity rather than detoxification. Uridine diphosphate glucuronyl transferases, which conjugate certain foreign and endogenous compounds with glucuronic acid, are demonstrable mainly in the endoplasmic reticulum of this region[2]. N-acetyl transferases which conjugate an acetyl moiety with the substrate's nitrogen group are found mainly in the pars recta of the proximal tubules. Likewise, the distribution of glutathione-S-transferases is primarily in the proximal tubules and, depending on the animal species, particularly in the S_3 segment[39,47]. β-Lyase, a pyridoxal phosphate-dependent enzyme which catalyses the conversion of cysteine conjugates to thiols, pyruvate, and ammonia[35], is again a cytosolic enzyme with a cortical distribution. In contrast to the aforementioned, prostaglandin endoperoxide synthetase-mediated co-oxidation has been proposed as an alternative pathway for the metabolism of xenobiotics in the inner medulla[26]. This enzymic system involves the synthesis of prostaglandins from arachidonic acid precursor, and comprises two distinct activities. The first step in the arachidonic acid cascade involves fatty acid cyclooxygenase-mediated synthesis of prostaglandin G_2. Prostaglandin hydroperoxidase then catalyses the formation of prostaglandin H_2 from G_2, and it is during this second step in the synthetic process that some foreign compounds may be co-oxidized, resulting in the formation of unstable intermediates.

DMN, a potent inducer of renal cell tumours in mature rats that have been dietarily preconditioned with high carbohydrate and no protein[55], is known to require metabolic activation in order to exert its toxic and carcinogenic effects[106], the liver playing the dominant functional role in the normal animal[103]. It has been generally accepted for some time that DMN metabolism is mediated by the microsomal mixed-function oxidase system via a cytochrome P-450-dependent pathway[99], although sound evidence now supports the existence of several different nitrosamine demethylases[6,91]. Furthermore, it is known that rat kidney does possess the capacity to metabolize DMN and that, under the dietary conditions of protein deprivation which enhance renal carcinogenesis, the proportion of the dose metabolized by this organ is substantially increased[166,167]. The exact location of DMN metabolism in the kidney has not been biochemically identified. However, the increased proliferation of SER visualized by electronmicroscopy in the S_2 segments of convoluted proximal tubules at 6 and 12 hours after a carcinogenic dose of DMN in rats suggests that this is the specific site for DMN metabolism in the kidney under the operative experimental conditions[62]. In the mouse, purified microsomal enzymes from kidney have been shown to generate mutagenic metabolites from DMN, and a strain difference in this capacity correlates with the varying renal tumour susceptibility of those strains to DMN[179]. The precise metabolic pathway for DMN in either liver or kidney is not known, but biotransformation by the cytochrome P-450 system is presumed to proceed first to the putative reactive metabolite, methylhydroxymethylnitrosamine, and ultimately to the methyl-diazonium cation which in turn might degrade to the evanescent methylcarbonium ion[104] (Chart II).

Amongst those organohalides which are recognized as renal carcinogens, chloroform appears to be metabolized by the cytochrome P-450 system also. Although there are no data concerning the metabolic mechanism for chloroform-induced renal carcinogenesis, recent studies suggest that acute nephrotoxicity produced by this compound may be associated with P-450 catalysed dechlorination in the renal cortex to trichloromethanol with further spontaneous dechlorination to phosgene, an electrophilic intermediate capable of reacting with nucleophilic sites on cellular macromolecules[8,160]. In distinction to the monooxygenase pathway, the available evidence indicates that HCBD nephrotoxicity is mediated in a quite different fashion. Mainly through the catalytic activity of a microsomal glutathione transferase, this compound becomes directly conjugated with glutathione in the liver[181], and is excreted as the conjugate through the biliary route. The biliary

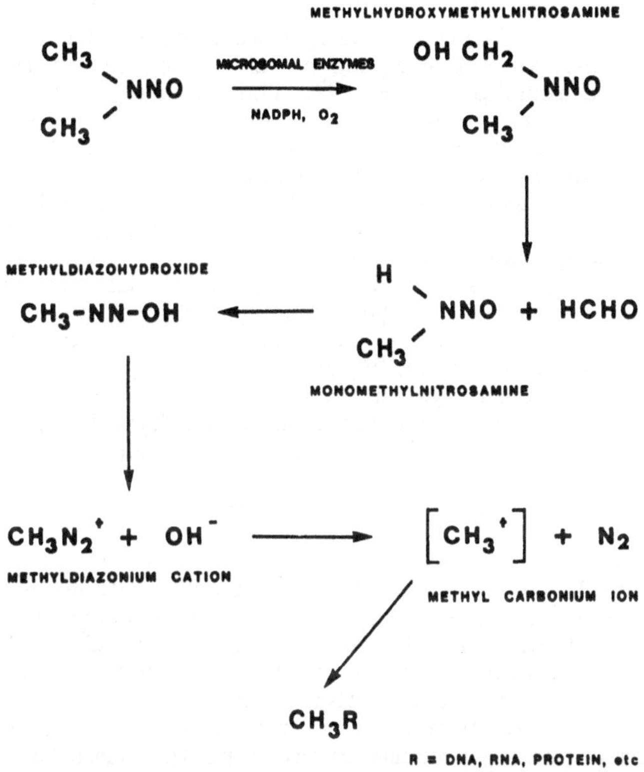

Chart II Putative pathway for the metabolism of DMN. (Modified from Magee, 1982[104].)

metabolites of HCBD are re-absorbed from the gut and excreted via the kidneys[122]. Studies from Lock's laboratory[122] have led to the proposal that the glutathione conjugate of HCBD is degraded to a cysteine conjugate by means of brush-border enzymes such as gamma-glutamyl transpeptidase and cysteinylglycinase. Identification of a urinary sulphenic acid metabolite of HCBD suggests that the cysteine-HCBD conjugate is cleared by the renal cortical enzyme, β-lyase, with subsequent generation of a nephrotoxic thiol[122].

Even less is known about the relevant renal metabolism of other kidney carcinogens. Inorganic lead, for instance, becomes sequestered as lead-protein complexes (inclusion bodies) in the nuclei of proximal tubules, but the role which these intracellular reservoirs of the metal play in the induction and development of renal cell neoplasia is unclear. Lead is a mitogen capable of stimulating cell replication[23] but it is also able to mediate the expression of specific new gene products within the renal tubule cells and the apparent repression of others[41], implying that the element may be in a dynamic state with respect to its intranuclear environment despite sequestration as an inclusion body.

In the inner medulla the mechanism of co-oxidation via the prostaglandin endoperoxide synthetase system is believed to be the

231

main pathway responsible for the activation of certain analgesics and N-[4-(5-nitro-2-furyl)-2-thiazolyl]formamide FANFT, which exert their nephrotoxic and carcinogenic effects on the urothelium of the papilla and renal pelvis[7,26,185]. The disparity in the primary locations of this enzyme system and tumours of the renal parenchyma suggests that medullary co-oxidation might play little in the way of a role in the activation of chemicals capable of inducing the cortical types of neoplasms. Nevertheless, prostaglandin-forming cyclo-oxygenase has been detected by immunohistochemical technique in collecting tubules of the renal cortex of several laboratory animal species[161], thus providing a metabolic basis for the renal carcinogenic action of 3-hydroxymethyl-1-{[3-(5-nitro-2-furyl)-allydidene]amino}hydantoin. This chemical induces epithelial tumours of the renal cortex[169] but it is not processed by the mixed-function oxidase system[184]. Zenser and co-workers[184] in fact have obtained data consistent with the hypothesis that the compound undergoes facilitated organic acid transport into cortical tubule epithelium with subsequent co-oxidative metabolism by prostaglandin endoperoxide synthetase, possibly generating an activated product which could act locally.

The fate of the carcinogenic hormone, DES, in hamster kidney is presently controversial. Liver metabolism studies have indicated that mono-oxygenases can convert DES to catechols, and to the 3,4-oxide, both of which are chemically reactive[115]. However, this activation pathway has been questioned as not altogether consistent with the carcinogenic activity data[95]. Peroxidases, on the other hand, yield β-dienestrol, a major in vivo metabolite of DES in several animal species, presumably involving the formation of reactive intermediates such as semiquinones and quinones in the process[116]. The most recent studies utilizing hamster kidney tissue re-implicate the renal microsomal mono-oxygenase system in oestrogen metabolism[95].

VIII. MOLECULAR MECHANISMS OF RENAL CARCINOGENESIS

Current views concerning the mechanisms whereby normal renal tubule cells are converted by renal carcinogens into the precursors of adenomas and adenocarcinomas are purely speculative. However most compounds which can induce renal cancer fit the concept pertaining to chemical carcinogens in general, namely that they are degraded to reactive electrophilic (electron-deficient) species which are capable of binding to nucleophilic (electron-rich) sites on cellular macromolecules including DNA, RNA, proteins and lipids[117]. In particular, binding to the informational macromolecule DNA is considered specifically relevant to the process of carcinogenesis.

Of all the renal carcinogens, probably more is known about the molecular interactions of nitrosamines in kidney than any other chemical class. The amount of information is nonetheless limited. Carcinogenic nitrosocompounds lead to the formation of alkylation products which represent a range of modified bases within DNA. Of the 12 primary alkylation sites identified on the bases of DNA[158], alkylation at the N-7 and O-6 positions are the major products and have been the most extensively studied in nitrosamine carcinogenesis. For kidney, DNA adduct formation has been investigated by using primarily the DMN renal tumour model. After single carcinogenic doses of this compound, both 7-methylguanine and O^6-methylguanine are formed in the rat renal tissue[123]. With protein-deprivation the amount of nucleic acid alkylation in this organ is increased by approximately 2 to 3 times when compared to

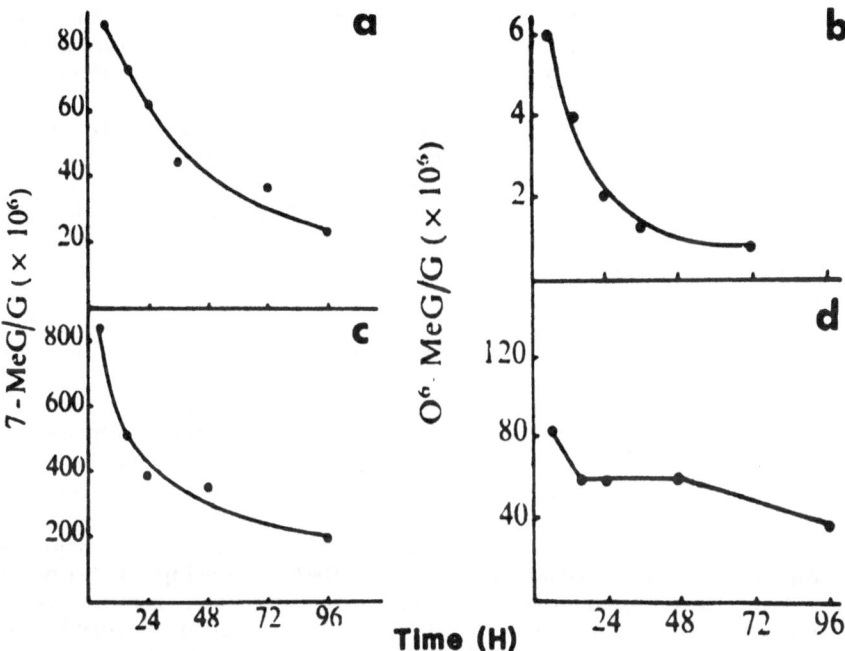

Chart III Formation and subsequent loss of 7-methylguanine (a and c) and O^6-methylguanine (b and d) in rat kidney DNA following administration of a non-carcinogenic 2.5 mg/kg dose of DMN (a and b) and a carcinogenic dose of 20 mg/kg of DMN (c and d). At the higher dose there is persistence of the O^6 adduct in contrast to the rapid loss of 7-methylguanine at either dose, or O^6-methylguanine at the low dose. (Reproduced in modified form with permission from Nature[123].)

the kidneys of rats fed a normal diet[166,167], thus correlating with the substantially enhanced renal tumour induction afforded by the special diet[59,112]. Furthermore, there is evidence to indicate that the rat kidney is capable of excision repair of the altered base damage[123,165]. Accordingly, a methyl-accepting protein which catalyses the removal of O^6-methylguanine in DNA by transfer of the methyl group to a cysteine residue on its own molecular structure with regeneration of guanine directly in the DNA, namely O^6-methylguanine-DNA methyltransferase, has recently been identified in rat kidney tissue[132]. In keeping with the currently accepted tenet that persistence of alkylated oxygen residues of DNA is the event which best correlates with organ-specific carcinogenesis rather than the rate of loss of 7-alkylguanine[130,157], the studies of Nicoll et al.[123] have also demonstrated a prolonged stability of O^6-methylguanine after a high carcinogenic dose of DMN, but rapid removal following a low dose not carcinogenic for kidney (Chart III). The persistence of substituents bound to DNA increases the likelihood of the alteration becoming inherited by cell progeny, and the O^6-product in particular has been shown to miscode and is therefore a potentially mutagenic lesion[42,100]. Alkylation of rat liver and kidney nucleic acids has also been measured following the oral administration of low levels of DMN[31,131] to compare the differential organ formation of the N-7 and O-6 DNA adducts under varied conditions of dosing. The results indicate that low doses of DMN absorbed from the intestine are so rapidly metabolized by the liver that very little of the carcinogen reaches the kidney for subsequent modification of renal DNA, thus contrasting with the high kidney levels of N-7 and O-6 alkylation produced after large, parenterally administered doses of DMN. In conjunction with the adduct persistence data gleaned by the study of Nicoll et al.[123], such results provide in part an explanation for the earlier observations of Magee and Barnes[105] that DMN, administered chronically as low doses in the diet, can produce liver cancer but not renal cancer, whereas the opposite effect is achieved with high doses of the carcinogen.

Structural damage caused by DMN to rat kidney DNA has also been evaluated by the techniques of BD-cellulose chromatography[163] and alkaline elution[13] using the single-dose regime. In both studies DNA damage in the form of single-stranded regions was observed shortly after the administration of DMN. The sequential study of Stewart and Brian[163] showed the pattern of damage to be biphasic, with maximal alteration to DNA occurring at 1 and 4 days after carcinogen administration. Although these results could be addressed to the role of cellular replication preceding completion of structural repair to DNA, it is now evident from recent ultrastructural data[62] that the peaks in single-strand breaks also coincide precisely with the biphasic manifestation of morphological damage to renal tubule epithelium.

With diethylnitrosamine, which like DMN, can induce tumours of the renal tubule epithelium after only one dose[120], single-stranded regions were demonstrated in renal DNA by the BD-cellulose chromatography technique[163] but not by alkaline elution[13]. The amount of DNA damage produced by DEN, as indicated by the highest increase of caffeine-eluted DNA, was calculated to be less than half the damage induced by an equitoxic dose of DMN, a difference attributed to the potency of the DMN renal carcinogenesis system[163].

In contrast to the nitrosocompounds, the covalent binding of the powerful hamster carcinogen, DES, to hamster kidney DNA is very low[101]. DNA-reactivity, expressed as the covalent binding index per unit dose, is so low in fact that mechanisms other than DNA modification need consideration in order to explain the renal carcinogenic effect of DES in hamsters. Most prominent amongst the various possibilities are hormone-mediated mechanisms. Li and Li[95] have summarized the hormonal foundations of the DES hamster renal adenocarcinoma system as (1) elevation of a specific oestrogen receptor in hamster kidney by prolonged oestrogen administration, (2) inhibition of the oestrogen receptor complex binding activity by anti-oestrogens, (3) induction by oestrogen of progesterone receptor in hamster kidney which also can be inhibited by androgens and anti-oestrogens, and (4) prevention of renal tumour induction by progesterone, androgens, and anti-oestrogens. Because hamster renal tumour development is suppressed significantly also by α-naphthoflavone, an inhibitor of the microsomal mono-oxygenase system, whereas oestrogens in turn, depress aryl hydrocarbon hydroxylase activity in hamster kidney, Li and Li[95] conclude that DES-renal carcinogenesis represents an interaction of both hormonal and carcinogenic mechanisms.

IX. RENAL CARCINOMA IN CELL CULTURE

Although an increasing number of cell lines have been successfully established from human renal cell carcinoma[180], in vitro representatives of chemically induced renal adenocarcinomas derived from experimental animals do not exist. Attempts have been made in the author's laboratory to propagate cell lines using adenocarcinomas induced in rats by DMN or DEN. In these studies, isolation of virtually pure populations of epithelial cells consistent with tubule epithelium, and subsequent early passage, was achieved. However by the eighth subculture the vigorously growing monolayers would undergo a lethal crisis (G.C. Hard, unpublished observations). The sudden nature of this event was not consistent with the process of senescence but suggested obligatory dependence on some physiological factor(s) not provided by the culture conditions. Similar experiences with rodent renal adenocarcinomas have been encountered in other laboratories, indicating that the fastidious in vitro requirements for these cell types are yet to be defined.

The only cell culture model reflecting chemically induced transformation in vivo of rodent renal cells is one designated TRKE-1, which has been produced by the means of the in vivo-in vitro system of isolation[58]. In this transformation system, cells are isolated from the target organ into culture after the animal has been exposed to an effective dose of carcinogen, thus permitting the purification of carcinogen-altered target cells consistent with the cancer type which would have developed in the intact animal[57]. TRKE-1 was derived from a 2-month-old Porton Wistar rat at 48 hours after treatment with a single 50 mg/kg intraperitoneal administration of DMN, using culture conditions which provided epithelium with a selective survival advantage over fibroblasts[58]. The cell line is characterized by cohesive growth behaviour typical for epithelium (Figure 13) and the formation of hemicysts (domes) at post-confluence as a manifestation of the differentiated function of transepithelial fluid transport. TRKE-1 cells are further characterized by structural features found in mammalian renal tubule epithelium in vivo, including microvilli, junctional complexes, endocytic vesicles, microfilament tracts and basolateral cellular interdigitations (Figure 14). The normal polarity of these structures is preserved in monolayer culture, identifying the cell line in particular with proximal tubule epithelium. When grown in suspension culture as multicellular tumour spheroids, TRKE-1 not only display microvillus-lined intracytoplasmic lumina recalling the features of renal carcinoma in vivo, but also a capacity for organoid differentiation into acinar structures[63]. Representing, as it does, in vivo chemically transformed renal epithelium, this cell line at the present time provides the only in vitro animal model which may be analogous to human renal cell carcinoma.

X.   MODULATION OF RENAL CELL CARCINOGENESIS

Since recognition of the initiation-promotion sequence which has been well studied in epidermal carcinogenesis[17], the search for chemicals with true promoting activity for neoplasia of internal organs has received impetus in recent years. Many such studies have been directed to liver carcinogenesis, but a number of reports also claim demonstration of tumour enhancement or promotion in the kidney. These examples are listed in Table 4.

Table 4 Two stage-carcinogenesis in rat kidney

Initiator	"Promoter"	Reference
DMN	NDPS	77
DEN	Nicotinamide	144
	Sodium arsenite	154
EHEN	β-Cyclodextrin	70
	DL-Serine	66
	Folic acid	155
	Lead acetate	69
	Trisodium nitrilotriacetate	71
Streptozotocin	NDPS	153
	Citrinin	152
FBPA	Lead acetate	168

In considering the purported instances of multistage renal carcinogenesis it becomes necessary to recall the specific properties of promoters as identified in the classic skin tumour model. Promoters lack significant carcinogenic activity themselves, but are chemicals which enable the development of tumours when administered repetitively after the administration of a single subcarcinogenic dose of an initiating agent, a compound that is a solitary or complete carcinogen at higher doses for the organ under study. True promoters do not enhance tumour induction when administered before the initiating agent, nor is the strategy successful when the interval between promoter applications is extended. Furthermore, the initiating event appears irreversible, whereas the promotion phase is characterized by reversibility. Thus the delay between the administration of the initiator and the first applications of promoter can be lengthy, but there is a temporal limit to the intervals between the individual applications of promoter[133]. Recent studies have defined some of the cellular effects of known skin promoters, identifying two substages in the promotion process: a rapid first phase which induces specific biochemical changes at the target cell membrane, and a prolonged second phase in which the initiated target cell population is selectively amplified[72]. In the various studies characterizing promoters, there is no hint that they are in themselves overt toxins for target cells. In contrast to promoters, co-carcinogens are factors which appear able to enhance tumour induction by solitary carcinogens in a more random fashion without dependence on the strict temporal sequence that characterizes promoters. Such factors include those capable of rendering injury to the target organ. Syncarcinogenesis, on the other hand, describes the situation in which two or more solitary carcinogens act in additive or synergistic fashion to enhance tumour expression[65].

From Table 4 it is clear that several agents with proposed promoting activity for renal cell carcinogenesis are themselves capable of inducing adenomas or adenocarcinomas at appropriate concentrations. Thus lead acetate, NTA, and citrinin could represent the process of syncarcinogenesis rather than promotion. On the other hand, NDPS, β-cyclodextrin, DL-serine and folic acid are known nephrotoxins, and may be enhancing renal cell tumour induction by the process of co-carcinogenesis. Certainly, none of these kidney tumour "promoters" have been tested sufficiently to determine whether the precise temporal restrictions that typify classical two-stage carcinogenesis apply. Of all the chemicals listed in Table 4, nicotinamide may represent the best prospect for a renal tumour promoter; it has not been demonstrated as nephrotoxic, nor does it appear to be a carcinogen for the rat or mouse[144,173]. However, the significance of this agent in renal tubular neoplasia needs further clarification in view of the fact that, in one study using streptozotocin as carcinogen, nicotinamide produced a reduction in kidney tumour incidence[136].

As noted earlier, and in Table 3, the single-dose, high-frequency system for renal tumour induction by DMN is dependent upon preconditioning of the rats with a high carbohydrate-no protein diet given for several days immediately before the treatment with carcinogen[59,112]. The apparent basis for the modifying effects of the diet leading to enhanced kidney tumour induction lies in a decreased microsomal enzyme activity in the liver permitting higher concentrations of carcinogen to reach the kidney for subsequent activation there[166]. For much the same reason, it seems, renal tumours of predominantly the cortical epithelial type are increased in rats subject to partial hepatectomy, particularly when DMN is administered 24 hours after the surgical procedure[38]. Partial hepatectomy and the time elapsing before carcinogen treatment also influence the frequency of DEN-induced renal cell tumours[113]. Both unilateral nephrectomy[76] and unilateral hydronephrosis[128] have been reported as increasing the incidence of cortical epithelial tumours by DMN in the contralateral kidney. The resultant proliferative stimulus afforded by organ ablation was believed to be the mechanism responsible for tumour enhancement.

Certain hormonal influences in DMN renal carcinogenesis have been suggested by the studies of Noronha and co-workers[124-127]. Following demonstration of a suppressing effect on DMN-induced cortical epithelial tumour in male mice by orchiectomy[124], these authors observed an increased frequency of the epithelial tumours associated with a single dose of DMN in the female rat when testosterone, with or without gonadectomy, was administered after the carcinogen treatment[125]. Oestrogen, on the other hand, was found to exert no influence on single-dose DMN renal epithelial carcinogenesis in male rats[126]. The hormone-related data obtained for chemical carcinogenesis of the renal parenchyma in rodents were considered by the authors as consistent with the levels of different steroid receptors found in human renal cell cancer, androgen receptors being detectable at significant levels, but oestrogen receptors absent[127]. Inconsistent with this idea of hormone regulation in chemically-induced renal carcinogenesis is the apparent inability of testosterone to influence the development of lead-associated renal cell tumours[143]. Unfortunately, some of the very diverse studies on modification of the renal tumour models described above have suffered from low sample size and/or marginal tumour frequency, thus compromising interpretation of the results.

An increasing amount of attention is now being devoted to the identification and study of chemical compounds, the so-called anticarcinogenic agents, that can inhibit the cancer process. Application of this concept of chemoprevention to carcinogenesis in the kidney has been recent. Antioxidants represented by butylated hydroxyanisole and ethoxyquin are known for their inhibitory effects in various systems of chemical carcinogenesis[178]. However, the evidence obtained in EHEN-induced renal carcinogenesis runs contrary to the general experience, as these compounds were found to enhance and not suppress the development of renal cell tumours of the rat[174].

The DMN model has also been used to determine whether chemopreventive agents proven in other systems have an effect on single-dose kidney carcinogenesis. Foremost amongst these are the vitamin A analogues which are effective inhibitors in various epithelial tumour models including the lower urinary tract[73]. Retinoids, whether administered during the latent period of development or for the phase of tumour growth as well, exerted no influence on DMN renal tumour incidence, histological type or grade of tumour, latency, or metastatic invasion[64]. Two additional anticarcinogens also proved negative in this tumour system, the immunopotentiating agent levamisole[52], and the hormone dehydroepiandrosterone (.T Ogiu, G.C. Hard and A. Schwartz, unpublished observations). Several explanations could be ventured for the null response of DMN carcinogenesis to chemopreventive agents, but a possibility that deserves serious consideration is the degree of potency of animal tumour models which are based on only one large dose of carcinogen. In the protein-deprived rat treated with a high dose of DMN, the carcinogen is not detectable in body tissues 19 hours after its administration[166], implying that in this type of model target cells are programmed for the later expression of transformation within a very brief time span, possibly within hours of initial exposure. It is perhaps because of an apparent independence of post-initiation events that DMN-induced kidney carcinogenesis is unresponsive to the modulating effects of various cancer inhibitory agents which tend to exert their action during the promotional phase of cancer induction.

XI.   CHEMICAL FACTORS IN THE AETIOLOGY OF HUMAN RENAL CELL CANCER

Discussion of chemically induced tumours of the renal parenchyma would not be complete without some consideration of the aetiology of human renal cell cancer. The only environmental factor that has been positively associated with kidney cancer in man is tobacco[16,111,183]. Indeed, a recent estimate suggests that 30% of renal cell cancers in males, and 24% amongst women, are due to smoking[111]. Amongst the numerous and diverse chemical compounds generated in tobacco smoke are volatile N-nitrosamines including the experimental renal carcinogens DMN and DEN[18].

In their population-based case-control study, McLaughlin et al.[111] also found a positive association between the long-term use of phenacetin-containing analgesics and renal cell cancer. Human phenacetin abuse correlates primarily with renal pelvic carcinoma, but it is interesting to note that, in rats, phenacetin induces not only transitional cell carcinomas of the pelvic urothelium but also adenocarcinomas of the cortical parenchyma in low incidence[80]. This compound therefore appears to represent a case where rodent carcinogenicity data extrapolate directly to man. Kidney cancer rates in males also show a positive correlation with the levels of trihalomethanes in drinking water[22], some of which are well-known renal carcinogens in rats and mice. This possible association clearly requires further investigation.

In the occupational setting there appears to be an increased risk of renal cell cancer for workers in the petroleum refining and petrochemical industries where there is exposure to petroleum, tar and pitch products[50,111,171]. An unusually high vulnerability to renal carcinoma has been identified for coke-oven workers in the steel milling industry[138], the overall relative risk being in the order of 7.5. On the other hand, the reported association of cadmium with renal cancer[90] appears tenuous[27].

Notably, epidemiological studies to date show no definitive evidence for an association of industrial exposure to inorganic lead with renal cell carcinoma[27,83]. This despite the fact that lead is a potent renal carcinogen in the rat, and provides the one rare example of environmental chemical cancer in wild animals, as discussed earlier[86]. Although the epidemiology is essentially negative, there are nevertheless two case reports of renal cell cancer occurring in lead workers[9,97]. In each instance there was evidence of high blood and/or tissue lead concentrations, as well as chronic lead nephropathy including, in one individual, presence of the characteristic lead-induced intranuclear inclusion bodies. Both patients had histories of prolonged occupational exposure, having worked in lead smelting companies for periods of 22 and 34 years in situations, particularly furnace tending, where the levels of lead

239

fumes or dust were high. In addition to these case reports a very recent retrospective analysis of the patterns of death in lead smelter workers not only found excess mortality from chronic renal disease but recorded six cases of death from renal cancer[149]. The standardized mortality ratio for the latter was elevated, particularly for workers exposed to high levels of lead, but the excess was not quite statistically significant. Such cases are suggestive, however, and a causal relationship between lead and human renal cancer, if it exists, needs to be demonstrated by further carefully planned epidemiological evaluations.

XII. CONCLUDING REMARKS

Numerous chemicals have been associated with the induction of cortical epithelial tumours in the kidneys of laboratory animals, and some of these constitute potent animal models for studying renal carcinogenesis, particularly in the rat. The morphology of chemically induced renal cell tumours in experimental animals clearly establishes their relationship to the renal cortical tubules, but it can be concluded from the various ultrastructural reports that most identify primarily with the proximal tubules. The evidence to date indicates that the precise sites of origin within this part of the nephron, though, may differ depending on the inducing chemical. The significance of proliferative lesions within single tubule profiles requires further investigation, as does the sequence of pathogenesis in general, in order to more fully define criteria for discriminating reversible hyperplasia from irreversible precursor foci of renal cell cancer. It is also necessary to fill the void which represents our poor understanding of the metabolic pathways of renal carcinogens within kidney tissue, and the molecular mechanisms responsible for the conversion and progression of normal tubule cells to neoplastic cell populations. Immortal in vitro cell lines derived directly from chemically induced animal renal cell tumours are non-existent, but, if developed, could contribute to an understanding of the role that oncogenes might play in epithelial renal carcinogenesis. On the other hand, the various in vivo models already available have stimulated increasing interest in identifying agents or factors which can modulate the renal cancer process. Finally, the role which chemical exposure plays in the causation of renal carcinoma in humans requires substantial clarification by improved clinical diagnosis associated with well-executed epidemiological enquiry.

ACKNOWLEDGEMENTS

During the preparation of this review the author was supported by grants CA-24216 and CA-12227 awarded by the National Cancer Institute, DHHS. Three colleagues who contributed illustrative material are gratefully acknowledged; Dr P. Bannasch, German Cancer Research Centre, Heidelberg, for Figures 4 and 7; Dr P.N. Magee, Fels Research Institute, Temple University School of Medicine, Philadelphia, for Chart II; and Dr A.E. Pegg, Department of Physiology, Pennsylvania State University, Hershey, for Chart III. Finally, the author wishes to thank the secretaries who were involved in typing the manuscript, namely Loretta Sucharski, Sherry Battaglia and Dorothy Wyszynski.

REFERENCES

1. Adamson, R.H. and Sieber, S.M., Chemical carcinogenesis studies in non-human primates, in Organ and Species Specificity in Chemical Carcinogenesis, Langenbach, R., Nesnow, S. and Rice, J.M., Eds., Plenum Publishing Corp., New York, 129-156, 1983.

2. Aitio, A. and Marnieni, J., Extrahepatic glucuronide conjugation, in Extrahepatic Metabolism of Drugs and other Foreign Compounds, Gram, T.E., Ed., Spectrum, New York, 365-387, 1980.

3. Alden, C.L. and Kanerva, R.L., The pathogenesis of renal cortical tumours in rats fed 2% trisodium nitrilotriacetate monohydrate, Food Chem. Toxicol., 20, 441-450, 1982.

4. Althoff, J. and Chesterman, F.C., Tumours of the kidney, in Pathology of Tumours in Laboratory Animals. Vol. III, Tumours of the Hamster, Turusov, V.S., Ed., IARC Scientific Publications, No. 34, 147-162, 1982.

5. Arai, M. and Hibino, T., Tumorigenicity of citrinin in male F344 rats. Cancer Lett., 17, 281-287, 1983.

6. Arcos, J.C., Davies, D.L., Brown, C.E.L. and Argus, M.F., Repressible and inducible enzymic forms of dimethylnitrosamine-demethylase, Z. Krebsforsch., 89, 181-199, 1977.

7. Bach, P.H. and Bridges, J.W., The role of metabolic activation of analgesics and non-steroidal anti-inflammatory drugs in the development of renal papillary necrosis and upper urothelial carcinoma. Prostaglandins Leukotrienes Med., 15, 251-274, 1984.

8. Baile, M.B., Smith, J.H., Newton, J.F. and Hook, J.B., Mechanism of chloroform nephrotoxicity. IV. Phenobarbital potentiation of in vitro chloroform metabolism and toxicity in rabbit kidneys, Toxicol. Appl. Pharmacol., 74, 285-292, 1984.

9. Baker, E.L., Goyer, R.A., Fowler, B.A., Khettry, U., Bernard, D.B., Adler, S., de Vere White, R., Babayan, R and Feldman, R.G., Occupational lead exposure, nephropathy, and renal cancer, Am. J. Ind. Med., 1, 139-148, 1980.

10. Bannasch, P., Krech, R. and Zerban, H., Morphogenese und Mikromorphologie epithelialer Nierentumoren bei Nitrosomorpholin-vergifteten Ratten. II. Tubuläre Glykogenose und die Genese von klar-oder acidophilzelligen Tumoren, Z. Krebsforsch., 92, 63-86, 1978.

11. Bannasch, P., Krech, R. and Zerban, H., Morphogenese und Mikromorphologie epithelialer Nierentumoren bei Nitrosomorpholin-vergifteten Ratten. III. Onkocytentubuli und Onkocytome, Z. Krebsforsch., 92, 87-104, 1978.

12. Bannasch, P., Krech, R. and Zerban, H., Morphogenese und Mikromorphologie epithelialer Nierentumoren bei Nitrosomorpholin-vergifteten Ratten. IV. Tubuläre Läsionen und basophile Tumoren, J. Cancer Res. Clin. Oncol., 98, 243-265, 1980.

13. Barbin, A., Béréziat, J-C. and Bartsch, H., Evaluation of DNA damage by the alkaline elution technique in liver, kidneys and lungs of rats and hamsters treated with N-nitrosodialkylamines, Carcinogenesis, 4, 541-545, 1983.

14. Bartsch, H. and Montesano, R., Relevance of nitrosamines to human cancer, Carcinogenesis, 5, 1381-1393, 1984.

15. Bennington, J.L., Cancer of the kidney - etiology, epidemiology, and

241

pathology, Cancer, 32, 1017-1029, 1973.

16. Bennington, J.L. and Laubsher, F.A., Association of renal adenocarcinoma with smoking, Cancer, 21, 1069-1071, 1968.

17. Berenblum, I. and Shubik, P., A new, quantitative approach to the study of the stages of chemical carcinogenesis in the mouse's skin, Brit. J. Cancer, 1, 383-391, 1947.

18. Brunnemann, K.D., Yu, L. and Hoffmann, D., Assessment of carcinogenic volatile N-nitrosamines in tobacco in mainstream and sidestream smoke from cigarettes, Cancer Res., 37, 3218-3222, 1977.

19. Butler, W.H., Acute toxicity of aflatoxin B_1 in rats, Brit. J. Cancer, 18, 756-762, 1964.

20. Butler, W.H., Greenblatt, M. and Lijinsky, W., Carcinogenesis in rats by aflatoxins B_1, G_1, and B_2, Cancer Res., 29, 2206-2211, 1969.

21. Butler, W.H. and Lijinsky, W., Acute toxicity of aflatoxin G_1 to the rat, J. Pathol., 102, 209-212, 1970.

22. Cantor, K.P., Hoover, R. and Manson, T.J., Association of cancer mortality with halomethanes in drinking water, J. Natl. Cancer Inst., 61, 979-985, 1978.

23. Choie, D.D. and Richter, G.W., Stimulation of DNA synthesis in rat kidney by repeated administration of lead, Proc. Soc. Exp. Biol. Med., 142, 446-449, 1973.

24. Claude, A., Adenocarcinome rénale endémique chez une souche pure de souris. Son effet sur la croissance, Rev. Franc. Etud. Clin. Biol., 3, 261-262, 1958.

25. Crain, R.C., Spontaneous tumors in the Rochester strain of the Wistar rat, Am. J. Pathol., 34, 311-336, 1958.

26. Davis, B.B., Mattammal, M.B. and Zenser, T.V., Renal metabolism of drugs and xenobiotics, Nephron, 27, 187-196, 1981.

27. Dayal, H. and Kinman, J., Epidemiology of kidney cancer, Semin. Oncol., 10, 366-377, 1983.

28. Dees, J.H., Heatfield, B.M., Reuber, M.D. and Trump, B.F., Adenocarcinoma of the kidney. III. Histogenesis of renal adenocarcinomas induced in rats by N-(4'-fluoro-4-biphenylyl)acetamide, J. Natl. Cancer Inst., 64, 1537-1545, 1980.

29. Dees, J.H., Heatfield, B.M. and Trump, B.F., Adenocarcinoma of the kidney. IV. Electron microscopic study of the development of renal adenocarcinomas induced in rats by N-(4'-fluoro-4-biphenylyl)acetamide, J. Natl. Cancer Inst., 64, 1547-1562, 1980.

30. Dees, J.H., Reuber, M.D. and Trump, B.F., Adenocarcinoma of the kidney. I. Ultrastructure of renal adenocarcinomas induced in rats by N-(4'fluoro-4-biphenylyl)acetamide, J. Natl. Cancer Inst., 57, 779-794, 1976.

31. Diaz Gomez, M.I., Swann, P.F. and Magee, P.N., The absorption and metabolism in rats of small oral doses of dimethylnitrosamine. Implication for the possible hazard of dimethylnitrosamine in human food, Biochem. J., 164, 497-500, 1977.

32. Eble, J.N. and Hull, M.T., Morphologic features of renal oncocytoma. A light and electron microscopic study, Human Pathol., 15, 1054-1061, 1984.

33. Eker, R. and Mossige, J., A dominant gene for renal adenomas in the rat, Nature, 189, 858-859, 1961.

34. Eker, R., Mossige, J., Johannessen, J.V. and Aars, H., Hereditary renal adenomas and adenocarcinomas in rats, Diag. Histopathol., 4, 99-110, 1981.

35. Elfarra, A.A. and Anders, M.W., Renal processing of glutathione conjugates. Role in nephrotoxicity, Biochem. Pharmacol., 33, 3729-3732, 1984.

36. Epstein, S.M., Bartus, B. and Farber, E., Renal epithelial neoplasms induced

in male Wistar rats by oral aflatoxin B_1, Cancer Res., 29, 1045-1050, 1969.

37. Ertürk, E., Cohen, S.M. and Bryan, G.T., Induction, histogenesis, and isotransplantability of renal tumors induced by formic acid 2-[4-(5-nitro-2-furyl)-2-thiazolyl]hydrazide in rats, Cancer Res., 30, 2098-2106, 1970.

38. Evarts, R.P., Brown, C.A. and Mostafa, M.H., Production of kidney tumors in rats with low dose of dimethylnitrosamine after partial hepatectomy, J. Natl. Cancer Inst., 68, 293-298, 1982.

39. Ford, S.M. and Hook, J.B., Biochemical mechanisms of toxic nephropathies, Semin. Nephrol., 4, 88-106, 1984.

40. Fortner, J.G., Spontaneous tumors, including gastrointestinal neoplasms and malignant melanomas, in the Syrian hamster, Cancer, 10, 1153-1156, 1957.

41. Fowler, B.A., Mistry, P. and Victery, W.W., Ultrastructural morphometric studies of lead intranuclear inclusion body formation in kidney proximal tubule cells: relationship to altered renal protein synthetic patterns, Toxicologist, 5, 53, 1985.

42. Gerchman, L.L. and Ludlum, D.B., The properties of O^6-methylguanine in templates for RNA polymerase, Biochim. Biophys. Acta, 308, 310-316, 1973.

43. Goodman, D.G., Ward, J.M., Squire, R.A., Chu, K.C. and Linhart, M.S., Neoplastic and non-neoplastic lesions in aging F344 rats, Toxicol. Appl. Pharmacol., 48, 237-248, 1979.

44. Goodman, D.G., Ward, J.M., Squire, R.A., Paxton, M.B., Reichardt, W.D., Chu, K.C. and Linhart, M.S., Neoplastic and non-neoplastic lesions in aging Osborne-Mendel rats, Toxicol. Appl. Pharmacol., 55, 433-447, 1980.

45. Goyer, R.A., Falk, H.L., Hogan, M., Feldman, D.D. and Richter, W., Renal tumors in rats given trisodium nitrilotriacetic acid in drinking water for 2 years, J. Natl. Cancer Inst., 66, 869-880, 1981.

46. Goyer, R.A. and Moore, J.F., Cellular effects of lead, Adv. Exp. Med. Biol., 48, 447-462, 1974.

47. Guder, W.G. and Ross, B.D., Enzyme distribution along the nephron, Kidney Int., 26, 101-111, 1984.

48. Gusek, W., Die Ultrastruktur Cycasin-induzierter Nierenadenome, Virchows Arch. A. Path. Anat. Histol., 365, 221-237, 1975.

49. Hamilton, J.M., Flaks, A., Saluja, P.G. and Maguire, S., Hormonally induced renal neoplasia in the male Syrian hamster and the inhibitory effect of 2-bromo-α-ergocryptine methanesulfonate, J. Natl. Cancer Inst., 54, 1385-1400, 1975.

50. Hanis, N.M., Holmes, T.M., Shallenberger, L.G. and Jones, K.E., Epidemiologic study of refinery and chemical plant workers, J. Occup. Med., 24, 203-212, 1982.

51. Hard, G.C., Autoradiographic analysis of proliferative activity in rat kidney epithelial and mesenchymal cell subpopulations following a carcinogenic dose of dimethylnitrosamine, Cancer Res., 35, 3762-3773, 1975.

52. Hard, G.C., Levamisole is without effect in modifying chemically-induced renal carcinogenesis, Cancer Lett., 3, 221-226, 1977.

53. Hard, G.C., Effect of age at treatment on incidence and type of renal neoplasm induced in the rat by a single dose of dimethylnitrosamine, Cancer Res., 39, 4965-4970, 1979.

54. Hard, G.C., Morphological correlates of irreversible tumour formation, in Mechanisms of Toxicity and Hazard Evaluation, Holmstedt, B., Lauwerys, R., Mercier, M. and Roberfroid, M., Eds., Elsevier/North Holland Biomedical Press, 231-240, 1980.

55. Hard, G.C., High frequency, single-dose model of renal adenoma/carcinoma induction using dimethylnitrosamine in Crl:(W)BR rats, Carcinogenesis, 5, 1047-1050, 1984.

56.   Hard, G.C., Identification of a high frequency model for renal carcinoma by
       the induction of renal tumors in the mouse with a single dose of streptozo-
       tocin, Cancer Res., 45, 703-708, 1985.

57.   Hard, G.C., Borland, R. and Butler, W.H., Altered morphology and behaviour
       of kidney fibroblasts in vitro, following in vivo treatment of rats with a
       carcinogenic dose of dimethylnitrosamine, Experientia, 27, 1208-1209, 1971.

58.   Hard, G.C., Brown, C. and King, H., Isolation of a morphologically-
       transformed epithelial cell-line from rat kidney following an in vivo dose
       of dimethylnitrosamine, Cancer Lett., 10, 277-283, 1980.

59.   Hard, G.C. and Butler, W.H., Cellular analysis of renal neoplasia: induction
       of renal tumors in dietary-conditioned rats by dimethylnitrosamine with a
       reappraisal of morphological characteristics, Cancer Res., 30, 2796-2805,
       1970.

60.   Hard, G.C. and Butler, W.H., Morphogenesis of epithelial neoplasms induced
       in the rat kidney by dimethylnitrosamine, Cancer Res., 31, 1496-1505, 1971.

61.   Hard, G.C. and Butler, W.H., Ultrastructural aspects of renal adenocarcinoma
       induced in the rat by dimethylnitrosamine, Cancer Res., 31, 366-372, 1971.

62.   Hard, G.C., Mackay, R.L. and Kochhar, O.S., Electron microscopic determina-
       tion of the sequence of acute tubular and vascular injury induced in the rat
       kidney by a carcinogenic dose of dimethylnitrosamine, Lab. Invest., 50, 659-
       672, 1984.

63.   Hard, G.C., Mackay, R.L., Martin, J.T. and Inoue, K., Differentiated fea-
       tures of a transformed epithelial cell line (TRKE-1) derived from
       dimethylnitrosamine-treated rat kidney, Cancer Res., 43, 6045-6056, 1983.

64.   Hard, G.C. and Ogiu, T., Null effects of vitamin A analogs on the dimethyl-
       nitrosamine kidney tumor model, Carcinogenesis, 5, 665-669, 1984.

65.   Hecker, E., Definitions and terminology in cancer (tumor) etiology. An
       analysis aiming at proposals for a current internationally standardized ter-
       minology, Z. Krebsforsch., 86, 219-230, 1976.

66.   Hiasa, Y., Enoki, N., Kitahori, Y., Konishi, N. and Shimoyama, T., DL-
       serine: promoting activity on renal tumorigenesis by N-ethyl-N-
       hydroxyethylnitrosamine in rats, J. Natl. Cancer Inst., 73, 297-299, 1984.

67.   Hiasa, Y., Lin, J-C., Konishi, N., Kitahori, Y., Enoki, N. and Shimoyama,
       T., Histopathological and biochemical analyses of transplantable renal
       adenocarcinoma in rats induced by N-ethyl-N-hydroxyethylnitrosamine, Cancer
       Res., 44, 1664-1670, 1984.

68.   Hiasa, Y., Ohshima, M., Iwata, C. and Tanikate, T., Histopathological
       studies on renal tubular cell tumors in rats treated with N-ethyl-N-
       hydroxyethylnitrosamine, Gann, 70, 817-820, 1979.

69.   Hiasa, Y., Ohshima, M., Kitahori, Y., Fujita, T., Yuasa, T. and Miyashiro,
       A., Basic lead acetate: promoting effect on the development of renal tubular
       cell tumors in rats treated with N-ethyl-N-hydroxyethylnitrosamine, J. Natl.
       Cancer Inst., 70, 761-765, 1983.

70.   Hiasa, Y., Ohshima, M., Kitahori, Y., Konishi, N., Fujita, T. and Yuasa, T.,
       β-Cyclodextrin: promoting effects on the development of renal tubular cell
       tumors in rats treated with N-ethyl-N-hydroxyethylnitrosamine, J. Natl. Can-
       cer Inst., 69, 963-967, 1982.

71.   Hiasa, Y., Kitahori, Y., Konishi, N., Enoki, N., Shimoyama, T. and
       Miyashiro, A., Trisodium nitrilotriacetate monohydrate: promoting effects on
       the development of renal tubular cell tumors in rats treated with N-ethyl-N-
       hydroxyethylnitrosamine, J. Natl. Cancer Inst., 72, 483-489, 1984.

72.   Hicks, R.M., Pathological and biochemical aspects of tumour promotion, Car-
       cinogenesis, 4, 1209-1214, 1983.

73.   Hill, D.L. and Grubbs, C.J., Retinoids as chemopreventive and anticancer

agents in intact animals (review), Anticancer Res., 2, 111-124, 1982.

74.   Hinton, D.E., Heatfield, B.M., Lipsky, M.M. and Trump, B.F., Animal model: chemically induced renal tubular carcinoma in rats, Am. J. Pathol., 100, 317-320, 1980.

75.   Horning, E.S. and Whittick, J.W., The histogenesis of stilboestrol-induced renal tumours in the male golden hamster, Brit. J. Cancer, 8, 451-457, 1954.

76.   Ito, N., Hiasa, Y., Tamai, A. and Yoshida, K., Effect of unilateral nephrectomy on the development of kidney tumor in rats treated with N-nitrosodimethylamine, Gann, 60, 319-327, 1969.

77.   Ito, N., Sugihara, S., Makiura, S., Arai, M., Hirao, K., Denda, A. and Nishio, O., Effect on N-(3,5-dichlorophenyl)succinimide on the histological pattern and incidence of kidney tumors in rats induced by dimethylnitrosamine, Gann, 65, 131-138, 1974.

78.   Jasmin, G. and Cha, J.W., Renal adenomas induced in rats by dimethylnitrosamine. An electron microscopic study, Arch. Pathol., 87, 267-278, 1969.

79.   Jasmin, G. and Riopelle, J.L., Renal carcinomas and erythrocytosis in rats following intrarenal injection of nickel subsulfide, Lab. Invest., 35, 71-78, 1976.

80.   Johannsen, S.L., Carcinogenicity of analgesics: long-term treatment of Sprague-Dawley rats with phenacetin, phenazone, caffeine and paracetamol, (acetamidophen), Int. J. Cancer, 27, 521-529, 1980.

81.   Jones, S.R. and Casey, H.W., Primary renal tumors in nonhuman primates, Vet. Pathol., 18 (Suppl. 6), 89-104, 1981.

82.   Kanisawa, M. and Suzuki, S., Induction of renal and hepatic tumors in mice by ochratoxin A, a mycotoxin, Gann, 69, 599-600, 1978.

83.   Kantor, A.F., Current concepts in the epidemiology and etiology of primary renal cell carcinoma, J. Urol., 117, 415-417, 1977.

84.   Kaufman, A.F. and Quist, K.D., Spontaneous renal carcinoma in a New Zealand white rabbit, Lab. Anim. Care, 20, 530-532, 1970.

85.   Khudoley, V.V. and Picard, J.J., Liver and kidney tumors induced by N-nitroso-dimethylamine in Xenopus borealis (Parker), Int. J. Cancer, 25, 679-683, 1980.

86.   Kilham, L., Low, R.J., Conti, S.F. and Dallenbach, F.D., Intranuclear inclusions and neoplasms in the kidneys of wild rats, J. Natl. Cancer Inst., 29, 863-885, 1962.

87.   Kirkman, H. and Bacon, R.L., Malignant renal tumors in male hamsters (Cricetus auratus) treated with estrogen, Cancer Res., 10, 122-124, 1950.

88.   Kluwe, W.M., Abdo, K.M. and Huff, J., Chronic kidney disease and organic chemical exposures: evaluations of causal relationships in humans and experimental animals, Fund. Appl. Toxicol., 4, 889-901, 1984.

89.   Kociba, R.J., Keyes, D.G., Jersey, G.C., Ballard, J.J., Dittenber, D.A., Quast, J.F., Wade, C.E., Humiston, C.G. and Schwartz, B.A., Results of a two year chronic toxicity study with hexachlorobutadiene in rats, Am. Ind. Hyg. Assoc. J., 38, 589-602, 1977.

90.   Kolonel, L.N., Association of cadmium with renal cancer, Cancer, 37, 1782-1787, 1976.

91.   Kroeger-Koepke, M.B. and Michejda, C.J., Evidence for several demethylase enzymes in the oxidation of dimethylnitrosamine and phenylmethylnitrosamine by rat liver fractions, Cancer Res., 39, 1587-1591, 1979.

92.   Kurokawa, Y., Hayashi, Y., Maekawa, A., Takahashi, M., Kokubo, T. and Odashima, S., Carcinogenicity of potassium bromate administered orally to F344 rats, J. Natl. Cancer Inst., 71, 965-972, 1983.

93.   Laqueur, G.L. and Spatz, M., Toxicology of cycasin, Cancer Res. 28, 2262-67,

245

1968.

94.   LePage, R.N. and Christie, G.S., Induction of liver tumours in the rabbit by feeding dimethylnitrosamine, Brit. J. Cancer, 23, 125-131, 1969.

95.   Li, J.J. and Li, S.A., Estrogen-induced tumorigenesis in hamsters: roles for hormonal and carcinogenic activities, Arch. Toxicol., 55, 110-118, 1984.

96.   Li, J.J., Li, S.A., Klicka, J.K., Parsons, J.A. and Lam, L.K.T., Relative carcinogenic activity of various synthetic and natural estrogens in the Syrian hamster kidney, Cancer Res., 43, 5200-5204, 1983.

97.   Lilis, R., Long-term lead exposure, chronic nephropathy, and renal cancer: a case report, Am. J. Ind. Med., 2, 293-297, 1981.

98.   Lombard, L.S., Rice, J.M. and Vesselinovitch, S.D., Renal tumors in mice: light microscopic observations of epithelial tumors induced by ethyl-nitrosourea, J. Natl. Cancer Inst., 53, 1677-1685, 1974.

99.   Lotlikar, P.D., Baldy, W.J. and Dwyer, E.N., Dimethylnitrosamine demethyla-tion by reconstituted liver microsomal cytochrome P-450 enzyme system, Biochem. J., 152, 705-708, 1975.

100. Loveless, A., Possible relevance of O-6 alkylation of deoxyguanosine to mutagenicity and carcinogenicity of nitrosamines and nitrosamides, Nature, 223, 206-207, 1969.

101. Lutz, W.K, Jaggi, W. and Schlatter, C., Covalent binding of diethylstil-bestrol to DNA in rat and hamster liver and kidney, Chem-Biol. Interact., 42, 251-257, 1982.

102. Maekawa, A., Kurokawa, Y., Takahashi, M., Kokubo, T., Ogiu, T., Onodera, H., Tanigawa, H., Ohno, Y., Furukawa, F. and Hayashi, Y., Spontaneous tumors in F-344/DuCrj rats, Gann, 74, 365-372, 1983.

103. Magee, P.N., Toxic liver injury. The metabolism of dimethylnitrosamine, Biochem. J., 64, 676-682, 1956.

104. Magee, P.N., Interaction of activated intermediates of chemical carcinogens with cellular DNA and its possible prevention, in Free Radicals, Lipid Peroxidation and Cancer, McBrien, D.C.H. and Slater, T.F., Eds., Academic Press, London, 353-369, 1982.

105. Magee, P.N. and Barnes, J.M., The experimental production of tumours in the rat by dimethylnitrosamine (N-nitroso dimethylamine), Acta Unio Intern. Con-tra Cancrum., 15, 187-190, 1959.

106. Magee, P.N., Montesano, R. and Preussmann, R., N-nitroso compounds and re-lated carcinogens, in Chemical Carcinogens, Searle, C.E., Ed., ACS Monograph Series No. 173, Washington, D.C., American Chemical Society, 491-625, 1976.

107. Mannweiler, K. and Bernhard, W., Recherches ultrastructurales sur une tumeur rénale expérimentale du hamster, J. Ultrastruct. Res., 1, 158-169, 1957.

108. Mao, P. and Molnar, J.J., The fine structure and histochemistry of lead-induced renal tumors in rats, Am. J. Pathol., 50, 571-603, 1967.

109. Matthews, J.J. and Walpole, A.L., Tumours of the liver and kidney induced in Wistar rats with 4'-fluoro-4-aminodiphenyl, Brit. J. Cancer, 12, 234-241, 1958.

110. McCoy, G.W., A preliminary report on tumors found in wild rats, J. Med. Res., 21, 285-296, 1909.

111. McLaughlin, J.K., Mandel, J.S., Blot, W.J., Schuman, L.M., Mehl, E.S. and Fraumeni, J.F., A population-based case-control study of renal cell car-cinoma, J. Natl. Cancer Inst., 72, 275-284, 1984.

112. McLean, A.E.M. and Magee, P.N., Increased renal carcinogenesis by dimethyl-nitrosamine in protein deficient rats, Brit. J. Exp. Pathol., 51, 587-590, 1970.

113. Meister, P. and Rabes, H., Nierentumoren durch Diäthylnitrosamin nach par-tieller Leberresektion: Morphologie und Wachstumsverhalten, Z. Krebsforsch.,

80, 169-178, 1973.

114.   Merkow, L.P., Epsein, S.M., Slifkin, M. and Pardo, M., The ultrastructure of renal neoplasms induced by aflatoxin B_1, Cancer Res., 33, 1608-1614, 1973.

115.   Metzler, M., Studies on the mechanism of carcinogenicity of diethyl-stilboestrol: role of metabolic activation, Fd. Cosmet. Toxicol., 19, 611-615, 1981.

116.   Metzler, M. and McLachlan, J.A., Peroxidase-mediated oxidation, a possible pathway for metabolic activation of diethylstilbestrol, Biochem. Biophys. Res. Comm., 85, 874-884, 1978.

117.   Miller, E.C. and Miller, J.A., Searches for ultimate chemical carcinogens and their reactions with cellular macromolecules, Cancer, 47, 2327-2345, 1981.

118.   Mitsumori, K., Maita, K., Saito, T., Tsuda, S. and Shirasu, Y., Car-cinogenicity of methylmercury chloride in ICR mice: preliminary note on renal carcinogenesis, Cancer Lett., 12, 305-310, 1981.

119.   Mohr, U., Haas, H. and Hilfrich, J., The carcinogenic effects of dimethyl-nitrosamine and nitrosomethylurea in European hamsters (Cricetus cricetus L.), Brit. J. Cancer, 29, 359-364, 1974.

120.   Mohr, U. and Hilfrich, J., Effect of a single dose of N-diethylnitrosamine on the rat kidney, J. Natl. Cancer Inst., 49, 1729-1731, 1972.

121.   Murphy, G.P., Mirand, E.A., Johnston, G.S., Schmidt, J.D. and Scott, W.W., Renal tumors induced by a single dose of dimethylnitrosamine: morphologic, functional, enzymatic and hormonal characterizations, Invest. Urol., 4, 39-56, 1966.

122.   Nash, J.A., King, L.J., Lock, E.A. and Green, T., The metabolism and dis-position of hexachloro-1:3-butadiene in the rat and its relevance to nephro-toxicity, Toxicol. Appl. Pharmacol., 73, 124-137, 1984.

123.   Nicoll, J.W., Swann, P.F. and Pegg, A.E., Effect of dimethylnitrosamine on persistence of methylated guanines in rat liver and kidney DNA, Nature, 254, 261-262, 1975.

124.   Noronha, R.F.X., The inhibition of dimethylnitrosamine-induced renal tumorigenesis in NZO/B1 mice by orchiectomy, Invest. Urol., 13, 136-141, 1975.

125.   Noronha, R.F.X. and Goodall, C.M., Enhancement by testosterone of dimethyl-nitrosamine carcinogenesis in lung, liver and kidney of inbred NZR/Gd female rats, Carcinogenesis, 4, 613-616, 1983.

126.   Noronha, R.F.X. and Goodall, C.M., The effects of estrogen on single dose dimethylnitrosamine carcinogenesis in male inbred Crl/CDF rats, Car-cinogenesis, 5, 1003-1007, 1984.

127.   Noronha, R.F.X., Rao, B.R. and Goodall, C.M., Significance of elevated androgen receptor levels in human renal adenocarcinoma, Proc. 13th Int. Can-cer Congr., Seattle, 1982, 345.

128.   Ohmori, T. and Tabei, R., Modulation of N-nitrosodimethylamine kidney tumorigenesis by unilateral hydronephrosis and multiple putrescine ad-ministrations, J. Natl. Cancer Inst., 71, 787-793, 1983.

129.   Ohmori, T., Hiasa, Y., Murata, Y. and Williams, G.M., Gamma glutamyl transpeptidase activity in carcinogen-induced epithelial lesions of rat kid-ney, Gann, 73, 543-548, 1982.

130.   Pegg, A.E., Formation and metabolism of alkylated purines: possible role in carcinogenesis by N-nitroso compounds and alkylating agents, Adv. Cancer Res., 25, 195-269, 1977.

131.   Pegg, A.E. and Perry, W., Alkylation of nucleic acids and metabolism of small doses of dimethylnitrosamine in the rat, Cancer Res., 41, 3128-3132, 1981.

247

132. Pegg, A.E. and Wiest, L., Regulation of O^6-methylguanine-DNA methyltransferase levels in rat liver and kidney, Cancer Res., 43, 972-975, 1983.

133. Pitot, H.C., Triggering the cellular change to neoplasia, Urology (April Suppl.), 23, 9-17, 1984.

134. Pour, P., Althoff, J., Salmasi, S.Z. and Stepan, K., Spontaneous tumors and common diseases in three types of hamsters, J. Natl. Cancer Inst., 63, 797-811, 1979.

135. Rabstein, L.S. and Peters, R.L., Tumors of the kidneys, synovia, exocrine pancreas, and nasal cavity in BALB/cf/Cd mice, J. Natl. Cancer Inst., 51, 999-1006, 1973.

136. Rakieten, N., Gordon, B.S., Beaty, A., Cooney, D.A., Schein, P.S. and Dixon, R.L., Modification of renal tumorigenic effect of streptozotocin by nicotinamide: spontaneous reversibility of streptozotocin diabetes, Proc. Soc. Exp. Biol. Med., 151, 356-361, 1976.

137. Rakieten, N., Gordon, B.S., Cooney, D.A., Davis, R.D. and Schein, P.S., Renal tumorigenic action of streptozotocin (NSC-85998) in rats, Cancer Chemother. Rep., 52, 563-567, 1968.

138. Redmond, C.K., Ciocco, A., Lloyd, J.W. and Rush, H.W., Long-term mortality study of steelworkers. VI. Mortality from malignant neoplasms among coke oven workers, J. Occup. Med., 14, 621-629, 1972.

139. Reichert, D., Spengler, V., Romen, W. and Henschler, D., Carcinogenicity of dichloroacetylene: an inhalation study, Carcinogenesis, 5, 1411-1420, 1984.

140. Reznik, G., Ward, J.M., Hardisty, J.F. and Russfield, A., Renal carcinogenic and nephrotoxic effects of the flame retardant tris(2,3-dibromopropyl) phosphate in F344 rats and (C57BL/6N X C3H/HeN)F_1 mice, J. Natl. Cancer Inst., 63, 205-212, 1979.

141. Ritchie, A.W.S. and Chisholm, G.D., The natural history of renal carcinoma, Semin. Oncol., 10, 390-400, 1983.

142. Ritchie, A.W.S., Kemp, I.W. and Chisholm, G.D., Is the incidence of renal carcinoma increasing?, Brit. J. Urol., 56, 571-573, 1984.

143. Roe, F.J.C., Boyland, E., Dukes, C.E. and Mitchley, B.C.V., Failure of testosterone or xanthopterin to influence the induction of renal neoplasms by lead in rats, Brit. J. Cancer, 19, 860-866, 1965.

144. Rosenberg, M.R., Novicki, D.L., Jirtle, R.L., Novotny, A. and Michalopoulos, G., Promoting effect of nicotinamide on the development of renal tubular cell tumors in rats initiated with diethylnitrosamine. Cancer Res., 45, 809-814, 1985

145. Ross, J., Hendrickson, M.R. and Kempson, R.L., The problem of the poorly differentiated sarcoma, Semin. Oncol., 9, 467-483, 1982.

146. Rush, G.F., Maita, K., Sleight, S.D. and Hook, J.B., Induction of rabbit renal mixed-function oxidases by phenobarbital: cell specific ultrastructural changes in the proximal tubule, Proc. Soc. Exp. Biol. Med., 172, 430-439, 1983.

147. Schmäl, D., Habs, M. and Ivankovic, S., Carcinogenesis of N-nitroso-diethylamine (DENA) in chickens and domestic cats, Int. J. Cancer, 22, 552-557, 1978.

148. Schmäl, D., Osswald, H. and Goerttler, K., Cancerogene Wirkung von Diäthylnitrosamin bei Schweinen, Z. Krebsforsch., 72, 102-104, 1969.

149. Selevan, S.G., Landrigan, P.J., Stern, F.B. and Jones, J.H., Mortality of lead smelter workers, Am. J. Epidemiol., 122, 673-683, 1985.

150. Selli, C., Hinshaw, W.M., Woodard, B.H. and Paulson, D.F., Stratification of risk factors in renal cell carcinoma, Cancer, 52, 899-903, 1983.

151. Sempronj, A. and Morelli, E., Carcinoma of the kidney in rats treated with

beta-anthraquinoline, Am. J. Cancer, 35, 534-537, 1939.

152. Shinohara, Y., Arai, M., Hirao, K., Sugihara, S., Nakanishi, K., Tsunoda, H. and Ito, N., Combination effect of citrinin and other chemicals on rat kidney tumorigenesis, Gann, 67, 147-155, 1976.

153. Shinohara, Y., Miyata, Y., Murasaki, G., Nakanishi, K., Yoshimura, T. and Ito, N., Effect of N-(3,5-dichlorophenyl)succinimide on the histological pattern and incidence of kidney tumors induced by streptozotocin in rats, Gann, 68, 397-404, 1977.

154. Shirachi, D.Y., Johansen, M.G., McGowan, J.P. and Tu, S-H., Tumorigenic effect of sodium arsenite in rat kidney, Proc. West. Pharmacol. Soc., 26, 413-415, 1983.

155. Shirai, T., Ohshima, M., Masuda, A., Tamano, S. and Ito, N., Promotion of 2-(ethylnitrosamino)ethanol-induced renal carcinogenesis in rats by nephrotoxic compounds: positive responses with folic acid, basic lead acetate, and N-(3,5-dichlorophenyl)succinimide but not with 2,3-dibromo-1-propanol phosphate, J. Natl. Cancer Inst., 72, 477-482, 1984.

156. Silverberg, E., Cancer statistics 1985, CA, 35, 19-35, 1983.

157. Singer, B., N-nitroso alkylating agents: formation and persistence of alkyl derivatives in mammalian nucleic acids as contributing factors in carcinogenesis, J. Natl. Cancer Inst., 62, 1329-1339, 1979.

158. Singer, B. and Kusmierek, J.T., Chemical mutagenesis, Ann. Rev. Biochem., 52, 655-693, 1982.

159. Slye, M., Holmes, H.F. and Wells, H.G., Primary spontaneous tumors in the kidney and adrenal of mice, J. Cancer Res., 6, 305-336, 1921.

160. Smith, J.H. and Hook, J.B., Mechanism of chloroform nephrotoxicity. III. Renal and hepatic microsomal metabolism of chloroform in mice. Toxicol. Appl. Pharmacol., 73, 511-524, 1984.

161. Smith, W.L. and Bell, T.G., Immunohistochemical localization of the prostaglandin-forming cyclooxygenase in renal cortex, Am. J. Physiol., 235, F451-F457, 1978.

162. Sternberg, S.S., Philips, F.S. and Cronin, A.P., Renal tumors and other lesions in rats following a single intravenous injection of Daunomycin, Cancer Res., 32, 1029-1036, 1972.

163. Stewart, B.W. and Brian, M.J., Evidence of carcinogen-induced replication of partially-repaired DNA in target cells during nitrosamine carcinogenesis, Europ. J. Cancer, 15, 251-256, 1979.

164. Sunderman, F.W., McCully, R.S. and Hopfer, S.M., Association between erythrocytosis and renal cancers in rats following intrarenal injection of nickel compounds, Carcinogenesis, 5, 1511-1517, 1984.

165. Swann, P.F., Magee, P.N., Mohr, U., Reznik, G., Green, U. and Kaufman, D.G., Possible repair of carcinogenic damage caused by dimethylnitrosamine in rat kidney, Nature, 263, 134-136, 1976.

166. Swann, P.F. and McLean, A.E.M., Cellular injury and carcinogenesis. The effect of protein-free high-carbohydrate diet on the metabolism of dimethylnitrosamine in the rat, Biochem. J., 124, 283-288, 1971.

167. Swann, P.F., Kaufman, D.G., Magee, P.N. and Mace, R., Induction of kidney tumors by a single dose of dimethylnitrosamine: dose response and influence of diet and benzo(a)pyrene pretreatment, Brit. J. Cancer, 41, 285-294, 1980.

168. Tanner, D.C. and Lipsky, M.M., Effect of lead acetate on N-(4'-fluoro-4-biphenyl)acetamide-induced renal carcinogenesis in the rat, Carcinogenesis, 5, 1109-1113, 1984.

169. Tekeli, S., Biava, C.G. and Price, J.M., The carcinogenic activity of 3-hydroxy-methyl-1-{[3-(5-nitro-2-furyl)allydidene]amino}hydantoin in rats, Cancer Res., 33, 2894-2897, 1973.

170. Terracini, B., Palestro, G., Gigliardi, R.M. and Montesano, R., Carcinogenicity of dimethylnitrosamine in Swiss mice, Brit. J. Cancer, 20, 871-876, 1966.

171. Thomas, T.L., Decoufle, P. and Moure-Eraso, R., Mortality among workers employed in petroleum refining and petrochemical plants, J. Occup. Med., 22, 97-103, 1980.

172. Thorhallsson, P. and Tulinius, H., Tumours in Iceland. 3. Malignant tumours of kidney. A histological classification, Acta Pathol. Microbiol. Scand., Sect. A., 89, 403-410, 1981.

173. Toth, B., Lack of carcinogenicity of nicotinamide and isonicotinamide following lifelong administration to mice, Oncology, 40, 72-75, 1983.

174. Tsuda, H., Sakata, T., Masui, T., Imaida, K. and Ito, N., Modifying effects of butylated hydroxyanisole, ethoxyquin and acetaminophen on induction of neoplastic lesions in rat liver and kidney initiated by N-ethyl-N-hydroxyethylnitrosamine, Carcinogenesis, 5, 525-531, 1984.

175. Tsuda, H., Sakata, T., Tamano, S., Okumura, M. and Ito, N., Sequential observations on the appearance of neoplastic lesions in the liver and kidney after treatment with N-ethyl-N-hydroxyethylnitrosamine followed by partial hepatectomy and unilateral nephrectomy, Carcinogenesis, 4, 523-528, 1983.

176. van Esch, G.J. and Kroes, R., The induction of renal tumours by feeding basic lead acetate to mice and hamsters, Brit. J. Cancer, 23, 765-771, 1969.

177. Ward, J.M., Goodman, D.G., Squire, R.A., Chu, R.C. and Linhart, M.S., Neoplastic and non-neoplastic lesions in aging (C57BL/6N X CH3/HeN)F_1 (B6C3F_1) mice, J. Natl. Cancer Inst., 63, 849-854, 1979.

178. Wattenberg, L.W., Inhibitors of chemical carcinogens, Adv. Cancer Res., 26, 197-226, 1978.

179. Weekes, U.Y., Metabolism of dimethylnitrosamine to mutagenic intermediates by kidney microsomal enzymes and correlation with reported host susceptibility to kidney tumors, J. Natl. Cancer Inst., 55, 1199-1201, 1975.

180. Williams, R.D., Human urologic cancer cell lines, Invest. Urol., 17, 359-363, 1980.

181. Wolf, C.R., Berry, P.N., Nash, J.A., Green, T. and Lock, E.A., The role of microsomal cytosolic glutathione-S-transferases in the conjugation of hexochloro-1:3-butadiene and its possible relevance to toxicity, J. Pharmacol. Exp. Ther., 228, 202-208, 1984.

182. Woolley, P.G. and Wherry, W.B., Notes on twenty-two spontaneous tumors in wild rats (M. norvegicus), J. Med. Res., 25, 205-215, 1911.

183. Wynder, E.L., Mabuchi, K. and Whitmore, W.F., Epidemiology of adenocarcinoma of the kidney, J. Natl. Cancer Inst., 53, 1619-1634, 1974.

184. Zenser, T.V., Balasubramanian, T.M., Mattammal, M.B. and Davis, B.B., Transport of the renal carcinogen 3-hydroxymethyl-1-{[3-(5-nitro-2-furyl)allydidene]amino}hydantoin by renal cortex and cooxidative metabolism by prostaglandin endoperoxide synthetase, Cancer Res., 41, 2032-2037, 1981.

185. Zenser, T.V. and Davis, B.B., Enzyme systems involved in the formation of reactive metabolites in the renal medulla: cooxidation via prostaglandin H synthase, Fund. Appl. Toxicol., 4, 922-929, 1984.

186. Zollinger, H.U., Durch chronische Bleivergiftung erzeugte Nieradenome und-carcinome bei Ratten und ihre Beziehungen zu den entsprechenden Neubildungen des Menschen, Virchows Archiv., 323, 694-710, 1953.

8

ASSESSMENT OF THE KIDNEY IN RELATION TO BLOOD PRESSURE REGULATION

J. ATKINSON

I.   INTRODUCTION

The kidney responds to wide variations in the external environment to maintain relatively constant ionic conditions around the cells. These changes in kidney function are aimed at maintaining homeostasis and can be brought about by several factors, the most important of which is a change in blood pressure. The interaction between the kidney and blood pressure is primarily mediated via changes in the excretory function of the kidney. Renal diseases, nephrotoxicity or experimental manipulations to the kidneys generally produce hypertension, but sometimes there are no changes in blood pressure. Such renal compromise very rarely leads to a decrease in blood pressure, and it can therefore be argued that if renal excretory function is impaired in any way, a compensatory increase in systemic arterial pressure will occur. Thus the kidney fulfils its homeostatic role at the expense of an increase in blood pressure. The "renal blood volume pressure regulatory system" or "the sodium homeostatic mechanism" fulfils such a role[1]. However the corollary of this is that renal dysfunction is the primary cause of hypertension, and this is one of the most enduring controversies of modern day pathophysiology.

   The systems involved in blood pressure control have been classified according to the speed with which they are called into play following a change in blood pressure and their feedback gains[1]. This latter parameter is a measure of the capacity of a given system to return the blood pressure to its original value. The various pressure control systems are shown in Figure 1. They can be divided into three categories.

(a)   The first systems to be set in motion involve the various reflexes of the nervous system which are stimulated by the baro- and chemoreceptors. These systems are characterized by their fast reaction times and by the fact that they adapt to prolonged changes in pressure. They are not effective as regulators of the overall pressure level, but they can buffer short-lived changes in blood pressure.

(b)   The second category consists of systems with an intermediate time course. These include (i) local vascular relaxation to increased tension on the vessel walls, (ii) the renin-angiotensin vasoconstrictor system, and (iii) a shift in extracellular fluid movement at the capillary level.

(c)   The third and final category consists of a renal system with a very long time course: "the renal blood volume-pressure regulatory system" or the "sodium homeostasis mechanism". This acts via a pressure-diuresis phenomenon whereby an increase in arterial pressure leads to an increase in sodium excretion. This slowly acting system is responsible for the long-term setting of the overall pressure level as it possesses an infinite feedback gain and does not adapt until sodium output is equal to input.

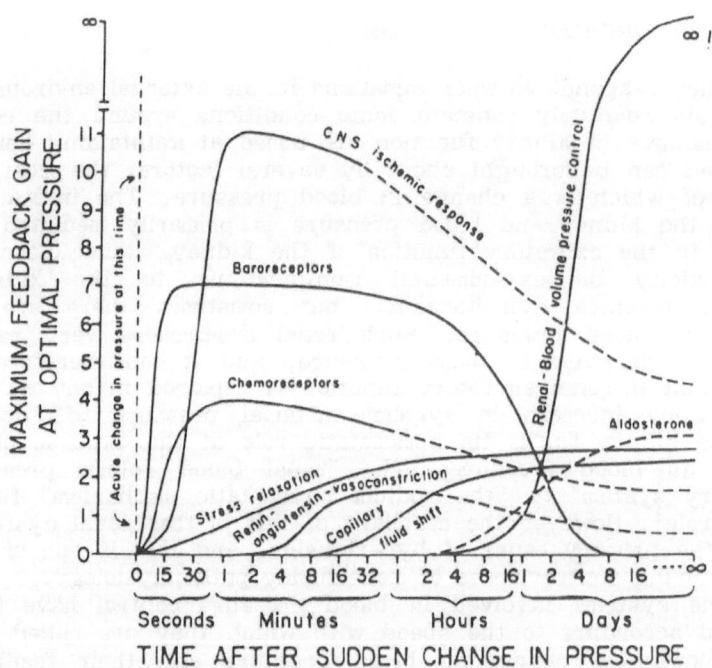

Figure 1 Degree of activation, expressed in terms of feedback gain, of different pressure control mechanisms following a sudden change in arterial pressure. (Reproduced from Guyton[1] with the permission of W.B. Saunders and Co. and the author.)

This chapter first describes the renal blood volume pressure regulatory system. It then considers three types of circulating factors - angiotensin, renomedullary lipids and natriuretic hormones - which modify the relationship between changes in arterial pressure and sodium excretion.

II. THE RENAL BLOOD VOLUME-PRESSURE REGULATORY SYSTEM

Following acute salt loading (i.e. an increase of salt input over salt output), there is an expansion of extracellular and blood volumes giving rise to increased cardiac output[2]. This increases blood pressure and leads to a shift in the balance between glomerular filtration rate and tubular sodium reabsorption towards sodium excretion. As a result of this, there is a fall in extracellular and blood volumes and finally a decrease in blood pressure (see Figure 2). As stated above, the system possesses an infinite feedback gain and does not adapt until sodium output is equal to input, i.e. sodium homeostasis is achieved.

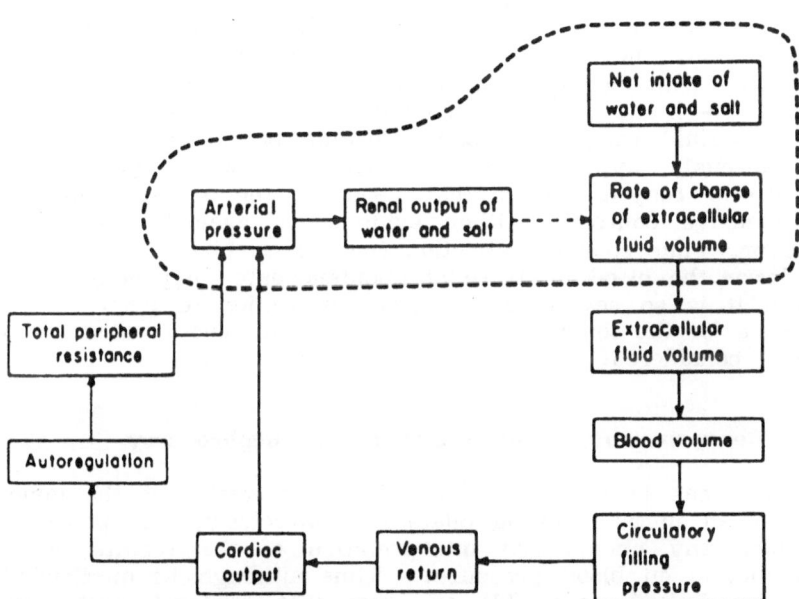

Figure 2 The feedback control loop of the renal body fluid arterial control mechanism. The dashed arrow indicates a negative effect. Those portions of the diagram in the heavy dashed enclosure represent the "determinants" of arterial pressure. Those outside the enclosure represent the variables of the system. (Reproduced from Guyton[2], with permission of The American Journal of Medicine and the authors.)

In the case of a positive sodium balance, i.e. sustained increase in salt intake and/or renal dysfunction in sodium excretion, blood pressure is permanently increased firstly by increased cardiac output and subsequently by an increase in peripheral resistance. Blood pressure is maintained at a level such that salt input and output are equal, and the homeostatic role of the kidney is assured[1-3]. In the established phase of hypertension the renal defect in sodium excretion may no longer be obvious as the increased blood pressure ensures sodium homeostasis.

The evidence for the existence of this mechanism has come from studies on renoprival states (see below). The term "renoprival" in its literal sense denotes removal of all kidney tissue. This limited use has been extended, however, to include states of partial nephrectomy produced by surgery and/or natural or artificial lesions of the kidney. The sodium homeostasis mechanism is also important in renovascular hypertension, i.e. hypertension arising from a modification of blood flow to the kidneys. In the spontaneous (essential or primary) hypertension, whether such a mechanism plays a roll is less certain[4]. In the spontaneously hypertensive rat (and in other types of primary hypertension), salt and water retention due to renal dysfunction may occur at a very early stage. This would lead to an increase in cardiac output and, by autoregulation, an increase in peripheral resistance[4]. There is some indirect evidence of this. Following withdrawal of antihypertensive therapy from spontaneously hypertensive rats, the ensuing rebound increase in blood pressure is associated with increased extracellular fluid volume[5]. Transplantation of the kidney of a hypertensive rat into a normotensive rat leads to fluid retention[6]. Saline loading of the adrenalectomized spontaneously hypertensive rat gives a smaller diuretic and natriuretic response than that seen in the Wistar-Kyoto non-hypertensive control[7]. Other evidence is against this theory, however. Thus sodium restriction (even from birth onwards) does not lower the blood pressure of spontaneously hypertensive rats unless it is so severe as to cause restriction of growth[8]. The evidence for the sodium homeostasis theory in renoprival states will now be considered.

A.   Renoprival hypertensive states: total nephrectomy

Research has been hindered by the deterioration of the general state of an animal following bilateral nephrectomy, a response that excludes any unequivocal interpretation of the results of this manipulation on blood pressure. Thus although Braun-Menéndez and von Euler[9] were able to show that bilateral nephrectomy produces a rise in blood pressure in 33% of the rats, long term observation was hindered by the fact that blood urea rose and the rats died after several days.

1.   Total nephrectomy and volume loading: evidence that
     hypertension is produced by the sodium
     homeostatic mechanism

One of the most conclusive pieces of evidence for any role of renal function in blood pressure regulation would stem from surgical removal of the kidneys. In order to avoid the complications of bilateral nephrectomy such as uraemia, other approaches (subtotal nephrectomy and parabiosis) have been attempted.

The early work on the effects of total nephrectomy on blood pressure have been summarized by Grollman et al.[10], Del Greco et al.[11] and by Ledingham[12]. There is evidence that anephric animals and man can remain normotensive in the absence of volume loading. The latter manipulation, however, generally leads to an increase in blood pressure. This increase can be explained on the basis of an interruption of the feedback control loop of the renal-body arterial pressure control mechanism (Figure 2). The sequence of events involved has been shown to occur in several species: in man[13,14], in dogs[15] and in sheep[16]. After overhydration in three anephric patients an initial increase in cardiac output occurred followed by an increase in total peripheral resistance and arterial pressure[13]. The increase in renal resistance leading to a modification of the renal function curve relating sodium excretion to arterial pressure is of primary importance. Increases in peripheral resistance elsewhere in the body are secondary[14]. In nephrectomized sheep, haemodialysis was used to increase extracellular fluid volume without changing sodium concentration, and in uninephrectomized sheep, dialysis and deoxycorticosterone acetate (DOCA) were used to change sodium without changing volume[16]. "High volume" sheep showed a marked increase in arterial pressure but the increase in "high sodium" sheep was only slight. Total exchangeable sodium was equal in the two groups. The authors concluded that "sodium retention causes hypertension almost entirely because of sodium-induced expansion of extracellular fluid volume"[16]. The possibility exists that the remaining kidney in the uni-nephrectomized sheep prevented the development of hypertension via some renal secretory, antihypertensive mechanism (see below). The authors discarded this possibility, as hypertension does occur following partial nephrectomy and salt loading if the volume is allowed to increase[17].

2.　　Total nephrectomy and volume loading: lack of correlation between volume loading and the increase in blood pressure

Some authors have shown that increases in blood pressure following salt loading in anephric patients are correlated (as predicted by the sodium homeostasis mechanism) with increases in parameters such as blood volume[18] and exchangeable sodium[19], but others have not found such clear-cut correlations. Part of the problem may be explained by differences in the time at which the changes occur. Thus Hampers and co-workers[20] provided evidence that the initial increase in blood pressure in the early renoprival state is linked to an increase in blood volume, but that a subsequent increase in peripheral resistance is required for the maintenance of an elevated blood pressure level.

Salt and water loading in anephric patients may not produce hypertension whatever the time course. In a group of previously normotensive anephric patients salt and water loading produced minor and inconsistent changes in blood pressure, cardiac output and peripheral resistance[21]. Such a result may be explained either by a peripheral vascular defect which hinders the retention of fluid by the circulatory system, or by cardiac failure which would prevent pressure rising in the face of increases in blood volume[21].

The increase in blood pressure following total nephrectomy can also be taken as evidence for the existence of renal secretory depressor systems which modulate the activity of the sodium homeostasis mechanism outlined above.

B. Renoprival hypertensive states: partial reduction of renal mass

1. Uninephrectomy

Uninephrectomy of the normotensive animal generally does not alter blood pressure[11,22]. The rat may be an exception to this rule. Thus Grollman and Halpert[23] found that, 3 months following uninephrectomy of normotensive rats from their stock colony, only 23% remained normotensive and 20% had developed marked hypertension. The degree of hypertension was correlated with the incidence of lesions in the kidney removed at the start of the experiment. The authors suggested that the renal lesions stemmed from dietary deficiences in early life and rendered the rat more susceptible to the hypertensive effects of uninephrectomy.

Uninephrectomy can potentiate the effects of other hypertension-inducing manipulations. Thus hypertension induced by excessive sodium intake and/or administration of DOCA was more pronounced following unilateral nephrectomy[24]. Sodium restriction does not alter blood pressure in normal rats[25], but if sodium restricted rats undergo unilateral nephrectomy there is an increase in blood pressure. The increase appears to be mediated by the renin-angiotensin system as it is blocked by intraperitoneal infusion of captopril[25].

2. Degree of reduction in functional renal mass and change in blood pressure

The frequency of hypertension following reduction of functional renal mass depends on the extent of reduction involved[26]. There was an incidence of 18% after unilateral nephrectomy and 45 to 69% in rats with two-thirds to four-fifths renal ablation. Hypertension in the latter group was often only moderate and slowly developing. Predictable levels of hypertension could be rapidly obtained when 1% saline was given[26].

3. Uninephrectomy plus removal of the poles of the remaining kidney (reduction of functional renal mass by 70-80%)

Reduction of renal mass by 70-80% produces only moderate hypertension in rats[26-28], and dogs[17] as long as the animals are not volume loaded. Upon giving the animals saline (0.9 or 1%) to drink or a diet high in sodium, salt (and therefore fluid) loading occurs and marked hypertension develops. Ylitalo et al.[28], showed that following removal of 70% of the functional renal mass of the rat a normal daily sodium intake of 1.8 to 3 mEq/rat produced an increase in blood pressure of 15 mmHg after 4-6 weeks. Feeding animals 10-15 mEq/rat a day produced a 64 mmHg increase, whereas rats maintained on a low sodium diet (0.002 to 0.004 mEq/rat per day) did not increase their blood pressure. Marked compensatory hypertrophy of the remaining kidney tissue occurred on the high sodium diet but, in spite of this, extracellular fluid volume and blood pressure increased. In the rats given a low sodium diet both the plasma and renal renin-angiotensin systems were stimulated, but as fluid equilibrium was maintained, hypertension did not occur. Thus the renin-angiotensin system alone cannot produce long lasting hypertension if fluid equilibrium is maintained.

4. Reduction of functional renal mass and volume loading:
    increase in blood pressure via the sodium
    homeostatic mechanism

The sequence of events which leads to hypertension following volume overload in the presence of reduced functional renal mass is summarized in Figure 2[1,17,29,30]. High saline intake with reduced functional renal mass produces positive fluid balance leading to an increase in blood and other extracellular fluid volumes. The increase in blood volume produces an increase in mean circulatory filling pressure, venous return, right atrial pressure and finally cardiac output. Increased cardiac output (with as yet no change in total peripheral resistance) produces an increase in arterial pressure which stimulates the baroreceptor reflex[31]. Elicitation of the baroreceptor reflex lowers heart rate and peripheral resistance in an attempt to lower blood pressure. The effect of the baroreceptor reflex diminishes as the reflex adapts to the higher pressure, and the baroreceptors are reset at a higher pressure level. The elevated arterial pressure level produces an increase in sodium and water excretion and so the mean circulatory pressure falls, as does cardiac output. Total peripheral resistance rises due to autoregulation as cardiac output falls[32]. In stable volume-loaded hypertension, peripheral resistance is increased but cardiac output is only slightly above normal. The increase in peripheral resistance, being mainly arteriolar in nature, is accompanied by a fall in capillary pressure leading to reabsorption of interstitial fluid back into the circulation. The extra fluid in the circulation is eliminated by the kidneys, and so extracellular fluid volumes return to normal. The high salt intake causes a marked decrease in the activity of the renin-angiotensin-aldosterone axis[29] but volume loading hypertension occurs in spite of this.

Factors modulating the kidney's blood volume-pressure regulatory system will now be considered starting with the renin-angiotensin system.

III. THE RENIN-ANGIOTENSIN SYSTEM

Renin secreted by the kidneys generates angiotensin I from circulating angiotensinogen, and this decapeptide is then split by the converting enzyme to produce the octapeptide, angiotensin II. Angiotensin II is a powerful vasoconstrictor. In the presence of excess amounts of the substrate, angiotensinogen, and a non-limiting converting enzyme activity (conditions which may not always be fulfilled[33]), the amount of renin liberated by the kidneys will be the rate-limiting step in the formation of the vasoconstrictor, angiotensin II. The rate of release of renin from the kidney is controlled by several factors, most prominent of which is blood pressure. Thus following a decrease in renal arterial pressure the degree of increase in systemic arterial pressure produced by angiotensinergic vasoconstriction will be inversely proportional to the fall in renal perfusion pressure[34]. Such a mechanism is called into play following acute changes in blood pressure. The role of the renin-angiotensin system in long-term blood pressure control involves the antinatriuretic - and not the vasoconstrictor - effect of angiotensin.

A.   Renovascular hypertensive states: induction of hypertension by ischaemia limited to the kidney

Ischaemia limited to the kidney produces permanent hypertension[35] due initially to the secretion by the ischaemic kidney of a circulating vasoconstrictor agent[36].

The clip or clamp technique developed by Goldblatt[37] was intended as a way of producing a disturbance of renal haemodynamics similar to that which preceded the development of hypertension. From the start workers found it easier to produce hypertension by this method in the rat, sheep and goat than in the dog. Removal of the contralateral kidney (one-kidney, one-clip hypertension) or destruction of the medulla of the contralateral kidney by ureteral ligation accentuated the hypertension.

According to Goldblatt[37] reduction in renal blood flow leads to liberation of renin into the circulation. Renin then acts upon angiotensinogen to form angiotensin, the active vasoconstrictor agent. Recent work has concentrated on the biochemistry of the renin-angiotensin system, the ubiquity of the system and the development of inhibitors[38,39]. This chapter will focus on the modification of the renal blood volume-pressure system by angiotensin, the role of this modification in renovascular hypertension and how this may relate to blood pressure changes following toxic injury. The subject has been reviewed extensively[1,27,40-48].

B.   The one-kidney, one-clip model

Renal clipping produces a shift in the kidney function curve relating arterial pressure to sodium excretion[49]. Arterial pressure increases in direct proportion to the decrease produced by the clip, such that renal function is restored at a higher systemic arterial pressure but at a "normal" intra-renal arterial pressure. In the early stages the renin-angiotensin system is stimulated by the fall in intra-renal arterial pressure. Blood pressure is increased due to the vasoconstrictor effect of angiotensin. The renin-angiotensin system is then switched off when the post-clip renal arterial pressure returns to normal. Inhibition of the renin-angiotensin system will delay the development of hypertension but will not prevent it, as the established hypertension is a type of volume loading hypertension (see Figure 3)[50-60].

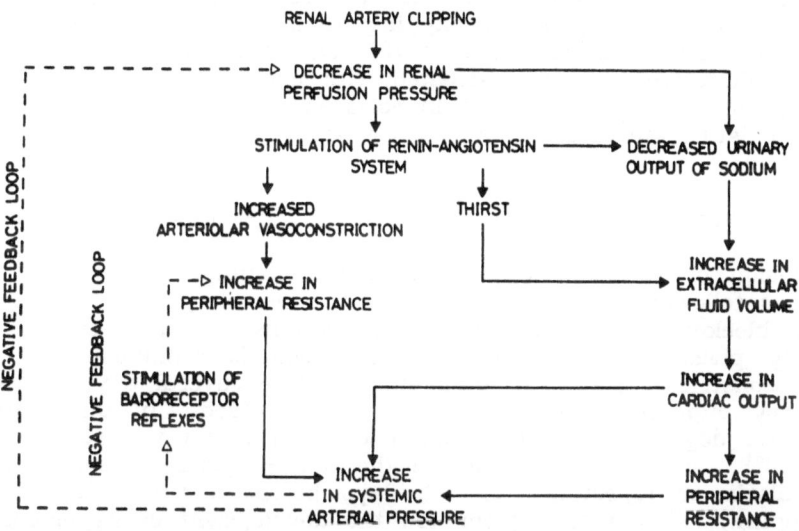

Figure 3 Events following renal artery clipping (with or without contralateral nephrectomy) leading to renovascular hypertension.

1. Changes in the renin-angiotensin system during the development of one-kidney, one-clip hypertension

Details of the changes following unilateral renal artery clipping after contralateral nephrectomy have been described by several workers[41,61-63]. During the hours following clipping, plasma renin concentration and blood pressure increase. The linear regression between the two is similar to that obtained following infusion of exogenous renin. Then plasma renin concentration decreases, sodium retention occurs and body fluid volumes increase. During the next stage cardiac output increases, whereas peripheral resistance decreases and finally sodium balance, body fluid volumes and plasma renin are normal, whereas peripheral resistance is increased. One-kidney, one-clip hypertension therefore has three phases: (a) an initial phase with increased angiotensin levels, (b) an intermediate phase with increased fluid volume and cardiac output and (c) a final phase with increased peripheral resistance. Hypertension in the one-kidney, one-clip model is basically a volume loading type of hypertension with, at its onset, stimulation of the renin-angiotensin system.

2. Physiological disruption of the renin-angiotensin system

Several weeks' unilateral renal artery constriction produces a decrease in the renin content of the contralateral kidney to 5% that of a normal kidney[64]. On removal of the clipped kidney, blood pressure falls but the rat is renin-depleted for several weeks. Such renin-depleted rats are incapable of renin secretion in the face of stimuli such as haemorrhage[65]. Clipping of the artery of the renin-depleted rat produces neither renin secretion nor an increase in blood pressure[64]. Complete recovery of the renin and blood pressure response to clipping occur when the renin content of the kidney has returned to 75% that of normal[64]. Clipping of uninephrectomized rats pretreated with cycloheximide showed that approximately half of the renin released came from a liberation of pre-existing stores and half from de novo protein synthesis[66].

3. Pharmacological disruption of the renin-angiotensin system

Infusion of saralasin (an angiotensin II antagonist) during the hours following clipping potentiated the rise in plasma renin level but blocked the increase in blood pressure[67]. Thus during the early phase of this model, hypertension is maintained by the vasoconstrictor action of angiotensin. After several days of renal artery clipping other mechanisms are involved. In uninephrectomized dogs in which the blood flow to the kidney was reduced by 55-60%[68], continuous blockade of the renin-angiotensin system with saralasin or teprotide (for 1-2 days before and 6-7 days after clipping), slowed and attenuated the development of hypertension but did not prevent it[50]. Discontinuation of the treatment with teprotide in clipped animals led to a further increase in blood pressure. The orally active converting enzyme inhibitor, captopril, gave similar results: prolonged administration of captopril delayed the development of hypertension in one-kidney, one-clip dogs but again did not prevent it[59]. The development of one-kidney, one-clip hypertension could be prevented only by a combination of interruption of the renin-angiotensin system (with captopril) and salt depletion[69].

Acute blockade of the renin-angiotensin system has little effect in established one-kidney, one-clip hypertension. Injections or infusions of short duration of angiotensin antagonists are without effect[70-71]. Several minutes infusion of teprotide produces a slight fall in blood pressure in established one-kidney, one-clip hypertensive rats, but this fall is no larger than that seen in normotensive rats[72]. Longer term blockade of converting enzyme activity lowers blood pressure. Captopril produced a significant decrease in blood pressure in one-kidney, one-clip rats with established hypertension after several days' infusion only. The blood pressure decrease was accompanied by an increase in urinary sodium excretion[73]. Thus in established hypertension the activity of the renin-angiotensin system is apparently normal, and pharmacological interruption of the system produces a slowly developing decrease in blood pressure following increased sodium excretion. The renin-angiotensin system thus plays a role in established one-kidney, one-clip hypertension via an action of angiotensin that is different from its extra-renal vasoconstrictor action.

Investigation of renal hormonal systems involved in blood pressure control is hampered by the difficulty involved in ablating the source of the system, the kidney. Thus pharmacological interruption is used. When interpreting data obtained with pharmacological blocking agents (and especially so with angiotensin converting enzyme inhibitors), it should not be forgotten that the fact that blood pressure falls following blockade of a certain renal particular system does not prove that a modification of this system is the primary underlying cause of the increase in blood pressure following a change of kidney function. Furthermore the results of experiments in which blocking agents are given for long periods are complicated by the secondary readjustments and adaptations which occur in renal and extra-renal systems not blocked by the agent used.

C. The two-kidney, one-clip model

This type of hypertension can also be divided into several phases[74]. During the first brief period hypertension is maintained by the peripheral vasoconstrictor effect of angiotensin only. During a second phase angiotensin-induced vasoconstriction plays a less important role and blood pressure is maintained by a slow pressor effect of angiotensin involving its antinatriuretic action (see later). Removal of the clipped kidney during these two stages normalizes blood pressure. After several months, uninephrectomy becomes a less and less efficient cure for hypertension as lesions of the vasculature of the contralateral kidney develop. Blood pressure is finally set according to the sodium homeostasis theory.

The mechanism involved is basically the same as that of the one-kidney, one-clip model (see Figure 3). The presence of the contralateral kidney complicates the picture, however. Although renal blood flow increases so as to compensate for the decrease in the clipped kidney[75], in the "second phase" increased circulating angiotensin levels "clip" the contralateral kidney. Therefore it cannot excrete the amount of sodium necessary to fully compensate for the diminished sodium level excretion of the physically clipped kidney, at least at a normal arterial pressure[76,77]. Arterial pressure therefore rises, and the contralateral kidney starts to compensate for the decrease in sodium excretion. Such partial compensation prevents the arterial pressure from reaching a high enough level such that the clipped kidney could by itself fully compensate for diminished sodium excretion[78]. Thus the renin-angiotensin system of the clipped kidney is not completely switched off as was the case in the one-kidney, one-clip model, and it plays a more important role in established hypertension in two-kidney, one-clip animals[79]. This role may be one of inter-renal or internephron communication. Ischaemic nephrons dampen the compensatory increase in sodium excretion by non-ischaemic nephrons such that arterial pressure rises and perfusion of the ischaemic nephrons is improved. Prolonged inhibition of the renin-angiotensin system prevents the development of hypertension in this model[80].

1.   Changes in the renin-angiotensin system during the
      development of two-kidney, one-clip hypertension

Chronic hypertension in dogs can be produced by unilateral renal
artery clipping leading to a decrease in renal blood flow of
80%[81],[82]. Plasma renin activity is elevated for the first 3-4 days
but arterial pressure is elevated for several months, until a col-
lateral circulation develops[83]. Short infusions of saralasin in the
chronic phase do not lower blood pressure unless the renin-
angiotensin system is stimulated by salt depletion prior to infusion.

Vasopressin, in the absence of the renin-angiotensin system,
appears to play a major role in blood pressure control[84] and in the
control of extracellular fluid sodium concentration[85]. It has also
been reported that angiotensin will stimulate vasopressin release[86].
Vasopressin, however, does not appear to be implicated in the effects of the renin-angiotensin system in renovascular
hypertension[87],[88].

2.   Physiological disruption of the renin-angiotensin system

Surgical removal of the clipped kidney will cure hypertension but
the degree of improvement depends upon the duration of the hypertension prior to nephrectomy[89]. Up to 3 weeks' duration there
is a substantial fall in blood pressure following nephrectomy, the
decrease being proportional to the duration of hypertension (from 3
days to 3 weeks). After 4 weeks removal of the clipped kidney
produces a very slight fall in blood pressure. Thus clipping induces slowly developing changes such that, after a certain time,
removal of the clipped kidney is not a permanent cure for hypertension.

Dogs are generally less susceptible to manipulations aimed at
producing hypertension than rats. Likewise they appear more susceptible to the beneficial effects of removal of the clipped kidney.
After 4 to 16 months, removal of the clipped kidney produces a fall
in blood pressure back to preclipping, normotensive values[81].

3.   Pharmacological disruption of the renin-angiotensin system

Acute infusion of angiotensin antagonists in dogs lowers blood
pressure in the early phase of hypertension but not in the chronic
phase[90]. Acute infusion of saralasin in rats with established two-
kidney, one-clip hypertension does not decrease blood pressure unless the renin-angiotensin system is stimulated by salt depletion[91].
Following prolonged administration of captopril to normal and
sodium-depleted rats and to one- and two-kidney benign and
malignant hypertensive rats, a biphasic fall in blood pressure was
observed[92]. The degree of the initial rapid decrease was proportional to the activity of the renin-angiotensin system. The slower
decrease in blood pressure was accompanied by natriuresis and
diuresis[92]. Thus the long-term effect of captopril in established
hypertension is via blockade of the intrarenal antinatriuretic effect

of the renin-angiotensin system.

It has been suggested that the long term therapeutic use of blockers of the renin-angiotensin system such as captopril may be limited by aggravation of renal failure owing to blockade of the renin-angiotensin system[93]. Postglomerular resistance is maintained by the vasoconstrictor action of angiotensin (see below) and blockade of its formation with captopril will lead to a fall in this resistance and in glomerular capillary pressure. The ensuing fall in filtration will be well tolerated if the contralateral kidney is capable of compensation. If, however, the complications of stenosis are bilateral (or there is one solitary kidney) then renal failure may occur[93].

4. Antinatriuretic effect of angiotensin

Several lines of evidence suggest that the initial extra-renal vasoconstrictor effect of angiotensin II is superseded in the later phases of renovascular hypertension by an antinatriuretic role for angiotensin II. In normal subjects perfusion of angiotensin produces marked sodium retention, stimulation of aldosterone levels and an increase in blood pressure[94]. When normotensive dogs were infused intravenously with 5 ng/kg per min of angiotensin II there was no immediate effect on blood pressure which increased slowly over 3 days or more. The degree of increase depended upon the sodium intake[95]. Urinary sodium output was the same in controls and dogs receiving angiotensin at all levels of sodium intake (see Figure 4). Thus angiotensin appeared to block the normal pressure natriuresis which should have occurred[96], without any increase in aldosterone levels. Angiotensin II shifted the curve relating urinary sodium output to blood pressure, to the right, indicating that angiotensin has a direct antinatriuretic effect. Escape from the antinatriuretic effect of angiotensin infusion can occur following a sufficient rise in renal perfusion pressure[97]. The final plateau levels of hypertension obtained after angiotensin perfusion were not modified by baroreceptor denervation[98]. In sodium-depleted dogs angiotensin infusion did not produce hypertension[99]. Increases in aldosterone levels occurred at the beginning of the infusion but aldosterone levels tended to decrease thereafter[99]. Following induction of hypertension by angiotensin infusion, the addition of aldosterone did not further increase blood pressure[100]. Further studies have shown that angiotensin conserves sodium independently of changes in aldosterone levels[101-103]. Angiotensin II is several times more potent than aldosterone in the long term control of sodium balance[104]. However, angiotensin infusion in adrenalectomized dogs produced an increase in blood pressure which was smaller than that observed in normal dogs[100]. On the whole the evidence suggests that stimulation of aldosterone plays a minor role in angiotensin-induced hypertension.

The direct antinatriuretic effect of angiotensin has been repeatedly demonstrated by perfusion of angiotensin into the renal artery. Low dose infusion (which caused an increase in angiotensin levels within the physiological range), into the renal artery of acutely denervated kidneys of volume-expanded dogs produced

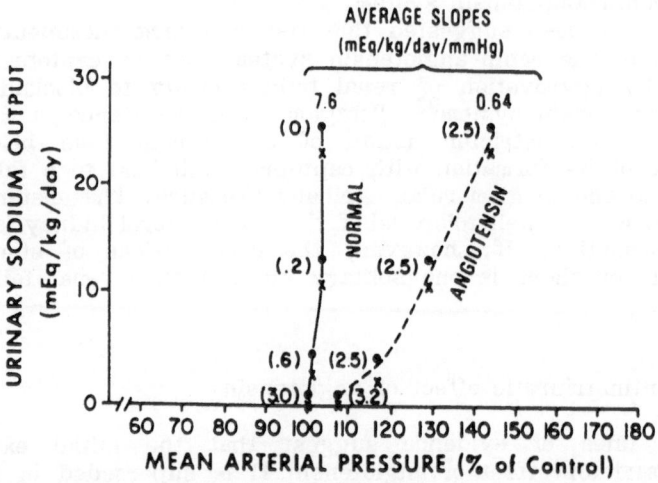

Figure 4 Curves representing the relationship between mean arterial pressure and urinary sodium output in normal and in angiotensin-infused dogs when the sodium intake was increased from a sodium-deficient level to a very high sodium intake level. (The numbers of parentheses represent the calculated relative levels of circulating angiotensin, considering the original control level to be 1.0. Reproduced from DeClue et al.[95], with permission of the American Heart Association and the authors.)

renal vasoconstriction, antinatriuresis and antikaliuresis[105]. Angiotensin infusion into the renal artery of intact kidneys of slightly volume-expanded dogs was antinatriuretic and antidiuretic at doses which did not alter glomerular filtration rate[106]. Intrarenal perfusion of the angiotensin antagonist, saralasin, produced natriuresis in sodium-depleted or dehydrated dogs in which the renin-angiotensin system was activated[107-109]. It appears that angiotensin II at physiological concentrations $(10^{-12}-10^{-10}\text{mol/l})$ stimulates proximal tubular sodium reabsorption while higher concentrations (10^{-7} mol/l) inhibit it[110].

It has been suggested that renin is released into the interstitium of the cortex and enters the renal circulation at the capillary level. This implies that the renin-angiotensin system has a primary intrarenal role[111]. Furthermore the renin-angiotensin system appears to play a key role in autoregulation of glomerular filtration rate and electrolyte excretion[112-114]. According to Thurau and Mason[115] the renin-angiotensin system may act primarily as an intrarenal system controlling glomerulotubular balance. Increased delivery of sodium to the macula densa stimulates the intrarenal renin-angiotensin system which in turn decreases filtration rate via its effect on afferent arterioles. Others have provided evidence, however, that the control of glomerular filtration rate by intrarenal angiotensin is via its effect on postglomerular vessels[116,117]. Whatever the mechanism involved, it would appear that in essential hypertension renal haemodynamics are adjusted so as to maintain a constant glomerular filtration rate[118].

In conclusion, the principal role of angiotensin II in the long term control of blood pressure appears to be an antinatriuretic one by which it modulates the renal blood volume-pressure regulatory system. Its extrarenal vasoconstrictor action appears to be limited to certain short-term situations.

IV.   RENOMEDULLARY FACTORS

A.   Antihypertensive effects of the kidney

Both renoprival and renovascular hypertensive states may be due to diminished activity of a renal antihypertensive secretory function which modifies the kidney blood volume-pressure regulatory system. Evidence for the existence of blood pressure lowering factors produced by the kidney has been reviewed by Muirhead[119], Muirhead and Pitcock[120] and Mandal[121]. Hamilton and Grollman[122], Grollman[123] and Page et al.[124,125] found that renal extracts would lower blood pressure in a wide variety of hypertension models including man. They did not isolate the active factor(s). More recently interest has centred on two types of renal antihypertensive factors: a factor control interstitial space compliance and vasodilator antihypertensive renomedullary lipids.

B.   A kidney hormone controlling interstitial space compliance

According to the hypothesis proposed by Floyer and co-workers, the kidney secretes a hormone which controls interstitial space compliance or capacity and so determines whether extracellular fluid overload will (or will not) be accompanied by hypertension[126]. Simple increase in volume will not increase blood pressure as fluid passes out of the circulation into the interstitial space. Only when interstitial space pressure rises to counteract this fluid movement (and maybe even force fluid into the circulation), will blood pressure rise.

Following unilateral nephrectomy and ureterocaval anastomosis, the remaining kidney retains its capacity to secrete a hormone which maintains interstitial space compliance although it loses its capacity to excrete sodium. Although extracellular fluid volume rises following injections of blood or saline drinking in such rats, blood pressure does not rise. The hormone allows the body to withstand the fluid overload by limiting plasma volume expansion[127,128]. Increases in extracellular fluid volume produced by the same manipulations in bilaterally nephrectomized rats produce hypertension.

The kidney therefore possesses at least two homeostatic mechanisms - the excretory, blood volume-pressure mechanism and a second secretory blood mechanism operating via movement of fluid between the interstitial space and the plasma. These two systems are complementary. The renal hormone alters the position, shape or slope of the volume/pressure curve of the interstitial space demonstrated by Guyton[129]. Furthermore, reduction in the compliance of the interstitial space cannot alone cause hypertension. Unless renal excretion of salt and water is reduced at the same time, equilibrium will occur with lower interstitial fluid volume and normal plasma volume[14,130].

This mechanism may also be involved not only in renoprival but also in renovascular hypertension[130]. After 60 days of renal artery clipping in the uninephrectomized rat, tissue and venous pressures and the ratio of plasma volume:interstitial fluid volume were increased. These changes were thought to be induced by a decreased secretion of a hormone controlling interstitial space compliance following renal artery clipping. Removal of the clip cured the rats of their hypertension, and at the same time plasma volume and the ratio of plasma volume:interstitial fluid volume fell. Interstitial fluid volume rose but tissue pressure fell, presumably due to increased compliance[130].

In further experiments on the declipping of one-kidney, one-clip hypertensive rats, blood pressure fell in spite of prevention of extrarenal fluid loss by administration of salt solution[131]. Kidney transplantation had similar effects[132]. Subpressor doses of angiotensin inhibited the blood pressure fall, whereas norepinephrine (noradrenaline) was without effect[132]. The renin-angiotensin system appears, therefore, to oppose the action of this hormone, possibly by inhibiting its release. A similar interaction between the renin angiotensin system and the renomedullary antihypertensive factors has been suggested by Muirhead[119] and Muirhead and Pitcock[120] (see below).

The "Floyer factor" has not yet been isolated, so we do not know whether it is similar to the "Muirhead factor" described below. The "Floyer factor" modulates the renal blood volume-pressure regulatory system by altering interstitial space compliance and so determining whether or not volume overload will induce hypertension. The "Muirhead factor" may act in a similar way but by changing vascular compliance, i.e. by inducing vasodilatation.

C.   Vasodilator antihypertensive renomedullary lipids

There is increasing evidence for the existence of vasodilator antihypertensive renomedullary lipids.

1.   Effects on blood pressure of non-excretory renal tissue

Early evidence was obtained from experiments on the antihypertensive effects of transplantation of non-excretory renomedullary tissue in binephrectomized animals. As hypertension can be induced following binephrectomy or ureterocaval anastomosis with or without volume expansion it was supposed that the primary factor was loss of renal antihypertensive secretory function[133,134]. Furthermore transplantation of non-excretory renal or renomedullary tissue induced a fall in blood pressure in the presence and in the absence of changes in extracellular fluid volume[134-137].

Subcutaneous transplants of normal or clipped kidneys lowered blood pressure to an equal extent in two kidney renovascular hypertensive rats[138,139]. Thus non-excretory kidney tissue can lower blood pressure. The transplant from the clipped kidney was equally capable of lowering blood pressure. These results can be interpreted as follows. Stenosis of the renal artery prevents the release of the antihypertensive factor, but following transplantation the medulla is able to release the antihypertensive factor(s). Following transplantation blood pressure was lowered but not normalized. Concomitant inhibition of the renin-angiotensin system (with teprotide or saralasin) was required before pressure could be normalized[138,139]. Thus during the development of hypertension following renal artery clipping, two hormone systems are involved: increased activity of the renin-angiotensin system and decreased release of antihypertensive medullary factors. Transplantation of renomedullary tissue has also been shown to lower blood pressure in the spontaneously hypertensive rat[140]. The authors suggested that there may be a deficiency of the renomedullary vasodepressor factor in the spontaneous hypertensive rat (SHR)[140].

2. Release of renomedullary antihypertensive factors and blood pressure fall following unclipping

Extracorporeal perfusion with the venous blood of acutely unclipped kidneys of chronic two-kidney, one-clip renal hypertensive rats produces marked falls in blood pressure in normotensive rats[141], possibly due to the release of depressor substances from the unclipped kidney. As the blood pressure fall is not accompanied by reflex tachycardia it was suggested that part of the depressor action was centrally mediated. On disconnecting the perfusion, the depressor action was very long-lasting[141]. The semi-purified antihypertensive renomedullary lipids of Muirhead (see below) have the same characteristics.

Renal venous blood was collected 5 hours after unclipping plus ureterocaval anastomosis following 6 months of one-kidney, one-clip hypertension[142]. An antihypertensive neutral renomedullary lipid was then isolated from the effluent and shown (a) to lower blood pressure in anaesthetized hypertensive rats, (b) to be free of prostaglandins and (c) to be the same as that isolated from renal medullary tissue[142]. As the kidney released its lipid into the venous blood, the interstitial cells of the renal papilla lost their lipid droplets.

Induction of papillary necrosis with bromoethanamine (see below) potentiates the hypertensive effect of unilateral renal artery clipping[143]. This observation suggests that two mechanisms are operating: stimulation of the renin-angiotensin pressor system and diminution of the activity of the renomedullary depressor system. The result, however, was at the limit of statistical significance and could not be reproduced by other workers[144,145]. Furthermore the reversal of two-kidney, one-clip hypertension by unclipping the renal artery is less marked following ablation of the papilla[145]. Thus the renal medulla produces a vasodepressor substance that maintains normal blood pressure and is responsible for the fall in blood pressure following reversal of Goldblatt hypertension[146,147]. This vasodepressor substance is probably not a prostaglandin or kallikrein as neither indomethacin nor aprotinin attenuated the fall in blood pressure upon reversal of Goldblatt hypertension[148].

267

There appears to be an interaction between the secretion of a renomedullary factor and the sodium volume status following unclipping[149,150]. This renomedullary hormonal system may therefore modulate the function of the renal blood volume-pressure regulatory system. After several months of one-kidney, one-clip hypertension, rats were unclipped and subject to (a) ureterocaval anastomosis, (b) ureteral ligation or (c) a sham operation. Some of the rats subjected to ureterocaval anastomosis were volume loaded by intravenous injections of saline. Following unclipping blood pressure returned to normal in 3 hours in rats with contracted body fluids (i.e. with normal urine flow), in 15-20 hours in rats with no change in body fluids (ureterocaval anastomosis), and in 45-50 hours in those with expanded body fluids (ureterocaval anastomosis plus saline loading). Thus the reduction in blood pressure following unclipping is due a combination of contraction of body fluids and secretion of renal antihypertensive factors. Unclipping combined with ureteral ligation produced a normalization of blood pressure in 45 hours. As ureteral ligation produces a form of papillary necrosis by pressure-induced ischaemia[151,152], it was suggested that the delayed fall in blood pressure in this group was due to diminished production of the renomedullary antihypertensive factor.

Further evidence of an interaction between renomedullary hormone(s) and sodium has been obtained with Dahl rats (see below). Renomedullary interstitial cells in culture from Dahl salt-resistant rats had more lipid droplets than those of salt-sensitive rats[153]. Transplantation of cells from salt-resistant rats had a greater antihypertensive effect than that of cells from salt-sensitive rats[153]. Thus several lines of evidence point to an interaction between the Muirhead factor and the renal blood volume-pressure regulatory system.

3.   Alterations in the medulla in hypertensive states

In rats with two-kidney, one-clip Goldblatt hypertension there is a reduction in the osmophilic lipid droplets of the interstitial cells of the renal papilla[154]. This is associated with a fall in the steep gradient of concentration for sodium between cortex and papilla generally seen in normotensive rats. Whether these two factors are functionally related, and what their relation is to the hypertensive state of the rat, is as yet unexplained. A reduction in the osmophilic droplets of the interstitial cells was also observed in DOCA-salt hypertension in the rat and in three patients with malignant nephrosclerosis[24,155]. The decrease in renal medullary interstitial cell droplets could, however, be a secondary phenomenon produced by a decrease in renal blood flow[24]. Renomedullary deficiency may be involved in the hypertensive state resulting from salt loading following partial nephrectomy[156]. Saline drinking in rats following ablations of 70-75% of renal mass produced a 47% increase in blood pressure compared to rats given water to drink after ablation. The increase in blood pressure in rats given saline was accompanied by a 74% increase in extracellular fluid volume and the number of droplets per renal interstitial cell fell by 117%. Transplants of the papillae from the partially nephrectomized, salt-loaded rats failed to lower blood pressure in one-kidney, one-clip Goldblatt hypertensive rats[156]. Thus renoprival hypertension may be due to a combination of volume loading and lack of a renomedullary hormone. Blood pressure rises following salt loading via the renal blood volume-pressure regulatory system only if the liberation of the antihypertensive renomedullary factor is decreased.

4.   Hypertension following selective destruction of the renal medulla

Further evidence of the importance of the renal medulla in blood pressure control has come from studies on selective destruction of this area. Muirhead et al.[157] showed that salt loading hypertension did not develop in dogs with ureterocaval anastomosis but did develop in dogs with ureteral ligation. The excretory function of the kidney was blocked in both cases, but ischaemic papillary necrosis developed in the latter but not in the former case. It was proposed that hypertension did not develop in dogs with ureterocaval anastomosis as the antihypertensive renomedullary system was left intact[157].

Selective papillary necrosis can be induced in the rat with a single dose of bromoethanamine[158,159]. This model, originally developed for its parallel with papillary necrosis following high intake of analgesic mixtures, is characterized by necrosis of the papilla and cortical scarring. Urine output is greatly increased. In spite of this, ablation of the renal medulla with bromoethanamine removes the depressor system of the kidney and hypertension occurs. In one report a single intravenous injection of bromoethanamine produced a 16 mmHg increase in blood pressure[143]. Other workers, however, were unable to reproduce this effect[145].

Taverner et al.[144] repeated the experiments with bromoethanamine injections in normotensive rats and showed that destruction of at least half of the papilla was associated with marked hypertension and polyuria. They suggested that their success in producing hypertension by this manipulation, after previous attempts had met with mixed success, was partly linked to the fact that they measured blood pressure by a direct method in awake rats. Chemical ablation of the medulla produces hypertension via a mechanism opposite to that of salt loading hypertension as there is a large sustained increase in urine volume[160,161]. There is a positive correlation between blood pressure and urine volume and a negative correlation between blood pressure and urinary PGE_2 excretion. The two factors are not causally related to blood pressure but are indicators of renal medullary damage. Sodium balance is initially negative following bromoethanamine and then returns to preinjection levels in spite of increased urinary volume. Plasma renin concentrations are similar in medullectomized and control rats, and there is no correlation between plasma renin concentration and blood pressure. The maintenance of a normal sodium balance in the face of increased urinary volume is assured by increased tubular reabsorption of sodium. Hypertension following destruction of the renal medulla is due to interference with the production of a vasodepressor substance by the renal medulla interstitial cells[160],[161].

5.   Effects of isolated renomedullary antihypertensive lipids

The steps in the isolation of antihypertensive lipids from the medulla of the kidney have been reviewed[162],[163]. Crude saline extracts of the renal medulla prevented renoprival hypertension in the dog[137] and in the rabbit[164]. The active fraction was a neutral lipid and was designated as antihypertensive neutral renomedullary lipid (ANRL). Following reduction and acetylation the active antihypertensive lipid became polar and was designated as antihypertensive polar renomedullary lipid (APRL). The latter is a semisynthetic derivative of ANRL, the endogenous hormone[165-167]. Single bolus i.v. injections of APRL to one-kidney, one-clip hypertensive rats produce a rapid fall in blood pressure back to normotensive levels followed by a rapid return to hypertensive levels (see Figure 5). Multiple doses of APRL produce a long-lasting decrease in blood pressure (see Figure 6)[162],[165]. The decrease in blood pressure produced by ANRL is slow in onset and development (see Figure 5). Thus at least part of the fall in blood

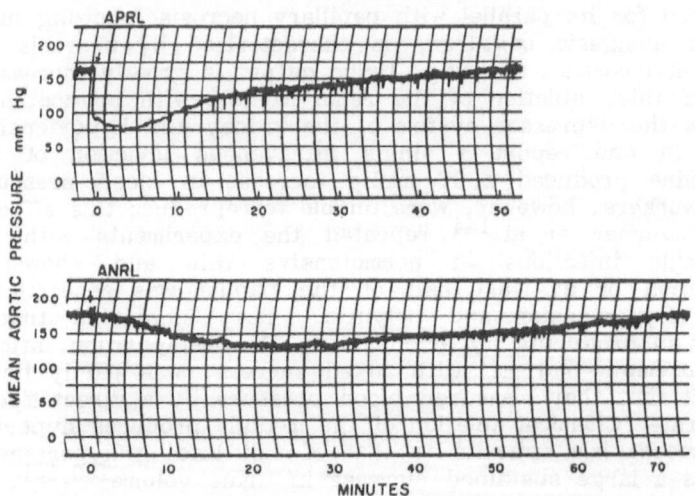

Figure 5 The responses of the mean arterial pressure to a bolus injection of the renomedullary lipids APRL and ANRL in an anaesthetized one-kidney one-clip hypertensive rat. Note the rapid and pronounced depressor effect evoked by APRL (from 160 to 75 mmHg) followed by recovery within 50 minutes. After ANRL injection there was a lag period of 3 minutes followed by a relatively slow and steady decline of the mean arterial pressure (from 175 to 130 mmHg within 20 minutes). The mean arterial pressure remained at 130 mmHg for 15 minutes, then steadily returned to the original level by 70 minutes. (Reproduced from Prewitt et al.[165], with permission of the American Heart Association and the authors.)

pressure could be due to a natriuretic effect of ANRL. The fall in blood pressure produced by ANRL is accompanied by a central and/or reflex suppression of sympathetic tone[166],[168]. However, its cardiovascular effects are probably not directly mediated through the central nervous system[169].

A greater sensitivity to APRL has been demonstrated in the spontaneously hypertensive rat. Superfusion of the microcirculation of the cremaster muscle produced three fold greater arteriolar dilation in SHR compared to their normotensive Wistar-Kyoto controls (WKY)[170]. Dose-response curves for the blood pressure lowering effect of intravenous injections of APRL showed a 25-fold shift to the left in SHR compared to WKY[170]. Blockade of endogenous dilating systems (cholinergic blocked with atropine, beta-adrenergic with propranolol, histaminergic with chlorpheniramine plus cimetidine, prostanoid with indomethacin and kinin with aprotinin) did not modify the effect of APRL[170]. Pressor responses to relatively high doses of norepinephrine (noradrenaline) (1 to 10 µg/kg, i.v.) were totally blocked by APRL, whereas the pressor

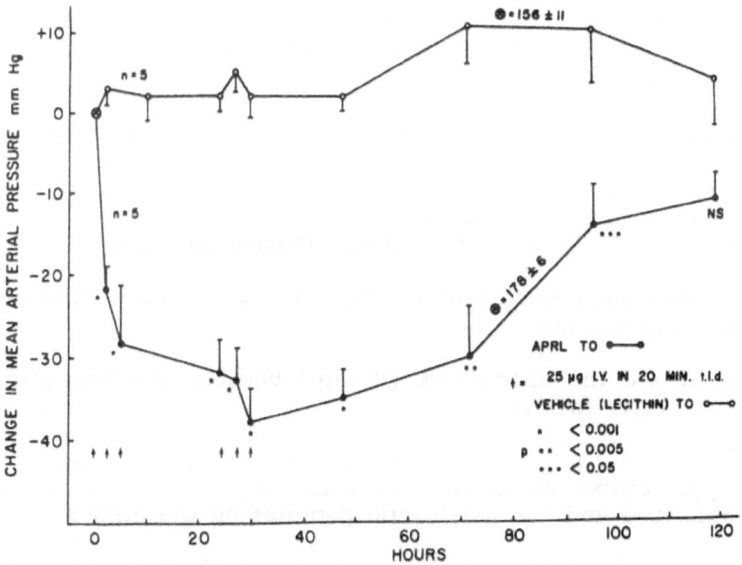

Figure 6 The prolonged depressor effect of APRL following three doses spaced 3 hours apart on two successive days is shown. Note that recovery, as compared to controls receiving the vehicle, did not occur until more than 60 hours after the last dose. (Reproduced from Prewitt et al.[165], with permission of the American Heart Association and the authors.)

responses to angiotensin II were not altered[170]. Further evidence of an interaction with the alpha-adrenergic nervous system came from studies showing that APRL interfered with binding of the selective alpha-adrenoceptor ligand [^{3}H]dihydroergocryptine. In aqueous solution APRL produced an increase in the dissociation constant (K_d) but no change in B_{max}; in solutions containing ethanol there was a substantial fall in B_{max} but no change in K_d[163]. It was suggested that insertion of the APRL into the cell membrane produced steric hindrance with the alpha adrenergic binding[163].

APRL has been tentatively identified as an alkyl ether phosphatidylcholine analogue[119]. Similar compounds prepared from choline plasmalogen of beef heart[171] have antihypertensive effects comparable to those of APRL in the one-kidney, one-clip hypertensive rat. Alkyl ether analogues of phosphatidylcholine were shown to be orally active in one-kidney, one wrap hypertensive rabbits[172]. Like the natural alkyl ether compounds derived from renomedullary tissue, they have an initial depressor action which is potentiated with repeated doses, and which is of long duration. These compounds are also potent platelet activators and it has been suggested that they are involved in the anaphylactic reaction[173]. While APRL and platelet activator are probably similar not only in their chemical structure but also in the fact that they produce a rapid fall in blood pressure, the endogenous hormone ANRL is different, as it produces a slowly developing fall in blood pressure.

In conclusion, determination of the true physiological role of renomedullary antihypertensive lipids awaits answers to the following questions:

(a)   What is the chemical nature of the endogenous compounds?

(b)   What is the mechanism of action of the blood pressure-lowering effect of the endogenous compounds? How does this mechanism relate to the sodium homeostasis theory?

(c)   Is decreased release of the factors a cause or a consequence of hypertension?

(d)   What are the differences (if any) between the Muirhead and the Floyer factors?

(e)   What are the relationships between the renomedullary antihypertensive lipids and the renin-angiotensin system on the one hand and the natriuretic peptides on the other?

The renin angiotensin system and the renomedullary antihypertensive lipid(s) have a "yin-yang" relationship[120] as shown in Figure 7. The renin-angiotensin system produces vasoconstriction and salt retention, and stimulates sympathetic activity, whereas the ANRL has the opposite effects. Furthermore high levels of angiotensin II suppress the activity of ANRL. The normal kidney is the site of an equilibrium between a prohypertensive system (angiotensin II) and an antihypertensive system (ANRL).

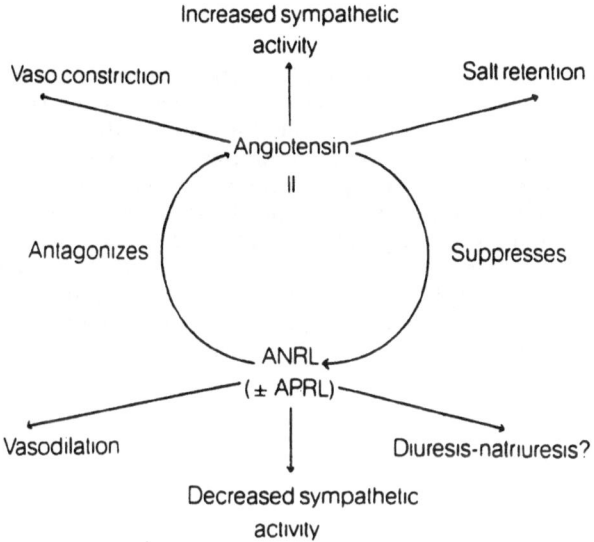

Figure 7 The proposed relationship between angiotensin II and the putative anti-hypertensive hormone of the renal papilla and its renomedullary interstitial cells (RIC). (Reproduced from Muirhead and Pitcock[120], with permission of the Journal of Hypertension and the authors.)

V.   NATRIURETIC FACTORS

The existence of extrarenally synthesized factors which control renal function, and directly or indirectly blood pressure, was postulated by Braun-Menéndez[174], who suggested the existence of a circulating protein "renotrophin" which regulates the functional capacity of the kidney. In situations where the kidney is unable to respond to renotrophin with an increase in functional capacity because of mechanical or pathological hindrance, hypertension develops. Thus renoprival hypertension would be caused by the failure of the kidney to react to, or to metabolize, an extrarenal factor. The recently described natriuretic factor(s) are representatives of such a class of factors[175-181].

Acute volume expansion produces natriuresis, an inhibition of sodium transport and an increase in vascular reactivity[180]. A natriuretic factor by definition produces natriuresis, but this does not necessarily mean that such a substance also induces the two other phenomena seen during acute volume expansion[180]. The only substance so far identified is the atrial natriuretic peptide or factor which does not inhibit sodium transport[182] and decreases vascular resistance[180]. It may be that the atrial natriuretic factor produces the natriuretic response, and that the second substance - possibly of hypothalamic origin[183] - is responsible for the inhibition of sodium transport and for the increase in vascular reactivity[180,184].

273

A. Hypothalamic factors

1. Salt sensitive rats

The existence of circulating factor(s) which alter sodium excretion by the kidney was suggested in early experiments on the effects of parabiosis on the induction of hypertension. Dahl and co-workers selected two strains of rats (R or resistant and S or sensitive) according to whether or not they developed hypertension when given a high salt diet[185]. The two strains have similar sensitivities to other hypertension-inducing procedures such as DOCA-salt and unilateral renal artery constriction[186], or cortisone administration following adrenalectomy[187]. The genetic background of the strain modifies its response to hypertension-inducing procedures. Parabiosis (surgical joining of the abdominal cavities) was carried

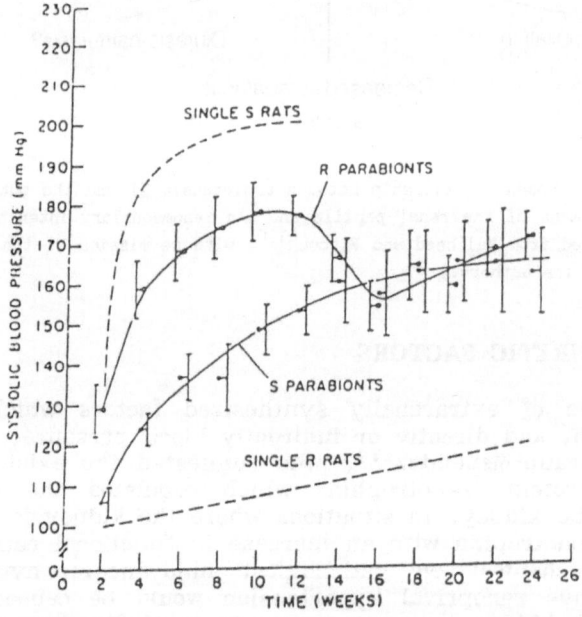

Figure 8 Increase in blood pressure in R and S parabionts given 8% NaCl compared to the increase in single R or single S rats. The symbols with open and closed circles represent mean ±1 standard deviation of B.P. obtained from R + S parabionts on 8% NaCl measured every 2nd week during the study, and demonstrate the anomalous development of B.P. in this group. The broken lines represent idealized average B.P. of large numbers of single S and R rats on 8% chow. The change in response to NaCl effected by parabiosis between rats, one from each strain, is apparent. From the 2nd through the 12th week the average B.P. of the R parabionts was higher (p<0.05) than that of their S partners at corresponding times. After the 12th week average B.P. in the two groups was not significantly different (p>0.05). Furthermore, only the average of the R parabionts at 16 weeks was significantly different from the average of this R group at 12 weeks; for this reason the curve shown for the R parabionts should be accepted with caution after the 12th week. (Reproduced from Dahl et al.[188], with permission of the Rockefeller University Press and the authors.)

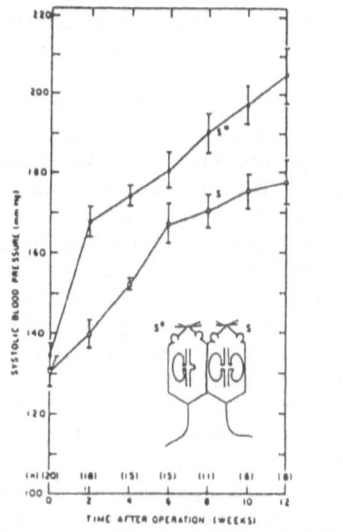

Blood pressure response of S*-S parabionts after Goldblatt procedure in only one rat (S*).

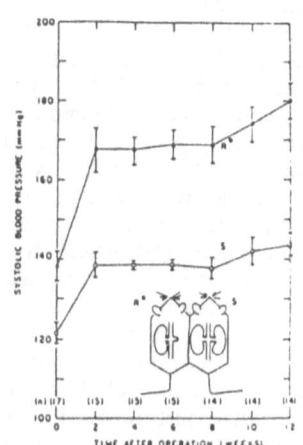

Blood pressure response of R*-S parabionts after Goldblatt procedure in only one rat (R*).

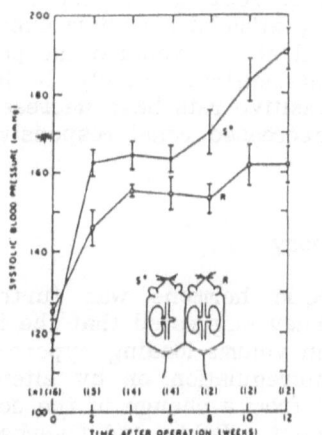

Blood pressure response of S*-R parabionts after Goldblatt procedure in only one rat (S*).

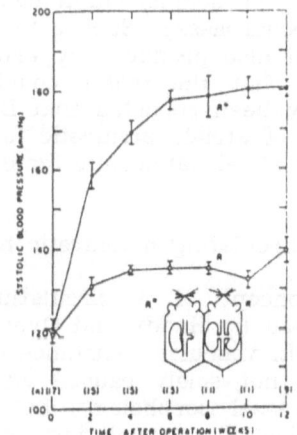

Blood pressure response of R*-R parabionts after Goldblatt procedure in only one rat (R*).

Figure 9 Blood pressure response of S*-S, R*-S, S*-R and R*-R parabionts after Goldblatt procedure in only one rat(*). (Reproduced from Dahl et al.[189], with permission of the Rockefeller University Press and the authors.)

out on weanlings and R+R, S+S and R+S parabiotic pairs produced[188]. The pairs were then given a low (0.4% NaCl) or a high (8% NaCl) salt diet. The R+S pair remained normotensive on the low salt diet, but when given a high salt diet both R and S members became hypertensive (see Figure 8). Thus a transmittable factor produced hypertension in the R rat when the latter was in parabiosis with an S rat and the pair were challenged with a high salt diet. In the S parabiont the rate of development and the average level of hypertension were lower than that of single S or S+S parabionts. Thus the R rat produced a transmittable (antihypertensive renomedullary lipid?) factor which partially protected the S rat from the hypertensive consequences of the high salt diet[188]. Similar results were obtained with another model of hypertension - renovascular hypertension[189]. Unilateral renal artery clipping of the S parabiont induced hypertension in the opposite partner (whether S or R), whereas clipping of the R parabiont induced hypertension in this rat only, and had little effect on the blood pressure of the partner (see Figure 9). It was suggested that in the S strain there were two pressor principles liberated in response to clipping. One factor was common to both strains and was probably angiotensin. This factor did not cross the parabiotic junction. The second factor was specific to the salt-prone strain, was transmittable and modified salt excretion. Compared to results in single animals, hypertension produced by clipping in parabionts was generally milder, the untouched partner again exercising a protective role as in the case of salt-induced hypertension.

In conclusion, a "sodium excreting hormone" is released in S rats in response to procedures which induce a change in the renal handling of sodium (high sodium intake or reduction in the functional renal mass). Such a factor not only stimulates sodium excretion but also produces hypertension. Dahl et al. excluded the possibility that the factor could be angiotensin[190]. Finally it has recently been reported that Dahl salt-sensitive rats have decreased release of atrial natriuretic factor and decreased renal responsiveness to atrial natriuretic factor[191].

2.   Circulating natriuretic hormone theory

The concept of a circulating natriuretic hormone was further developed by Haddy and Overbeck[192]. They suggested that the increase in vascular resistance occurring in volume loading hypertension is not solely caused either by autoregulation or by altered blood vessel morphology, but may result from a change in the concentration of a circulating vasoactive agent. Haddy and Overbeck eliminated many of the known agents (angiotensin, vasopressin, kinins, prostaglandins and catecholamines) as either (a) the changes in their plasma levels in response to volume loading were opposite to those predicted, or (b) their haemodynamic actions did not fit with those predicted. They retained four substances: potassium ions, methylguanidine and its analogues, adrenal steroids and natriuretic factor(s). Although we do not know the chemical identity of the factors, compounds such as the sesquiterpenoid derivative, urodiolenone, may act as a natriuretic factor as this substance is a potent Na-K,ATPase inhibitor and it is found in the urine of hypertensive patients[193].

The hypothesis that a circulating agent inhibits the Na-K,ATPase of the cardiovascular system, and so produces a rise in blood pressure in volume-expanded hypertension, is apparently not in agreement with the fact that long term treatment with cardiac glycosides generally does not produce hypertension. As blood volume falls during such treatment (due to concomitant diuretic therapy and the natriuretic action of the glycosides themselves) this presumably obliterates any tendency for blood pressure to rise following the increase in peripheral resistance that they produce[194].

The hypothesis is also in apparent disagreement with the observations that blood pressure returns to normal following unclipping in the one-kidney, one-clip model when a fall in extracellular fluid volume is prevented by ureterocaval anastomosis or fluid replacement[131,149,195]. Floyer[195] interpreted the fall in blood pressure following unclipping with ureterocaval anastomosis as being due to re-establishment of the renal circulation and the ability of the kidney to inactivate an extrarenal pressor factor. Haddy and Overbeck, on the other hand, suggested that in such situations renomedullary antihypertensive factors may be involved.

A link between sodium balance, blood pressure and extracellular fluid was proposed by Borst and Borst-de Geus[196] after a re-examination of Starling's theory of fluid balance and circulatory homeostasis. They proposed that "hypertension is part of a homeostasis reaction to deficient renal sodium output. When sodium output is insufficient at a normal arterial pressure, accumulation of extracellular fluid will raise the pressure to the abnormally high level required for re-establishment of sodium balance; thus a seemingly normal sodium output is maintained at the expense of hypertension". Such ideas are very similar to those proposed in the sodium homeostasis theory.

3.   Sodium and intracellular calcium

The increase in peripheral resistance caused by a natriuretic hormone can be explained on the basis of the Blaustein hypothesis[197], which developed the following argument:

(a)   there is a large gradient of calcium from the extracellular to the intracellular compartments;

(b)   extrusion of intracellular calcium is coupled with movement of sodium from the extracellular to the intracellular compartment;

(c)   the intracellular concentration of calcium in vascular smooth muscle is above the threshold for development of tension, and slight increases in the intracellular concentration of calcium will cause increases in the resting tone of the vascular smooth muscle;

(d)   sodium-calcium exchange plays a critical role in resting tone, i.e. muscle contractility depends upon extracellular sodium concentration;

(e)   natriuretic hormone causes an increase in sodium excretion via inhibition of renal Na-K,ATPase. In parallel, it also inhibits other Na-K,ATPases such as that of vascular smooth muscle;

(f)   inhibition of vascular Na-K,ATPase will cause an increase in intracellular sodium and hence an increase in intracellular calcium;

(g)   the increase in intracellular calcium will produce an increase in tone and so in blood pressure.

It should be noted that there is no direct evidence as yet that this sodium-calcium exchange mechanism plays an important role in maintaining increased vascular resistance in hypertension[198,199].

4.   Role of the hypothalamic factors in hypertension

On the basis of the above postulates, De Wardener and MacGregor[178,200] and others[201] suggested that a hypothalamic natriuretic hormone may be a connecting link in the triad of salt intake, extracellular fluid volume and blood pressure . The underlying genetic lesion of essential hypertension is a defect in sodium excretion by the kidney. This defect becomes more apparent when salt intake is increased. There is a transient increase in extracellular fluid volume, blood volume and especially intrathoracic blood volume. The latter stimulus causes the hypothalamus to liberate the natriuretic hormone which restores sodium balance. Inhibition of vascular sodium transport causes an increase in vascular tone by the Blaustein mechanism[197]. Reconsidering the sodium homeostatic theory in the light of the hypothesis of De Wardener and MacGregor, we see that whereas Guyton proposed that the increase in peripheral resistance following salt loading with decreased functional renal mass was the result of autoregulation, for De Wardener and MacGregor the increase in peripheral resistance would be a "side-effect" of the hypothalamic natriuretic hormone (see Figure 10.

This theory hinges upon the idea that blood contains a circulating hormone which will inhibit sodium transport, and that the level of this hormone is altered by changes in salt intake or in blood pressure. Several lines of evidence suggest that this is so. Plasma obtained from healthy subjects given a high sodium diet caused a 25-fold greater decrease in the Na-K,ATPase activity of guinea pig kidney slices than that produced by plasma from the same subjects given a low sodium diet[202]. Plasma from essential hypertensive patients caused a decrease in the active sodium transport of white blood cells from normotensive subjects[203]. Using stimulation of renal glucose-6-phosphate dehydrogenase in vitro as

278

an indicator of inhibition of Na-K,ATPase[204], further evidence of the ability of plasma from essential hypertensive patients to inhibit sodium transport was obtained[205,206]. The ability to stimulate glucose-6-phosphate dehydrogenase was significantly correlated with diastolic blood pressure[205,206]. Natriuretic substances have also been detected in the urine of salt-loaded men[207]. Recently a non-peptide factor which binds to ouabain sites, inhibits Na-K,ATPase and increases myocardial contractility has been isolated

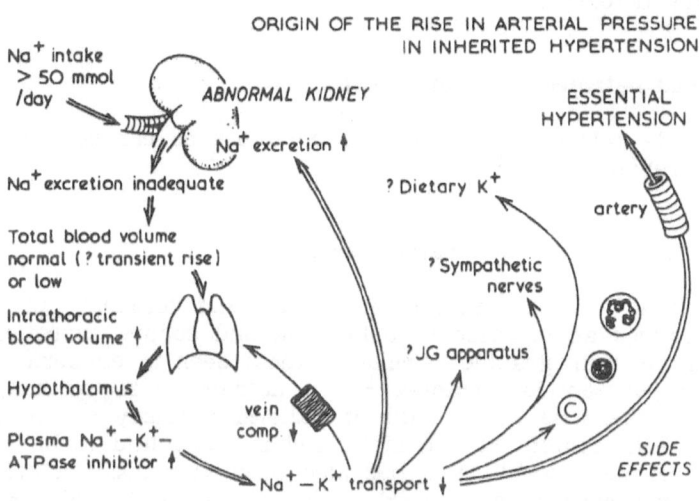

ORIGIN OF THE RISE IN ARTERIAL PRESSURE
IN INHERITED HYPERTENSION

Figure 10 Sequence of events to explain a postulated inherited defect in the kidney's ability to excrete sodium, the observed rise in concentration of a circulating sodium-transport inhibitor, salt intake, and the rise in peripheral resistance in essential hypertension (JG = juxtaglomerular; vein comp. = vein compliance). (Reproduced from De Wardener and MacGregor[178], with permission of the Lancet and the authors.)

from the plasma of rats[208]. There was, however, no significant difference in plasma levels between Sabra hypertensive and normotensive rats, and no demonstration of whether the substance was natriuretic or not[208].

A defect in sodium transport has been observed in some animal models such as the SHR. There was an increase in intracellular sodium and a decrease in the rate constant for sodium efflux[209]. In the low renin Goldblatt hypertensive rat the evidence is contradictory[210,211]. The defect in ion transport associated with essential hypertension may not be limited to cations, and anions such as chloride may also be involved[212].

De Wardener and co-workers have provided evidence that the hypothalamus is the source of the circulating sodium transport inhibitor[213]. Acetone extracts from several rat tissues were tested for their ability to stimulate renal glucose-6-phosphate dehydrogenase as an indicator of inhibition of Na-K,ATPase. The only tissue extract found to be active was that of the hypothalamus. They then showed that this extract directly inhibited Na-K,ATPase. The activity in one hypothalamus was 10,000 to 100,000 times that of 1 ml of plasma from the same animal. Levels of the inhibitor in the hypothalamus of rats on a high sodium diet were 150 times those found in rats on a low sodium diet. Plasma levels increased 6 times under the same conditions. It should be noted, however, that whilst natriuretic substances may be produced in the brain, we lack definite evidence as to whether the sodium transport inhibitor extracted from the brain is the natriuretic factor[180].

B.   Atrial natriuretic factors (ANF)

The possible role of atrial natriuretic factors as cardiac hormones has been reviewed[214-216].

1.   Atrial receptors and natriuresis

Stimulation of receptors in the left atrium and terminal pulmonary veins produces an increase in urine flow and sodium excretion[217]. Atrial cells contain granules similar to those seen in endocrine cells producing polypeptide hormones[218]. A natriuretic factor has been detected in the atria using a direct radioimmunoassay[219]. Interestingly the ANF content of the right atrium was found to be higher than that of the left[219]. ANF has also been visualized in atria by immunocytochemical techniques[220]. The number of atrial granules varies with changes in fluid and electrolyte balance[221,222]. Water deprivation and sodium deficiency give hypergranulation, whereas DOCA and 2% salt drinking produce degranulation. The increase in the number of granules produced by water deprivation is accompanied by a decrease in the acid-extractable diuretic and natriuretic activities[223]. Thus the number of atrial granules may not provide a direct indication of the natriuretic potency of an atrial extract[223]. Using an improved bioassay for ANF activity, Johnson has shown that extracts of atria of water-deprived Long Evans rats and diabetes insipidus rats contain more natriuretic activity than those of control Long Evans rats[224].

Increases in extracellular volume and sodium load stimulate an atrial receptor which releases an atrial natriuretic factor into the blood stream[180], possibly via activation of an inositol triphosphate second messenger[225]. This hormone then increases sodium excretion and so indirectly provokes a fall in extracellular fluid volume (see Figure 11)[179,226]. Recent evidence has shown that ANF is indeed a circulating hormone[227-232] with a relatively short half-life[233]. It may be catabolized by kallikrein and by converting enzyme[233,234]. Other lines of evidence suggest that ANF has an important physiological role. The BIO 14.6 strain of hamster, which are deficient in ANF, are susceptible to congestive heart failure and oedema. This can be partly cured by parabiosis with normal hamsters[235]. SHR have a reduced atrial ANF content and it has been suggested that this may stem from exaggerated chronic release which may play a role in the development of their hypertension[236]. ANF secretion in the Dahl salt-sensitive rat is increased whilst sensitivity of the natriuretic response is decreased[191,237]. The relationship of these phenomena to the development of hypertension following salt loading in Dahl salt sensitive rats is as yet unclear. Finally, following atrial appendectomy the diuretic and natriuretic responses to acute volume overload were reduced[238].

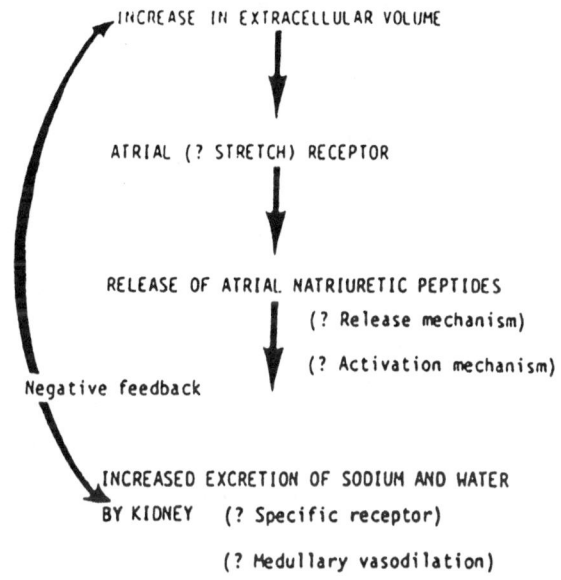

Figure 11 Hypothetical scheme for release and action of atrial natriuretic factor. (Reproduced from Sagnella and MacGregor[179], with permission of Macmillan Journals Limited and the authors.)

2. Atrial natriuretic factors

Supernatants of the homogenates of rat atrium produce marked diuresis, natriuresis and kaliuresis when injected into anaesthetized bioassay rats[239]. There is a fall in blood pressure with a rise in haematocrit, but no change in heart rate. The fall in blood pressure may be due to fluid loss. As the atrial extract did not modify glomerular filtration rate, the natriuretic effect was ascribed to a specific effect on sodium transport and not to renal vasodilatation. The inhibition of sodium transport by atrial extracts is not due to inhibition of Na-K,ATPase[223,240].

Recently several atrial natriuretic peptides have been chemically identified (see Figure 12). They have very similar structures, the rat peptides differing from the human peptides by one amino acid only[179]. They have been called atrial natriuretic factor[241], cardionatrin[242], auriculin[243] or atriopeptin[226]. The active peptides appear to be derived from a high molecular weight precursor[226,244]. Their biological selectivity and potency depends on the degree of cleavage at the C terminal[226,245]. All require an intact disulphide bridge for full expression of their biological activity[243,246,247] and appear to take on a round structure[246,248]. The configuration of the N-terminal appears to be important for their vasorelaxant activity[249].

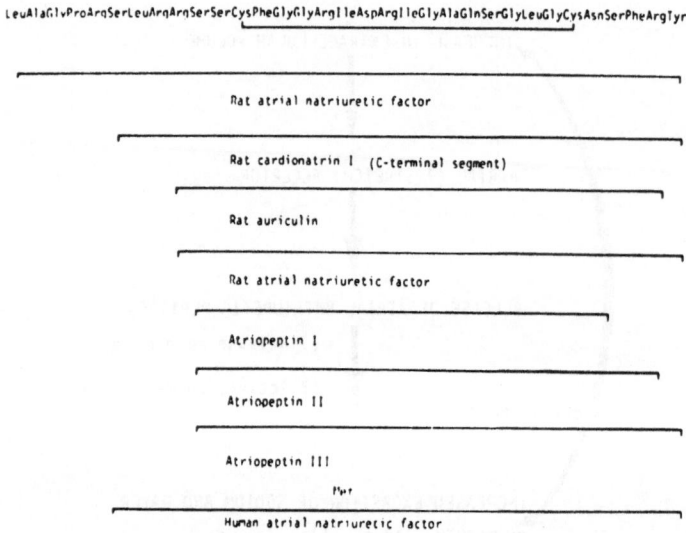

Figure 12 Amino acid sequences and proposed names of rat and human atrial natriuretic peptides (above) and organisation of their precursors (below). (Reproduced from Sagnella and MacGregor[179], with permission of MacMillan Journals Limited and the authors.)

3. Effects of atrial natriuretic factors

These peptides are natriuretic[223,226,239,246,250,251] at very low doses and an intact disulphide bridge is essential for this activity[246]. It is less certain if their natriuretic effect is the result of a direct renal action such as an inhibition of tubular sodium transport[227,252-257] or of a modification of renal haemodynamics[243,255,256,258-260]. Differences in the results obtained may be due to the use of different species, anaesthesia, etc.[261], but other factors may also be involved. Whereas low doses of ANF inhibit sodium transport, higher doses have an effect on renal blood flow[253]. Inhibition of sodium transport by the atrial natriuretic factor depends on the state of the extracellular fluid volume of the test animal[254]. Although ANF increases renal blood flow and glomerular filtration rate[243,255,256,258-260] and increased sodium excretion is highly correlated with increased renal blood flow in animals treated with natriuretic factor[256] it is possible that the two effects are dissociated. If this is the case it is suprising that the renal vascular bed appears to be exquisitely sensitive to the dilator effects of the atrial natriuretic factor[255,262]. The natriuretic effect may be the result of some other action such as inhibition of renin release[263]. Furthermore, although ANF stimulates vasopressin release in vitro[264], increases in ANF in plasma and atria are associated with decreases in hypothalamic ANF[265] thus there may be an inverse relationship between the cerebral and peripheral ANF systems. ANF-containing neurons have been found throughout the brain, especially in the anteroventral third ventricle, an area critically involved in hypertension and in fluid and electrolyte balance[266]. ANF will relax isolated blood vessels (rabbit aorta seems the most sensitive) which are vasoconstricted with epinephrine, histamine, angiotensin II, carbachol or potassium[243,246,250,251,267-269]. In vivo the blood pressure lowering effect is slow in onset[259,270] and may therefore be the result of the natriuretic effect[239]. Peripheral vasodilation and inhibition of the renin angiotensin system may, however, also play a role[270]. Specific binding sites have been found in vascular smooth muscle cells in vitro[271,272] and in culture[273]. These receptors appear to be coupled to activation of guanylate cyclase and/or inhibition of cGMP phosphodiesterase[273-276]. An inhibition of adenylate cyclase has also been reported[277]. Other authors have shown that synthetic atrial natriuretic factors lower blood pressure in different hypertensive states[278-282].

4. Atrial natriuretic factors and the renin-angiotensin aldosterone system

ANF will decrease plasma renin[259,260,270] and aldosterone[259,283]. As renin secretion was suppressed in spite of a fall in blood pressure[260] we may suggest that the inhibition of renin secretion stems from the increased delivery of sodium to the macula densa[284]. A direct effect on zona glomerulosa cells cannot be excluded[260]. ANF inhibits aldosterone synthesis[256,285,286] and angiotensin II, ACTH and potassium-stimulated aldosterone release[279,287-289]. The ANF receptor coupled to inhibition of adrenal steroidogenesis has been characterized[290].

In conclusion natriuretic peptides represent another class of compounds which can modulate the renal blood volume-pressure regulator system that acts as link between the cardiovascular system and the kidney. Like the renomedullary factors, there is an antagonism between the natriuretic peptides and the antinatriuretic renin angiotensin system.

CONCLUSION

In both normotension and renoprival and renovascular hypertension the kidney sets the long term blood pressure at a level such that sodium output and input are in equilibrium and sodium homeostasis of the body is assured. It does this by the renal blood volume-pressure regulatory system. Following a change in sodium balance there is a parallel change in extracellular fluid volume. Provided that the compliance of the cardiovascular system is not altered in a compensatory fashion, the change in extracellular fluid volume causes arterial pressure to alter firstly by a modification of cardiac output and afterwards by a change in peripheral resistance. The change in arterial pressure then provokes a modification of the renal excretion of sodium via the pressure-diuresis phenomenon. The function of this central control system can be modified by several factors such as angiotensin, the renomedullary factors and the natriuretic factors (Table 1). The role of angiotensin in long term blood pressure control is one of antinatriuresis. The role of the renomedullary factors is less well defined. They may represent the means by which the kidney can control the compliance of the cardiovascular system and so determine whether or not changes in extracellular fluid volume are accompanied by changes in arterial pressure. The natriuretic factors appear to serve a double function. Non-peptide factors, possibly of hypothalamic origin, increase blood pressure and so may restore sodium homeostasis via pressure diuresis. Peptides from the atria are natriuretic and vasodilator. Establishment of sodium homeostasis at a given blood pressure depends on the effects and interactions of these (and presumably other) factors.

Table 1 Factors modulating the kidney blood volume-pressure regulatory system

Level	Factor[a]	Origin	Target	Action
Renal output of salt and water	RAS	Kidney	Kidney	Antinatriuretic
	HF	Brain	Kidney	Natriuretic?
	ANF	Circulation	Kidney	Natriuretic
	RMF	Kidney	Kidney	Natriuretic?
Total peripheral resistance	RAS	Kidney	Circulation	Vasoconstrictor
	HF	Brain	Circulation	Vasoconstrictor
	ANF	Circulation	Circulation	Vasodilator
	RMF	Kidney	Circulation	Vasodilator plus increase in compliance

[a]RAS = renin angiotensin system; HF = hypothalamic factor; ANF = atrial natriuretic factor; RMF = renomedullary factor.

REFERENCES

1. Guyton, A.C., Arterial Pressure and Hypertension, W.B. Saunders, Philadelphia, 1980.
2. Guyton, A.C., Coleman, T.G., Cowley, A.W., Jr., Scheel, K.W., Manning, R.D., Jr. and Norman, R.A., Jr., Arterial pressure regulation. Overriding dominance of the kidneys in long-term regulation and in hypertension. Am.

J. Med., 52, 584, 1972.

3. Guyton, A.C., Manning, R.D., Lohmeier, T.E. and Hall, J.E., The kidney and hypertension, in Dopamine Receptor Agonists, Poste, G. and Crooke, S.T., Eds., Plenum, New York, 1984, 237.

4. Coleman, T.G., Manning, R.D., Jr., Norman, R.A., Jr. and DeClue, J., The role of the kidney in spontaneous hypertension, Am. Heart J., 89, 94, 1975.

5. Freis, E.D., Ragan, D., Pillsbury, H., III and Mathews, M., Alteration of the course of hypertension in the spontaneously hypertensive rat, Circ. Res., 31, 1, 1972.

6. Bianchi, G., Fox, U., Di Francesco, G.F., Bardi, U. and Radice, M., The hypertensive role of the kidney in spontaneously hypertensive rats, Clin. Sci. Mol. Med., 45, 135s, 1973.

7. Kenyon, C.J., DeConti, G.A., Cupolo, N.A. and Morris, D.J., The role of aldosterone in the development of hypertension in spontaneously hypertensive rats, Endocrinology, 109, 1841, 1981.

8. Toal, C.B. and Leenen, F.H.H., Dietary sodium restriction and development of hypertension in spontaneously hypertensive rats, Am. J. Physiol., 245, H1081, 1983.

9. Braun-Menéndez, E. and Von Euler, U.S., Hypertension after bilateral nephrectomy in the rat, Nature, 160, 905, 1947.

10. Grollman, A., Muirhead, E.E. and Vanatta, J., Role of the kidney in pathogenesis of hypertension as determined by a study of the effects of bilateral nephrectomy and other experimental procedures on the blood pressure of the dog, Am. J. Physiol., 157, 21, 1949.

11. Del Greco, F., Grollman, A., Ledingham, J.M., Merrill, J.P. and Muirhead, E.E., Renoprival hypertension, in Renal Hypertension, Page, I.H. and McCubbin, J.W., Eds., Year Book Medical Publ., Chicago, 1968, 276.

12. Ledingham, J.M., Blood-pressure regulation in renal failure, J. R. Coll. Phys. Lond., 5, 103, 1971.

13. Coleman, T.G., Bower, J.D., Langford, H.G. and Guyton, A.C., Regulation of arterial pressure in the anephric state, Circulation, 42, 509, 1970.

14. Guyton, A.C., Coleman, T.G., Bower, J.D. and Granger, H.J., Circulatory control in hypertension, Circ. Res., 26/27 (Suppl. 2), 135, 1970.

15. Houck, C.R., Problems in maintenance of chronic bilaterally nephrectomized dog, Am. J. Physiol., 176, 175, 1954.

16. Nordman, R.A., Jr., Coleman, T.G., Wiley, T.L., Jr., Manning, R.D., Jr. and Guyton, A.C., Separate roles of sodium ion concentration and fluid volumes in salt-loading hypertension in sheep, Am. J. Physiol., 229, 1068, 1975.

17. Langston, J.B., Guyton, A.C., Douglas, B.H. and Dorsett, P.E., Effect of changes in salt intake on arterial pressure and renal function in partially nephrectomized dogs, Circ. Res., 12, 508, 1963.

18. Dustan, H.P. and Page, I.H., Some factors in renal and renoprival hypertension, J. Lab. Clin. Med., 64, 948, 1964.

19. Wilkinson, R., Scott, D.F., Uldall, P.R., Kerr, D.N.S. and Swinney, J., Plasma renin and exchangeable sodium in the hypertension of chronic renal failure, Q. J. Med., 39, 377, 1970.

20. Hampers, C.L., Skillman, J.J., Lyons, J.H., Olsen, J.E. and Merrill, J.P., A hemodynamic evaluation of bilateral nephrectomy and hemodialysis in hypertensive man, Circulation, 35, 272, 1967.

21. Onesti, G., Kim, K.E., Greco, J.A., Del Guercio, E.T., Fernandes, M. and Swartz, C., Blood pressure regulation in end-stage renal disease and anephric man, Circ. Res., 36/37 (Suppl. 1), 145, 1975.

22. Essadki, A., Le Système rénine-angiotensine et la régulation de la pression artérielle chez le rat, Thèse, Université de Lausanne, Suisse, 1983.

23. Grollman, A. and Halpert, B., Renal lesions in chronic hypertension induced by unilateral nephrectomy in the rat, Proc. Soc. Exp. Biol. Med., 71, 394, 1949.

24. Muehrcke, R.C., Mandal, A.K., Epstein, M. and Volini, F.I., Cytoplasmic granularity of the renal medullary interstitial cells in experimental hypertension, J. Lab. Clin. Med., 73, 299, 1969.

25. Seymour, A.A., Davis, J.O., Freeman, R.H., DeForrest, J.M., Rowe, B.P., Stephens, G.A. and Williams, G.M., Hypertension produced by sodium depletion and unilateral nephrectomy: A new experimental model, Hypertension, 2, 125, 1980.

26. Koletsky, S. and Goodsitt, A.M., Natural history and pathogenesis of renal ablation hypertension, AMA Arch. Pathol., 69, 654, 1960.

27. Gross, F., The renin-angiotensin system and hypertension, Ann. Intern. Med., 75, 777, 1971.

28. Ylitalo, P., Hepp, R., Oster, P., Möhring, J. and Gross, F., Effects of varying sodium intake on blood pressure and renin-angiotensin system in subtotally nephrectomized rats, J. Lab. Clin. Med., 88, 807, 1976.

29. Manning, R.D., Jr., Coleman, T.G., Guyton, A.C., Norman, R.A., Jr. and McCaa, R.E., Essential role of mean circulatory filling pressure in salt-induced hypertension, Am. J. Physiol., 236, R40, 1979.

30. Manning, R.D., Jr., Cowley, A.W., Jr. and Coleman, T.G., Effects of baroreceptor denervation on volume loading hypertension in anephric dogs, Hypertension, 7, 562, 1985.

31. Cowley, A.W. and Guyton, A.C., Baroreceptor reflex effects on transient and steady-state hemodynamics of salt-loading hypertension in dogs, Circ. Res., 36, 536, 1975.

32. Coleman, T.G. and Guyton, A.C., Hypertension caused by sodium loading in the dog. III. Onset transients of cardiac output and other circulatory variables, Circ. Res., 25, 152, 1969.

33. Gardes, J., Bouhnik, J., Clauser, E., Corvol, P. and Menard, J., Role of angiotensinogen in blood pressure homeostasis, Hypertension, 4, 185, 1982.

34. Cowley, A.W., Jr., Miller, J.P. and Guyton, A.C., Open-loop analysis of the renin-angiotensin system in the dog, Circ. Res., 28, 568, 1971.

35. Goldblatt, H., Lynch, L., Hanzal, R.F. and Summerville, W.W., Studies on experimental hypertension. I. The production of persistent elevation of systolic blood pressure by means of renal ischemia, J. Exp. Med., 59, 347, 1934.

36. Fasciolo, J.C., Houssay, B.A. and Taquini, A.C., The blood-pressure raising secretion of the ischaemic kidney, J. Physiol. (Lond.), 94, 281, 1938.

37. Goldblatt, H., The renal origin of hypertension, Physiol. Rev., 27, 120, 1947.

38. Hsueh, W.A., Components of the renin system: an update, Am. J. Nephrol., 3, 109, 1983.

39. Atlas, S.A., Niarchos, A.P. and Case, D.B., Inhibitors of the renin-angiotensin system. Effects on blood pressure, aldosterone secretion and renal function, Am. J. Nephrol., 3, 118, 1983.

40. Rossier, B.C., Geering, K., Atkinson, J. and Roch-Ramel, F., Renal receptors, in The Kidney: Physiology and Pathophysiology, Seldin, D.W. and Giebisch, G., Eds., Raven Press, New York, 1985, 775.

41. Ferrario, C.M. and Carretero, O.A., Hemodynamics of experimental renal hypertension, in Handbook of Hypertension, Vol. 4: Experimental and Genetic Models of Hypertension, De Jong, W., Ed., Elsevier, Amsterdam, 1984, 55.

42. Davis, J.O., The pathogenesis of chronic renovascular hypertension, Circ. Res., 40, 439, 1977.

43. Gross, F., Schaechtelin, G., Brunner, H. and Peters, G., The role of the renin-angiotensin system in blood pressure regulation and kidney function, Can. Med. Assoc. J., 90, 258, 1964.

44. Kotchen, T.A. and Guthrie, G.P., Jr., Renin-angiotensin-aldosterone and hypertension, Endocrine Rev., 1, 78, 1980.

45. Atlas, S.A. and Case, D.B., Renin in essential hypertension, Clin. Endocrinol. Metab., 10, 537, 1981.

46. Laragh, J.H., Sealey, J.E., Bühler, F.R., Vaughan, E.D., Brunner, H.R., Gavras, H. and Baer, L., The renin axis and vasoconstriction volume analysis for understanding and treating renovascular and renal hypertension, Am. J. Med., 58, 4, 1975.

47. Textor, S.C., Pathophysiology of renovascular hypertension, Urol. Clin. North. Am., 11, 373, 1984.

48. Perloff, D. and Schambelan, M., Renovascular hypertension, Clin. Endocrinol. Metab., 10, 513, 1981.

49. Norman, R.A., Jr., Enobakhare, J.A., DeClue, J.W., Douglas, B.H. and Guyton, A.C., Renal function curves (RFC) in Goldblatt and spontaneously hypertensive rats, Fed. Proc., 36, 531, 1977.

50. Watkins, B.E., Davis, J.O., Freeman, R.H., DeForrest, J.M. and Stephens, G.A., Continuous angiotensin II blockade throughout the acute phase of one-kidney hypertension in the dog, Circ. Res., 42, 813, 1978.

51. Norman, R.A., Jr., Enobakhare, J.A., DeClue, J.W., Douglas, B.H. and Guyton, A.C., Arterial pressure-urinary output relationship in hypertensive rats, Am. J. Physiol., 234, R98, 1978.

52. Hedwall, P.R., Effect of rabbit antibodies against angiotensin-II on the pressor response to angiotensin-II and renal hypertension in the rat, Br. J. Pharmacol., 34, 623, 1968.

53. Weiser, R.A., Johnson, A. G. and Hoobler, S.W., The effect of antirenin on the blood pressure of the rat with experimental renal hypertension, Lab. Invest., 20, 326, 1969.

54. Eide, I. and Aars, H., Renal hypertension in rabbits immunized with angiotensin, Nature, 222, 571, 1969.

55. Eide, I. and Aars, H., Renal hypertension in rabbits immunized with angiotensin-II, Scand. J. Clin. Lab. Invest., 25, 119, 1970.

56. Johnston, C.I., Hutchinson, J.S. and Mendelsohn, F.A., Biological significance of renin angiotensin immunization, Circ. Res., 26/27 (Suppl. 2), 215, 1970.

57. Macdonald, G.J., Louis, W.J., Renzini, V., Boyd, G.W. and Peart, W.S., Renal-clip hypertension in rabbits immunized against angiotensin II, Circ. Res., 27, 197, 1970.

58. Oates, H.F., Stokes, G.S., Storey, B.G., Glover, R.G. and Snow, B.F., Renal hypertension in rats immunized against angiotensin I and angiotensin II, J. Exp. Med., 139, 239, 1974.

59. Watkins, B.E., Davis, J.O., Freeman, R.H., Stephens, G.A. and DeForrest, J.M., Effects of the oral converting enzyme inhibitor (SQ 14225) on one-kidney hypertension in the dog, Proc. Soc. Exp. Biol. Med., 157, 245, 1978.

60. Bengis, R.G. and Coleman, T.G., Antihypertensive effect of prolonged blockade of angiotensin formation in benign and malignant, one- and two-kidney Goldblatt hypertensive rats, Clin. Sci., 57, 53, 1979.

61. Bianchi, G., Tilde Tenconi, L. and Lucca, R., Effect in the conscious dog of constriction of the renal artery to a sole remaining kidney on haemodynamics sodium balance, body fluid volumes, plasma renin concentration and pressor responsiveness to angiotensin, Clin. Sci., 38, 741, 1970.

62. Brown, T.C., Davis, J.O., Olichney, M.J. and Johnston, C.I., Relation of

plasma renin to sodium balance and arterial pressure in experimental renal hypertension, Circ. Res., 18, 475, 1966.

63. Harris, R.C. and Ayers, C.R., Renal hemodynamics and plasma renin activity after renal artery constriction in conscious dogs, Circ. Res., 31, 520, 1972.

64. Atkinson, J., Kirchertz, E.J., Peters-Haefeli, L. and Lüthi, P., The role of plasma and renal renin in the rise in blood pressure following unilateral renal artery constriction, Renal Physiol., 5, 235, 1982.

65. Essadki, A. and Atkinson, J., Renin release by renin-depleted rats following hypotensive haemorrhage and anesthetics, Pfluegers Arch., 392, 46, 1981.

66. Atkinson, J., Luthi, P. and Boillat, N., Cycloheximide and renin release following renal artery constriction, J. Pharmacol. (Paris), 14, 161, 1983.

67. Atkinson, J., Lüthi, P., Péra-Bally, R. and Peters-Haefeli, L., Interaction between the renin-angiotensin and beta adrenergic nervous systems in drinking and pressor responses after renal artery constriction, J. Pharmacol. Exp. Ther., 221, 453, 1982.

68. Watkins, B.E., Davis, J.O., Freeman, R.H. and Stephens, G.A., Production of renovascular hypertension in adrenalectomized dogs, Physiologist, 19, 405, 1976.

69. Seymour, A.A., Davis, J.O., Freeman, R.H., DeForrest, J.M., Rowe, B.P., Stephens, G.A. and Williams, G.M., Sodium and angiotensin in the pathogenesis of experimental renovascular hypertension, Am. J. Physiol., 240, H788, 1981.

70. Miller, E.D., Jr., Samuels, A.I., Haber, E. and Barger, A.C., Inhibition of angiotensin conversion and prevention of renal hypertension, Am. J. Physiol., 228, 448, 1975.

71. Miller, E.D., Jr., Samuels, A.I., Haber, E. and Barger, A.C., Inhibition of angiotensin conversion in experimental renovascular hypertension, Science, 177, 1108, 1972.

72. Coleman, T.G. and Guyton, A.C., The pressor role of angiotensin in salt deprivation and renal hypertension in rats, Clin. Sci. Mol. Med., 48, 45s, 1975.

73. Bengis, R.G., Coleman, T.G., Young, D.B. and McCaa, R.E., Long-term blockade of angiotensin formation in various normotensive and hypertensive rat models using converting enzyme inhibitor (SQ 14,225), Circ. Res., 43 (Suppl. 1), 45, 1978.

74. Riegger, A.J.G., Tree, M., Bean, B.L., Casals-Stenzel, J., Brown, J.J., Fraser, R., Lever, A.F., Morton, J.J. and Robertson, J.I.S., Does angiotensin II act in two ways to raise blood pressure in renal artery stenosis?, in The Kidney in Arterial Hypertension, Bianchi, G. and Bazzato, G., Eds., Bunge Scientific Publ., Utrecht, 1979, 100.

75. Zimmerman, B.G. and Mommsen, C., Renal blood flow changes in contralateral kidney Goldblatt hypertensive dog, Am. J. Physiol., 241, H145, 1981.

76. Thompson, J. and Dickinson, C.J., A cross perfusion study of the rabbit kidney to assess the possibilities of long term blood pressure regulation by the kidney, Eur. J. Clin. Invest., 3, 272, 1973.

77. Masaki, Z., Ferrario, C.M. and Bumpus, F.M., Effects of SQ 20,881 on the intact kidney of dogs with two-kidney, one clip hypertension, Hypertension, 2, 649, 1980.

78. DeForrest, J.M., Davis, J.O., Freeman, R.H., Watkins, B.E. and Stephens, G.A., Separate renal function studies in conscious dogs with renovascular hypertension, Am. J. Physiol., 235, F310, 1978.

79. Hashimoto, H., Hiwada, K. and Kokubu, T., Different mechanisms maintaining high blood pressure in chronic one-kidney, one-clip, and two-kidney, one

clip hypertensive rats, Clin. Exp. Hypert., Part A, 5, 429, 1983.

80. Freeman, R.H., Davis, J.O. and Watkins, B.E., Angiotensin blockade with a new converting enzyme inhibitor (SQ 14,225) in rats and dogs with renovascular hypertension, IRCS Med. Sci., Cardiovasc. Syst./Physiology/Kidneys Urinary System, 5, 470, 1977.

81. Lupu, A.N., Maxwell, M.H., Kaufman, J.J. and White, F.N., Experimental unilateral renal artery constriction in the dog, Circ. Res., 30, 567, 1972.

82. Lupu, A.N., Maxwell, M.H. and Kaufman, J.J., Mechanisms of hypertension during the chronic phase of the one-clip, two-kidney model in the dog, Circ. Res., 40 (Suppl. 1), 57, 1977.

83. Watkins, B.E., Davis, J.O., Hanson, R.C., Lohmeier, T.E. and Freeman, R.H., Incidence and pathophysiological changes in chronic two-kidney hypertension in the dog, Am. J. Physiol., 231, 954, 1976.

84. Cowley, A.W., Jr., Switzer, S.J. and Guinn, M.M., Evidence and quantification of the vasopressin arterial pressure control system in the dog, Circ. Res., 46, 58, 1980.

85. Young, D.B., Pan, Y.J. and Guyton, A.C., Control of extracellular sodium concentration by antidiuretic hormone-thirst feedback mechanism, Am. J. Physiol., 232, R145, 1977.

86. Share, L., Interrelations between vasopressin and the renin-angiotensin system, Fed. Proc., 38, 2267, 1979.

87. Cowley, A.W., Jr., Guinn, M., Quillen, E.W. and Hockel, G.M., Vasopressin and thirst response to chronic I.V. angiotensin II infusion in dogs, Fed. Proc., 38, 967, 1979.

88. Ben, L.K., Maselli, J., Keil, L.C. and Reid, I.A., Role of the renin-angiotensin system in the control of vasopressin and ACTH secretion during the development of renal hypertension in dogs, Hypertension, 6, 35, 1984.

89. Koletsky, S. and Rivera-Velez, J.M., Factors determining the success or failure of nephrectomy in experimental renal hypertension, J. Lab. Clin. Med., 76, 54, 1970.

90. Masaki, Z., Ferrario, C.M., Bumpus, F.M., Bravo, E.L. and Khosla, M.C., the course of arterial pressure and the effect of Sar^1-Thr^8-angiotensin II in a new model of two-kidney hypertension in conscious dogs, Clin. Sci. Mol. Med., 52, 163, 1977.

91. Gavras, H., Brunner, H.R., Thurston, H. and Laragh, J.H., Reciprocation of renin dependency with sodium volume dependency in renal hypertension, Science, 188, 1316, 1975.

92. McCaa, R.E., McCaa, C.S., Bengis, R.G. and Guyton, A.C., Role of aldosterone in experimental hypertension, J. Endocrinol., 81, 69P, 1979.

93. Hollenberg, N.K., Renal hemodynamics in essential and renovascular hypertension, Am. J. Med., 76, 22, 1984.

94. Ames, R.P., Borkowski, A.J., Sicinski, A.M. and Laragh, J.H., Prolonged infusions of angiotensin II and norepinephrine and blood pressure, electrolyte balance, and aldosterone and cortisol secretion in normal man and in cirrhosis with ascites, J. Clin. Invest., 44, 1171, 1965.

95. DeClue, J.W., Guyton, A.C., Cowley, A.W., Jr., Coleman, T.G., Norman, R.A., Jr. and McCaa, R.E., Subpressor angiotensin infusion, renal sodium handling, and salt-induced hypertension in the dog, Circ. Res., 43, 503, 1978.

96. Lohmeier, T.E. and Cowley, A.W., Jr., Hypertensive and renal effects of chronic low level intrarenal angiotensin infusion in the dog, Circ. Res., 44, 154, 1979.

97. Hall, J.E., Granger, J.P., Hester, R.L., Coleman, T.G., Smith, M.J., Jr. and Cross, R.B., Mechanisms of escape from sodium retention during angiotensin II hypertension, Am. J. Physiol., 246, F627, 1984.

98.   Cowley, A.W., Jr. and DeClue, J.W., Quantification of baroreceptor influence on arterial pressure changes seen in primary angiotensin-induced hypertension in dogs, Circ. Res., 39, 779, 1976.

99.   Cowley, A.W., Jr. and McCaa, R.E., Acute and chronic dose-response relationships for angiotensin, aldosterone, and arterial pressure at varying levels of sodium intake, Circ. Res., 39, 788, 1976.

100. Lohmeier, T.E., Cowley, A.W., Jr., DeClue, J.W. and Guyton, A.C., Failure of chronic aldosterone infusion to increase arterial pressure in dogs with angiotensin-induced hypertension, Circ. Res., 43, 381, 1978.

101. Hall, J.E., Guyton, A.C., Smith, M.J., Jr. and Coleman, T.G., Blood pressure and renal function during chronic changes in sodium intake: role of angiotensin, Am. J. Physiol., 239, F271, 1980.

102. Hall, J.E., Guyton, A.C., Salgado, H.C., McCaa, R.E. and Balfe, J.W., Renal hemodynamics in acute and chronic angiotensin II hypertension, Am. J. Physiol., 235, F174, 1978.

103. Hall, J.E., Guyton, A.C., Smith, M.J., Jr. and Coleman, T.G., Long-term regulation of arterial pressure, glomerular filtration and renal sodium reabsorption by angiotensin II in dogs, Clin. Sci., 59, 87s, 1980.

104. McCaa, R.E., Role of the renin-angiotensin-aldosterone and kallikrein-kinin systems in the control of fluid and electrolyte metabolism, renal function, and arterial blood pressure, Clin. Exp. Hypert., Part A, 4, 1593, 1982.

105. Waugh, W.H., Angiotensin II: Local renal effects of physiological increments in concentration, Can. J. Physiol. Pharmacol., 50, 711, 1972.

106. Fagard, R.H., Cowley, A.W., Jr., Navar, L.G., Langford, H.G. and Guyton, A.C., Renal responses to slight elevations of renal arterial plasma angiotensin II concentration in dogs, Clin. Exp. Pharmacol. Physiol., 3, 531, 1976.

107. Hall, J.E., Guyton, A.C., Trippodo, N.C., Lohmeier, T.E., McCaa, R.E. and Cowley, A.W., Jr., Intrarenal control of electrolyte excretion by angiotensin II, Am. J. Physiol., 232, F538, 1977.

108. Trippodo, N.C., Hall, J.E., Lohmeier, T.E. and Guyton, A.C., Intrarenal role of angiotensin II in controlling sodium excretion during dehydration in dogs, Clin. Sci. Mol. Med., 52, 545, 1977.

109. Lohmeier, T.E., Cowley, A.W., Jr., Trippodo, N.C., Hall, J.E. and Guyton, A.C., Effects of endogenous angiotensin II on renal sodium excretion and renal hemodynamics, Am. J. Physiol., 233, F388, 1977.

110. Harris, P.J. and Navar, L.G., Tubular transport responses to angiotensin, Am. J. Physiol., 248, F621, 1985.

111. Morgan, R. and Davis, J.M., Renin secretion at the individual nephron level, Pfluegers Arch., 359, 23, 1975.

112. Regoli, D., Studies on the intrarenal action of the renin-angiotensin system, in Hypertension - 1972, Genest, J. and Koiw, E., Eds., Springer, Berlin, 1972, 72.

113. Hall, J.E., Guyton, A.C. and Cowley, A.W., Jr., Dissociation of renal blood flow and filtration rate autoregulation by renin depletion, Am. J. Physiol., 232, F215, 1977.

114. Hall, J.E., Coleman, T.G., Guyton, A.C., Balfe, J.W. and Salgado, H.C., Intrarenal role of angiotensin II and [des-Asp[1]] angiotensin II, Am. J. Physiol., 236, F252, 1979.

115. Thurau, K. and Mason, J., Renin-angiotensin: a local determinant for glomerular filtration, in Mechanisms of Hypertension, Sambhi, M.P., Ed., Excerpta Medica, Amsterdam, Elsevier, New York, 1973, 32.

116. Hall, J.E., Guyton, A.C., Jackson, T.E., Coleman, T.G., Lohmeier, T.E. and Trippodo, N.C., Control of glomerular filtration rate by renin-angiotensin

system, Am. J. Physiol., 233, F366, 1977.

117. Hall, J.E. and Granger, J.P., Renal hemodynamic actions of angiotensin II: interaction with tubuloglomerular feedback, Am. J. Physiol., 245, R166, 1983.

118. Ljungman, S., Aurell, M., Hartford, M., Wikstrand, J., Wilhelmsen, L. and Berglund, G., Blood pressure and renal function, Acta. Med. Scand., 298, 17, 1980.

119. Muirhead, E.E., Antihypertensive functions of the kidney, Hypertension, 2, 444, 1980.

120. Muirhead, E.E. and Pitcock, J.A., The renal antihypertensive hormone, J. Hypert., 3, 1, 1985.

121. Mandal, A.K., The renal papilla and hypertension. An up-to-date review, Pathol. Annu., 16, 295, 1981.

122. Hamilton, J. G. and Grollman, A., The preparation of renal extracts effective in reducing blood pressure in experimental hypertension, J. Biol. Chem., 233, 528, 1958.

123. Grollman, A., Pathogenesis of hypertension and implications for its therapeutic management, Clin. Pharmacol. Ther., 10, 755, 1969.

124. Page, I.H., Helmer, O.M., Kohlstaedt, K.G., Kempf, G.F., Gambill, W.D. and Taylor, R.D., The blood pressure reducing property of extracts of kidneys in hypertensive patients and animals, Ann. Intern. Med., 15, 347, 1941.

125. Page, I.H., Helmer, O.M., Kohlstaedt, K.G., Fouts, P.J. and Kempf, G.F., Reduction of arterial blood pressure of hypertensive patients and animals with extracts of kidneys, J. Exp. Med., 73, 7, 1941.

126. Floyer, M.A., Renal control of interstitial space compliance: a physiological mechanism which may play a part in the etiology of hypertension, Clin. Nephrol., 4, 152, 1975.

127. Green, J.A., Lucas, J. and Floyer, M.A., The effect of the kidney in altering the response of the circulation to fluid loading, Clin. Sci., 38, 4P, 1970.

128. Lucas, J. and Floyer, M.A., Renal control of changes in the compliance of the interstitial space: A factor in the aetiology of renoprival hypertension, Clin. Sci., 44, 397, 1973.

129. Guyton, A.C., Interstitial fluid pressure. II. Pressure-volume curves of interstitial space, Circ. Res., 16, 452, 1965.

130. Lucas, J. and Floyer, M.A., Changes in body fluid distribution and interstitial tissue compliance during the development and reversal of experimental renal hypertension in the rat, Clin. Sci. Mol. Med., 47, 1, 1974.

131. Neubig, R.R. and Hoobler, S.W., Reversal of chronic renal hypertension: Role of salt and water excretion, Proc. Soc. Exp. Biol. Med., 150, 254, 1975.

132. Hoobler, S.W., Eto, T., Welk, R. and Burge, H., Antihypertensive effect of transplant of rat kidney or its unclipping. Hemodynamic effects and control mechanisms, Hypertension, 3 (Suppl. 2), 200, 1981.

133. Muirhead, E.E., Jones, F. and Graham, P., Hypertension following bilateral nephrectomy of the dog. The influence of dietary protein on its pathogenesis with emphasis on its development in the absence of "extracellular fluid" expansion, Circ. Res., 1, 439, 1953.

134. Muirhead, E.E., Stirman, J.A., Lesch, W. and Jones, F., The reduction of postnephrectomy hypertension by renal homotransplant, Surg. Gynaecol. Obst., 103, 673, 1956.

135. Muirhead, E.E., Brooks, B. and Brosius, W.L., Renomedullary deficiency, Arch. Pathol., 95, 77, 1973.

136. Susic, D., Sparks, J.C. and Machado, E.A., Salt-induced hypertension in rats with hereditary hydronephrosis: the effect of renomedullary transplantation,

J. Lab. Clin. Med., 87, 232, 1976.

137. Muirhead, E.E., Jones, F. and Stirman, J.A., Antihypertensive property in renoprival hypertension of extract from renal medulla, J. Lab. Clin. Med., 56, 167, 1960.

138. Manthorpe, T., Antihypertensive and hypertensive effects of the kidney: elucidated by treatment with medullary transplants and with blockade either of the renin angiotensin-system or of the prostaglandin biosynthesis, Acta Pathol. Microbiol. Scand., Sect. A, 83, 395, 1975.

139. Manthorpe, T., The effect on renal hypertension of subcutaneous isotransplantation of renal medulla from normal or hypertensive rats: including studies on spontaneous variations in blood pressure in normal and hypertensive rats, Acta. Pathol. Microbiol. Scand., Sect. A, 81, 725, 1973.

140. Manger, W.M., Van Praag, D., Weiss, R.J., Hart, C.J., Hulse, M., Rock, T.W. and Farber, S.J., Effect of transplanting renomedullary tissue into spontaneously hypertensive rats (SHR), Fed. Proc., 35, 556, 1976.

141. Göthberg, G., Lundin, S. and Folkow, B., Acute vasodepressor effect in normotensive rats following extracorporal perfusion of the declipped kidney of two-kidney, one clip hypertensive rats, Hypertension, 4 (Suppl. 2), 101, 1982.

142. Muirhead, E.E., Byers, L.W., Desiderio, D.M., Jr., Pitcock, J.A., Brooks, B., Brown, P.S. and Brosius, W.L., Derivation of antihypertensive neutral renomedullary lipid from renal venous effluent, J. Lab. Clin. Med., 99, 64, 1982.

143. Heptinstall, R.H., Salyer, D.C. and Salyer, W.R., Experimental hypertension. The effects of chemical ablation of the renal papilla on the blood pressure of rats with and without silver-clip hypertension, Am. J. Pathol., 78, 297, 1975.

144. Taverner, D., Bing, R.F., Fletcher, A., Russell, G., Swales, J.D. and Thurston, H., Hypertension produced by chemical renal medullectomy: evidence for a renomedullary vasodepressor function in the rat, Clin. Sci., 67, 521, 1984.

145. Bing, R.F., Russell, G.I., Swales, J.D., Thurston, H. and Fletcher, A., Chemical renal medullectomy; effect upon reversal of two-kidney, one-clip hypertension in the rat, Clin. Sci., 61, 335s, 1981.

146. Russell, G.I., Taverner, D., Jackson, J., Bing, R.F., Swales, J.D. and Thurston, H., Role of the renal medulla in experimental hypertension, in Contributions to Nephrology, Karger, Basel, vol. 41, 1984, 163.

147. Muirhead, E.E., Pitcock, J.A., Nasjlett, A., Brown, P. and Brooks, B., The antihypertension function of the kidney. Its elucidation by captopril plus unclipping, Hypertension, 7 (Suppl. 1), 127, 1985.

148. Russell, G.I., Bing, R.F., Swales, J.D. and Thurston, H., Indomethacin or aprotinin infusion: effect on reversal of chronic two-kidney, one-clip hypertension in the conscious rat, Clin. Sci., 62, 361, 1982.

149. Muirhead, E.E., Leach, B.E., Byers, L.W., Brooks, B. and Pitcock, J.A., Renomedullary interstitial cells and the antihypertensive renomedullary hormone, Clin. Res., 24, 474A, 1976.

150. Muirhead, E.E. and Brooks, B., Reversal of one-kidney, one-clip hypertension by unclipping: The renal, sodium-volume relationship reexamined, Proc. Soc. Exp. Biol. Med., 163, 540, 1980.

151. Muirhead, E.E., Vanatta, J. and Grollman, A., Papillary necrosis of the kidney. A clinical and experimental correlation, J. Am. Med. Assoc., 142, 627, 1950.

152. Muirhead, E.E. and Stirman, J.A., Dietary protein and hypertension of dog: Protection by uretero-caval anastomosis with a study of kidneys so treated,

Am. J. Pathol., 34, 561, 1958.

153.   Pitcock, J.A., Brown, P.S., Brooks, B., Rapp, J.P., Rightsel, W. and Muir-head, E.E., The morphology and antihypertensive effect of renomedullary in-terstitial cells derived from Dahl sensitive and resistant rats, Exp. Mol. Pathol., 42, 29, 1985.

154.   Ishii, M. and Tobian, L., Interstitial cell granules in renal papilla and the solute composition of renal tissue in rats with Goldblatt hypertension, J. Lab. Clin. Med., 74, 47, 1969.

155.   Muehrcke, R.C., Mandal, A.K. and Volini, F.I., A pathophysiological review of the renal medullary interstitial cells and their relationship to hyper-tension, Circ. Res., 26/27 (Suppl. 1), 109, 1970.

156.   Pitcock, J.A., Brown, P.S., Brooks, B., Clapp, W.L., Brosius, W.L. and Muir-head, E.E., Renomedullary deficiency in partial nephrectomy-salt hyperten-sion, Hypertension, 2, 281, 1980.

157.   Muirhead, E.E., Jones, F. and Stirman, J.A., Hypertensive cardiovascular disease of dog, Arch. Pathol., 70, 108, 1960.

158.   Murray, G., Wyllie, R.G., Hill, G.S., Ramsden, P.W. and Heptinstall, R.H., Experimental papillary necrosis of the kidney. I. Morphologic and func-tional data, Am. J. Pathol., 67, 285, 1972.

159.   Axelsen, R.A., Healed experimental renal papillary necrosis and cortical scarring in the rat from 2-bromoethylamine hydrobromide, Virchows Arch., A: Pathol. Anat. Histol., 381, 63, 1978.

160.   Bing, R.F., Russell, G.I., Thurston, H., Swales, J.D., Godfrey, N., Lazarus, Y. and Jackson, J., Chemical renal medullectomy. Effect on urinary pros-taglandin E_2 and plasma renin in response to variations in sodium intake and in relation to blood pressure, Hypertension, 5, 951, 1983.

161.   Chen, P.S., Caldwell, R.M. and Hsu, C.H., Role of renal papillae in the regulation of sodium excretion during acute elevation of renal perfusion pressure in the rat, Hypertension, 6, 893, 1984.

162.   Muirhead, E.E., Case for a renomedullary blood pressure lowering hormone, in Contributions to Nephrology, Vol. 12: Vasoactive Renal Hormones, Eisenbach, G.M. and Brod, J., Eds., Karger, Basel, 1978, 69.

163.   Smith, K.A., Cornett, L.E., Norris, J.S., Byers, L.W. and Muirhead, E.E., Blockade of alpha-adrenergic receptors by analogues of phosphatidylcholine, Life Sci., 31, 1891, 1982.

164.   Muirhead, E.E., Leach, B.E., Brooks, B., Shaw, P.H., Brosius, W.L., Jr., Daniels, E.G. and Hinman, J.W., Antihypertensive renomedullary lipid in the hypertensive rabbit, Rev. Franc. Etud. Clin. Biol., 12, 893, 1967.

165.   Prewitt, R.L., Leach, B.E., Byers, L.W., Brooks, B., Lands, W.E.M. and Muir-head, E.E., Antihypertensive polar renomedullary lipid, a semisynthetic vasodilator, Hypertension, 1, 299, 1979.

166.   Muirhead, E.E., Folkow, B., Byers, L.W., Desiderio, D.M., Jr., Thorén, P., Göthberg, G., Dow, A.W. and Brooks, B., Cardiovascular effects of antihyper-tensive polar and neutral renomedullary lipids, Hypertension, 5 (Suppl. 1), 112, 1983.

167.   Muirhead, E.E., Byers, L.W., Folkow, B., Göthberg, G., Thorén, P. and Brooks, B., Antihypertensive polar and neutral renopapillary lipids. Which is a hormone?, Hypertension, 5 (Suppl. 5), 61, 1983.

168.   Muirhead, E.E., Folkow, B., Byers, L.W., Aus, G., Friberg, P., Göthberg, G., Nilsson, H. and Thoren, P., Cardiovascular effects of antihypertensive renomedullary lipids (APRL and ANRL), Acta Physiol. Scand., 117, 465, 1983.

169.   Faber, J.E., Barron, K.W., Bonham, A.C., Lappe, R., Muirhead, E.E. and Brody, M.J., Regional hemodynamic effects of antihypertensive renomedullary lipids in conscious rats, Hypertension, 6, 494, 1984.

293

170. Smith, K.A., Prewitt, R.L., Jr., Byers, L.W. and Muirhead, E.E., Analogs of phosphatidylcholine: α-adrenergic antagonists from the renal medulla, Hypertension, 3, 460, 1981.

171. Blank, M.L., Snyder, F., Byers, L.W., Brooks, B. and Muirhead, E.E., Antihypertensive activity of an alkyl ether analog of phosphatidylcholine, Biochem. Biophys. Res. Commun., 90, 1194, 1979.

172. Muirhead, E.E., Byers, L.W., Desiderio, D., Jr., Smith, K.A., Prewitt, R.L. and Brooks, B., Alkyl ether analogs of phosphatidylcholine are orally active in hypertensive rabbits, Hypertension, 3 (Suppl. 1), 107, 1981.

173. McManus, L.M., Hanahan, D.J., Demopoulos, C.A. and Pinckard, R.N., Pathobiology of the intravenous infusion of acetyl glyceryl ether phosphorylcholine (AGEPC), a synthetic platelet-activating factor (PAF), in the rabbit, J. Immunol., 124, 2919, 1980.

174. Braun-Menéndez, E., The prohypertensive and antihypertensive actions of the kidney, Ann. Intern. Med., 49, 717, 1958.

175. De Wardener, H.E. and MacGregor, G.A., The natriuretic hormone and hypertension, J. Chron. Dis., 34, 233, 1981.

176. Marx, J.L., Natriuretic hormone linked to hypertension, Science, 212, 1255, 1981.

177. De Wardener, H.E. and MacGregor, G.A., Dahl's hypothesis that a saluretic substance may be responsible for a sustained rise in arterial pressure: Its possible role in essential hypertension, Kidney Int., 18, 1, 1980.

178. De Wardener, H.E. and MacGregor, G.A., The natriuretic hormone and essential hypertension, Lancet, 1, 1450, 1982.

179. Sagnella, G.A. and MacGregor, G.A., Cardiac peptides and the control of sodium excretion, Nature, 309, 666, 1984.

180. De Wardener, H.E. and Clarkson, E.M., Concept of natriuretic hormone, Physiol. Rev., 65, 658, 1985.

181. Mills, I.H., Atrial natriuretic factor: a new hormone?, Br. Med. J., 289, 210, 1984.

182. Trippodo, N.C., Cole, F.E. and MacPhee, A.A., Atrial natriuretic factor: sodium transport in human erythrocytes, Clin. Sci., 67, 403, 1984.

183. Sagnella, G.A. and MacGregor, G.A., Endogenous digitalis: true or false?, Trends Pharmacol. Sci., 6, 393, 1985.

184. Pamnani, M.B., Clough, D.L., Chen, J.S., Link, W.T. and Haddy, F.J., Effects of rat atrial extract on sodium transport and blood pressure in the rat, Proc. Soc. Exp. Biol. Med., 176, 123, 1984.

185. Dahl, L.K., Knudsen, K.D., Heine, M.A. and Leitl, G.J., Effects of chronic excess salt ingestion. Modification of experimental hypertension in the rat by variations in the diet, Circ. Res., 22, 11, 1968.

186. Dahl, L.K., Heine, M. and Tassinari, L., Effects of chronic excess salt ingestion. Role of genetic factors in both DOCA-salt and renal hypertension, J. Exp. Med., 118, 605, 1963.

187. Dahl, L.K., Heine, M. and Tassinari, L., Effects of chronic excess salt ingestion. Further demonstration that genetic factors influence the development of hypertension: Evidence from experimental hypertension due to cortisone and to adrenal regeneration, J. Exp. Med., 122, 533, 1965.

188. Dahl, L.K., Knudsen, K.D., Heine, M. and Leitl, G., Effects of chronic excess salt ingestion. Genetic influence on the development of salt hypertension in parabiotic rats: Evidence for a humoral factor, J. Exp. Med., 126, 687, 1967.

189. Iwai, J., Knudsen, K.D., Dahl, L.K., Heine, M. and Leitl, G., Genetic influence on the development of renal hypertension in parabiotic rats, J. Exp. Med., 129, 507, 1969.

190. Dahl, L.K., Knudsen, K.D. and Iwai, J., Humoral transmission of hypertension: Evidence from parabiosis, Circ. Res., 24/25 (Suppl. 1), 21, 1969.

191. Snajdar, R.M. and Rapp, J.P., Atrial natriuretic factor in Dahl rats. Atrial content and renal and aortic responses, Hypertension, 7, 775, 1985.

192. Haddy, F.J. and Overbeck, H.W., The role of humoral agents in volume expanded hypertension, Life Sci., 19, 935, 1976.

193. Neufeld, E., Sklarz, B., Goldberg, S., Gilad, S., Goldfarb, H., Laurian, L., Silverberg, D.S. and Chayen, R., Observations on the chemical and physiological properties of urodiolenone, an urinary compound found in hypertension, Nephron, 39, 146, 1985.

194. Mason, D.T. and Braunwald, E., Studies on digitalis. X. Effects of ouabain on forearm vascular resistance and venous tone in normal subjects and in patients in heart failure, J. Clin. Invest., 43, 532, 1964.

195. Floyer, M.A., Further studies on the mechanism of experimental hypertension in the rat, Clin. Sci., 14, 163, 1955.

196. Borst, J.G.G. and Borst-De Geus, A., Hypertension explained by Starling's theory of circulatory homeostasis, Lancet, 1, 677, 1963.

197. Blaustein, M.P., Sodium ions, calcium ions, blood pressure regulation, and hypertension: A reassessment and a hypothesis, Am. J. Physiol., 232, C165, 1977.

198. Brading, A.F. and Lategan, T.W., Na-Ca exchange in vascular smooth muscle, J. Hypert., 3, 109, 1985.

199. Shore, A.C., Beynon, G.W., Jones, J.C., Markandu, N.D., Sagnella, G.A. and MacGregor, G.A., Mononuclear leucocyte intracellular free calcium: Does it correlate with blood pressure?, J. Hypert., 3, 183, 1985.

200. De Wardener, H.E., The concept of the natriuretic hormone and its relation to hypertension, Clin. Exp. Hypert., Part A, 7, 647, 1985.

201. Haddy, F.J. and Pamnani, M.B., Evidence for a circulating sodium-potassium pump inhibitor in low renin hypertension, Clin. Exp. Hypert., Part A, 7, 633, 1985.

202. De Wardener, H.E., MacGregor, G.A., Clarkson, E.M., Alaghband-Zadeh, J., Bitensky, L. and Chayen, J., Effect of sodium intake on ability of human plasma to inhibit renal Na^+-K^+-adenosine triphosphatase in vitro, Lancet, 1, 411, 1981.

203. Poston, L., Sewell, R.B., Wilkinson, S.P., Richardson, P.J., Williams, R., Clarkson, E.M., MacGregor, G.A. and De Wardener, H.E., Evidence for a circulating sodium transport inhibitor in essential hypertension, Br. Med. J., 282, 847, 1981.

204. Fenton, S., Clarkson, E.M., MacGregor, G.A., Alaghband-Zadeh, J. and De Wardener, H.E., An assay of the capacity of biological fluids to stimulate renal glucose-6-phosphate dehydrogenase activity in vitro as a marker of their ability to inhibit sodium potassium-dependent adenosine triphosphatase activity, J. Endocrinol., 94, 99, 1982.

205. MacGregor, G.A., Fenton, S., Alaghband-Zadeh, J., Markandu, N., Roulston, J.E. and De Wardener, H.E., Evidence for a raised concentration of a circulating sodium transport inhibitor in essential hypertension, Br. Med. J., 283, 1355, 1981.

206. MacGregor, G.A., Fenton, S., Alaghband-Zadeh, J., Markandu, N.D., Roulston, J.E. and De Wardener, H.E., An increase in a circulating inhibitor of Na^+,K^+-dependent ATPase: a possible link between salt intake and the development of essential hypertension, Clin. Sci., 61, 17s, 1981.

207. Clarkson, E.M., Raw, S.M. and De Wardener, H.E., Two natriuretic substances in extracts of urine from normal man when salt-depleted and salt-loaded,

Kidney Int., 10, 381, 1976.

208. Lichtstein, D., Minc, D., Shimoni, Y., Deutsch, J., Mekler, J. and Ben-Ishay, D., Demonstration of a ouabainlike plasma compound in hypertension prone and hypertension resistant rats, Hypertension, 7, 729, 1985.

209. Jones, R.B., Patrick, J. and Hilton, P.J., Increased sodium content and altered sodium transport in thymocytes of spontaneously hypertensive rats, Clin. Sci., 61, 313, 1981.

210. Pamnani, M.B., Buggy, J., Huot, S.J. and Haddy, F.J., Studies on the role of a humoral sodium-transport inhibitor and the anteroventral third ventricle (AV3V) in experimental low-renin hypertension, Clin. Sci., 61, 57s, 1981.

211. Mason, J.C., Poston, L. and Hilton, P.J., Sodium pump activity in thymocytes of rats with Goldblatt hypertension, Clin. Sci., 68, 11, 1985.

212. Zidek, W., Losse, H., Lange-Asschenfeldt, H. and Vetter, H., Intracellular chloride in essential hypertension, Clin. Sci., 68, 45, 1985.

213. Alaghband-Zadeh, J., Fenton, S., Hancock, K., Millett, J. and De Wardener, H.E., Evidence that the hypothalamus may be a source of a circulating Na^+-K^+-ATPase inhibitor, J. Endocrinol., 98, 221, 1983.

214. Blaine, E.H., Emergence of a new cardiovascular control system: atrial natriuretic factor. An introduction, Clin. Exp. Hypert., Part A, 7, 839, 1985.

215. Maack, T., Camargo, M.J.F., Kleinert, H.D., Laragh, J.H. and Atlas, S.A., Atrial natriuretic factor: Structure and functional properties, Kidney Int., 27, 607, 1985.

216. Needleman, P., Adams, S.P., Cole, B.R., Currie, M.G., Geller, D.M., Michener, M.L., Saper, C.B., Schwartz, D. and Standaert, D.G., Atriopeptins as cardiac hormones, Hypertension, 7, 469, 1985.

217. Henry, J.P., Gauer, O.H. and Reeves, J.L., Evidence of the atrial location of receptors influencing urine flow, Circ. Res., 4, 85, 1956.

218. De Bold, A.J., Raymond, J.J. and Bencosme, S.A., Atrial specific granules of the rat heart: light microscopic staining and histochemical reactions, J. Histochem. Cytochem., 26, 1094, 1978.

219. Gutkowska, J., Thibault, G., Januszewicz, P., Cantin, M. and Genest, J., Direct radioimmunoassay of atrial natriuretic factor, Biochem. Biophys. Res. Commun., 122, 593, 1984.

220. Cantin, M., Gutkowska, J., Thibault, G., Milne, R.W., Ledoux, S., MinLi, S., Chapeau, C., Garcia, R., Hamet, P. and Genest, J., Immunocytochemical localization of atrial natriuretic factor in the heart and salivary glands, Histochemistry, 80, 113, 1984.

221. De Bold, A.J., Heart atria granularity effects of changes in water-electrolyte balance, Proc. Soc. Exp. Biol. Med., 161, 508, 1979.

222. Pollock, D.M. and Banks, R.O., Influence of dietary sodium on the natriuretic activity of atrial tissue, Mineral Electrolyte Metab., 10, 337, 1984.

223. Thibault, G., Garcia, R., Cantin, M. and Genest, J., Atrial natriuretic factor. Characterization and partial purification, Hypertension, 5 (Suppl. 1), 75, 1983.

224. Johnson, M.D., An improved bioassay method for determining natriuretic activity of atrial extracts, Am. J. Physiol., 248, F314, 1985.

225. Sonnenberg, H. and Veress, A.T., Cellular mechanism of release of atrial natriuretic factor, Biochem. Biophys. Res. Commun., 124, 443, 1984.

226. Currie, M.G., Geller, D.M., Cole, B.R., Siegel, N.R., Fok, K.F., Adams, S.P., Eubanks, S.R., Galluppi, G.R. and Needleman, P., Purification and sequence analysis of bioactive atrial peptides (atriopeptins), Science, 223, 67, 1984.

227. Gutkowska, J., Horky, K., Thibault, G., Januszewicz, P., Cantin, M. and Genest, J., Atrial natriuretic factor is a circulating hormone, Biochem. Biophys. Res. Commun., 125, 315, 1984.

228. Dietz, J.R., Release of natriuretic factor from rat heart-lung preparation by atrial distension, Am. J. Physiol., 247, R1093, 1984.

229. Veress, A.T. and Sonnenberg, H., Right atrial appendectomy reduces the renal response to acute hypervolemia in the rat, Am. J. Physiol., 247, R610, 1984.

230. Tikkanen, I., Fyhrquist, F., Metsärinne, K. and Leidenius, R., Plasma atrial natriuretic peptide in cardiac disease and during infusion in healthy volunteers, Lancet, 2, 66, 1985.

231. Lang, R.E., Thölken, H., Ganten, D., Luft, F.C., Ruskoaho, H. and Unger, T., Atrial natriuretic factor: a circulating hormone stimulated by volume loading, Nature, 314, 264, 1985.

232. Inagami, T., Misono, K.S., Grammer, R.T., Fukumi, H., Maki, M., Tanaka, I., McKenzie, J.C., Takayanagi, R., Pandey, K.N. and Parmentier, M., Biochemical studies of rat atrial natriuretic factor, Clin. Exp. Hypert., Part A, 7, 851, 1985.

233. Tang, J., Webber, R.J., Chang, D., Chang, J.K., Kiang, J. and Wei, E.T., Depressor and natriuretic activities of several atrial peptides, Regul. Pept., 9, 53, 1984.

234. Thibault, G., Garcia, R., Cantin, M. and Genest, J., Atrial natriuretic factor and urinary kallikrein in the rat: antagonistic factors?, Can. J. Physiol. Pharmacol., 62, 645, 1984.

235. Chimoskey, J.E., Spielman, W.S., Brandt, M.A. and Heidemann, S.R., Cardiac atria of BIO 14.6 hamsters are deficient in natriuretic factor, Science, 223, 820, 1984.

236. Sonnenberg, H., Milojevic, S., Chong, C.K. and Veress, A.T., Atrial natriuretic factor: Reduced cardiac content in spontaneously hypertensive rats, Hypertension, 5, 672, 1983.

237. Hirata, Y., Ganguli, M., Tobian, L. and Iwai, J., Dahl S rats have increased natriuretic factor in atria but are markedly hyporesponsive to it, Hypertension, 6 (Suppl. 1), 148, 1984.

238. Kobrin, I., Kardon, M.B., Trippodo, N.C., Pegram, B.L. and Frohlich, E.D., Renal response to acute volume overload in conscious rats with atrial appendectomy, J. Hypert., 3, 145, 1985.

239. De Bold, A.J., Borenstein, H.B., Veress, A.T. and Sonnenberg, H., A rapid and potent natriuretic response to intravenous injection of atrial myocardial extract in rats, Life Sci., 28, 89, 1981.

240. Sagnella, G.A., Nolan, D.A., Shore, A.C. and MacGregor, G.A., Effects of synthetic atrial natriuretic peptides on sodium-potassium transport in human erythrocytes, Clin. Sci., 69, 223, 1985.

241. Seidah, N.G., Lazure, C., Chrétien, M., Thibault, G., Garcia, R., Cantin, M., Genest, J., Nutt, R.F., Brady, S.F., Lyle, T.A., Paleveda, W.J., Colton, C.D., Ciccarone, T.M. and Veber, D.F., Amino acid sequence of homologous rat atrial peptides: Natriuretic activity of native and synthetic forms, Proc. Natl. Acad. Sci. U.S.A., 81, 2640, 1984.

242. Flynn, T.G., De Bold, M.L. and De Bold, A.J., The amino acid sequence of an atrial peptide with potent diuretic and natriuretic properties, Biochem. Biophys. Res. Commun., 117, 859, 1983.

243. Atlas, S.A., Kleinert, H.D., Camargo, M.J., Januszewicz, A., Sealey, J.E., Laragh, J.H., Schilling, J.W., Lewicki, J.A., Johnson, L.K. and Maack, T., Purification, sequencing and synthesis of natriuretic and vasoactive rat atrial peptide, Nature, 309, 717, 1984.

244. Seidman, C.E., Duby, A.D., Choi, E., Graham, R.M., Haber, E., Homcy, C.,

Smith, J.A. and Seidman, J.G., The structure of rat preproatrial natriuretic factor as defined by a complementary DNA clone, Science, 225, 324, 1984.

245. Garcia, R., Thibault, G., Seidah, N.G., Lazure, C., Cantin, M., Genest, J. and Chrétien, M., Structure-activity relationships of atrial natriuretic factor (ANF). II. Effect of chain-length modifications on vascular reactivity, Biochem. Biophys. Res. Commun., 126, 178, 1985.

246. Misono, K.S., Fukumi, H., Grammer, R.T. and Inagami, T., Rat atrial natriuretic factor: Complete amino acid sequence and disulfide linkage essential for biological activity, Biochem. Biophys. Res. Commun., 119, 524, 1984.

247. Geller, D.M., Currie, M.G., Wakitani, K., Cole, B.R., Adams, S.P., Fok, K.F., Siegel, N.R., Eubanks, S.R., Galluppi, G.R. and Needleman, P., atriopeptins: A family of potent biologically active peptides derived from mammalian atria, Biochem. Biophys. Res. Commun., 120, 333, 1984.

248. Misono, K.S., Grammer, R.T., Fukumi, H. and Inagami, T., Rat atrial natriuretic factor: Isolation, structure and biological activities of four major peptides, Biochem. Biophys. Res. Commun., 123, 444, 1984.

249. Thibault, G., Garcia, R., Carrier, F., Seidah, N.G., Lazure, C., Chrétien, M., Cantin, M. and Genest, J., Structure-activity relationships of atrial natriuretic factor (ANF). I. Natriuretic activity and relaxation of intestinal smooth muscle, Biochem. Biophys. Res. Commun., 125, 938, 1984.

250. Currie, M.G., Geller, D.M., Cole, B.R., Boylan, J.G., YuSheng, W., Holmberg, S.W. and Needleman, P., Bioactive cardiac substances: Potent vasorelaxant activity in mammalian atria, Science, 221, 71, 1983.

251. Grammer, R.T., Fukumi, H., Inagami, T. and Misono, K.S., Rat atrial natriuretic factor. Purification and vasorelaxant activity, Biochem. Biophys. Res. Commun., 116, 696, 1983.

252. Sonnenberg, H., Cupples, W.A., DeBold, A.J. and Veress, A.T., Intrarenal localization of the natriuretic effect of cardiac atrial extract, Ann. N.Y. Acad. Sci., 372, 213, 1981.

253. Briggs, J.P., Steipe, B., Schubert, G. and Schnermann, J., Micropuncture studies of the renal effects of atrial natriuretic substance, Pfluegers Arch., 395, 271, 1982.

254. Pollock, D.M. and Banks, R.O., Effect of atrial extract on renal function in the rat, Clin. Sci., 65, 47, 1983.

255. Oshima, T., Currie, M.G., Geller, D.M. and Needleman, P., An atrial peptide is a potent renal vasodilator substance, Circ. Res., 54, 612, 1984.

256. Needleman, P., Currie, M.G., Geller, D.M., Cole, B.R. and Adams, S.P., Atriopeptins: potential mediators of an endocrine relationship between heart and kidney, Trends Pharmacol. Sci., 5, 506, 1984.

257. Keeler, R. and Azzarolo, A.M., Effects of atrial natriuretic factor on renal handling of water and electrolytes in rats, Can. J. Physiol. Pharmacol., 61, 996, 1983.

258. Koike, H., Sada, T., Miyamoto, M., Oizumi, K., Sugiyama, M. and Inagami, T., Atrial natriuretic factor selectively increases renal blood flow in conscious spontaneously hypertensive rats, Eur. J. Pharmacol., 104, 391, 1984.

259. Maack, T., Marion, D.N., Camargo, M.J., Kleinert, H.D., Laragh, J.H., Vaughan, E.D., Jr. and Atlas, S.A., Effects of auriculin (atrial natriuretic factor) on blood pressure, renal function, and the renin-aldosterone system in dogs, Am. J. Med., 77, 1069, 1984.

260. Burnett, J.C., Jr., Granger, J.P. and Opgenorth, T.J., Effects of synthetic atrial natriuretic factor on renal function and renin release, Am. J. Physiol., 247, F863, 1984.

261. Seymour, A.A., Renal and systemic effects of atrial natriuretic factor,

Clin. Exp. Hypert., Part A, 7, 887, 1985.

262.   Aalkjaer, C., Mulvany, M.J. and Nyborg, N.C.B., Atrial natriuretic factor causes specific relaxation of rat renal arcuate arteries, Br. J. Pharmacol., 86, 447, 1985.

263.   Reinhardt, H.W., Kaczmarczyk, G., Mohnhaupt, R. and Simgen, B., Atrial natriuresis under the condition of a constant renal perfusion pressure. Experiments on conscious dogs, Pfluegers Arch., 389, 9, 1980.

264.   Januszewicz, P., Gutkowska, J., De Lean, A., Thibault, G., Garcia, R., Genest, J. and Cantin, M., Synthetic atrial natriuretic factor induces release (possibly receptor-mediated) of vasopressin from rat posterior pituitary, Proc. Soc. Exp. Biol. Med., 178, 321, 1985.

265.   Tanaka, I., Misono, K.S. and Inagami, T., Atrial natriuretic factor in rat hypothalamus, atria and plasma: Determination by specific radioimmunoassay, Biochem. Biophys. Res. Commun., 124, 663, 1984.

266.   Jacobowitz, D.M., Skofitsch, G., Keiser, H.R., Eskay, R.L. and Zamir, N., Evidence for the existence of atrial natriuretic factor-containing neurons in the rat brain, Neuroendocrinology, 40, 92, 1985.

267.   Winquist, R.J., Faison, E.P. and Nutt, R.F., Vasodilator profile of synthetic atrial natriuretic factor, Eur. J. Pharmacol., 102, 169, 1984.

268.   Garcia, R., Thibault, G., Cantin, M. and Genest, J., Effect of a purified atrial natriuretic factor on rat and rabbit vascular strips and vascular beds, Am. J. Physiol., 247, R34, 1984.

269.   Kleinert, H.D., Maack, T., Atlas, S.A., Januszewicz, A., Sealey, J.E. and Laragh, J.H., Atrial natriuretic factor inhibits angiotensin-, norepinephrine-, and potassium-induced vascular contractility, Hypertension, 6 (Suppl. 1), 143, 1984.

270.   Garcia, R., Thibault, G., Gutkowska, J., Hamet, P., Cantin, M. and Genest, J., Effect of chronic infusion of synthetic atrial natriuretic factor (ANF 8-33) in conscious two-kidney, one-clip hypertensive rats, Proc. Soc. Exp. Biol. Med., 178, 155, 1985.

271.   Napier, M.A., Vandlen, R.L., Albers-Schönberg, G., Nutt, R.F., Brady, S., Lyle, T., Winquist, R., Faison, E.P., Heinel, L.A. and Blaine, E.H., Specific membrane receptors for atrial natriuretic factor in renal and vascular tissues, Proc. Natl. Acad. Sci. U.S.A., 81, 5946, 1984.

272.   Winquist, R.J., Napier, M.A., Vandlen, R.L., Arcuri, K., Keegan, M.E., Faison, E.P. and Baskin, E.P., Pharmacology and receptor binding of atrial natriuretic factor in vascular smooth muscle, Clin. Exp. Hypert., Part A, 7, 869, 1985.

273.   Hirata, Y., Tomita, M., Yoshimi, H. and Ikeda, M., Specific receptors for atrial natriuretic factor (ANF) in cultured vascular smooth muscle cells of rat aorta, Biochem. Biophys. Res. Commun., 125, 562, 1984.

274.   Winquist, R.J., Faison, E.P., Waldman, S.A., Schwartz, K., Murad, F. and Rapoport, R.M., Atrial natriuretic factor elicits an endothelium-independent relaxation and activates particulate guanylate cyclase in vascular smooth muscle, Proc. Natl. Acad. Sci. U.S.A., 81, 7661, 1984.

275.   Waldman, S.A., Rapoport, R.M. and Murad, F., Atrial natriuretic factor selectively activates particulate guanylate cyclase and elevates cyclic GMP in rat tissues, J. Biol. Chem., 259, 14332, 1984.

276.   Hamet, P., Tremblay, J., Pang, S.C., Garcia, R., Thibault, G., Gutkowska, J., Cantin, M. and Genest, J., Effect of native and synthetic atrial natriuretic factor on cyclic GMP, Biochem. Biophys. Res. Commun., 123, 515, 1984.

277.   Anand-Srivastava, M.B., Franks, D.J., Cantin, M. and Genest, J., Atrial natriuretic factor inhibits adenylate cyclase activity, Biochem. Biophys.

Res. Commun., 121, 855, 1984.

278. Seymour, A.A., Marsh, E.A., Mazack, E.K., Stabilito, I.I. and Blaine, E.H., Synthetic atrial natriuretic factor in conscious normotensive and hypertensive rats, Hypertension, 7 (Suppl. 1), 35, 1985.

279. Chartier, L., Schiffrin, E., Thibault, G. and Garcia, R., Atrial natriuretic factor inhibits the stimulation of aldosterone secretion by angiotensin II, ACTH and potassium in vitro and angiotensin II-induced steroidogenesis in vivo, Endocrinology, 115, 2026, 1984.

280. Marsh, E.A., Seymour, A.A., Haley, A.B., Whinnery, M.A., Napier, M.A., Nutt, R.F. and Blaine, E.H., Renal and blood pressure responses to synthetic atrial natriuretic factor in spontaneously hypertensive rats, Hypertension, 7, 386, 1985.

281. Kihara, M., Nakayama, K., Nakao, K., Sugawara, A., Morii, N., Sakamoto, M., Suda, M., Shimokura, M., Kiso, Y., Imura, H. and Yamori, Y., Accelerated natriuresis induced by synthetic atrial natriuretic polypeptide in spontaneously hypertensive rats, Clin. Exp. Hypert., Part A, 7, 539, 1985.

282. Richards, A.M., Nicholls, M.G., Espiner, E.A., Ikram, H., Yandle, T.G., Joyce, S.L. and Cullens, M.M., Effects of α-human atrial natriuretic peptide in essential hypertension, Hypertension, 7, 812, 1985.

283. Volpe, M., Odell, G., Kleinert, H.D., Müller, F., Camargo, M.J., Laragh, J.H., Maack, T., Vaughan, E.D., Jr. and Atlas, S.A., Effect of atrial natriuretic factor on blood pressure, renin, and aldosterone in Goldblatt hypertension, Hypertension, 7 (Suppl. 1), 43, 1985.

284. Keeton, T.K. and Campbell, W.B., The pharmacologic alteration of renin release, Pharmacol. Rev., 31, 81, 1981.

285. Goodfriend, T.L., Elliott, M.E. and Atlas, S.A., Actions of synthetic atrial natriuretic factor on bovine adrenal glomerulosa, Life Sci., 35, 1675, 1984.

286. De Léan, A., Racz, K., Gutkowska, J., Nguyen, T.T., Cantin, M. and Genest, J., Specific receptor-mediated inhibition by synthetic atrial natriuretic factor of hormone-stimulated steroidogenesis in cultured bovine adrenal cells, Endocrinology, 115, 1636, 1984.

287. Atarashi, K., Mulrow, P.J., Franco-Saenz, R., Snajdar, R. and Rapp, J., Inhibition of aldosterone production by an atrial extract, Science, 224, 992, 1984.

288. Chartier, L., Schiffrin, E. and Thibault, G., Effect of atrial natriuretic factor (ANF)-related peptides on aldosterone secretion by adrenal glomerulosa cells: Critical role of the intramolecular disulphide bond, Biochem. Biophys. Res. Commun., 122, 171, 1984.

289. Kudo, T. and Baird, A., Inhibition of aldosterone production in the adrenal glomerulosa by atrial natriuretic factor, Nature, 312, 756, 1984.

290. De Léan, A., Gutkowska, J., McNicoll, N., Schiller, P.W., Cantin, M. and Genest, J., Characterization of specific receptors for atrial natriuretic factor in bovine adrenal zona glomerulosa, Life Sci., 35, 2311, 1984.

9
RENAL SLICES
AND PERFUSION

W.O. BERNDT

I. INTRODUCTION

No attempt will be made to review all aspects of renal in vitro
techniques.   The focus will be on renal slices and perfusion techniques as they apply to toxicological problems.   For broader
coverage of in vitro procedures, especially physiological studies
the reader is referred to several reviews[1,2].   In addition, extensive reviews of renal slices and renal perfusion and other techniques have been published[3-5].

Both of these procedures offer the general advantages associated with in vitro techniques.   Difficulties associated with undesirable changes in renal haemodynamics, generalized changes in
cardiovascular function, problems of maintenance of whole animal
body temperature, etc., are obviated by isolated tissue.   In
general, better temperature control, more precise regulation of the
perfusing or bathing solution, etc., is possible when isolated
tissue preparations are examined.   Since the use of these techniques will be presented in the context of toxicological investigations, it is noteworthy that using isolated tissues may obviate discovery of important effects of xenobiotics, albeit indirect effects on
renal function.   Alterations in cardiovascular function, for example, may be caused by certain chemicals and such effects could
be translated into a perturbation of renal function.   This would
not be observed when the isolated tissue techniques are used.
Hence, in general, the advantages of the in vitro procedures are
to enhance precision and control, and a disadvantage is the loss of
breadth of study.

No attempt will be made here to offer a complete review of
renal physiology or anatomy, but a few words pertaining to renal
function are necessary.   For example, for an appropriate understanding of the power of the renal slice technique, it is important
to appreciate which of the normal physiological processes can be
assessed and how those data can be interpreted.   Further, the

isolated perfusion kidney technique will be better appreciated if some aspects of renal haemodynamics as well as transport characteristics of the kidney are at hand. Hence, a few introductory comments will be offered with the understanding that details will have to be gleaned from the published literature. The comments here can serve merely as a guide to which aspects of renal physiology and biochemistry are important.

II. RENAL SLICES

Various studies have been undertaken to demonstrate the utility of the renal slice technique to monitor organic anion and organic cation transport. These studies have been directed at a better understanding of those processes involved in the active tubular secretion of diverse chemical substances[5,6]. In general, the transport mechanism located on the peritubular side of proximal tubule cells is sufficiently effective to permit the rapid movement of certain organic substances such as p-aminohippuric acid (PAH) into the cells and their ultimate passive movement from the cells into the tubular fluid. The efficiency of this process is appreciated when it is realized that the clearance of a compound like PAH can be used to monitor total renal blood flow, given an estimate of the haematocrit. Similarly, various organic bases such as tetraethylammonium (TEA) can be transported equally rapidly and can also be used to monitor renal blood flow, although the latter is usually not done for various technical and analytical reasons.

Various studies, starting with those of Cross and Taggart[7] and Mudge and Taggart[8], demonstrated the correlation of the in vivo secretory activities with a renal slice accumulation of those substances[4,6]. Net accumulation of these model ions by renal slices provides a quantitative assessment of the magnitude of the transport process and these uptake data correlate qualitatively with the active tubular secretion of the same compounds. Hence, in vitro studies can be used to monitor the effects of various xenobiotics on these important transport functions. Since these functions occur in the proximal tubule and since many nephrotoxins exert their primary effect on that tubule section, the renal slice procedure can be used to assess nephrotoxic actions in well controlled in vitro experiments. In some experiments, important mechanisms of action may also be investigated, although in general the technique is most useful for assessment of the likelihood of a chemical effect on renal function. As indicated above, in all probability the utility of this procedure rests with the fact that most nephrotoxins appear to exert a primary action on one or another segment of the proximal tubular epithelium where organic ion transport occurs.

III. ISOLATED PERFUSED KIDNEY

The intent of this procedure is to allow the investigator to examine intact organ function under rather rigidly controlled in vitro conditions. Accordingly, it is important to develop techniques which will allow intact organ function to remain as near physiological as possible. Hence it is critical that the investigator appreciate various aspects of renal physiology, particularly those pertaining to haemodynamic considerations, oxygenation requirements, etc.

Intrarenal haemodynamics are complicated since the vascular network which supplies the glomerulus is the same network which supplies oxygen and nutrients to the actively functioning proximal tubular and distal tubular cells. The capillaries which form the glomerulus are not "classical" in that the efferent vessel is an artery. With respect to proximal tubular function, it is this efferent arteriole which initiates the network of vessels bathing the cells of the proximal tubule. Hence these complex anatomical relationships more than usual for an isolated system, dictate that one achieve appropriate physiological parameters with respect to flow and oxygen delivery, since both glomerular and tubular function depend on this blood supply. This requirement is dictated by virtue of the fact that in the intact animal the kidneys, which comprise less than 1% of body weight, receive nearly 25% of the cardiac output. Clearly, this high blood delivery represents nothing more or less than the requirement for high oxygen delivery by an organ with both high metabolic and transport activity.

In addition, the unusual intra-organ distribution of blood is an important consideration in the ability of the kidney to produce a concentrated urine given that other physiological parameters are appropriate. The absence of an adequate medullary flow (which comes from cortical areas) will greatly limit the concentrating ability of the kidney and compromise overall renal function. Indeed, in the intact animal a very early sign of the development of nephrotoxicity is the failure of the renal concentrating mechanism, although it must be admitted that the mechanism or mechanisms by which nephrotoxins exert this effect is (are) poorly understood. It is an effect which might be mediated through an alteration in renal haemodynamics perhaps related to as yet poorly defined actions of nephrotoxic substances on the proximal tubular blood flow network.

The proximal tubular areas of the nephron are metabolically very active. In addition, the epithelial cells transport into intracellular compartments a variety of amino acids and other nutrients, the metabolism of which may in some situations support specific transport functions[9]. Hence, under in vitro conditions it is critical to assure that appropriate nutrients are supplied to the renal tubular cells in addition to adequate oxygenation.

IV. RENAL SLICES

A. History

Tissue slices from various organs have been used for decades to study physiological and biochemical processes. In the 1920's and 30's slices of liver, for example, were utilized to assess oxygen consumption and other biochemical parameters (see Berndt[6] for a review). By the 1940's Forster[10] had developed an isolated renal slice technique to examine the transport of organic ions. Although this original work was with fish kidneys, Forster's approach established the usefulness of the isolated renal tissue procedure for assessment of renal function, at least in some aspects. Adaptation of this procedure to mammalian kidney required the view of another group and the application to renal slices of certain analytical techniques used in renal clearance experiments. Cross and Taggert[7] used renal slices of various mammals and studied the accumulation of PAH for the first time. Subsequently, various changes in these original techniques have yielded more refined procedures valuable in the assessment of xenobiotic actions on renal function. Further, the same procedures have proven useful in predicting the transport ability of new chemicals and drugs by kidney. Mudge[11] took the procedure one step further in demonstrating its applicability to the measurement of the transport of inorganic ions such as sodium or potassium.

B. The preparation and use of renal slices

Several procedures are available for the preparation of renal slices which are useful in metabolic and transport studies. The oldest technique for the preparation of renal slices is the free-hand method. Although suggestions have been made that this technique yields slices of non-uniform thickness, its worth has been proven over the years. Although this procedure may require more practice than some of the others, slices of 0.2 to 0.5 mm in thickness can be prepared routinely. Regardless of which animal may be used for these studies, renal cubes of 1 to 1.5 cm^2 are prepared and slices taken from each cube. The cube is placed on a block and gentle pressure applied to the top of the cube with a microscope slide, and a razor blade held in a haemostat is drawn through the tissue underneath the slide. Sufficient practice allows one to become proficient at the preparation of slices of uniform thickness and of approximately the same size so that necessary quantities of tissue (e.g. 100 mg per 4 ml of bathing solution) can be available for uptake experiments.

The Stadie-Riggs microtome is also available and will allow the preparation of uniform tissue slices. This procedure relies on the use of a Plexiglas device wherein the thickness of the slices determined is by the proper milling of the Plexiglas tissue holder. Details have been provided by Berndt[6].

Mechanized devices such as the McIlwain tissue chopper also are available. This device can permit the preparation of tissue pieces of uniform thickness and size, depending upon the tissue section from which the pieces are prepared. Thickness of the tissue section is determined by a micrometer and the cutting is done by the repetitious action of a mechanical arm attached to which is a razor blade. This will permit the rapid preparation of large numbers of tissue segments.

Recently, a mechanical device has been developed which will allow preparation of tissue while submerged in an oxygenated medium[12]. The suggested utility of this device is that the tissue is never exposed to a situation wherein poor oxygenation is experienced as long as the medium is oxygenated thoroughly.

However, a functional demonstration is still lacking to show that this procedure yields tissue slices or fragments that are more satisfactory than those prepared by the other methods.

Once prepared, 100 or more milligrams of tissue are transferred to beakers or flasks containing oxygenated buffer in a metabolic shaker. These uptake experiments are usually performed at 25 °C, since this temperature seems to provide for better tissue survival than a higher temperature, i.e. 37 °C. Usually, the tissue slices are shaken at the appropriate temperature in the presence of 100% oxygen or 95% oxygen/5% CO_2, depending on the buffer, for approximately 15 or 20 min before the addition of the transport substrate. Once the transport substrate (i.e. PAH, TEA, etc.) is added to the beaker, an additional 90 to 120 min of incubation ensues. At the end of that time, the tissue slices are removed, blotted thoroughly on moist filter paper, weighed, and an appropriate analysis is performed for the transport substrate in question. This may involve chemical analysis (e.g. for PAH see Smith[13]) or radiochemical analysis. Similarly, transport substrate concentration in the bathing solution is assessed. The uptake data are expressed as the slice to medium ratio (S/M ratio), i.e., concentration of the transport substrate of tissue per unit weight divided by the concentration of the transport substrate per unit volume of bathing solution.

In general, the medium used for these experiments is a phosphate buffer with a relatively high potassium concentration (see Cross and Taggert[7]). Potassium stimulates organic anion uptake, has no detrimental effect on organic cation uptake, and has therefore been used relatively routinely. Although bicarbonate buffer has been used in some experiments, mostly phosphate is used, and there seems to be little difference in tissue slice performance depending on buffer. Almost all studies have been done on renal cortical slices, although a few have been done with renal medullary slices (Berndt and Miller[14]). Renal medullary slices are much more poorly understood with respect to their "physiological" function and deserve more study. Various substrates have been used to enhance renal cortical slice organic anion or cation uptake, and although the effects of lactate, acetate, etc., are clear, underlying mechanisms still lack definition. Metabolic effects may be involved, but probably the actions are much more specific. In any event, lactate or acetate enhance slice accumulation of organic anions in most species while having little or no effect on organic cation uptake.

C. Advantages and disadvantages of renal slices

The general advantages of in vitro techniques over their in vivo counterparts were discussed earlier. The specific advantages relate to the utility of this technique for the study of organic ion accumulation and/or efflux and the relationship of these accumulation or efflux processes to overall renal function. Large numbers of samples can be managed in a single experiment which will permit assessment of the effects of a variety of xenobiotics on the accumulation of various endogenous (e.g. uric acid[15,16]) and/or exogenous transport substrates. Indeed, with careful planning and appropriate techniques the transport of more than one substance can be assessed in a single sample, e.g. through the use of tritium-labelled and C-14 labelled transport substrates or one chemical and one radiochemical analysis. In addition, along with substrate accumulation, oxygen uptake can be monitored (e.g. with a Clark electrode) as can bathing solution pH, etc.

There are disadvantages and limitations to the use of the renal slice technique. Certainly the problems associated with any in vitro procedure pertain to the renal slice technique as well. Although a good correlation has been demonstrated between in vivo renal tubular secretion of certain organic substances and renal slice uptake of these compounds (summarized by Berndt[6]), generalizations about whole organ function are difficult. Further, relationships between discrete biochemical events which can be studies in vitro and intact physiological functions are difficult to establish. It is unclear how many of these difficulties pertain to the disruption of anatomical or structural relationships within the kidney. Although it is possible that some superficial intact nephrons may persist in slices, there is little doubt that nephron fragments also exist. Further, the relationship of one nephron to another will clearly have been disrupted by the slicing technique. Of course, there are no clear data to establish the importance of these structural relationships for organic ion transport, but to whatever extent they are important, their disruption represents a significant disadvantage in the use of renal slices.

D. Examples of the use of renal slices

The use of renal slices in the assessment of physiological functions has been alluded to above. The remarkable correlation between renal slice accumulation of PAH and TEA and the in vivo secretory activity of the proximal tubule is noteworthy. Further, the effects of various organic acids such as acetate or lactate to stimulate the transport of PAH in vivo has an exact counterpart in vitro. The enhanced net accumulation of PAH in response to acetate or lactate has been reported by many workers, although exact mechanisms are far from clear cut. Whatever the specific mechanisms, the substrate stimulation has served to strengthen the correlation between the in vitro and in vivo procedures.

As with organic anion accumulation, mechanisms underlying the substrate enhancement of accumulation by potassium ion in potassium-depleted slices[9,17,18] are poorly understood. The relationship may pertain to the striking requirement for inorganic cations in the organic anion accumulation process[7,15,16], but definitive data are lacking.

Renal slices have also been used to examine the steady state distribution of inorganic electrolytes. For example, citrinin[19] and acute anoxia[20] were studied for effects on tissue slice sodium and potassium concentrations, extracellular water (inulin space) and total tissue water. These data, as well as oxygen consumption data, give generally useful information about tissue slice viability rather than specific evaluations of renal function or transport.

From the point of view of toxicology, renal slices have been used extensively. Studies have been undertaken after pretreatment of animals with presumed nephrotoxins and at varying periods of time after pretreatment the kidneys were removed and a slice uptake experiment performed. Other studies have been done wherein the presumed nephrotoxins have been added directly to fresh renal cortex slices prepared from untreated animals. In the first instance, one is capable of defining a clear time course for the onset of a nephrotoxic effect on renal slice transport, but this does not illustrate whether or not the substance has a direct action on the transport mechanism. That is to say, the effect could be mediated through alterations in blood flow, etc. By the addition of nephrotoxins directly to renal cortex slices from untreated animals, one can determine whether or not there are direct effects upon the kidney. Again, this procedure would not necessarily delineate an action of a toxin directly on the transport mechanism, since an action may be mediated through an interruption of metabolism. Nonetheless, in the latter case a direct effect on the kidney can be demonstrated whereas with administration of a nephrotoxin to an animal the action might be one mediated through indirect mechanisms. Hirsch[21], Kacew and Hirsch[22] and Berndt[4] have discussed these and other aspects of the use of slices in toxicological studies. In particular, specific references to the use of slices to study the effects of heavy metals, various organic ions, drugs and other chemicals are available in those reviews.

In addition to the use of slices to examine renal transport mechanisms, they have also been used to study certain metabolic functions within the kidney. In particular, alterations in gluconeogenesis and ammoniagenesis have been studied by several workers. For example, Preuss[23] reported that α-methylglutamate not only reduced ammonia excretion by rats, but also reduced ammonia production by renal slices from treated rats. Gluconeogenesis has been shown to be altered by gentamicin[24] or cephaloridine[25] after administration of these substances to the intact animal. Slices removed from those animals showed a reduced level of gluconeogenesis.

These examples of the usefulness of slices serve to highlight an important point. There is little doubt that slices will continue to serve a useful function in the assessment of potential nephrotoxic effects by a variety of chemicals. The scientific experience would suggest that substances which can alter organic ion transport can also have dramatic effects on overall renal function, so that slice studies can serve a predictive function. However, these more or less routine uses of slices will only occasionally be helpful in understanding mechanisms of nephrotoxic events. This is not to suggest that slices have no utility in mechanistic studies. On the contrary, at varying levels of sophistication renal slices have helped us understand toxic events at a mechanistic level[26,27], or at the very least to give clear direction for future studies of a mechanistic nature[28]. Nonetheless, such studies have not been a major thrust for the use of slices, and their continued use as valuable predictors for possible nephrotoxic events will probably remain their major use. Clearly, however, extending their use into more mechanistic areas would broaden the base of scientific information obtainable from these procedures and allow the technique a more important role in understanding nephrotoxicity.

V.   ISOLATED PERFUSED KIDNEY

A.   History

The basic concept of the use of an isolated perfused organ, whether kidney or otherwise, is not new. Among others, Brodie[29] described an isolated organ perfusion in a 1903 publication. More recent interest in isolated perfused organs is demonstrated by the works of Diczfalusy[30], Ritchie and Hardcastle[31] and Ross[32]. Regardless of the organ under study, an essential consideration in the development of these techniques is the desirability of separating a given organ from other organs within the animal to permit the study of the responses of the physiology and biochemistry of that organ independent of other homeostatic influences.   Such reasoning is also important when studying the effects of externally added chemicals.   That is to say, the toxicologist wants to know whether or not a given substance has a direct effect on a particular organ,   even if it might also have an effect mediated through an action on another organ.

One of the earliest studies involving the use of the isolated perfused kidney was conducted by Weiss et al.[33]. The techniques used by Weiss et al. were relatively rudimentary and the autoregulation studies at different pressures had many difficulties. Bauman et al.[34] paid much closer attention to the functional integrity of the isolated perfused kidney and attempted to improve its function by perfusing it with heparinized blood.   Bauman's studies showed that there were difficulties with using blood as a perfusate, but remarkably near physiological function could be achieved at least for short periods of time.   Nishiitsutsuji-Uwo et al.[35] were the first to define an erythrocyte-free artificial perfusate that permitted the isolated perfused organ to function near physiological levels.   The organ in these studies was used to study biochemical events, e.g. gluconeogenesis, and the artificial perfusate permitted the addition of a variety of substrates for these studies.   Other refinements to the perfusion technique were developed by Ross and colleagues[36] for a recirculating system. Such refinements as the use of two pumps instead of one and the introduction of filters in the perfusate line helped improve the performance of the isolated perfused kidney.   Many of the developments for improved organ function must be acknowledged to have come from various studies with other isolated organs.   In particular, the work of Miller et al.[37] and Schimassek[38] gave clear direction to the efforts of those using the isolated kidney.   For example, these studies helped direct the research into artificial perfusates and the selection of the smaller more convenient rat as the animal of choice.

B. The preparation and use of the isolated perfused kidney

The apparatus used for these preparations has been described by several workers[32,39,40]. Various refinements are involved in these procedures, but all of the apparatus include a pump for movement of the perfusate, an oxygenation device (e.g. membrane oxygenators, glass lung, etc.), a mechamism for control of temperature and so forth. Some procedures permit the perfusate to flow through the kidney under gravity, while others employ a second pump to actually perfuse the organ. It is also possible to monitor in-line pH, oxygen content of the perfusate, and perfusion pressure. In general it would appear that the type of equipment used will largely be a matter of individual choice and availability since many different types of equipment have been used with approximately the same degree of success.

As with the particular apparatus to be used, the surgical techniques involved in the isolation of the organ are generally well understood as originally described by Ross[32]. Very detailed descriptions of these surgical techniques are available in the review by Mehendale[40] and by Newton and Hook[39]. All of these describe surgical procedures whereby the catheter (19 gauge, thin wall cannula or specifically designed glass cannula) is inserted through the superior mesenteric artery, across the aorta and into the right renal artery of the rat. This approach is important since it allows for continuous perfusion of the organ during the isolation process. A second consideration which deserves emphasis is the speed with which the surgical procedure is undertaken once the abdominal cavity is opened. Experience suggests that the more rapidly the kidney is cannulated and isolated the greater the likelihood of success in achieving an organ with function near physiological. Of course, before the actual cannulation takes place it is necessary to tie off a variety of other small vessels in the surgical area. Although not mentioned by all investigators, many believe it is important to inject an adequate amount of heparin into the animal just prior to the cannulation process. It is argued that the availability of the heparin will tend to minimize the formation of small clots which might obstruct the intrarenal vessels and interfere with the perfusion process. Once the kidney has been removed from the animal to the apparatus, a 15 or 20 minute "equilibration" period is usually allowed for organ function to stabilize. If an artificial medium is used (see below), it is wise to measure the perfusion flow rate going through the organ after this equilibration period has taken place. High perfusion rates are essential with the artificial medium to insure adequate oxygenation. An organ which is not receiving a flow rate of the order of 25 to 35 ml per min will probably show poor function.

The choice of the perfusion medium has proven to be extremely important in the development of a physiologically functioning isolated perfused kidney. Nizet[41] discussed in detail the problems associated with the use of blood as the perfusion medium. For a variety of reasons it would appear that the presence of blood in the perfusate more often lead to a compromised renal function than does the use of an artificial medium. Such problems as embolization of fat droplets and formation of small clots are examples

309

of the difficulties. In addition, even when using the rat as the experimental animal approximately 100 ml of perfusate will be required. Hence, a large number of blood donors would be necessary in order to perfuse a single kidney if undiluted rat blood was to be used.

Most of the defined media are a modification of a Krebs-Ringer buffer. Various means are used to supply appropriate oncotic pressure. For example, the plasma expander Haemaccel, dextran, fluorocarbons as well as bovine serum albumin have all been used by one or another investigator[36,42,43]. Varying degrees of success have been reported with the different colloidal materials, but albumin seems to have been the most widely used. Newton and Hook[39] comment on the different brands of bovine serum albumin available and the possibility of obtaining different results with the different preparations. In any event, it is probably important to try more than one preparation of albumin and use the one which yields the better results in a particular laboratory setting. In general, it is the Fraction V albumin that is used regardless of the supplier. Preparation of the albumin solution for perfusion may also affect the functioning of the kidney, and athough there seems to be no standard procedure for its dialysis before use, all workers would agree that dialysis is necessary. Further, it is generally agreed that it is important to filter the perfusate through very small Millipore-type filters before use. Of course, such filtration will not remove bacterial toxins, so preparation of the perfusate under as near sterile conditions as possible is wise. The concentration of albumin in the perfusate appears to vary depending upon the particular batch of albumin, but a concentration in the range of 6.5 to 7% seems to be appropriate for must perfusion systems. Many workers now believe that the perfusate should be appropriately supplemented with amino acids[44]. The availability of a complete amino acid supplement appeared to improve the physiological functioning of the isolated perfused kidney dramatically over that seen with a perfusate containing only glucose. Not only were quantitative measures of physiological function improved, but in addition the duration of performance of the isolated perfused kidney was enhanced greatly. Epstein's group also examined the question of whether the three amino acid precursors to glutathione were sufficient to support a better functioning kidney and concluded that these were not sufficient. Indeed, although sodium reabsorption seems to be sustained better in the presence of these three amino acids, other function was not adequately sustained and at no time did the kidney perform as well as with all the amino acids present.

The presence of albumin in the perfusate may be important for studies in toxicology. Obviously, as in the physiological situation, protein binding of drugs, other xenobiotics, their metabolites, etc., may be important in various toxicological studies, and that binding will occur with the isolated perfused kidney as well. If protein binding is to be eliminated as a consideration in the studies, some other colloid would have to be used.

Although most investigators have not had great success with the use of blood as a perfusate, this procedure cannot be completely discounted. Recent evidence suggests that with the isolated rabbit kidney, homologous blood may work quite adequately if properly prepared before use[43]. These investigators found that homologous blood deprived of platelets, leukocytes, floating lipoproteins, microclots, etc., did not cause vasoconstriction of the vessels in the isolated kidney and permitted a superior physiological performance over artificial media.

C. Advantages and disadvantages of the isolated perfused kidney

Most workers agree that an evaluation of renal function necessitates retention of the relationship of nephrons to each other, and of nephrons to non-nephron elements within the kidney. The isolated perfused kidney affords this advantage which allows the investigator to isolate the organ from the influences of other organs. In addition, the investigator has the advantage with the isolated kidney of being able to control many variables which are known to alter renal function in the intact animal, such as renal perfusion pressure, etc. As with the intact animal, both quantitative and qualitative techniques can be applied to assess renal function. Standard clearance calculations are possible and mass balance studies can be undertaken. In addition, and very important from a toxicological viewpoint, the isolated perfused kidney can be used to assess metabolic activities of this organ independent of influences from, for example, the liver.

There are several disadvantages in the use of the isolated perfused kidney, many of which are applicable to all isolated perfused organs. For example, a disadvantage of whole organ studies is that mechanisms of drug or toxin action are hard to assess since to a large extent specific cellular sites of action cannot be delineated. A similar problem exists with the isolated perfused kidney. The perfusion process extracts whole organ information and does not allow one to discern with great reliability specific actions on specific nephron sections. Indeed, with the isolated perfused organ, as with the intact animal, one is assessing the nephron population behaviour.

Many of the other disadvantages to the use of the isolated perfused kidney seem to pertain to technical matters. The isolated perfused kidney remains functional for only a relatively short period of time. Even with amino acid supplementation[44], 3 hours of function appeared to be maximal. Most workers agree that 90 minutes of function is about the best that can be achieved without amino acid supplementation. Obviously the short time with which relatively normal physiological behavior occurs is a significant disadvantage.

The isolated perfused kidney does not concentrate the urine well. Whatever the cause of this difficulty, amino acid supplementation appears to help somewhat, but this is still a deficiency and highlights the fact that the kidney never achieves a true physiological performance. If one is to use the isolated perfused kidney to study the effects of drugs and chemicals it may be difficult to interpret the results obtained if the drugs and chemicals are being used on an organ that is deteriorating from the outset.

Finally, it must be appreciated that using an isolated per-

Finally, it must be appreciated that using an isolated perfused kidney is a technically difficult procedure which requires some considerable practice and expertise. It is not a simple procedure which can be learned readily and applied with impunity.

D. Criteria for assessing the viability of the isolated perfused kidney

Various approaches have been adopted to assess the viability of the isolated organ and, although many workers use the same criteria, there has been no general agreement on what constitutes a satisfactorily functioning isolated kidney. Blood flow through an intact kidney in vivo can reach 6 to 7 ml/min-gram of tissue depending upon perfusion pressures and so forth. With the artificial, low viscosity medium, perfusion flow rates of 20 to 50 ml/min can be achieved at approximately the same perfusion pressures as seen in the intact animal. Most workers agree that it is essential that the flow rate of medium be sufficiently high to support tissue respiration and that probably means flow rates are needed in excess of 25 ml/min.

Various renal function parameters have also been examined as criteria. In general, urinary concentrating ability is compromised in the isolated perfused kidney. However, the higher the urinary concentration obtained, presumably the better the function. Maintenance of a glomerular filtration rate (i.e. inulin clearance) near 1 ml/min-gram is generally viewed as evidence of a well functioning organ. Similarly, reabsorption of 97 or 98% of the filtered sodium and minimal potassium loss by the organ are also important criteria.

There does not appear to be any single criterion which will describe an adequately functioning isolated perfused kidney. Rather, the investigator should use several criteria (sodium reabsorption, filtration rate, etc.) as evidence that the organ is functioning well. In addition, morphological criteria can be used, as can biochemical (e.g. maintenance of tissue glutathione). Both morphology and tissue glutathione content were improved greatly by amino acid supplementation[44].

E. Examples of the use of the isolated perfused kidney

The bulk of the isolated perfused kidney work has been to examine physiological functions. Many of these important studies have been summarized by Nizet[41].

From the point of view of toxicology and pharmacology, most of the studies with the isolated perfused kidney have been directed at renal metabolism. Summerfield et al.[46] examined conjugating reactions involved in the elimination of bile acids in the urine. These findings supported the hypothesis that synthesis of some sulphate conjugates by kidney may account for some of the bile acid sulphates present in the urine. Tark and colleagues[47] examined substrate metabolism in the isolated dog kidney and demonstrated that fatty acids could serve as substrates for sodium precisely at toxicological mechanisms, similar kinds of approaches certainly could be used for such studies even directed at toxic events altering sodium reabsorption. Many other endogenous substances are also metabolized by the kidney, and many of the studies using the isolated perfused organ have been summarized by Bach and Lock[3].

A variety of exogenous substances also are metabolized by the isolated perfused kidney and this technique has been used to demonstrate important events related to toxicology. For example, Mitchell et al.[48] demonstrated that the isolated perfused rat kidney destroyed or removed certain antibiotics from the perfusate. Gentamicin, for example, tended to be removed from the perfusate, but it was not clear whether this represented organ sequestration of the drug or actual metabolism to inactive metabolites. Szefler and Acara[49] demonstrated not only the transport of isoproterenol, but also its metabolism with the isolated perfused kidney. Tange et al.[50] used the isolated perfused kidney to demonstrate the initial biochemical effects involved with the nephrotoxicity of p-aminophenol. Several investigators have used the isolated perfused kidney to demonstrate the important renal metabolism of acetaminophen involved in the production of nephrotoxicity by this important drug[51-53].

Although studies have been done to examine the effects of various xenobiotics on the function of the isolated perfused kidney, these studies have been mostly descriptive in nature. Specific investigations to help us better define mechanisms of nephrotoxicity directed at renal function have been no more successful with the isolated perfused organ than with the intact animal. Some such studies have been summarized by Bach and Lock[3].

VI. SUMMARY

The renal slice procedure has been used more extensively for investigations of renal biochemistry and pharmacology than has the isolated perfused kidney. The renal slice studies are very useful in the demonstration of potential nephrotoxic effects or other drug effects on kidney. Slices have not been particularly useful in defining clear cut mechanisms of toxicity except for a few examples where metabolism has been disrupted.

Using isolated perfused kidney is a considerably more complex technique than renal slices, but can yield more powerful data. With respect to renal metabolism, this procedure has revealed several important processes which might explain or at least underlie certain nephrotoxicities. It would appear that a combination of renal slice studies with the isolated perfused kidney especially directed at xenobiotic effects on metabolism, or the metabolism of xenobiotics, would be a powerful combination of techniques for our better understanding of the role of the kidney in metabolism and the consequences for the renal metabolism of exposure to various chemicals.

REFERENCES

1.   Orloff, J. and Breliner, P.H.,   Renal Physiology, Handbook of Physiology. American Physiological Society, Washington, D.C., 1973. Chapters 6, 7.

2.   Brenner, B.M. and Rector, F.C., Jr., The Kidney. Vol. I and II, 2nd edition, W.B. Saunders Company, New York, 1981.

3.   Bach, P.H. and Lock, E.A., The use of renal slices, perfusion and infusion techniques to assess nephrotoxicity related changes, in Nephrotoxicity, Assessment and Pathogenesis, Bach, P.H., Bonner, F.W., Bridges, J.W. and Lock, E.A., Eds., John Wiley and Sons, New York, 1982, 128.

4.   Berndt, W.O., Renal methods in toxicology, in Principles and Methods of Toxicology, Hayes, A.W., Ed., Raven Press, New York, 1982, 447.

5.   Berndt, W.O., Use of renal function tests in the evaluation of nephrotoxic effects, in Toxicology of the Kidney, Hook, J.B., Ed., Raven Press, New York, 1981, 1.

6.   Berndt, W.O., Use of renal slice technique for evaluation of renal tubular transport process. Environ. Health Perspect., 15, 73, 1976.

7.   Cross, R.J. and Taggart, J.V., Renal tubular transport: accumulation of p-aminohippurate by rabbit kidney slices, Am. J. Physiol., 161, 181, 1950.

8.   Mudge, G.H. and Taggart, J.V., Effect of acetate on renal excretion of p-aminohippurate in dog, Am. J. Physiol., 161, 191, 1950.

9.   Cohen, J.J., Chesney, R.W., Brand, P.H., Neville, H.F. and Blanchard, C.F., Metabolism and K^+ uptake by dog kidney slices, Am. J. Physiol., 217, 161, 1969.

10.   Forster, R.P., Use of thin kidney slices and isolated renal tubules for direct study of cellular transport kinetics, Science, 108, 65, 1948.

11.   Mudge, G.H., Electrolyte and water metabolism of rabbit kidney slices: effect of metabolic inhibitors, Am. J. Physiol., 167, 206, 1951.

12.   Krumdieck, C.L., dos Santos, J.E. and Ho, K.J., A new instrument for the rapid preparation of tissue slices. Anal. Biochem., 104, 118, 1980.

13.   Smith, H.W., Principles of Renal Physiology. Oxford University Press, New York, 1956, 212.

14.   Berndt, W.O. and Miller, R.K., The accumulation and metabolism of ^{14}C-hypoxanthine by slices of rabbit renal medulla. Biochem. Biophys. Acta, 266, 453, 1972.

15.   Berndt, W.O. and Beechwood, E.C., Influence of inorganic electrolytes and ouabain on uric acid transport, Am. J. Physiol., 208, 642, 1965.

16.   Platts, M.M. and Mudge, G.H., Accumulation of uric acid by slices of kidney cortex, Am. J. Physiol., 200, 387, 1961.

17.   Berndt, W.O. and LeSher, D.A., Effects of substrate on potassium accumulation by rabbit kidney cortex, Am. J. Physiol., 200, 111, 1961.

18.   Selleck, B.H. and Cohen, J.J., Specific localization of alpha-ketoglutarate uptake to dog kidney and liver in vivo, Am. J. Physiol., 208, 24, 1965.

19.   Berndt, W.O. and Hayes, A.W., Effects of citrinin on renal transport processes, J. Environ. Pathol. Toxicol., 1, 93, 1977.

20.   Berndt, W.O., Effects of acute anoxia on renal transport processes, J. Tox. Environ. Hlth, 2, 1, 1976.

21.   Hirsch, G.H., Differential effects on nephrotoxic agents on renal transport and metabolism by use of in vitro techniques, Environ. Hlth Perspect., 15, 89, 1976.

22.   Kacew, S. and Hirsch, G., Evaluation of nephrotoxicity of various compounds by means of in vitro methods, in Toxicology of the Kidney , J.B. Hook and R. Dixon, eds. Raven Press, New York, 1981, 77.

23.   Pruess, H.G., The effects of α-methylglutamate on ammonium excretion and

renal ammonia production in rats, Toxicol. Appl. Pharmacol., 54, 454, 1980.

24. Kluwe, W.M. and Hook, J.B., Functional nephrotoxicity of gentamicin in the rat, Toxicol. Appl. Pharmacol., 45, 163, 1978.

25. Wold, J.S., Turnipseed, S.A. and Miller, B.L., The effect of renal cation transport inhibition on cephaloridine nephrotoxicity, Toxicol. Appl. Pharmacol., 47, 115, 1979.

26. Berndt, W.O. and Hayes, A.W., Effect of probenecid on citrinin-induced nephrotoxicity, Toxicol. Appl. Pharmacol., 64, 118, 1982.

27. Meisner, H. and Selanik, P., Inhibition of renal gluco- neogenesis in rats by ochratoxin, Biochem. J., 180, 681, 1979.

28. Carpenter, H.M. and Mudge, G.H., Acetaminophen nephrotoxicity: Studies on renal acetylation and deacetylation, J. Pharmacol. Exp. Therap., 218, 161, 1981.

29. Brodie, T.G., The perfusion of surviving organs. J. Physiol. Lond., 24, 266, 1903.

30. Diczfalusy, E., Perfusion Techniques, Karolinska Institute, Stockholm, Sweden, 1971.

31. Ritchie, H.D. and Hardcastle, J.D., Isolated Organ Perfusion, University Park Press, Baltimore, 1973.

32. Ross, B.D., Perfusion Techniques in Biochemistry, Clarendon Press, Oxford, 1974.

33. Weiss, C., Passow, H. and Rothstein, A., Autoregulation of flow in isolated rat kidney in the absence of red cells, Am. J. Physiol., 196, 1115, 1959.

34. Bauman, A.W., Clarkson, T.W. and Miles, E.M., Functional evaluation of isolated perfused rat kidney, J. Appl. Physiol., 18, 1239, 1963.

35. Nishiitsutsuji-Uwo, J.M., Ross, B.D. and Krebs, H.A., Metabolic activities of the isolated perfused rat kidney, Biochem. J., 103, 852, 1967.

36. Ross, B.D., Epstein, F.H. and Leaf, A., Sodium reabsorption in the perfused rat kidney, Am. J. Physiol., 225, 1165, 1973.

37. Miller, L.L., Bly, C.G., Watson, M.L. and Bolo, W.F., The dominant role of the liver in plasma protein synthesis, J. Exp. Med., 94, 431, 1959.

38. Schimassek, H., Metabolite der Kohlenhydratstoffwechsels der isoliert perfuudierten rattenleber, Biochem. Z., 336, 460, 1963.

39. Newton, J.F., Jr. and Hook, J.B., Isolated perfused rat kidney, Meth. Enzymol., 77, 94, 1981.

40. Mehendale, H.M., Application of isolated organ techniques in toxicology, in Methods in Toxicology, Hayes, A.W., Ed., Raven Press, New York, 1982.

41. Nizet, A., The isolated perfused kidney: possibilities, limitations and results, Kidney Int., 7, 1, 1975.

42. Franke, H. and Weiss, C., The O_2 supply of the isolated cell-free perfused rat kidney, Adv. Exp. Med. Biol., 75, 425, 1976.

43. Koschier, F.J. and Acara M., Transport of 2,4,5-trichlorophenoxyacetate in the isolated perfused rat kidney, J. Pharmacol. Exp. Therap., 208, 287, 1979.

44. Epstein, F.H., Brosnan, J.T., Tange, J.D. and Ross, B.D., Improved function with amino acids in the isolated perfused kidney, Am. J. Physiol., 243, F284, 1982.

45. Pacini, A.B. and Bocci, V., Analysis of the optimal conditions for perfusing an isolated rabbit kidney with homologous blood, Renal Physiol., Basel, 6, 72, 1983.

46. Summerfield, J.A., Gollan, J.L. and Billing, B.H., Synthesis of bile acid monophosphate by the isolated perfused rat kidney, Biochem. J., 156, 339, 1976.

47. Tark, M., Randall, H.M., Jr. and Hoffer, T.L., Substrate metabolism in the

isolated perfused kidney, Invest. Urol., 14, 132, 1976.

48. Mitchell, C.J., Bullock, S. and Ross, B.D., Renal handling of gentamicin and other antibiotics by the isolated perfused rat kidney: mechanism of nephro-toxicity, J. Antimicrob. Chemother., 3, 593, 1977.

49. Szefler, S.J. and Acara, M., Isoproterenol excretion and metabolism in the isolated perfused rat kidney, J. Pharmacol. Exp. Therap., 210, 195, 1979.

50. Tange, J.D., Ross, B.D. and Ledingham, J.G., Effects of analgesics and re-lated compounds on renal metabolism in rats, Clin. Sci. Mol. Med., 53, 485, 1977.

51. Emslie, K.R., Smail, M.C., Calder, I.C., Hart, S.J. and Tange, J.D., Paracetamol and the isolated perfused kidney: metabolism and functional ef-fects, Xenobiotica, 11, 43, 1981.

52. Hart, S., Calder, I., Ross, B. and Tange, J., Renal metabolism of paracetamol: studies in the isolated perfused rat kidney, Clin. Sci., 58, 379, 1980.

53. Newton, J.F., Kluwe, W.M. and Hook, J.B., Acetaminophen (APAP)-induced glutathione depletion in the isolated perfused kidney, Toxicol. Appl. Phar-macol., 48, A19, 1979.

10

THE USE OF SINGLE NEPHRON TECHNIQUES IN RENAL TOXICITY STUDIES

J. DIEZI AND F. ROCH-RAMEL

I.   INTRODUCTION

The use of techniques to measure specific transport and functional lesions at the single tubule level goes back many decades, but their systematic and broad application is more recent. Both "in vivo" micropuncture and, more recently, "in vitro" microperfusion of defined nephron segments have contributed considerably to our knowledge of the tubular localization of physiological processes along the nephron, especially the cellular transport mechanisms of fluid, electrolytes and organic compounds. These techniques have been applied much less frequently to investigate the tubular effects and handling of foreign compounds in renal pharmacology and toxicology, with the exception of the mechanisms and sites of action of the diuretics, and glomerular and tubular changes associated with acute renal failure. This is explained by the fact that exogenous compounds sometimes alter the function of the kidney so extensively that single tubule techniques cannot be applied reliably. The analytical techniques in microsamples have often been difficult to develop, and satisfactory answers have frequently been provided on the whole kidney using specific antagonists of transport or clearance or stop flow methods to define tubular sites of organic compound transport. These single tubule techniques (as shown below) are therefore valuable because they can provide information on the transport and effect of exogenous chemicals, and also limited in their applicability to renal pharmacology and toxicology, because of the nature of the functional changes induced by some toxic chemicals (e.g. transient blood flow redistribution, or non-homogeneity of tubular lesions). The present chapter aims at describing the main characteristics of single tubule methods and reviewing published observations on the renal transport or toxic effects of various chemicals.

II.   SINGLE TUBULE FUNCTION: METHODS OF STUDY

Single tubule studies may be carried out either:

1.   In vivo, using micropuncture to obtain tubular fluid samples, in anaesthetized animals, from various parts of the nephron, after puncture of the tubular wall with glass micropipets (Figure 1). Several variations of this basic technique have been developed, and will be described below.

2.   In vitro, where tubule segments are first quickly dissected from the kidney, and are studied in conditions where the initial composition of the fluids both bathing the tubule and perfused through its lumen can be precisely controlled.

Sites of Micropuncture

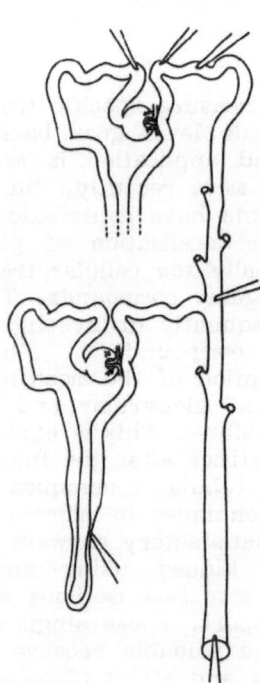

Figure 1 Tubular sites accessible to micropuncture "in vivo", in surface and juxtamedullary nephrons. In some animal strains, surface glomeruli are also accessible to puncture. (Reprinted with permission from Int. J. Biochem. 12; G.Giebisch, Methods of localizing transport processes using micropuncture techniques - Evidence for nephron heterogeneity; 1980, Pergamon Journals Ltd.).

A. In vivo micropuncture

This technique has been used frequently in rats, desert rats, dogs and Necturus[1,2], but rarely in monkeys[3-6], rabbits[7,8], cats[9], pigs[10], frogs[11,12] and Amphiuma[13,14]. Some strains of rats have been used for specific purposes, e.g. the Munich-Wistar strain[15,16], in which glomeruli are accessible to micropuncture at the surface of the kidney, or the Brattleboro strain with heredit- ary neurogenic diabetes insipidus[17].

A brief description of the micropuncture technique will be given here, with special reference to the rat preparation. More ex- tensive information can be found in a number of books or chap- ters[1,2,18-23].

Micropunctures at the surface of the kidney are performed in anaesthetized animals, in which one kidney has been freed from its connective attachments. The kidney is usually kept in a plastic cup and its ureter cannulated, care being taken to avoid any compres- sion of the vascular pedicle. Proximal and distal tubules at the kidney surface can be recognized by inspection through a stereo- scope with 10-40 x magnification. The use of dyes, such as lissamine green, helps to distinguish between proximal and distal segments of the nephron since, following i.v. injection, the dye accumulates transiently and successively along the nephron. Sharpened glass micropipettes, with a tip diameter varying between 4 and 12 μm (according to the size of the tubule to be punctured) are filled with coloured mineral oil. The pipette is mounted in a holder and, using a micromanipulator, the tip is introduced into the selected tubule. Depending on the experimental protocol, native tubular fluid can be collected and analysed (free-flow micropunctures); or small amounts of an artificial fluid of known initial composition can be perfused or injected into the tubule lumen, and re-collected through a second micropipette in the same tubule or in pelvic urine (microperfusion, microinjection).

1. Free-flow micropunctures

In free-flow micropunctures a quantitative collection of tubular fluid is obtained by blocking the tubular lumen downstream from the site of impalement, and by applying a gentle initial suction into the pipette. Typically, the rate of sampling is calculated from the absolute amount of fluid obtained and the duration of the collection (usually 2-3 min). Single nephron filtration rate (SNGFR) can be calculated if an appropriate glomerular marker (e.g. inulin) is in- fused into the animal. Measurement of the concentration ratio (tubule/plasma) of inulin and any other solute(s) allows you to determine the net transport of fluid and solute(s) to the site of puncture. Several tubular sites can be reached by this technique (Figure 1). The function of juxtamedullary nephrons can be es- timated by puncture of descending or ascending limbs of Henle's loop located at the surface of the papilla, which is possible in only some animal species (desert rodents[24], hamsters[25], young rats[26], or after special surgical preparation[27]).

The use of the re-collection technique has proved useful in

situations where, for instance, the effects of a drug on tubule function has to be investigated[28]. In such a case fluid samples are obtained from the same puncture sites before and after administration of the compound. This approach helps to eliminate the usually large intertubular functional variability. The site of puncture and fluid collection along the nephron can be precisely identified by filling the punctured tubule with latex, after completion of the sampling, and subsequent dissection of the filled tubules following maceration of the kidney in concentrated hydrochloric acid. It is then possible to measure the distance between the glomerulus and the site of puncture.

Free-flow micropuncture techniques have proved fruitful for assessing the localization and importance of net tubular transports of a variety of endogenous and exogenous solutes along the nephron[2,23]. Furthermore, the development of micropressure transducer systems has allowed the glomerular ultrafiltration dynamics to be characterized, and the study of the role of Starling forces in the control of proximal isotonic fluid reabsorption[29,30]. In the field of pharmacology and toxicology more specifically, they have been used to investigate the tubular transport of drugs and chemicals, and in the study of the mechanisms of acute renal failure[31].

2. Microperfusion

In microperfusion studies, specific segments of the nephron (proximal and distal tubules, loop of Henle) can be perfused in vivo, using a micropump delivering an artificial fluid of known composition in the nl/min range. The perfusion and collection micropipettes must be isolated by proximal and distal oil blocks to avoid any contamination originating from tubular fluid. Changes in the composition of the original fluid following contact with the tubular cell membrane permit an assessment of the bidirectional transport of a solute.

In the stationary microperfusion technique a small fluid droplet, containing a solute to be studied, is placed in the lumen of a specific tubular segment between two oil columns. If reabsorption of the fluid droplet is prevented by addition of an non-permeant compound (e.g. raffinose), information on the tubular transport of the solute under study can be derived from measurements of its concentration changes and steady-state distribution across various parts of the nephron. Based on a similar technique, measurements of the rate of disappearance (reabsorption) of an isotonic saline droplet (without addition of an non-permeant solute) have been used to study isotonic fluid reabsorption in mammalian and amphibian kidneys, and to characterize the influence of various factors, such as diuretics or extracellular volume expansion, on reabsorption in proximal tubules[2].

Both continuous and stationary tubular microperfusions can be carried out during simultaneous microperfusion of peritubular capillaries. This method allows a better control of the initial composition of the peritubular and luminal environment. The amphibian kidney has been used extensively, since its anatomy is such that the blood supplies to the glomeruli and the tubules originate from different vessels. Thus, the luminal and the peritubular sides of such kidneys can be perfused independently with appropriate artificial solutions[13,14,32].

3. Microinjections

In tubular and capillary microinjections, a small droplet (typically 10-20 nl) of fluid containing the (radiochemically labelled) solute to be studied, and an non-permeant labelled compound (e.g. inulin) is injected into the lumen of a surface tubule. Starting with the microinjection, serial collections, each lasting 30-60 s, of ureteral urine are carried out, in order to obtain a time-related profile of the excretion of the labelled compound. A simultaneous measurement of the recovery of radioactive inulin is used both to check the technical quality of the microinjection (inulin recovery should exceed 90-95%) and to compare with the tubular handling of the solute under study. A similar technique can be used for microinjections into peritubular capillaries. Continuous, low-rate microinfusion of the labelled solutes, followed by urine analysis, may be preferred to rapid microinjection, since it would be expected to cause the least disturbance to tubular hydrodynamics.

B. Electrophysiology of the nephron

Methods for applying electrical measurements to renal tubules have only been used extensively in the past 10-20 years. They will not be described here in detail, since they do not appear to have been applied in the field of renal toxicology. It is noteworthy, though, that various chemicals and drugs (such as diuretics) have been used as probes to help delineate tubular cell and membrane functions related to the transport of ions[1].

Measurements of transepithelial potentials and specific resistances have been carried out in most segments of the nephron from many animal species, using both in vivo and in vitro preparations. Fine-tipped (< 1 μm) glass electrodes (Ling-Gerard type), filled with a concentrated electrolyte solution have been used, while attempts to circumvent the problem of liquid junction potentials have used micropipettes with larger diameter tips (2-11 μm) for transepithelial electrical measurements. These techniques have, for instance, been used to characterize the driving forces acting on single ions, and the relative permeability coefficients of specific ions[33]. Very fine-tipped electrodes have also been used to measure electrochemical potential gradients and electrical resistances across single tubule cell membranes in amphibian and mammalian kidneys, and in isolated tubule preparations. Such approaches have been useful for assessing passive and active transport of ions across individual tubular cell membranes, and the role of paracellular shunt pathways in net ion transport across the epithelium of specific tubular segments. Furthermore, the recent development of ion-selective electrodes, filled with liquid ion exchangers, has allowed the intracellular activities of specific ions to be measured in proximal and distal tubules of several animal species[34]. Such measurements can, in principle, yield information on the electromotive forces characterizing individual ion species, and can also be used to show how these are changed by the exposure of cells to toxic chemicals.

C.   Limitations of micropuncture and microperfusion techniques

As already pointed out, micropuncture and microperfusion methods have contributed to our understanding of the function of the nephron, by allowing the tubular sites of individual transport processes to be mapped, the rate of solute transport along single nephron segments to be quantified, and the driving forces involved in transport to be characterized. Such techniques, however, have clear limitations and drawbacks, which must be kept in mind[20,22]. Besides the obvious changes of kidney function resulting from general anaesthesia and extensive surgery, problems arise from the fact that in vivo micropuncture can only be carried out in some species. Similarly, it is only the most superficial tubules that are studied, which do not necessarily represent the whole nephron population. In addition, technical artifacts may result from tubular punctures, such as increased intratubular pressure due to oil blocks, entailing reductions of single nephron filtration rate; creation of inter-nephron fistulae with artifactual increase of tubular flow rate; alterations of epithelial permeability characteristics near the puncture site, etc. Changes of tubular fluid composition as a function of the puncture site along the nephron can be assessed by free-flow micropuncture techniques. Clearly, however, inter-nephron and interindividual variations are large, and changes of small magnitude (e.g. resulting from a low-level exposure to a toxic agent) would be difficult to identify. Recollection techniques may obviate some of these difficulties.

Free-flow collection methods are also open to technical artifacts, such as downstream fluid contamination which occurs particularly during sample collections in distal tubules at high tubular pressures. Furthermore, changes in fluid composition between two sites of collection must be interpreted cautiously if tubular urine originating from other nephrons also contributes to the downstream sample, e.g. along the papillary collecting ducts.

The microinjection technique has the advantage of relative technical simplicity, and can be well controlled. However, it only provides information on unidirectional transport, necessitates intravenous infusion of large amounts of fluid (to enhance tubular fluid flow rate), and requires the availability of labelled compounds of both high specific activity and chemical purity. The continuous microperfusion allows bidirectional solute fluxes to be discriminated, but is technically demanding and fraught with artifacts such as fluid leaks and contamination.

D.   Microperfusion of isolated tubules "in vitro"

This technique, described in detail in several recent reviews, 34,35,36, has allowed the study of nearly all tubular segments (such as the descending and ascending limbs of the loop of Henle, the cortical collecting tubules and various parts of juxtamedullary nephrons) which are not accessible by in vivo micropuncture studies[37,38]. In addition, the composition of the bathing and perfusing fluids can be controlled precisely, in contrast to most other types of micropuncture studies. Nearly all tubular segments isolated and perfused have been obtained from the rabbit kidney[39], but some tubular segments can also be obtained from man, mouse, rat, hamster, amphibian and snake kidneys[1,34].

The tubule segments are dissected free-hand, under a stereoscope (20-40% magnification) with the help of fine needles and forceps, at 4 °C. After dissection, the tubules are transferred into a small chamber filled with an appropriate fluid and are observed through an inverted microscope (magnification 40-400 x). With the help of micromanipulators, one end of the tubule is then gently aspirated into a holding pipette sliding on a "V track", and restrained against a small constriction of the pipet (Figure 2).

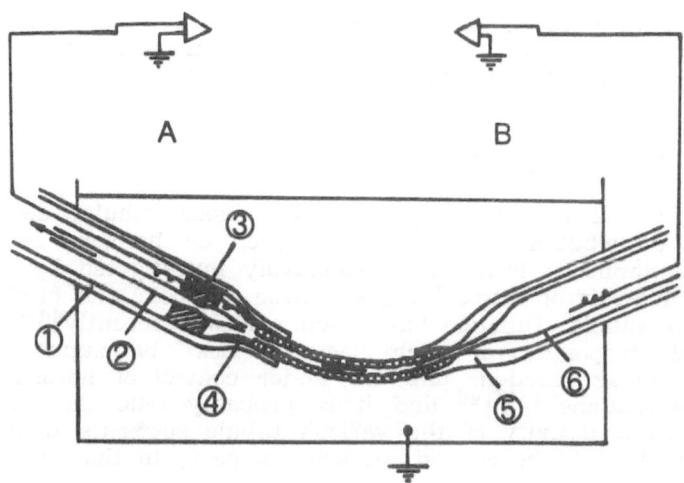

Figure 2 Schematic representation of tubular microperfusion "in vitro". The set of pipettes for fluid perfusion is on the right side (B), for fluid collection on the left side (A). 1 and 5 illustrate the holding pipettes (with constriction in 5), collecting and perfusing pipettes (2 and 6 , respectively). The Sylgar seal at the end of the tubule on the collecting side is represented in 4 , the paraffin oil to prevent evaporation in 3. Electrophysiological measurements can also be carried out.

An inner pipette, precisely centred within the holding pipette and connected to a reservoir or a micropump, can then be introduced into the lumen of the tubule and is used as a perfusion pipette. The other end of the tubule is aspirated into another holding pipette fixed to a second "V-track" and is sealed by using a thick silicon oil (Sylgar). With the help of a second micromanipulator (fixed on the "V-track"), a volumetric pipette is introduced near the end of the segment for collection of the perfused fluid.

Evaporation of the collected fluid is prevented by paraffin oil, the collection pipette being introduced through the oil layer. The observation of the displacement of the fluid/oil meniscus allows the measurement of the fluid collection rate. Functional capacities of tubule segments can be assessed by measurements of unidirectional fluxes (bath to lumen or lumen to bath) and net transports, using radioactively labelled compounds or ion-sensitive electrodes, electron probe analysis, etc. Measurements of transepithelial electrical potential and resistance are also used to assess ion transport[40]. More refined techniques applied to the study of isolated tubules include intracellular electrical measurements and the patch-clamp method[41]. The addition of radiolabelled inulin to the perfusion fluid is used to evaluate water movements, and to assess the technical success of the preparation by the absence of inulin leaks.

This sophisticated technique has still not been widely used in toxicological studies. However, it has been applied (see below) to the study of early functional changes in specific tubular segments after ischaemic injury. The method is more difficult to use in chronic nephrotoxicity studies, or during the recovery stages following an acute lesion, because the tubule dissection is markedly hampered by the extreme fragility of the tissue[42,43].

E.   Study of non-perfused single tubules

The biochemical heterogeneity between various tubular segments, and the distribution of enzyme activities or hormone receptors along the nephron, have been extensively investigated by dissection and analysis of single tubules. These metabolic and biochemical aspects of tubular function have been reviewed recently[44-46]. The functional properties of each segment must be supported by energy-yielding reactions and are under control of hormonal and neural regulations[44,47,48] and it is probably true that the differences in sensitivity of the various tubule segments to nephrotoxic agents might be related, at least in part, to the distribution of specific enzyme activities.

Segments of proximal tubules have higher activities of gluconeogenic enzymes (glucose-6-phosphatase, fructose 1,6-biphosphatase, phosphoenol-pyruvatekinase), but lower glycolytic enzyme activities (hexokinase, phosphofructokinase, pyruvatekinase) than the thick ascending limbs of Henle's loop, distal tubules or collecting ducts[49]. As predicted from this enzyme distribution, proximal tubules are producing glucose, while glucose utilization occurs at more distal sites[50]. Fructokinase and enzymes of fructose metabolism, as well as glycerolkinase, are found only in proximal tubules[49]. Proximal tubules are also characterized by high levels of enzymes of the tricarboxylic cycle, in contrast with distal tubules. The role of these enzymes in cell metabolism and substrate utilization has been reviewed[45,51], and will not be discussed here.

Adenylate cyclase activity is found in most parts of the nephron[52], but its hormonal regulation varies between the different tubular segments[44,47,53]. The characteristics of this hormonal control have been reported for vasopressin[54], parathyroid hormone[55], calcitonin[56], glucagon[57], and α- or β-adrenergic agents[58-60].

The distributions of Na,K-ATPase activity[61-63], aldosterone binding sites[64-66], and ouabain sensitivity[67] along the nephron have been delineated, and the specific effects of thyroid hormone on Na,K-ATPase have been recognized[68]. The enzymes involved in 1,25-dihydroxycholecalciferol production[69] and prostaglandin synthesis[70], as well as tubular α-adrenoceptors[71] and glucagon binding sites[72] are distributed specifically in distinct tubular segments. Kallikrein and kininogenase are found only in specific parts of the convoluted distal tubule (granular portion) and the cortical collecting tubule (granular portion)[73].

Many other enzymes have been found to be heterogeneously distributed along the nephron. Lysosomal enzymes (e.g. β-galactosidase and N-acetyl-β-D-glucosaminidase), and peroxisomal enzymes are mainly found in proximal tubules[49]. The activity of enzymes of glutathione metabolism, of hydrogen peroxide and NADH formation, and cytochrome P-450 are highest in the straight part of proximal tubule[49,74]. This segment appears to be an important site for the metabolism of xenobiotics such as anaesthetics, insecticides, carcinogens and analgesics[75]. The high sensitivity of the straight part of proximal tubules to nephrotoxicants might result from these metabolic characteristics. In contrast, glucuronidation, which decreases drug toxicity, appears to predominate in the convoluted part of the proximal tubules, as shown by morphine metabolism[76].

In a somewhat different perspective, the approach used by Biber et al.[77] and Kramp et al.[78] is also of interest, where tubular dissection and histological observation were carried out on nephrons which had been previously investigated functionally by micropuncture techniques. Such an approach has allowed the heterogeneity of functional and structural alterations of the nephrons after acute or chronic toxic injury to be delineated.

The integrity of proximal tubule function can be estimated by measuring the intracellular accumulation, and transepithelial secretion, of organic ions, a specific function of proximal tubules. It has been shown that the accumulation of organic anions (e.g. p-amino-hippurate (PAH)) in proximal tubule cells is very sensitive to metabolic alterations, anoxia, Na,K-ATPase inhibition[79] and requires reduced sulphydryl groups[80] and normal Ca transport[81,82]. The technique used in such experiments is basically similar to that using incubations of renal cortical slices, but allows obviously a more precise localization of the tubular alteration.

III. ACUTE RENAL FAILURE

Micropuncture studies aimed at investigating the pathophysiology of acute renal failure (ARF) have provided valuable information on functional changes in individual nephrons and glomeruli shortly after exposure to toxic compounds or ischaemia, which induce decreases of glomerular filtration rate (GFR). The most significant contributions from these techniques to our understanding of the mechanisms of ARF will be summarized. The current interpretations on the pathophysiology of ARF are based on a much larger body of experimental studies using many technical approaches, the discussion of which is beyond the scope of this chapter, but have been reviewed[83-89].

Micropuncture techniques are well suited for the investigation of the contribution of various tubular and vascular changes to the decreased GFR which characterizes ARF. Several experimental models of ARF make use of heavy metal ions (mercuric chloride, uranyl nitrate, potassium dichromate), drugs (aminoglycoside antibiotics, cisplatin), and other compounds (glycerol, folic acid, lysine, p-aminophenol, Bence-Jones protein). Some of these agents are further discussed in Section V of this chapter. In addition, many single nephron studies have investigated the mechanisms of ischaemic ARF following renal artery occlusion or norepinephrine infusion.

The most important mechanisms of renal injury leading to filtration failure and oligo-anuria which have been investigated in micropuncture studies include tubular obstruction, altered epithelial permeability, reduced ultrafilterability across glomerular capillaries and vasoconstriction of afferent glomerular arterioles, possibly through activation of the tubuloglomerular feedback.

A.   Tubular obstruction

Tubular obstruction has been usually assessed by measuring intraluminal hydraulic pressure. It must be stressed that apparently normal tubular hydraulic pressures may still be observed despite tubular obstruction, if primary filtration failure or abnormal tubular permeability (resulting from epithelial damage) occur concomitantly. Such appear to be the case in the maintenance phase of mercuric chloride-induced ARF, where tubular pressure was not consistenly changed[90] despite tubular obstruction by cell debris and casts[77,91], and in ARF following cisplatin injection[92]. Similarly, in the model of uranyl nitrate-induced ARF, proximal tubule hydrostatic pressures were found close to or lower than control values[90,93-95], except for transient increases shortly after the administration of the toxic agent. This observation was not considered to be related to tubular obstruction[95]. No evidence of tubular obstruction, as manifest by changes of tubular pressures, was obtained in the early phases of methaemoglobin or glycerol-induced ARF[96,97], but intraluminal casts and increased hydrostatic pressure, observed at later stages of renal failure, may also play a role in this model[90,98]. Average intratubular pressures were not increased after 4 mg/kg gentamicin[99], but higher doses caused morphological and functional heterogeneity of surface nephrons. This suggests a wide degree of luminal obstruction, as indicated by the large scatter[100], or mean increase[99,101] of proximal tubule hydrostatic pressures. In contrast, significantly increased intraluminal hydrostatic pressure has been reported following the administration of large doses of folic acid[102], p-aminophenol[103], glaphenine[104], lysine[105] or Bence-Jones protein[106].

The role of tubular obstruction in ischaemic ARF has been investigated in a number of studies[84,86], which have frequently recorded increased tubular pressures following reflow after tem-

porary renal artery occlusion. The presence, or quantitative importance, of these changes were dependent on various factors such as
the time which had elapsed since the acute injury and/or the duration of ischaemia. No significant tubular pressure changes were recorded in the first hours of reflow following a 45 min ischaemia[90],
but increased pressures were measured (occasionally after several
days) in studies where occlusion lasted 60 min or more[107-110], or
after intra-arterial infusion of norepinephrine[111,112].

B.   Back-leak of ultrafiltrate

The outflow of abnormal amounts of ultrafiltrate through the
damaged tubular epithelium may contribute to the apparent
decrease of GFR in several experimental models of ARF. This back-
leak has usually been assessed by the fractional recovery in the
pelvic urine of small amounts of radioactive inulin microinjected into
proximal tubules. A decreased ipsilateral recovery and an increased
contralateral excretion of the marker suggest nephron damage.
Direct observation of abnormal proximal outflux of dyes such as
lissamine green, or apparent decreases of single nephron
glomerular filtration rate (SNGFR) measured at different sites along
the surface tubules have also been used as arguments for tubular
epithelial injury in ARF. Some studies assigned a major role to increased back-flux of filtrate in mercuric chloride ARF, as shown
by reduced inulin recovery[113], or abnormally enhanced reabsorption of an intraluminal saline droplet in some surface tubules[114],
while in other studies back-leak could not be detected, or was only
of marginal importance[91,115-117]. Similarly, the literature provides
contradictory evidence for increased out-flux of filtrate in the
pathogenesis of uranyl nitrate-induced ARF: inulin recovery has
been shown to be markedly reduced in some studies[94,95], while
others concluded that epithelial leak was absent[93]. On the other
hand, increased tubular permeability has been demonstrated or
suspected after the administration of various other nephrotoxic
agents such as amphotericin B[118], cisplatin[92] or gentamicin at
high[100,119] but not low[99] doses. Increased back-leak has been
frequently found in ischaemic experimental renal
injury[108,110,120,121]; the degree of functional leak, though,
depends on the duration of the ischaemia[116,121] and the lesion was
not detected in the norepinephrine model of ARF[111,112].

Thus, tubular back-leak of filtrate appears to play a significant role in several different models of ARF, though technical
artifacts may lead to overestimating its importance[116]. The role of
back-leak is likely to be important when tubular necrosis has
developed[86], as suggested by investigations on the urinary
clearance of dextrans of graded size in human ARF, indicating an
occurrence of filtrate back-leak in the more severe forms of post-
ischaemic renal injury[122].

C.   Ultrafiltration coefficient

Determinants of glomerular filtration include the glomerular capillary ultrafiltration coefficient and the mean effective filtration pressure. The former can be calculated from direct measurements of SNGFR and of capillary and tubular hydraulic and oncotic pressures. Such measurements have been made possible in particular by the use of a rat strain with surface glomeruli and by the development of micropuncture techniques allowing precise pressure recordings in single vessels and tubules at the kidney surface[123]. Such methods have allowed the possible role of altered glomerular ultrafiltration coefficient (K_f) as a cause of decreased GFR to be investigated. Thus, 2 hours after administration of uranyl nitrate (15 or 25 mg/kg), a significant, dose-related reduction of K_f was observed, but decrease of SNGFR was only observed at the highest dose[95]. It must be noted that this reduction may result from a decrease of either the filtering surface area or the glomerular permeability (or both), since K_f is derived from the product of the two terms.

Similar observations have been made following gentamicin administration (4 or 40 mg/kg, 10 days), where nearly identical decreases of K_f were measured at the two doses used. Although significant reductions of SNGFR occurred, the glomerular plasma flow rate remained unaffected at the lower dose[99]. Electron microscopy of the kidneys of treated animals failed to reveal glomerular damage. Decreased K_f values have also been reported in ischaemic ARF in some[83], but not all[84] investigations.

The reduction of K_f may be mediated in part by hormones such as angiotensin II[124], as suggested by the fact that the decrease of K_f (and of SNGFR and glomerular plasma flow) following gentamicin (40 mg/kg, 10 days) could be prevented by concomitant administration of captopril, a converting enzyme inhibitor[125]. K_f values have been shown to decrease during infusion of angiotensin II[126], and of a variety of other endogenous vasoactive compounds[124]. One possible mechanism for this effect may involve contraction of glomerular mesangial cells (through activation of specific receptors or a cAMP mediated pathway) resulting in reduced filtering surface area[124].

D.   Renal blood flow and tubuloglomerular feedback

Marked decreases of renal blood flow have been frequently, though not constantly, recorded in the various models of experimental ARF, in the initiation as well as in the maintenance phases of renal failure. It is also well established that reductions of GFR may persist well beyond the return of renal blood flow to near-normal levels at later stages of injury. These findings may be ascribed to various changes of resistance to flow in afferent and efferent arterioles which, particularly at early stages, might be mediated by hormones such as angiotensin II and prostaglandins[124]. Increases of afferent and efferent arteriolar resistances, resulting in reduced glomerular blood flow with relative constancy of SNGFR, have been documented by micropuncture techniques during infusion of noradrenaline or angiotensin II[127]. However, for most of the experimental models of ARF, the changes of flow resistance in specific renal arteriolar and glomerular vessels, and the mechanisms by which they are induced, remain to be investigated.

The existence of a single-nephron tubulo-glomerular feedback pathway, where SNGFR is controlled in part by the electrolyte composition or delivery of tubular fluid at the macula densa, has been demonstrated in a number of micropuncture experiments, and its probable role in several conditions of normal or altered renal functions has been recognized[128-130]. Since reduced reabsorption of fluid and electrolyte has been measured at tubular sites upstream of the macula densa in several models of ARF, an activation of the feedback pathway in such circumstances might be expected. The resulting decrease of GFR could be considered as a useful response by the kidney to preserve extracellular volume[128]. However, there is currently no definitive experimental evidence to support a major role for such a feedback mechanism when GFR is reduced during ARF. Thus, although this mechanism appears functionally intact at early stages of several experimental models of ARF (i.e. the flow rate in early proximal tubules of either normal or damaged kidneys is decreased in similar proportions when NaCl concentrations at the macula densa site are increased)[131], administration of furosemide at doses sufficient to inhibit the feedback mechanism failed to prevent or correct the GFR decreases consecutive to ischaemic insult, and improved renal function in toxic models of ARF by mechanisms unrelated to feedback inhibition[132]. The tubuloglomerular feedback, on the other hand, was found to play a minimal role at best in the reduction of SNGFR occurring after 24 hour tubular obstruction[133]. Experimental evidence, therefore, obtained from micropuncture methodology or other techniques do not favour the assumption of a major role of tubuloglomerular feedback in ischaemic ARF and post-obstructive decreases of GFR. It remains possible, however, that this system might be involved in some types of renal injury, or at some specific times in the development of the renal failure. Thus, in the initiation phase of uranyl nitrate-induced ARF, changes of early distal tubular fluid composition were found. This might suggest a possible involvment of tubuloglomerular feedback[134]. On the other hand, serum from patients with ARF asociated with hepatic injury was reported to contain an undefined factor which appears to activate the tubuloglomerular feedback in superficial rat nephrons[135].

E.   Tubular dysfunction in ARF

Toxic or ischaemic renal injuries may result in impairment of specific tubular functions. In some instances these alterations have been characterized by micropuncture techniques.

Salts of heavy metals, such as mercuric chloride or uranyl nitrate, inhibit the active Na transport across the turtle urinary bladder epithelium in vitro[136]. A similar impairment may occur in the mammalian nephron, since both compounds reduce tubular fluid and Na reabsorption. Thus, 48 hours after uranyl nitrate administration, fractional fluid reabsorption was decreased in proximal superficial tubules in dogs[94] and rats[93]. Even earlier alterations of epithelial function could be detected beyond the convoluted part of proximal tubules, as shown by a decrease of absolute fluid reabsorption to distal tubule puncture sites[93] and a marked increase of Na concentration in distal fluid[137], 6 h after uranyl nitrate. Administration of mercuric chloride was followed by decreases of absolute[115] and fractional tubular fluid reabsorption[77]. A direct demonstration of the toxic effects of mercuric chloride on epithelial transport was obtained in the experiments of Huguenin et al., using the stationary microperfusion ("split-drop") technique 48 h after mercuric chloride, where significant reductions of isotonic fluid reabsorption in (non-necrotic) proximal tubules could be observed[114]. However, at earlier stages (5-13 h after mercuric chloride), the diluting capacity of ascending limbs of Henle's loops remained unaltered[138]. Cisplatin did not appear to affect fluid reabsorption in superficial proximal tubules 3-4 days after injection, despite severe renal functional impairment[92,139]. However, damage to tubule segments not accessible to micropuncture (e.g. the pars recta) may contribute to the reduction of maximal urine concentrating ability by decreasing the corticopapillary osmolality gradient[139]. Further aspects of cisplatin tubular toxicity are discussed later in this chapter.

During glycerol-induced ARF, free-flow micropunctures indicated decreased fractional fluid reabsorption in proximal tubules during the established phase of the renal failure (i.e. 24 h after glycerol), while stationary microperfusions suggested an impairment of proximal reabsorption within the first 4 h after glycerol injection[97]. However, as stressed by Oken et al.[97], these changes reflected the function of the tubules with the least abnormal appearance, and in which complete filtration failure had not occurred. An additional impairment of Na reabsorption in collecting ducts has also been reported after glycerol injection[84].

Decreased proximal fluid reabsorption was also measured by stationary microperfusion after administration of large doses of folic acid. These alterations, occurring within 2 h after injection of large doses of the toxic agent, were ascribed by the authors to the intratubular obstruction and increased luminal hydrostatic pressure due to precipitation of folic acid crystals[102].

Alterations of tubule functions after renal ischaemia have been characterized by both "in vivo" micropunctures and "in vitro" microperfusions. Not unexpectedly, the severity of the functional lesions can be related to the duration of ischaemia. Thus, a 25-min ischaemia entailed a reduction of absolute and fractional Na reabsorption in proximal superficial tubules during the first hours following reflow. Tubular function and morphology returned to normal after 7-8 h[140]. Similarly, within the first hours of reflow after 60 min of ischaemia, net fluid reabsorption, measured by stationary microperfusion, was reduced in proximal tubules, and the diluting capacity of the ascending limbs of Henle's loops was compromised[138]. Isolated tubule studies have also provided direct evidence of severe transport defects in different segments of rabbit tubules studied after 60 min of renal ischaemia[141]. Thus, fluid reabsorption was decreased in convoluted and straight portions of the proximal tubule, diluting ability of the ascending limb of Henle's loop was impaired, and the response of the cortical collecting tubule to the hydrosmotic effect of vasopressin was markedly reduced[43]. Administration of mannitol or furosemide before the insult partially protected against ischaemic damage in the proximal tubules[42].

F.   ARF and nephron functional heterogeneity

Marked nephron function heterogeneity has been observed in various models of ARF that have been investigated by micropuncture techniques. This functional heterogeneity has been suggested both by marked internephron variations of superficial tubules and by the frequently reported discrepancy between severe reductions of whole kidney GFR and only moderate decreases of superficial SNGFR. Although this variability might represent the non-homogeneity of nephron damage, the possible role of technical artifacts must be considered.

Apparent heterogeneity among superficial tubules revealed by visual inspection of the kidney surface has occasionally been reported following acute renal injury, and was found to be effectively related to differing functional properties[109,114,115,142]. However, as shown by a specific study using the noradrenaline-induced ischaemic model[112], technical artifacts may significantly contribute to an apparent scattering of surface nephron SNGFR if more than one mechanism of filtration failure is operating concomitantly. Thus, in this model where tubular obstruction is an important but not unique pathogenic mechanism, the scatter of SNGFR values was reduced when fluid sampling was carried out at hydrostatic pressures prevailing before fluid collection.

Apparent functional heterogeneity between surface and deep nephrons is suggested by the frequent observation in experimental ARF that SNGFR is much less reduced than kidney GFR. Such a finding may indicate an actual intrarenal redistribution of function among different nephron populations, but may also potentially result from several artifacts. Thus, biased selection of punctured surface tubules, excessive reduction of intratubular pressure during fluid collection, or the occurrence of an abnormal epithelial "leak" localized beyond the tubular puncture site are potential sources of error that need to be considered in the interpretation of discrepancies between whole kidney and single nephron filtration rates. The use of other techniques may be required. For example, Mason et al.[143] studied the post-ischaemic model of ARF and used a variety of methods to investigate the intrarenal distribution of SNGFR and blood flow in the first hours following reflow. It was concluded from this study that the function of deeper nephrons is indeed the most severely compromised in this experimental model of post-ischaemic ARF, and that the data obtained from micropuncture of the relatively well preserved surface tubules obviously do not apply to other nephron populations.

IV.   CHRONIC RENAL INJURY AND NEPHRON ADAPTATION

A few micropuncture studies have investigated the function of the nephrons at late stages (several weeks) after acute toxic injury[78,144]. A marked functional heterogeneity of superficial

331

nephrons in rats was observed 3-4 weeks after acute toxic injury induced by injection of potassium dichromate and mercuric chloride[78]. Extreme values of SNGFR varied by a factor of more than 20, as compared to about 3 in normal kidneys. Glomerulotubular balance was, however, well maintained in these nephrons, as indicated by the similarity of fractional fluid reabsorption in proximal tubules. No abnormal permeability of the tubule to microinjected inulin was noted. In a similar experimental model, the characteristics of tubular glucose reabsorption were investigated by microinjection techniques. Saturation of glucose reabsorption was observed in both normal and "damage-adapted" nephrons, but the scatter of reabsorptive rates and average maximal transport were larger in the latter. These functional properties were related to the compensatory hypertrophy in the adapted tubules, and were characterized by a markedly enhanced capacity of the terminal, straight portion of the proximal tubules to reabsorb glucose[144].

Most studies on single nephron segments in chronic renal failure have been carried out in animals where uraemia was induced by subtotal surgical nephrectomy. Under these circumstances nephrons show relatively homogeneous functional properties, rather than a wide scatter of functional and morphological lesions typical of toxic injury.

Functional changes in the adapted nephrons of remnant kidneys have been reviewed[145]. These changes result both from intrinsic adaptation of tubular transport mechanisms (as shown for instance by in vitro studies of hypertrophic single tubules) and from increases of nephron plasma flow, glomerular filtration and luminal flow rate. These adaptive changes include, notably, enhancement of proximal tubule fluid reabsorption and increased SNGFR, which result in the maintenance of glomerulotubular balance; a reduction of Na reabsorption in the collecting duct system, possibly mediated through the effect of endogenous natriuretic factors, and enhanced K secretion capacity in the cortical collecting tubules. Several other adaptive changes relating to proton secretion, divalent cations and organic anions handling have also been described in single nephron studies. In addition, it is noteworthy that hyperfiltration in the glomeruli of remnant nephrons and the attending changes of glomerular blood flow and pressures[146] probably initiate the progressive functional and morphological glomerular damage which is known to occur in kidneys with reduced populations of nephrons[145].

V.   DRUGS AND CHEMICALS INDUCING ALTERATIONS OF NEPHRON FUNCTION

A.   Antibiotics and related compounds

1. Aminoglycosides

The renal transport of gentamicin and netilmicin and the renal toxicity of netilmicin and tobramycin have been investigated by micropuncture techniques[99,125,147-152]. Tubular transport of gentamicin and netilmicin were evaluated in rats by tubular and capillary microinjections[147,149,151] and by free-flow micropunctures[147,150,152]. After injection into early proximal tubules of a droplet containing a low or a high concentration of gentamicin, the fraction of the antibiotic reabsorbed by tubular cells down to the pelvic urine was found to range between 14% (high concentration) and 30% (low concentration)[149]. The recovery was larger after late proximal microinjection, and the microinjected drug was almost completely recovered after distal micro-injection[149,151]. These observations indicate tubular absorption of gentamicin along the convoluted part of the proximal tubule and the loop of Henle, presumably in the straight portion of the proximal tubule, where it was saturable[149]. Similar observations have been made with regard to netilmicin, which was found to be reabsorbed in the pars recta of proximal tubules, but not in the distal nephron[147]. The fractional recoveries of netilmicin in pelvic urine after microinjections in early and late proximal tubules amounted to 82% and 91%, respectively, and to 99% after microinjec-tion into early distal tubules[147].

Microinjection experiments do not provide information on the relative importance of the reabsorptive fluxes in the overall han-dling of aminoglycosides by the proximal tubule. Thus, if a secretory flux of gentamicin or netilmicin occurs simultaneously at the same tubular sites, the net result could be secretion as well as reabsorption. In fact, evidence for net tubular reabsorption and secretion of gentamicin and netilmicin has been obtained by free-flow micropuncture experiments[147,149,150,152], and will be dis-cussed below.

To assess the tubular handling of these compounds, both in free-flow micropuncture and clearance studies, the measurement of their glomerular ultrafilterability is required to calculate the fil-tered loads, and tubular fractional and absolute reabsorptions. In vitro measurements indicated that 83% of gentamicin was ultra-filterable[152]. Ultrafilterability of gentamicin and netilmicin was also measured in Munich-Wistar rats by direct punctures of surface glomeruli and analysis of inulin and gentamicin or netilmicin con-centrations in fluid from Bowman's space, and in plasma. The Bowman's space to plasma gentamicin concentration ratio was 0.85 (netilmicin: 0.86), a ratio close to that predicted by the Donnan equilibrium for the passive distribution of polycations across a semipermeable membrane[148].

The fractional reabsorption of gentamicin along the con-voluted part of superficial proximal tubules has been measured by free-flow micropunctures. This represents 25-40% of the filtered amount, depending on the experimental condition, for example reabsorption is larger in the non-diuretic state than in saline-loaded rats. Furthermore, a net reabsorption, corresponding to 15-30% of the filtered load, occurred along late proximal and early dis-tal tubules of superficial nephrons. In contrast net secretion of gentamicin appeared to occur in deep (juxtamedullary) nephrons, as indicated by a delivery of more than the filtered load at the tip of the loop of Henle[152]. These findings suggest some nephron heterogeneity with respect to gentamicin transport. The different handling of gentamicin by superficial and deep nephrons results in a final excreted load which is close to the filtered amount of the drug. The net secretion appears to be enhanced by extracellular volume expansion[152]. However, in a previous report no trans-epithelial secretion of gentamicin had been observed, using peritubular capillary microinjections[149]. The method of capillary microinjection is, however, less reliable than free flow micropuncture technique, and negative results from microinjection studies do not constitute a definitive answer.

Free-flow micropuncture studies showed net secretion of netilmicin along the convoluted part of the proximal tubule. The fractional excretion of the aminoglycoside measured in early proximal tubules was larger than unity, and remained the same down to late proximal segments. In contrast, there was net reab-sorption between the late proximal and early distal tubule (most probably along the pars recta), as shown by the fact that the delivery of netilmicin to distal tubules was lower than that measured at the end of proximal segments. Since the fractional excretion was larger in the final urine than that measured in late superficial distal tubules, it is reasonable to assume that netilmicin secretion was greater in deep than in the superficial nephrons.

It appears from these data that both gentamicin and netil-micin are reabsorbed and secreted along the proximal tubule, reab-sorption of gentamicin being somewhat larger than that of netil-micin. Vandewalle et al.[153] injected radioactively labelled genta-micin to rabbits in vivo and dissected the nephron segments to show that the cells of the pars recta had accumulated more gen-tamicin than cells of the pars convoluta in proximal tubules, while almost no gentamicin was measured in the distal nephron. These data are consistent with the results from micropuncture studies in-dicating the occurrence of a secretory transport of gentamicin be-sides a luminal uptake.

The nature of the carrier system involved in gentamicin reabsorption was investigated by Frommer et al.[151] using tubular microinjection experiments. A common carrier appeared to be shared by gentamicin and tobramycin, as suggested by the in-creased excretion of one antibiotic when the other was added to the microinjectate. Phospholipase A and spermine, a polyamine, also increased the recovery of gentamicin when added to the microin-jected solution. It was concluded that the carrier might be a phos-pholipid with high affinity for polyamines. In the same experi-ments, cephalothin had no effect on gentamicin reabsorption. Surprisingly, gentamicin reabsorption was decreased by probenecid, an organic anion, but was not inhibited by quinine, although both compounds are organic cations at physiological pH. The mechanisms involved in cellular transport of gentamicin are still unclear.

The nephrotoxic effects of aminoglycoside antibiotics, par-ticularly their influence on glomerular ultrafiltration dynamics, have been investigated in Munich-Wistar rats by micropuncture in vivo. It was found that a dose-related drop of SNGFR following gentamicin injection (4 or 40 mg/kg per day during 10 days) resulted predominantly from a decrease of the glomerular capillary ultrafiltration coefficient[99]. Tobramycin (40 mg/kg per day during 10 days) was shown to impair glomerular filtration much less than gentamicin at the same dose levels[125]. The decrease of the ultrafiltration coefficient and nephron plasma flow induced by gentamicin were nearly completely prevented by captopril, a converting enzyme inhibitor, given before and during the exposure to gentamicin. Angiotensin II may therefore be involved in the glomerular impairment due to gentamicin. Captopril, however, did not prevent the occurrence of morphological damage in the proximal tubule epithelium[125].

These observations suggest that a fall of GFR might be secondary to an initial effect of gentamicin on renal blood flow, as proposed by Klotman and Yarger[154]. These authors found in rats that a fall of renal blood flow occurred 24 h after a single injection of gentamicin (100 mg/kg), and preceded any change of GFR. Furthermore, the tubuloglomerular feedback mechanism appeared functional, as shown by the measurement of lower SNGFR values in distal than in proximal tubules.

Chronic exposure of adult or immature rabbits to gentamicin (30 mg/kg per day during 28-31 days) was also found to reduce ultrafiltration coefficient in glomeruli studied in vitro, where filtration was induced by a transcapillary oncotic gradient[155]. However, in spite of this alteration detected in vitro, no decrease of GFR could be measured in immature rabbits in vivo. Thus, a fall of ultrafiltration coefficient might not be sufficient in itself to reduce SNGFR. Savin et al.[155] suggested that the fall of ultrafiltration coefficient might be compensated for, in young rabbits, by increases of glomerular perfusion and ultrafiltration pressure. The decrease of GFR measured in older animals would result from several mechanisms, including a reduction of ultrafiltration coefficient.

Large doses of gentamicin (100-150 mg/kg per day during 10-14 days) resulted in a severe decrease of whole-kidney GFR[119]. A marked heterogeneity of superficial tubule appearance and function was observed, as shown by the wide internephron variation of SNGFR. Similar evidence of tubular function heterogeneity during gentamicin administration has been obtained by other authors[100,101].

Tubular functional defects were also induced by gentamicin, where repeated administration of high doses of the drug caused a transepithelial leak of inulin, while a reduction of proximal fluid reabsorption with increased delivery to the distal nephron was measured[119]. An inhibition of fluid reabsorption could be detected as early as 1 day after a single, high dose of gentamicin[154]. In the same study, chloride concentration was reduced in late proximal and early distal tubules, a finding thought to indicate an impaired proximal bicarbonate reabsorption. Other proximal functions are also altered during gentamicin toxicity, as shown by the reduced ability of rabbit proximal tubule cells to accumulate PAH following drug administration at 30 mg/kg per day. In both mature and immature rabbits, the impairment of tubular PAH accumulation correlated with the degree of GFR reduction[155].

2.   Amphotericin B

The nephrotoxicity of amphotericin B is well recognized, and has been shown to involve glomerular, proximal and distal tubular functions. In an attempt to delineate mechanisms of toxicity, Cheng et al.[118] used micropuncture-microinjection techniques to investigate the effects of single (1 mg/kg i.v.) or repeated (10 mg/kg per day i.p. over 4 days) doses of amphotericin B on glomerular and tubular function in rats. Whole-kidney GFR and plasma flow were reduced by the drug. These alterations were associated with a 20-25% decrease of glomerular capillary pressure, estimated by measurements of arterial oncotic pressure and proximal intratubular pressure in stop flow conditions. The fractional recovery in final urine of radiolabelled inulin microinjected into proximal tubules, following i.v. amphotericin B administration, amounted to 45%, though no evidence of histological lesions could be detected. Thus, amphotericin B altered renal function by at least two mechanisms: (1) increased vascular resistance, and (2) abnormal permeability of proximal tubules resulting in back-leak of luminal fluid, particularly after i.v. administration.

3.   Cyclosporin A

The immunosuppressant cyclosporin A has shown dose-related nephrotoxicity, with glomerular and tubular, functional and morphological lesions[156,157]. Some of these lesions appear to develop in human kidneys only[156]. Several micropuncture-microperfusion studies investigating the mechanisms of the cyclosporin A nephrotoxicity have been reported. Dieperink et al.[158] failed to detect specific alterations in proximal or distal tubules after administration of cyclosporin A (25 mg/kg per day during 13 days, or 12.5 mg/kg as a single i.v. dose). The functional nephrotoxicity induced by the drug (decreased whole kidney GFR; decreased absolute, but increased fractional, fluid reabsorption in proximal tubules, reduced proximal intratubular pressure) were considered to result from haemodynamic effects and not from direct tubular toxicity. Müller-Suur et al.[159] investigated the effects of cyclosporin A in a microperfusion study in rats given a dose of 15 mg/kg per day during 5-7 days. No significant changes of net reabsorption of water, Na, K, Cl, Ca or Mg were detected in Henle's loop epithelium (i.e. the segment between end-proximal and early distal tubules). In contrast, a micropuncture study[160] showed an impaired diluting ability of the ascending limb of Henle's loop, as indicated by increased salt concentrations at early distal tubular sites following cyclosporin A (15 mg/kg per day during 10 days, or 5 mg/kg as a single i.v. dose). Gnutzmann et al. suggested that these changes of luminal fluid composition might contribute to the decreased GFR by activation of the tubuloglomerular feedback mechanism[160].

As shown by these partially contradictory micropuncture studies (and by other investigations using different experimental approaches), the pathogenesis of cyclosporin A-induced nephrotoxicity remains unclear. Recent experimental evidence, however, underscores the important role of cyclosporin A-induced activation of the sympathetic nervous system, resulting in renal vaso-constriction[161] and salt and water retention[162]. Such alterations might represent the initial pathogenic steps, leading subsequently to more extensive drug-induced nephrotoxicity, although it is noteworthy that the development and characteristics of the renal alterations caused by cyclosporin A appear to differ between humans and animal models[156].

B. Metal ions: renal handling and toxicity

Several metal ions that induce tubular necrosis have been used as probes to study the pathogenesis of acute renal failure, and have already been discussed above. Several of these compounds have been investigated by single nephron techniques to characterize their specific toxic effects or their handling.

1. Aluminium

The ultrafilterability of aluminium was investigated "in vivo" by Bowman's space micropuncture in Munich-Wistar rats infused with large doses of $AlCl_3$[163]. A maximum of 8-9% (range: 1.7-8.4%) of plasma aluminium was found to cross the glomerular barrier in these conditions. These values were used to calculate fractional excretion of aluminium in clearance experiments, during hydropenia, volume expansion or administration of furosemide. About 60% of ultrafiltered aluminium was found to be reabsorbed in hydropenic conditions and after furosemide. In contrast, aluminium fractional reabsorption was decreased to nearly 15% during volume expansion, a finding which led the authors to suggest that aluminium is reabsorbed mostly along the proximal tubules.

2. Arsenate

The characteristics and mechanisms of arsenate toxicity were inves-tigated by in vitro microperfusion of rabbit proximal tubules[164]. Arsenate (10 μmol/l to 5 mmol/l) added to the perfusate inhibited, in a dose-dependent manner, fluid and phosphate reabsorption, but was without effect when present at the peritubular side. In con-trast, arsenate did not affect PAH secretion, and caused only a marginal decrease in glucose reabsorption. Parallel metabolic studies on proximal tubule suspensions suggested that the toxic ef-fect was related to uncoupling of oxidative phosphorylation, which resulted in differential inhibition of Na-dependent proximal transport systems.

3. Cadmium

The tubular handling of Cd was studied by microinjection tech-niques in rats[165]. About 70% of inorganic 109 Cd (1 mmol/l) microinjected into the lumen of proximal tubules was found to be taken up by epithelial cells, while the recovery in final urine was nearly complete after distal microinjection. Proximal uptake of Cd was further enhanced when equimolar concentrations of cysteine were added to the microinjectate. In contrast, the Cd-pentetic acid chelate was quantitatively recovered in final urine after injection into proximal tubules. The tubular uptake of Cd-metallothionein, for similar amounts of Cd in the microinjected solution, was found to be much lower (up to 17% of the injected load) than that of inorganic Cd (unpublished observations). No evidence for a secretory movement of Cd was found. Thus, inorganic Cd ions appear to be taken up quickly and extensively at the apical membrane of proximal tubule cells, but the mechanisms of binding or transport await elucidation.

4.   Cisplatin

Cisplatin-induced acute renal failure in rats has been shown to be associated with tubular fluid "backleak", decreased glomerular ultrafiltration and possibly tubular obstruction[92]. Other aspects of the tubular toxicity of cisplatin have also been studied in rats by micropuncture techniques. Thus, an attempt was made by free-flow micropunctures to investigate the mechanisms of magnesium wasting known to accompany cisplatin nephrotoxicity[166]. Administration of the drug during 3 weeks (2.5 mg/kg per day i.p.) entailed an increase of Mg urinary excretion, but Mg transport in the proximal and distal superficial tubules appeared unaltered. The functional injury must therefore be located in other (deep nephrons, or late distal) nephron segments. An electrophysiological study in rat distal superficial tubules has been performed to investigate cisplatin-induced modifications of transepithelial potential differences[167]. Cisplatin administration (2 mg/kg per hour i.v.) resulted in marked increases of late-distal transepithelial potential differences. This effect was suppressed by amiloride, suggesting that the potential difference increase induced by cisplatin is consecutive to an enhanced apical Na conductance, via amiloride-sensitive Na channels. These changes may, in part, explain the findings of electrolyte, most notably potassium, wasting in cisplatin toxicity.

5.   Lead

A free-flow micropuncture study investigated the effects of oral exposure to lead acetate (1% in drinking water) of young rats during 6 weeks since weaning[168]. Clearance and micropuncture investigations were carried out 3 and 16 weeks after the end of exposure, when blood lead levels amounted to 56 and 24 µg/dl respectively. Lead was found to reduce both whole kidney GFR and SNGFR of superficial tubules by nearly 30%. Renal blood flow was also reduced, while arterial pressure was significantly increased in exposed animals. The toxic effects of lead on renal function appeared to be relatively selective, and did not seem to result only from the general toxic action of the heavy metal, such as growth failure.

338

6.   Lithium

Lithium is reabsorbed along proximal tubules[169], and probably through paracellular pathways[170]. Lithium, however, can compete with Na on the apical membrane carrier system involved in Na-H exchange in proximal tubules, as indicated by membrane vesicle studies[171]. No net lithium reabsorption could be measured beyond the early distal tubule[169].

Lithium is known to cause a number of renal functional lesions, notably a decrease of tubular Na reabsorption, an impairment of urinary acidification and potassium excretion[172]. Evidence for lithium-induced decreases of Na reabsorption at several nephron sites has been obtained by free-flow micropuncture experiments after both single i.v. or repeated i.p. lithium administration, resulting in plasma concentrations averaging respectively 2-3 mmol/l[173], or 0.6 mmol/l[174]. Decreased Na tubular reabsorption may play a role in the concentrating defect resulting from Li administration[175]. However, inhibitory effects of lithium on the maximal concentrating ability have generally been considered to be the result of an impairment of the action of vasopressin on hydro-osmotic water flow in the distal nephron. Cogan and Abramow investigated these inhibitory effects of lithium (10 mmol/l) directly on the rabbit collecting tubule in vitro[176]. These authors reported that lithium significantly reduced both basal diffusional permeability to water and vasopressin-induced hydro-osmotic response, by 30% and 50% respectively. Lithium was effective only when added at the luminal border, and appeared to impair the vasopressin-induced adenylate cyclase stimulation from the cytoplasmic side since the increase of osmotic water flow caused by cAMP remained unaffected by lithium. It is worth noting that lithium was also shown to inhibit adenylate cyclase activity stimulated by vasopressin in unperfused, microdissected medullary-collecting tubules from rat kidneys[177].

7.   Mercury

A luminal (proximal tubules) and peritubular capillary microinjection study in rats[178] was carried out to characterize the tubular handling of $^{203}HgCl_2$. A large fraction (>90%) of intraluminally injected mercuric ions was taken up by tubular cells, while no tracer appeared in pelvic urine after peritubular microinjection. The luminal uptake was not decreased by known metabolic inhibitors, suggesting that the mercuric ion is not actively transported across the tubular epithelium.

8.   Vanadate

Orthovanadate ions inhibit Na,K-ATPase activity, and promote marked diuresis and natriuresis in experimental animals[179]. Several tubular effects of this ion have been investigated by single nephron techniques. In a free flow micropuncture study in rats, vanadate (0.5 or 1 μmol as i.v. bolus) decreased fractional and absolute fluid reabsorption in proximal tubules by about 30%, without significant alterations of SNGFR[180]. These findings were confirmed and extended in a study on isolated, in vitro perfused rabbit proximal tubules[181]. Vanadate was found to inhibit reversibly fluid reabsorption in S_1, but not S_2 segments of proximal tubules, by an average of 30% (1 or 10 μmol/l in the perfusate were equally effective). Vanadate also inhibited PAH tubular secretion in a dose-dependent manner, in both S_1 and S_2 segments. These experiments further indicated that inhibitory effects of vanadate on both fluid reabsorption and PAH secretion result from Na,K-ATPase inhibition following intracellular entry. Vanadate was more effective when added on the luminal side, and its effects were enhanced by increasing extracellular potassium concentration. Additional effects of vanadate ions have been described in the isolated cortical collecting tubule[182]. In that part of the nephron, vanadate impaired markedly in a dose-dependent manner, the induction of the hydro-osmotic effects of vasopressin or cyclic AMP, and reduced the transepithelial potential difference. In contrast to the observations made in proximal tubules, the ion was more effective when added on the peritubular side. Both effects on the cortical collecting tubule could be interpreted as a consequence of Na,K-ATPase inhibition, as shown by the fact that ouabain produced effects similar to those of vanadate.

C.   Analgesics

Chronic interstitial nephritis and papillary necrosis characterize analgesic nephropathy. A number of experimental studies have been carried out to unravel the pathogenesis of these injuries[183]; most of them were designed at investigating the biochemical mechanisms of the nephropathy rather than the functional defects at the single tubule level.

Early functional changes induced by p-aminophenol (400 mg/kg as i.v. bolus) were investigated by clearance and micropuncture techniques in rats[103]. The compound, a toxic metabolite resulting from deacetylation of phenacetin and acetaminophen, is known to damage the last third of proximal tubule[184]. Hydrostatic pressure in superficial proximal and distal tubules started to increase simultaneously about 40 min after injection of p-aminophenol. Glomerular filtration rate decreased markedly despite the maintenance of renal blood flow, and fractional Na excretion increased. Early morphological changes appeared in parallel with functional injury and remained localized to proximal tubules, the S_3 segment being more severely affected. Thus the authors suggested that early p-aminophenol injury results in metabolic cell damage associated with decreased fluid reabsorption in proximal tubules. This effect, together with the development of increased resistance to tubular flow in late distal parts of the nephron, would lead to the observed increase of intratubular hydrostatic pressures.

The tubular toxicity of p-aminophenol and acetaminophen probably results from a metabolic activation of the chemicals through the renal mixed function oxidase-cytochrome P450 system. The resulting reactive electrophilic intermediates bind covalently to cellular macromolecules and depletes glutathione[185,186], which is required for detoxification of reactive intermediates[187]. Endou et al.[188] demonstrated that cytochrome P450 activity could be detected in proximal tubules only. The presence of both cytochrome P450 and NADH-cytochrome-c reductase together in proximal tubules indicates that this part of the nephron contains the P450 monooxygenase system. Its activity appears to predominate in the straight portion of the proximal tubule, an observation which might explain the specific lesions entailed by acetaminophen in this nephron segment. It is of interest that glutathione-S-transferase, which is also essentially localized in proximal tubules[49], might play an important role, together with glutathione, in protecting the tubular cells against chemical aggression. Other tubular lesions induced by acetaminophen might result from co-oxidation with arachidonic acid through prostaglandin endoperoxide synthetase[189,190]. This enzyme is found in medullary collecting ducts, but not in medullary thick ascending limbs of Henle's loop[70]. Indomethacin and aspirin inhibit the arachidonic acid-dependent co-oxidation of acetaminophen.

The tubular fate of salicylate has been investigated in free-flow micropuncture experiments and in isolated tubule microperfusion. Net secretion of salicylate in the early part of the proximal tubule (fractional delivery: 125%) was found to occur in rats infused with salicylate (plasma concentration averaging 0.6 mmol/l). Salicylate reabsorption was measured at more distal segments, most notably between late proximal and early distal sites, where 85% of the filtered amount was reabsorbed. Further reabsorption occurred in the distal nephron, the urinary excretion averaging 0.5% of the amount filtered[191]. Alkalosis increased the concentration of salicylate in proximal tubules by 30%. This increase is less than would be expected from pH in proximal tubule fluid if non-ionized salicylate were the only permeant form of the drug[191]. The mechanisms involved in salicylate reabsorption were further investigated in proximal tubular S_2 segments perfused in vitro[192]. Salicylate reabsorption was shown to depend on proton secretion. The addition of ethoxyzolamide (an inhibitor of carbonic anhydrase activity) to the bathing medium completely abolished salicylate reabsorption. Although the mechanisms involved are still not completely understood, it is conceivable that an anion-exchange process may play a role either at the luminal or at the basolateral membrane[192].

In a free-flow micropuncture study in the rat, the effects of two organic anions, PAH and pyrazinoate, on the tubular transport of salicylate were investigated[193]. It was shown that both anions inhibited proximal net salicylate secretion. In addition, pyrazinoate appeared also to inhibit salicylate reabsorption. These various single nephron studies clearly indicate that salicylate ions are transported by diffusion and by carrier-mediated mechanisms.

D.   Urate toxicity and transport

Sudden and marked increases of urate plasma or urine levels may induce acute renal failure, which, in the clinical setting is a well-known possible complication of leukaemia chemotherapy or of uricosuric agents. The pathogenesis of this injury has been investigated by micropuncture studies in rats made hyperuricaemic by the administration of urate and/or oxonate, an inhibitor of urate degradation by uricase[194-197]. These studies indicated that urate-induced ARF probably resulted from a variety of pathogenic events, such as luminal obstruction in the late distal nephron, impairment of capillary blood flow by intravascular deposits of urate and uric acid, and/or possibly from a decrease of glomerular capillary pressure. Acute renal injury associated with hyperuricaemia could be prevented when tubular flow rates in rats were high (i.e. in Brattleboro rats, or by furosemide-induced diuresis), a finding which suggests that tubular obstruction plays a major pathogenic role.

Micropuncture, microperfusion and microinjection techniques have all been used to investigate the characteristics of the tubular transport of urate. As reviewed[198-200], both secretory and reabsorptive transports occur across the proximal tubule epithelium, and recent studies with plasma cell membrane vesicles have defined the role of anion exchange processes in the epithelial handling of urate at both luminal and basolateral membranes[200].

E.   Maleic acid-induced nephropathy

Parenteral administration of large doses (e.g. 100-200 mg/kg) of maleic acid increases the urinary excretion of water and various solutes - most notably Na, phosphate, bicarbonate, glucose, amino acids - and also induces a proximal renal tubular acidosis. This experimental nephropathy, which is reminiscent of the human Toni-Debré-Fanconi syndrome, has been investigated in several micropuncture studies. The initial reports by Bergeron et al.[201,202] 2-24 h after i.p. maleic acid, suggested that increased epithelial permeability was the major effect of the toxic agent, resulting in enhanced back-flux (blood to lumen) of glucose, phosphate and amino acids most notably in the distal nephron, while proximal tubule active reabsorption of the same solutes did not appear affected. Subsequent experiments using microinjection and free-flow micropuncture techniques supported these data and showed abnormal epithelial "leaks" to inulin and lissamine green dye in late proximal tubules (and at more distal sites,) 20 h after s.c. injection of maleic acid (200 mg/kg). Such alterations might explain the decrease of net Na and phosphate reabsorption in the superficial proximal tubules[203]. By contrast, other studies have detected major alterations of tubular electrolyte and amino acids reabsorption following administration of maleic acid. Thus, Günther et al.[204], using free-flow micropunctures and "in vivo" tubular microperfusions in rats to study the effects of maleic acid, injected i.p. 1-6 h before the experiments, observed a marked inhibition of amino acid reabsorption along proximal tubules, without evidence for increased passive permeability and back-flux. Similarly, a maleate-induced defect of Na, Cl and bicarbonate reabsorption along proximal tubules was found by microperfusion experiments "in vivo" (200 mg/kg of maleic acid, 60-90 min before experiments), and no evidence for increased epithelial permeability to inulin or bicarbonate was obtained[205]. In other experiments, proximal Na and phosphate reabsorption, studied by free-flow micropunctures, was significantly reduced after maleate (100 mg/kg per hour i.v.)[206]. Decreased proximal Na reabsorption was also considered to be the most likely explanation for the occurrence of a reduced secretory rate of protons that had been demonstrated by stationary microperfusion techniques in proximal tubules after maleate (200 mg/kg 15 min before experiments followed by continuous infusion of 42 mg/h)[207].

The micropuncture data on maleic acid tubular toxicity appear contradictory. These discrepancies may be related to the different times between maleate injection and the micropuncture experiments[205].

VI.   ORGANIC IONS: TUBULAR TRANSPORT AND METABOLISM

Both specific and non specific tubular transport mechanisms determine the renal excretory pattern of the many drugs and chemicals that are weak electrolytes. The studies on these transports and specific carriers systems have been reviewed recently[208]. Results obtained by the use of single tubule techniques will be briefly summarized here (data on organic ions such as urate, salicylate or aminoglycoside antibiotics have been discussed above).

A.   Organic anions

The predominant sites of net tubular transport of organic anions along the proximal tubules have been characterized in micropuncture and microperfusion studies. The secretory rate of PAH has been found to be the highest in the pars recta[209](mostly the S_2 segment[210]) of the rabbit proximal tubule. This distribution, however, differs between animal species. In the pig kidney, for instance, the highest PAH secretory rate was found in early proximal segments[211].

The net secretion of PAH results from an uphill transport inside the cell at the basolateral membrane, followed by luminal exit at the brush border membrane[209]. Investigations on transport at the single membrane level have been carried out on non-perfused tubules and membrane vesicle preparations[212-214]. These studies have indicated that the basolateral uptake of PAH is mediated by a saturable transport process which can be competitively inhibited, and which may function by an exchange process with intracellular anions or by a cotransport with Na. While the exact mechanisms remain unclear, Na and K gradients across the basolateral membrane appear important for the normal function of the transporter[208]. Similarly, the occurrence of brush border PAH carrier system (most likely an anion exchanger), which would transport PAH into the lumen down its concentration gradient[215], has been suggested. The renal toxicity of cephaloridine, associated with high intracellular concentrations of the antibiotic, may result from an inability of the anion to be transported by the luminal carrier system following basolateral uptake, as suggested by the absence of net cephaloridine secretion[216]. In contrast, micropuncture studies have shown that both benzylpenicillin and carbenicillin are secreted into the lumen of rat proximal tubules[217].

The tubular handling of pyrazinoate, a metabolite of the tuberculostatic drug pyrazinamide which may induce hyperuricaemia in man, has been investigated by single tubule techniques. Pyrazinoate is both secreted and reabsorbed by the mammalian kidney[218]. In microperfusion experiments on isolated rabbit tubules (S_2 segment), it was shown that secretion but not reabsorption of pyrazinoate could be inhibited by probenecid, while ouabain, in contrast, inhibited both fluxes[219]. These results indicate that a normal Na,K-ATPase activity is required to allow the secretion of pyrazinoate, and other organic anions as well[208]. It also appears that pyrazinoate reabsorption at the luminal step may depend on concomitant Na reabsorption. The inhibition of pyrazinoate reabsorption by lactate in the luminal fluid suggests that pyrazinoate might be reabsorbed by the Na-lactate reabsorptive mechanism[219]. The basolateral uphill transport of pyrazinoate, i.e. the initial "secretory" step, was investigated by measuring the cellular uptake of the anion by non-perfused S_2 proximal segments of the rabbit[220]. It was observed that this uptake could be inhibited only partially by probenecid or PAH. It has therefore been suggested that basolateral transport of pyrazinoate occurs through two transport systems, characterized by different affinities for probenecid and PAH. Urate and salicylate also showed some affinity for these carrier systems, though the inhibitory effects of salicylate resulted in part also from non-specific, metabolic alterations[220].

Some aspects of the tubular toxicity of ochratoxin A, a mycotoxin often contaminating various cereals[221], have been investigated by Endou et al.[222], using isolated, non-perfused proximal segments from rat kidneys. The tubular toxicity of the compound, most marked in the straight portion of the proximal tubule and revealed by the release of membrane-bound enzymes (e.g. alanine-aminopeptidase) into the incubation medium after addition of ochratoxin A (0.1 mmol/l), was prevented when probenecid was added simultaneously (0.4 mmol/l). These findings suggest that ochratoxin A is transported via the anion transport system that is inhibited by probenecid at the basolateral membrane, and exerts its tubular toxic effects after intracellular accumulation.

B.   Organic cations

The transport of exogenous organic cations is probably mediated by the mechanisms involved in the transport of endogenous compounds such as choline, catecholamines or N_1-methylnicotinamide[223]. Whereas micropuncture studies in rats have confirmed the occurrence of proximal transport of endogenous cations such as choline[224] or N_1-methylnicotinamide[225], no in vivo studies at the single tubule level have examined the handling of cationic xenobiotics. In contrast, a few in vitro studies have been carried out in isolated rabbit tubules.

Cimetidine, procainamide and morphine are examples of drugs

which are excreted by the kidney by the mechanisms involved in the secretion of organic cations[76,226,227]. The studies of McKinney et al.[226,227] demonstrated that the proximal secretion of cimetidine and procainamide could be inhibited by quinine and quinidine, two other organic cations, and by ouabain or hypothermia. Cimetidine and procainamide also compete for their own secretion[226,228]. It thus appears that both compounds are secreted through an active process, subjected to competitive inhibition by other organic cations. Furthermore, a marked heterogeneity in proximal transport of procainamide was demonstrated, as shown by the differences of the secretory rates between various proximal segments, and between superficial and juxtamedullary tubules[228]. The secretory transport was the lowest in the S_3 segments from both nephron populations, while transport in the S_2 segment was higher in juxtamedullary than in cortical nephrons. This distribution was clearly different from that of PAH[228]. Morphine has been shown to be accumulated by tubular cells of proximal, non-perfused segments of rabbits studied in vitro[76]. The drug was in part metabolized to form a glucuronide conjugate, the metabolic activity being the lowest in the S_3 and the highest in the S_1 segments. The effects of three other organic cations (N_1-methylnicotinamide, quinine and mepiperphenidol) on morphine accumulation were investigated: only the latter two compounds reduced morphine uptake. Since N_1-methylnicotinamide had been found unequivocally to be secreted by the rabbit kidney[229], it was concluded that more than one transport system for organic cations must exist in the proximal tubules of this species[76].

The secretion of tetraethylammonium into the lumen of perfused rabbit cortical nephrons was found to be the lowest in S_3 and the highest in S_1 segments, as for procainamide[230]. In contrast, the magnitude of intracellular accumulation of tetraethylammonium in non-perfused segments was similar in the three segments. These findings suggest that the basolateral uptake of the cation is of similar magnitude along the whole proximal tubule, whereas the transport rates at the luminal membrane differ between the proximal segments.

VII. CONCLUSIONS

Micropuncture and microperfusion techniques have been used in the field of renal toxicology mostly to investigate three main areas: the pathophysiology of oligoanuria associated with acute renal failure, the tubular sites of transport of various exogenous compounds, and some specific functional alterations caused by exogenous chemicals. Clearly, these techniques have been, and will remain, essential to delineate the sites of transport and toxicity of xenobiotics. They are fraught with limitations which have been stressed in this review, most notably in conditions where toxic agents induce severe functional alterations which compromise the reliability of these techniques. Complementary methods must therefore be considered and used in all studies on the toxic effects of chemical agents on renal tubule and cell function. This includes biochemical investigations on single tubule segments, which have allowed a detailed mapping of the enzymatic activities characteristic of specific parts of the nephron, and the elucidation of the effects of many endogenous and exogenous agents on these processes. Clearly, renal functional alterations result from the interaction of toxic agents with specific binding sites, transport systems or receptors in the kidney. Progress in the elucidation of the molecular properties of these putative "receptors" should therefore contribute to the understanding of the mechanisms of renal toxicity of foreign chemicals. In this respect the current developments in the "in vitro" culture of differentiated renal cells of defined tubular origin may provide useful models to characterize some fundamental mechanisms of renal toxicity. It must be stressed, however, that whatever the promises and successful outcome of approaches using morphological, biochemical, immunological and the most recent cell physiology or molecular biology techniques, micropuncture and microperfusion investigations at the single tubule level will remain essential for the overall assessment of normal and altered nephron function.

ACKNOWLEDGMENTS

The authors gratefully acknowledge the collaboration of Mrs N. Benmazari and Mrs M. Nenniger in the preparation of the manuscript. Work carried out in the author's laboratory is supported by the Swiss Science Foundation.

REFERENCES

1. Ullrich, K.J. and Greger, R., Approaches to the study of tubule transport functions, in The Kidney: Physiology and Pathophysiology, Vol. 1, Seldin, D.W. and Giebisch, G., Eds., Raven Press, New York, 1985, 427.

2. Quamme, G.A. and Dirks, J.H., Micropuncture techniques, Kidney Int., 30, 152, 1986.

3. Bennett, C.M., Brenner, B.M. and Berliner, R.W., Micropuncture study of nephron function in the Rhesus monkey, J. Clin. Invest., 47, 203, 1968.

4. Maddox, D.A., Deen, W.M. and Brenner, B.M., Dynamics of glomerular ultrafiltration: VI. Studies in the primate, Kidney Int., 5, 271, 1974.

5. Roch-Ramel, F., Diezi-Chométy, F., Roth, L. and Weiner, I.M., A micropuncture study of urate excretion by Cebus monkeys employing high performance liquid chromatography with amperometric detection of urate, Pfluegers Arch., 383, 203, 1980.

6. Wong, N.L.M., Reitzik, M. and Quamme, G.A., Micropuncture study of the superficial nephron of Cercopithecus aethiops, Renal Physiol., 9, 29, 1986.

7. Roch-Ramel, F., de Rougemont, D., Peters, G. and Weiner, I.M., Micropuncture study of urate excretion by the kidney of the rat, the Cebus monkey and the rabbit, in Amino Acid Transport and Uric Acid Transport, Silbernagl, S., Lang, F. and Greger, R., Eds., Thieme, Stuttgart, 1976, 188.

8. Chonko, A.M., Osgood, R.W., Nickel, A.E., Ferris, T.F. and Stein, J.H., The measurement of nephron filtration rate and absolute reabsorption in the proximal tubule of the rabbit kidney, J. Clin. Invest., 56, 232, 1975.

9. Friedman, P.A. and Roch-Ramel, F., Micropuncture study of fluid handling in

the cat kidney, Pfluegers Arch., 372, 239, 1977.

10. Roch-Ramel, F., White, F., Vowles, L., Simmonds, H.A. and Cameron, J.S., Micropuncture study of tubular transport of urate and PAH in the pig kidney, Am. J. Physiol., 239, F107, 1980.

11. Richards, A.N. and Walker, A.M., Methods of collecting fluid from known regions of the renal tubules of amphibia and of perfusing the lumen of a single tubule, Am. J. Physiol., 118, 111, 1937.

12. Fujimoto, M., Naito, K. and Kubota, T., Electrochemical profile for ion transport across the membrane of proximal tubular cells, Membrane Biochem., 3, 67, 1980.

13. Wiederholt, M. and Hansen, L.L., Amphiuma kidney as a model for distal tubular transport studies, in Contributions to Nephrology, Vol. 19: Research Animals and Experimental Design in Nephrology, Stolte, H. and Alt, J., Eds., Karger, Basel, 1980, 28.

14. Oberleithner, H. and Giebisch, G., Mechanism of potassium transport across distal tubular epithelium of Amphiuma, in Epithelial Ion and Water Transport, Macknight, A.D.C. and Leader, J.P., Eds., Raven Press, New York, 1981, 97.

15. Brenner, B.M., Troy, J.L. and Daugharty, T.M., The dynamics of glomerular ultrafiltration in the rat, J. Clin. Invest., 50, 1776, 1971.

16. Hackbarth, H., Büttner, D., Jarck, D., Pothmann, M., Messow, C. and Gärtner, K., Distribution of glomeruli in the renal cortex of Munich Wistar Frömter (MWF) rats, Renal Physiol., 6, 63, 1983.

17. Valtin, H. and Schroeder, H.A., Familial hypothalamic diabetes insipidus in rats (Brattleboro strain), Am. J. Physiol., 206, 425, 1964.

18. Windhager, E.E., Micropuncture Techniques and Nephron Function, Butterworths, London, 1968.

19. Giebisch, G.H., Ed., Renal Micropuncture Techniques: a Symposium, Yale J. Biol. Med., 45, No 3-4, 191, 1972.

20. Gottschalk, C.W. and Lassiter, W.E., Micropuncture methodology, in Handbook of Physiology, Section 8: Renal Physiology, Orloff, J. and Berliner, R.W., Eds., American Physiological Society, Washington, 1973, 129.

21. Andreucci, V.E., Ed., Manual of Renal Micropuncture, Idelson, Naples, 1978.

22. Lang, F., Greger, R., Lechene, C. and Knox, F.G., Micropuncture techniques, in Methods in Pharmacology, Vol. 4B: Renal Pharmacology, Martinez-Maldonado, M., Ed., Plenum Press, New York, 1978, 75.

23. Roch-Ramel, F. and Peters, G., Micropuncture techniques as a tool in renal pharmacology, Annu. Rev. Pharmacol. Toxicol., 19, 323, 1979.

24. De Rouffignac, C. and Morel, F., Micropuncture study of water, electrolyte and urea movements along the loops of Henle in Psammomys, J. Clin. Invest., 48, 474, 1969.

25. Marsh, D.J., Solute and water flows in thin limbs of Henle's loop in the hamster kidney, Am. J. Physiol., 218, 824, 1970.

26. Lassiter, W.E., Mylle, M. and Gottschalk, C.W., Micropuncture study of urea transport in rat renal medulla, Am. J. Physiol., 210, 965, 1966.

27. Sakai, F., Jamison, R.L. and Berliner, R.W., A method for exposing the rat renal medulla in vivo: micropuncture of the collecting duct, Am. J. Physiol., 209, 663, 1965.

28. Knox, F.G. and Marchand, G.R., Study of renal action of diuretics by micropuncture techniques, in Methods in Pharmacology, Vol. 4A: Renal Pharmacology, Martinez-Maldonado, M., Ed., Plenum Press, New York, 1976, 73.

29. Blantz, R.C. and Tucker, B.J., Measurements of glomerular dynamics, in Methods in Pharmacology, Vol. 4B: Renal Pharmacology, Martinez-Maldonado, M., Ed., Plenum Press, New York, 1978, 141.

30. Dworkin, L.D. and Brenner, B.M., Biophysical basis of glomerular filtration, in The Kidney: Physiology and Pathophysiology, Seldin, D.W. and Giebisch, G., Eds., Raven Press, New York, 1985, 397.

31. Diezi, J. and Roch-Ramel, F., The use of single nephron, micropuncture and microcannulation techniques in assessing renal function and malfunction, in Monographs in Applied Toxicology, No 1: Nephrotoxicity, Assessment and Pathogenesis, Bach, P.H., Bonner, F.W., Bridges, J.W. and Lock, E.A., Eds., Wiley, Chichester, 1982, 144.

32. Boulpaep, E.L. and Giebisch, G., Electrophysiological measurements on the renal tubule, in Methods in Pharmacology, Vol. 4B: Renal Pharmacology, Martinez-Maldonado, M., Ed., Plenum Press, New York, 1978, 165.

33. Frömter, E., The electrophysiological analysis of tubular transport, Kidney Int., 30, 216, 1986.

34. Burg, M.B. and Knepper, M.A., Single tubule perfusion techniques, Kidney Int., 30, 166, 1986.

35. Chonko, A.M. and Grantham, J.J., The use of the isolated tubule preparation for the investigation of diuretics, in Methods in Pharmacology, Vol. 4A: Renal Pharmacology, Martinez-Maldonado, M., Ed., Plenum Press, New York, 1976, 47.

36. Chonko, A.M., Irish III, J.M. and Welling, D.J., Microperfusion of isolated tubules, in Methods in Pharmacology, Vol. 4B: Renal Pharmacology, Martinez-Maldonado, M., Ed., Plenum Press, New York, 1978, 221.

37. Jacobson, H.R. and Kokko, J.P., Eds., Isolated perfused tubule symposium, Kidney Int., 22, No 5, 415, 1982.

38. Jacobson, H.R., Functional segmentation of the mammalian nephron, Am. J. Physiol., 241, F203, 1981.

39. Knepper, M. and Burg, M., Organization of nephron function, Am. J. Physiol., 244, F 579, 1983.

40. Koeppen, B.M. and Giebisch, G., Electrophysiology of mammalian renal tubules: Inferences from intracellular microelectrode studies, Annu. Rev. Physiol., 45, 497, 1983.

41. Greger, R., Application of electrical measurements in the isolated in vitro perfused tubule, Molec. Physiol., 8, 11, 1985.

42. Hanley, M.J. and Davidson, K., Prior mannitol and furosemide infusion in a model of ischemic acute renal failure, Am. J. Physiol., 241, F556, 1981.

43. Hanley, M.J., Isolated nephron segments in a rabbit model of ischemic acute renal failure, Am. J. Physiol., 239, F17, 1980.

44. Morel, F. and Doucet, A., Hormonal control of kidney functions at the cell level, Physiol. Rev., 66, 377, 1986.

45. Wirthensohn, G. and Guder, W.G., Renal substrate metabolism, Physiol. Rev., 66, 469, 1986.

46. Kurokawa, K., Use of isolated single nephron segments to study metabolic heterogeneity of the nephron, Mineral Electrolyte Metab., 9, 260, 1983.

47. Morel, F., Sites of hormone action in the mammalian nephron, Am. J. Physiol., 240, F159, 1981.

48. Imai, M., Torikai, S., Takeda, K., Mutou, S., Tabei, K., Kusano, E. and Asano, Y., The location and function of receptors along the nephron, in Monographs in Applied Toxicology, No 2: Renal Heterogeneity and Target Cell Toxicity, Bach, P.H. and Lock, E.A., Eds., Wiley, Chichester, 1985, 47.

49. Guder, W.G. and Ross, B.D., Enzyme distribution along the nephron, Kidney Int., 26, 101, 1984.

50. Klein, K.L., Wang, M.S., Torikai, S., Davidson, W.D. and Kurokawa, K., Substrate oxidation by isolated single nephron segments of the rat, Kidney Int., 20, 29, 1981.

51. Guder, W.G., Wagner, S. and Wirthensohn, G., Metabolic fuels along the nephron: Pathways and intracellular mechanisms of interaction, Kidney Int., 29, 41, 1986.

52. Imbert, M., Chabardès, D., Montégut, M., Clique, A. and Morel, F., Adenylate cyclase activity along the rabbit nephron as measured in single isolated segments, Pfluegers Arch., 354, 213, 1975.

53. Chabardès, D., Gagnan-Brunette, M., Imbert-Teboul, M., Gontcharevskaia, O., Montégut, M., Clique, A. and Morel, F., Adenylate cyclase responsiveness to hormones in various portions of the human nephron, J. Clin. Invest., 65, 439, 1980.

54. Imbert, M., Chabardès, D., Montegut, M., Clique, A. and Morel, F., Vasopressin dependent adenylate cyclase in single segments of rabbit kidney tubule, Pfluegers Arch., 357, 173, 1975.

55. Chabardès, D., Imbert, M., Clique, A., Montégut, M. and Morel, F., PTH sensitive adenyl cyclase activity in different segments of the rabbit nephron, Pfluegers Arch., 354, 229, 1975.

56. Chabardès, D., Imbert-Teboul, M., Montégut, M., Clique, A. and Morel, F., Distribution of calcitonin-sensitive adenylate cyclase activity along the rabbit kidney tubule, Proc. Natl. Acad. Sci. USA, 73, 3608, 1976.

57. Bailly, C., Imbert-Teboul, M., Chabardès, D., Hus-Citharel, A., Montégut, M., Clique, A. and Morel, F., The distal nephron of rat kidney: A target site for glucagon, Proc. Natl. Acad. Sci. USA, 77, 3422, 1980.

58. Umemura, S., Marver, D., Smyth, D.D. and Pettinger, W.A., α_2-adrenoceptors and cellular cAMP levels in single nephron segments from the rat, Am. J. Physiol., 249, F28, 1985.

59. Umemura, S., Smyth, D.D. and Pettinger, W.A., Regulation of renal cellular cAMP levels by prostaglandins and α_2-adrenoceptors: Microdissection studies, Kidney Int., 29, 703, 1986.

60. Chabardès, D., Imbert-Teboul, M., Montégut, M., Clique, A. and Morel, F., Catecholamine sensitive adenylate cyclase activity in different segments of the rabbit nephron, Pfluegers Arch., 361, 9, 1975.

61. Doucet, A. and Katz, A.I., High-affinity Ca-Mg-ATPase along the rabbit nephron, Am. J. Physiol., 242, F346, 1982.

62. Katz, A.I., Distribution and function of classes of ATPases along the nephron, Kidney Int., 29, 21, 1986.

63. Hersey, R.M., Gattone, V.H. and Weisz, J., [Na-K]ATPase activity in proximal and distal tubules of the rat kidney: Modification and application of a quantitative cytochemical technique, Cell Biochem. Function, 3, 255, 1985.

64. Doucet, A. and Katz, A.I., Mineralocorticoid receptors along the nephron: [^{3}H]aldosterone binding in rabbit tubules, Am. J. Physiol., 241, F605, 1981.

65. Farman, N. and Bonvalet, J.P., Aldosterone binding in isolated tubules. III. Autoradiography along the rat nephron, Am. J. Physiol., 245, F606, 1983.

66. Farman, N., Vandewalle, A. and Bonvalet, J.P., Autoradiographic determination of dexamethasone binding sites along the rabbit nephron, Am. J. Physiol., 244, F325, 1983.

67. Doucet, A. and Barlet, C., Evidence for differences in the sensitivity to ouabain of NaK-ATPase along the nephrons of rabbit kidney, J. Biol. Chem., 261, 993, 1986.

68. Garg, L.C. and Tisher, C.C., Effects of thyroid hormone on Na-K-adenosine triphosphatase activity along the rat nephron, J. Lab. Clin. Med., 106, 568, 1985.

69. Kawashima, H. and Kurokawa, K., Metabolism and sites of action of vitamin D in the kidney, Kidney Int., 29, 98, 1986.

70. Jackson, B.A., Edwards, R.M. and Dousa, T.P., Vasopressin-prostaglandin

interactions in isolated tubules from rat outer medulla, J. Lab. Clin. Med., 96, 119, 1980.

71.   Kusano, E., Nakamura, R., Asano, Y. and Imai, M., Distribution of alpha-adrenergic receptors in the rabbit nephron, Tohoku J. Exp. Med., 142, 275, 1984.

72.   Butlen, D. and Morel, F., Glucagon receptors along the nephron: [^{125}I]glucagon binding in rat tubules, Pfluegers Arch., 404, 348, 1985.

73.   Omata, K., Carretero, O.A., Scicli, A.G. and Jackson, B.A., Localization of active and inactive kallikrein (kininogenase activity) in the microdissected rabbit nephron, Kidney Int., 22, 602, 1982.

74.   Endou, H., Cytochrome P-450 monooxygenase system in the rabbit kidney: its intranephron localization and its induction, Jpn. J. Pharmacol., 33, 423, 1983.

75.   Hook, J.B., McCormack, K.M. and Kluwe, W.M., Biochemical mechanisms of nephrotoxicity, in Reviews in Biochemical Toxicology, Hodgson, E., Bend, J.R. and Philpot, R.M., Eds., Elsevier/North-Holland, New York, 1979, 53.

76.   Schäli, C. and Roch-Ramel, F., Transport and metabolism of [3H]morphine in isolated, nonperfused proximal tubular segments of the rabbit kidney, J. Pharmacol. Exp. Ther., 223, 811, 1982.

77.   Biber, T.U.L., Mylle, M., Baines, A.D., Gottschalk, C.W., Oliver, J.R. and MacDowell, M.C., A study by micropuncture and microdissection of acute renal damage in rats, Am. J. Med., 44, 664, 1968.

78.   Kramp, R.A., MacDowell, M., Gottschalk, C.W. and Oliver, J.R., A study by microdissection and micropuncture of the structure and the function of the kidneys and the nephrons of rats with chronic renal damage, Kidney Int., 5, 147, 1974.

79.   Weiner, I.M., Transport of weak acids and bases, in Handbook of Physiology, Section 8: Renal Physiology, Orloff, J. and Berliner, R.W., Eds., American Physiological Society, Washington, 1973, 521.

80.   Dantzler, W.H. and Bentley, S.K., Effects of sulfhydryl reagent, p-chloromercuribenzoate, on p-aminohippurate transport by isolated, perfused snake renal tubules, Renal Physiol., 6, 209, 1983.

81.   Dantzler, W.H. and Brokl, O.H., Effects of low [Ca^{2+}] and La^{3+} on PAH transport by isolated perfused renal tubules, Am. J. Physiol., 246, F175, 1984.

82.   Dantzler, W.H. and Brokl, O.H., Verapamil and quinidine effects on PAH transport by isolated perfused renal tubules, Am. J. Physiol., 246, F188, 1984.

83.   Stein, J.H., Lifschitz, M.D. and Barnes, L.D., Current concepts on the pathophysiology of acute renal failure, Am. J. Physiol., 234, F171, 1978.

84.   Hostetter, T.H., Wilkes, B.M. and Brenner, B.M., Renal circulatory and nephron function in experimental acute renal failure, in Acute Renal Failure, Brenner, B.M. and Lazarus, J.M., Eds., Saunders, Philadelphia, 1983, 99.

85.   Solez, K. and Whelton, A., Eds., Kidney Disease, Vol. 4: Acute Renal Failure: Correlations Between Morphology and Function, Dekker, New York, 1984.

86.   Brezis, M., Rosen, S. and Epstein, F.H., Acute renal failure, in The Kidney, Vol. 1, 3rd ed., Brenner, B.M. and Rector, F.C. Jr., Eds., Saunders, Philadelphia, 1986, 735.

87.   Porter, G.A. and Bennett, W.M., Nephrotoxic acute renal failure due to common drugs, Am. J. Physiol., 241, F1, 1981.

88.   Oken, D.E, Pathogenetic mechanisms in acute renal failure, in Toxicology of the Kidney, Hook, J.B., Ed., Raven Press, New York, 1981, 117.

89.   Thurau, K., Mason, J. and Gstraunthaler, G., Experimental acute renal

failure, in The Kidney: Physiology and Pathophysiology, Seldin, D.W. and Giebisch, G., Eds., Raven Press, New York, 1985, 1885.

90.   Mason, J., Olbricht, C., Takabatake, T. and Thurau, K., The early phase of experimental acute renal failure. 1. Intratubular pressure and obstruction, Pfluegers Arch., 370, 155, 1977.

91.   Flamenbaum, W., McDonald, F.D., DiBona, G.F. and Oken, D.E., Micropuncture study of renal tubular factors in low dose mercury poisoning, Nephron, 8, 221, 1971.

92.   Chopra, S., Kaufman, J.S., Jones, T.W., Hong, W.K., Gehr, M.K., Hamburger, R.J., Flamembaum, W. and Trump, B.F., Cis-diamminedichlorplatinum-induced acute renal failure in the rat, Kidney Int., 21, 54, 1982.

93.   Flamenbaum, W., Huddleston, M.L., McNeil, J.S. and Hamburger, R.J., Uranyl nitrate-induced acute renal failure in the rat: Micropuncture and renal hemodynamic studies, Kidney Int., 6, 408, 1974.

94.   Stein, J.H., Gottschall, J., Osgood, R.W. and Ferris, T.F., Pathophysiology of a nephrotoxic model of acute renal failure, Kidney Int., 8, 27, 1975.

95.   Blantz, R.C., The mechanism of acute renal failure after uranyl nitrate, J. Clin. Invest., 55, 621, 1975.

96.   Ruiz-Guiñazú, A., Coelho, J.B. and Paz, R.A., Methemoglobin-induced acute renal failure in the rat, Nephron, 4, 257, 1967.

97.   Oken, D.E., Arce, M.L. and Wilson, D.R., Glycerol-induced hemoglobinuric acute renal failure in the rat. 1: Micropuncture study of the development of oliguria, J. Clin. Invest., 45, 724, 1966.

98.   Cushner, H.M., Barnes, J.L., Stein, J.H. and Reineck, H.J., Role of volume depletion in the glycerol model of acute renal failure, Am. J. Physiol., 250, F315, 1986.

99.   Baylis, C., Rennke, H.R. and Brenner, B.M., Mechanisms of the defect in glomerular ultrafiltration associated with gentamicin administration, Kidney Int., 12, 344, 1977.

100. De Rougemont, D., Oeschger, A., Konrad, L., Thiel, G., Torhorst, J., Wenk, M., Wunderlich, P. and Brunner, F.P., Gentamicin-induced acute renal failure in the rat. Effect of dehydration, DOCA-saline and furosemide, Nephron, 29, 176, 1981.

101. Neugarten, J., Aynedjian, H.S. and Bank, N., Role of tubular obstruction in acute renal failure due to gentamicin, Kidney Int., 24, 330, 1983.

102. Huguenin, M.E., Birbaumer, A., Brunner, F.P., Thorhorst, J., Schmidt, U., Dubach, U.C. and Thiel, G., An evaluation of the role of tubular obstruction in folic acid-induced acute renal failure in the rat. A micropuncture study, Nephron, 22, 41, 1978.

103. Davis, J.M., Emslie, K.R., Sweet, R.S., Walker, L.L., Naughton, R.J., Skinner, S.L. and Tange, J.D., Early functional and morphological changes in renal tubular necrosis due to p-aminophenol, Kidney Int., 24, 740, 1983.

104. Ganeval, D., Grünfeld, J.P., Eloy, L., Lacour, B., Russo-Marie, F., Noël, L.H. and Anagnostopoulos, T., Glaphenine-induced acute renal failure in the rat: a new experimental model, Am. J. Physiol., 243, F416, 1982.

105. Racusen, L.C., Finn, W.F., Whelton, A. and Solez, K., Mechanisms of lysine-induced acute renal failure in rats, Kidney Int., 27, 517, 1985.

106. Weiss, J.H., Williams, R.H., Galla, J.H., Gottschall, J.L., Rees, E.D., Bhathena, D. and Luke, R.G., Pathophysiology of acute Bence-Jones protein nephrotoxicity in the rat, Kidney Int., 20, 198, 1981.

107. Tanner, G.A. and Sophasan, S., Kidney pressures after temporary renal artery occlusion in the rat, Am. J. Physiol., 230, 1173, 1976.

108. Arendshorst, W.J., Finn, W.F. and Gottschalk, C.W., Pathogenesis of acute renal failure following temporary renal ischemia in the rat, Circ. Res., 37,

558, 1975.

109. De Rougemont, D., Brunner, F.P., Torhorst, J., Wunderlich, P.F. and Thiel, G., Superficial nephron obstruction and medullary congestion after ischemic injury: Effect of protective treatments, Nephron, 31, 310, 1982.

110. Parekh, N., Esslinger, H.U. and Steinhausen, M., Glomerular filtration and tubular reabsorption during anuria in postischemic acute renal failure, Kidney Int., 25, 33, 1984.

111. Burke, T.J., Cronin, R.E., Duchin, K.L., Peterson, L.N. and Schrier, R.W., Ischemia and tubule obstruction during acute renal failure in dogs: mannitol in protection, Am. J. Physiol., 238, F305, 1980.

112. Conger, J.D., Robinette, J.B. and Kelleher, S.P., Nephron heterogeneity in ischemic acute renal failure, Kidney Int., 26, 422, 1984.

113. Bank, N., Mutz, B.F. and Aynedjian, H.S., The role of "leakage" of tubular fluid in anuria due to mercury poisoning, J. Clin. Invest., 46, 695, 1967.

114. Huguenin, M., Thiel, G. and Brunner, F.P., $HgCl_2$-induced acute renal failure studied by split drop micropuncture technique in the rat, Nephron, 20, 147, 1978.

115. Flanigan, W.J. and Oken, D.E., Renal micropuncture study of the development of anuria in the rat with mercury-induced acute renal failure, J. Clin. Invest., 44, 449, 1965.

116. Olbricht, C., Mason, J., Takabatake, T., Hohlbrugger, G. and Thurau, K., The early phase of experimental acute renal failure. II. Tubular leakage and the reliability of glomerular markers, Pfluegers Arch., 372, 251, 1977.

117. Vanholder, R.C., Praet, M.M., Pattyn, P.A., Leusen, I.R. and Lameire, N.H., Dissociation of glomerular filtration and renal blood flow in $HgCl_2$-induced acute renal failure, Kidney Int., 22, 162, 1982.

118. Cheng, J.T., Witty, R.T., Robinson, R.R. and Yarger, W.E., Amphotericin B nephrotoxicity: Increased renal resistance and tubule permeability, Kidney Int., 22, 626, 1982.

119. Safirstein, R., Miller, P. and Kahn, T., Cortical and papillary absorptive defects in gentamicin nephrotoxicity, Kidney Int., 24, 526, 1983.

120. Tanner, G.A., Sloan, K.L. and Sophasan, S., Effects of renal artery occlusion on kidney function in the rat, Kidney Int., 4, 377, 1973.

121. Donohoe, J.F., Venkatachalam, M.A., Bernard, D.B. and Levinsky, N.G., Tubular leakage and obstruction after renal ischemia: Structural-functional correlations, Kidney Int., 13, 208, 1978.

122. Myers, B.D. and Moran, S.M., Hemodynamically mediated acute renal failure, New Engl. J. Med., 314, 97, 1986.

123. Brenner, B.M., Dworkin, L.D. and Ichikawa, I., Glomerular ultrafiltration, in The Kidney, Vol. 1, 3rd ed., Brenner, B.M. and Rector, F.C. Jr., Eds., Saunders, Philadelphia, 1986, 124.

124. Dworkin, L.D., Ichikawa, I. and Brenner, B.M., Hormonal modulation of glomerular function, Am. J. Physiol., 244, F95, 1983.

125. Schor, N., Ichikawa, I., Rennke, H.G., Troy, J.L. and Brenner, B.M., Pathophysiology of altered glomerular function in aminoglycoside-treated rats, Kidney Int., 19, 288, 1981.

126. Blantz, R.C., Konnen, K.S. and Tucker, B.J., Angiotensin II effects upon the glomerular microcirculation and ultrafiltration coefficient of the rat, J. Clin. Invest., 57, 419, 1976.

127. Myers, B.D., Deen, W.M. and Brenner, B.M., Effects of norepinephrine and angiotensin II on the determinants of glomerular ultrafiltration and proximal tubule fluid reabsorption in the rat, Circ. Res., 37, 101, 1975.

128. Wright, F.S. and Briggs, J.P., Feedback control of glomerular blood flow, pressure and filtration rate, Physiol. Rev., 59, 958, 1979.

129. Schnermann, J. and Briggs, J., Concentration-dependent sodium chloride transport as the signal in feedback control of glomerular filtration rate, Kidney Int., 22, Suppl. 12, S-82, 1982.

130. Blantz, R.C. and Pelayo, J.C., A functional role for the tubuloglomerular feedback mechanism, Kidney Int., 25, 739, 1984.

131. Mason, J., Takabatake, T., Olbricht, C. and Thurau, K., The early phase of experimental acute renal failure. III. Tubuloglomerular feedback, Pfluegers Arch., 373, 69, 1978.

132. Mason, J., Kain, H., Welsch, J. and Schnermann, J., The early phase of experimental acute renal failure. VI. The influence of furosemide, Pfluegers Arch., 392, 125, 1981.

133. Tanner, G.A., Tubuloglomerular feedback after nephron or ureteral obstruction, Am. J. Physiol., 248, F688, 1985.

134. Flamenbaum, W., Kaufman, J., Chopra, S., Gehr, M. and Hamburger, R., Heavy metal models of experimental acute renal failure, in Nephrotoxic Mechanims of Drugs and Environmental Toxins, Porter, G.A., Ed., Plenum, New York, 1982, 65.

135. Wunderlich, P., Tubuloglomerular feedback in the rat initiated by serum activity in patients with acute renal failure, Kidney Int., 22, Suppl. 12, S-219, 1982.

136. Schwartz, J.H., Effect of heavy metals on sodium transport in vitro, in Nephrotoxic Mechanisms of Drugs and Environmental Toxins, Porter, G.A., Ed., Plenum, New York, 1982, 25.

137. Flamenbaum, W., Hamburger, R. and Kaufman, J., Distal tubule [Na+] and juxtaglomerular apparatus renin activity in uranyl nitrate induced acute renal failure in the rat. An evaluation of the role of tubuloglomerular feedback, Pfluegers Arch., 364, 209, 1976.

138. Mason, J., Gutsche, H.U., Moore, L. and Müller-Suur, R., The early phase of experimental acute renal failure. IV: The diluting ability of the short loops of Henle, Pfluegers Arch., 379, 11, 1979.

139. Safirstein, R., Miller, P., Dikman, S., Lyman, N. and Shapiro, C., Cisplatin nephrotoxicity in rats: defect in papillary hypertonicity, Am. J. Physiol., 241, F175, 1981.

140. Venkatachalam, M.A., Bernard, D.B., Donohoe, J.F. and Levinsky, N.G., Ischemic damage and repair in the rat proximal tubule: Differences among the S_1, S_2 and S_3 segments, Kidney Int., 14, 31, 1978.

141. Hanley, M.J., Studies on acute disease models, Kidney Int., 22, 536, 1982.

142. Thiel, G., de Rougemont, D., Torhorst, J., Kaufmann, A., Peters-Haefeli, L. and Brunner, F.P., Importance of tubular obstruction and its prevention in ischemic acute renal failure in the rat, in Renal Pathophysiology, Leaf, A., et al., Eds., Raven Press, New York, 1980, 223.

143. Mason, J., Welsch, J. and Takabatake, T., Disparity between surface and deep nephron function early after renal ischemia, Kidney Int., 24, 27, 1983.

144. Kramp, R.A. and Lorentz, W.B., Glucose transport in chronically altered rat nephrons, Am. J. Physiol., 243, F393, 1982.

145. Harris, R.C., Meyer, T.W. and Brenner, B.M., Nephron adaptation to renal injury, in The Kidney, Vol. 1, 3rd ed., Brenner, B.M. and Rector, F.C. Jr., Eds., Saunders, Philadelphia, 1986, 1553.

146. Hostetter, T.H., Olson, J.L., Rennke, H.G., Venkatachalam, M.A. and Brenner, B.M., Hyperfiltration in remnant nephrons: a potentially adverse response to renal ablation, Am. J. Physiol., 241, F85, 1981.

147. Pastoriza-Munoz, E., Timmerman, D. and Kaloyanides, G.J., Renal transport of netilmicin in the rat, J. Pharmacol. Exp. Ther., 228, 65, 1984.

148. Pastoriza-Munoz, E., Timmerman, D., Feldman, S. and Kaloyanides, G.J.,

Ultrafiltration of gentamicin and netilmicin in vivo, J. Pharmacol. Exp. Ther., 220, 604, 1982.

149. Pastoriza-Munoz, E., Bowman, R.L. and Kaloyanides, G.J., Renal tubular transport of gentamicin in the rat, Kidney Int., 16, 440, 1979.

150. Senekjian, H.O., Knight, T.F. and Weinman, E.J., Micropuncture study of the handling of gentamicin by the rat kidney, Kidney Int., 19, 416, 1981.

151. Frommer, J.P., Senekjian, H.O., Babino, H., Weinman, E.J., Intratubular microinjection study of gentamicin transport in the rat, Mineral Electrolyte Metab., 9, 108, 1983.

152. Sheth, A.U., Senekjian, H.O., Babino, H., Knight, T.F. and Weinman, E.J., Renal handling of gentamicin by the Munich-Wistar rat, Am. J. Physiol., 241, F645, 1981.

153. Vandewalle, A., Farman, N., Morin, J.P., Fillastre, J.P., Hatt, P.Y. and Bonvalet, J.P., Gentamicin incorporation along the nephron: Autoradiographic study on isolated tubules, Kidney Int., 19, 529, 1981.

154. Klotman, P.E. and Yarger, W.E., Reduction of renal blood flow and proximal bicarbonate reabsorption in rats by gentamicin, Kidney Int., 24, 638, 1983.

155. Savin, V., Karniski, L., Cuppage, F., Hodges, G. and Chonko, A., Effect of gentamicin on isolated glomeruli and proximal tubules of the rabbit, Lab. Invest., 52, 93, 1985.

156. Thiel, G., Nephrotoxicity of ciclosporin, Trends Pharmacol. Sci., 7, 167, 1986.

157. Myers, B.D., Ross, J., Newton, L., Luetscher, J. and Perlroth, M., Cyclosporine-associated chronic nephropathy, New Engl. J. Med., 311, 699, 1984

158. Dieperink, H., Leyssac, P.P., Starklint, H. and Kemp, E., Nephrotoxicity of cyclosporin A. A lithium clearance and micropuncture study in rats, Eur. J. Clin. Invest., 16, 69, 1986.

159. Müller-Suur, R. and Davis, S.D., Effect of cyclosporine A on renal electrolyte transport: whole kidney and Henle loop study, Clin. Nephrol., 25, Suppl. 1, S-57, 1986.

160. Gnutzmann, K.H., Hering, K. and Gutsche, H.U., Effect of cyclosporine on the diluting capacity of the rat kidney, Clin. Nephrol., 25, Suppl. 1, S-51, 1986.

161. Murray, B.M., Paller, M.S. and Ferris, T.F., Effect of cyclosporine administration on renal hemodynamics in conscious rats, Kidney Int., 28, 767, 1985.

162. Moss, N.G., Powell, S.L. and Falk, R.J., Intravenous cyclosporine activates afferent and efferent renal nerves and causes sodium retention in innervated kidneys in rats, Proc. Natl. Acad. Sci. USA, 82, 8222, 1985.

163. Burnatowska-Hledin, M.A., Mayor, G.H. and Lau, K., Renal handling of aluminium in the rat: clearance and micropuncture studies, Am. J. Physiol., 249, F192, 1985.

164. Brazy, P.C., Balaban, R.S., Gullans, S.R., Mandel, L.J. and Dennis, V.W., Inhibition of renal metabolism. Relative effects of arsenate on sodium, phosphate and glucose transport by the rabbit proximal tubule, J. Clin. Invest., 66, 1211, 1980.

165. Bosco, E., Porta, N. and Diezi, J., Renal handling of cadmium: A study by tubular microinjections, Arch. Toxicol., Suppl. 7, 371, 1984.

166. Mavichak, V., Wong, N.L.M., Quamme, G.A., Magil, A.B., Sutton, R.A.L. and Dirks, J.H., Studies on the pathogenesis of cisplatin-induced hypomagnesemia in rats, Kidney Int., 28, 914, 1985.

167. Allen, G.G. and Barratt, L.J., Effect of cisplatin on the transepithelial potential difference of rat distal tubule, Kidney Int., 27, 842, 1985.

168. Aviv, A., John, E., Bernstein, J., Goldsmith, D.I. and Spitzer, A., Lead intoxication during development: Its late effects on kidney function and blood pressure, Kidney Int., 17, 430, 1980.

169. Hayslett, J.P. and Kashgarian, M., A micropuncture study of the renal handling of lithium, Pfluegers Arch., 380, 159, 1979.

170. Corman, B., Roinel, N. and de Rouffignac, C., Dependence of water movement on sodium transport in kidney proximal tubule: A microperfusion study substituting lithium for sodium, J. Membrane Biol., 62, 105, 1981.

171. Mahnensmith, R.L. and Aronson, P.S., Interrelationships among quinidine, amiloride and lithium as inhibitors of the renal Na^+-H^+ exchanger, J. Biol. Chem., 260, 12586, 1985.

172. Myers, J.B., Morgan, T.O., Carney, S.L. and Ray, C., Effects of lithium on the kidney, Kidney Int., 18, 601, 1980.

173. Hecht, B., Kashgarian, M., Forrest, J.N. Jr. and Hayslett, J.P., Micropuncture study on the effects of lithium on proximal and distal tubule function in the rat kidney, Pfluegers Arch., 377, 69, 1978.

174. Carney, S.L., Wong., N.L.M. and Dirks, J.H., Effect of lithium treatment on rat renal tubule function. Evidence against impaired antidiuretic hormone action, Nephron, 25, 293, 1980.

175. Carney, S., Rayson, B. and Morgan, T., The effect of lithium on the permeability response induced in the collecting duct by antidiuretic hormone, Pfluegers Arch., 366, 19, 1976.

176. Cogan, E. and Abramow, M., Inhibition by lithium of the hydroosmotic action of vasopressin in the isolated perfused cortical collecting tubule of the rabbit, J. Clin. Invest., 77, 1507, 1986.

177. Jackson, B.A., Edwards, R.M. and Dousa, T.P., Lithium-induced polyuria: Effect of lithium on adenylate cyclase and adenosine 3',5'-monophosphate phosphodiesterase in medullary ascending limb of Henle's loop and in medullary collecting tubules, Endocrinology, 107, 1693, 1980.

178. Cikrt, M. and Heller, J., Renal tubular handling of $^{203}Hg^{2+}$ in the dog: A microinjection study, Environ. Res., 21, 308, 1980.

179. Balfour, W.E., Grantham, J.J. and Glynn, I.M., Vanadate-stimulated natriuresis, Nature, 275, 768, 1978.

180. Higashi, Y. and Bello-Reuss, E., Effects of sodium orthovanadate on whole kidney and single nephron function, Kidney Int., 18, 302, 1980.

181. Edwards, R.M. and Grantham, J.J., Effect of vanadate on fluid absorption and PAH secretion in isolated proximal tubules, Am. J. Physiol., 244, F367, 1983.

182. Edwards, R.M. and Grantham, J.J., Inhibition of vasopressin action by vanadate in the cortical collecting tubule, Am. J. Physiol., 245, F772, 1983.

183. Duggin, G.G., Mechanisms in the development of analgesic nephropathy, Kidney Int., 18, 553, 1980.

184. Rush, G.F., Newton, J.F. and Hook, J.B., Metabolic activation of chemicals and toxic nephropathies, in Monographs in Applied Toxicology, No 2: Renal Heterogeneity and Target Cell Toxicity, Bach, P.H. and Lock, E.A., Eds., Wiley, Chichester, 1985, 107.

185. Newton, J.F., Braselton, W.E. Jr., Kuo, C.H., Kluwe, W.M., Gemborys, M.W., Mudge, G.H. and Hook, J.B., Metabolism of acetaminophen by the isolated perfused kidney, J. Pharmacol. Exp. Ther., 221, 76, 1982.

186. Mudge, G.H., Gemborys, M.W. and Duggin, G.G., Covalent binding of metabolites of acetaminophen to kidney protein and depletion of renal glutathione, J. Pharmacol. Exp. Ther., 206, 218, 1978.

187. McMurty, R.J., Snodgrass, W.R. and Mitchell, J.R., Renal necrosis,

glutathione depletion and covalent binding after acetaminophen, Toxicol. Appl. Pharmacol., 46, 87, 1978.

188. Endou, H., Koseki, C., Hasumura, S., Kakuno, K., Hojo, K. and Sakai, F., Renal cytochrome P450 ; its localization along a single nephron and its induction, in INSERM Symposium, No 21: Biochemistry of Kidney Functions, Morel, F., Ed., Elsevier, Amsterdam, 1982, 319.

189. Mohandas, J., Duggin, G.G., Horvath, J.S. and Tiller, D.J., Metabolic oxidation of acetaminophen (paracetamol) mediated by cytochrome P-450 mixed-function oxidase and prostaglandin endoperoxide synthetase in rabbit kidney, Toxicol. Appl. Pharmacol., 61, 252, 1981.

190. Boyd, J.A. and Eling, T.E., Prostaglandin endoperoxide synthetase-dependent cooxidation of acetaminophen to intermediates which covalently bind in vitro to rabbit renal medullary microsomes, J. Pharmacol. Exp. Ther., 219, 659, 1981.

191. Roch-Ramel, F., Roth, L., Arnow, J. and Weiner, I.M., Salicylate excretion in the rat; free flow micropuncture experiments, J. Pharmacol. Exp. Ther., 207, 737, 1978.

192. Schild, L. and Roch-Ramel, F., Mechanisms involved in the reabsorption of salicylate in the proximal tubule of rabbits, in Progress in Clinical and Biological Research, Vol. 164: Information and Energy Transduction in Biological Membranes, Bolis, C.L., Helmreich, E.J.M. and Passow, H., Eds., A.R. Liss, New York, 1984, 417.

193. Ferrier, B., Martin, M. and Roch-Ramel, F., Effects of p-aminohippurate and pyrazinoate on the renal excretion of salicylate in the rat: A micropuncture study, J. Pharmacol. Exp. Ther., 224, 451, 1983.

194. Spencer, H.W., Yarger, W.E. and Robinson, R.R., Alterations of renal function during dietary-induced hyperuricemia in the rat, Kidney Int., 9, 489, 1976.

195. Conger, J.D., Falk, S.A., Guggenheim, S.J. and Burke, T.J., A micropuncture study of the early phase of acute urate nephropathy, J. Clin. Invest., 58, 681, 1976.

196. Conger, J.D. and Falk, S.A., Intrarenal dynamics in the pathogenesis and prevention of acute urate nephropathy, J. Clin. Invest., 59, 786, 1977.

197. Cook, M.A. and Adkinson, J.T., A micropuncture study of a dietary induced, hyperuricemic model of acute renal failure in the rat, Proc. Soc. Exp. Biol. Med., 163, 187, 1980.

198. Roch-Ramel, F. and Peters, G., Urinary excretion of uric acid in nonhuman mammalian species, in Handbook of Experimental Pharmacology, Vol. 51: Uric Acid, Kelley, W.N. and Weiner, I.M., Eds., Springer, Berlin, 1978, 211.

199. Weiner, I.M., Urate transport in the nephron, Am. J. Physiol., 237, F85, 1979.

200. Kahn, A.M. and Weinman, E.J., Urate transport in the proximal tubule: in vivo and vesicle studies, Am. J. Physiol., 249, F789, 1985.

201. Bergeron, M. and Vadeboncoeur, M., Microinjections of L-leucine into tubules and peritubular capillaries of the rat. II. The maleic acid model, Nephron, 8, 367, 1971.

202. Bergeron, M., Dubord, L. and Hausser, C., Membrane permeability as a cause of transport defects in experimental Fanconi syndrome. A new hypothesis, J. Clin. Invest., 57, 1181, 1976.

203. Maesaka, J.K. and McCaffery, M., Evidence for renal tubular leakage in maleic acid-induced Fanconi syndrome, Am. J. Physiol., 239, F507, 1980.

204. Günther, R., Silbernagl, S. and Deetjen, P., Maleic acid induced aminoaciduria, studied by free flow micropuncture and continuous microperfusion, Pfluegers Arch., 382, 109, 1979.

205. Bank, N., Aynedjian, H.S. and Mutz, B.F., Microperfusion study of proximal tubule bicarbonate transport in maleic acid-induced renal tubular acidosis, Am. J. Physiol., 250, F476, 1986.

206. Brewer, E.D., Senekjian, H.O., Ince, A. and Weinman, E.J., Maleic acid-induced reabsorptive dysfunction in the proximal and distal nephron, Am. J. Physiol., 245, F339, 1983.

207. Rebouças, N.A., Fernandes, D.T., Elias, M.M., de Mello-Aires, M. and Malnic, G., Proximal tubular HCO_3, H^+ and fluid transport during maleate-induced acidification defect, Pfluegers Arch., 401, 266, 1984.

208. Weiner, I.M., Organic acids and bases and uric acid, in The Kidney: Physiology and Pathophysiology, Vol. 2, Seldin, D.W. and Giebisch, G., Eds., Raven Press, 1985, 1703.

209. Tune, B.M., Burg, M.B. and Patlak, C.S., Characteristics of p-aminohippurate transport in proximal renal tubules, Am. J. Physiol., 217, 1057, 1969.

210. Woodhall, P.B., Tisher, C.C., Simonton, C.A. and Robinson, R.R., Relationship between para-aminohippurate secretion and cellular morphology in rabbit proximal tubules, J. Clin. Invest., 61, 1320, 1978.

211. Roch-Ramel, F., White, F., Vowles, L., Simmonds, H.A. and Cameron, J.S., Micropuncture study of tubular transport of urate and PAH in the pig kidney, Am. J. Physiol., 239, F107, 1980.

212. Schäli, C. and Roch-Ramel, F., Accumulation of [^{14}C]urate and [^{3}H]PAH in isolated proximal tubular segments of the rabbit kidney, Am. J. Physiol., 239, F222, 1980.

213. Schäli, C. and Roch-Ramel, F., Uptake of [^{3}H]PAH and [^{14}C]urate into isolated proximal tubular segments of the pig kidney, Am. J. Physiol., 241, F591, 1981.

214. Berner, W. and Kinne, R., Transport of p-aminohippuric acid by plasma membrane vesicles isolated from rat kidney cortex, Pfluegers Arch., 361, 269, 1976.

215. Guggino, S.E., Martin, G.J. and Aronson, P.S., Specificity and modes of the anion exchanger in dog renal microvillus membranes, Am. J. Physiol., 244, F612, 1983.

216. Tune, B.M. and Fravert, D., Mechanisms of cephalosporin nephrotoxicity: A comparison of cephaloridine and cephaloglycin, Kidney Int., 18, 591, 1980.

217. Bergeron, M.G., Gennari, F.J., Barza, M., Weinstein, L., Cortell, S., Renal tubular transport of penicillin G and carbenicillin in the rat, J. Infect. Dis., 132, 374, 1975.

218. Weiner, I.M. and Tinker, J.P., Pharmacology of pyrazinamide: Metabolic and renal function studies related to the mechanism of drug-induced urate retention, J. Pharmacol. Exp. Ther., 180, 411, 1972.

219. Besseghir, K. and Roch-Ramel, F., Pyrazinoate transport in the isolated perfused rabbit proximal tubule, Pfluegers Arch., 1986, 407, 643

220. Mosig, D., Schäli, C. and Roch-Ramel, F., Uptake of pyrazinoate (PZA) by isolated, nonperfused proximal renal tubules of rabbit, Experientia, 39, 682, 1983.

221. Krogh, P., Hald, B. and Pedersen, E.J., Occurrence of ochratoxin A and citrinin in cereals associated with mycotoxic porcine nephropathy, Acta Pathol. Microbiol. Scand., B81, 689, 1973.

222. Endou, H., Obara, T. and Ueno, Y., Use of isolated nephron segments and isolated renal cells for the evaluation of nephrotoxicity, in Monographs in Applied Toxicology, No 2: Renal Heterogeneity and Target Cell Toxicity, Bach, P.H. and Lock, E.A., Eds., Wiley, Chichester, 1985, 535.

223. Rennick, B.R., Renal tubule transport of organic cations, Am. J. Physiol., 240, F83, 1981.

224. Acara, M., Roch-Ramel, F. and Rennick, B., Bidirectional renal tubular transport of free choline: a micropuncture study, Am. J. Physiol., 236, F112, 1979.

225. Ross, C.R., Diezi-Chométy, F. and Roch-Ramel, F., Renal excretion of N^1-methylnicotinamide in the rat, Am. J. Physiol., 228, 1641, 1975.

226. McKinney, T.D., Myers, P. and Speeg, K.V. Jr., Cimetidine secretion by rabbit renal tubules in vitro, Am. J. Physiol., 241, F69, 1981.

227. McKinney, T.D. and Speeg, K.V. Jr., Cimetidine and procainamide secretion by proximal tubules in vitro, Am. J. Physiol., 242, F672, 1982.

228. McKinney, T.D., Heterogeneity of organic base secretion by proximal tubules, Am. J. Physiol., 243, F404, 1982.

229. Besseghir, K., Pearce, L.B. and Rennick, B., Renal tubular transport and metabolism of organic cations by the rabbit, Am. J. Physiol., 241, F308, 1981.

230. Schäli, C., Schild, L., Overney, J. and Roch-Ramel, F., Secretion of tetraethylammonium by proximal tubules of rabbit kidneys, Am. J. Physiol., 245, F238, 1983.

11
PROSTAGLANDINS AND OTHER EICOSANOIDS

K. CROWSHAW

INTRODUCTION

The biosynthetic capacity of the mammalian kidney to produce prostaglandins is exceeded only by the seminal vesicles. Although the medulla is the major site of synthesis in the kidney, an appreciable and physiologically important synthesis also occurs in the glomeruli, arterioles and collecting ducts. Aspirin and the non-steroidal anti-inflammatory (NSAI) agents are potent inhibitors of prostaglandin synthase[1,2]. Vane[1] suggested that most of the side effects produced by this class of drugs were a consequence of the decreased tissue production of specific prostaglandins, which normally exerted protective effects[3]. It has since been assumed that the renal toxicity of NSAIs arises from the inhibition of renal prostaglandin production. Accordingly, renal prostaglandins should also protect the kidney from the effects of non-NSAI drug or disease-induced renal damage. In recent years other metabolites of arachidonic acid have been discovered with a wide range of biological activities. The diversity of products complicates our understanding of their role in renal function, especially when we try to explore their role in nephrotoxicity. In this chapter our present understanding of the function of the renal prostaglandins will be reviewed, and related to various animal models of nephrotoxicity and human renal disease.

RENAL EICOSANOIDS

Prostaglandins are autocoids (local hormones) which are synthesized near their site of action and then enzymatically inactivated. Arachidonic acid is the major substrate for the synthesis of prostaglandins. This essential fatty acid is an important constituent of cell membrane phospholipids, where it is present in high concentrations. Arachidonic acid can be released by the action of two calcium-dependent phospholipases; phospholipase A_2 which acts on phosphatidylcholine and phospholipase C which acts on phosphatidylinositol[4]. The two major pathways for the conversion of the arachidonic acid to prostaglandins and other products are shown in Figure 1. In recent years these products have been termed eicosanoids, and include all the oxygenated products of arachidonic acid produced both from the cyclo-oxygenase[4] and lipoxygenase pathways[5]. More recently a series of epoxygenase enzymes have been identified in the cells of the thin ascending limb of Henle which form a series of stable arachidonic acid epoxides and their related dihydroxy-arachidonic acids[6]. Since the biological actions of these products have not yet been fully defined, they will not be discussed.

The cyclo-oxygenase enzyme converts arachidonic acid to two very potent endoperoxides, PGG_2 and PGH_2. Although these two compounds have biological activities[4] their physiological importance is that they are short-lived intermediates, with a half-life of several minutes, and are substrates for the three different enzymes which form the prostaglandins (PGE_2, PGD_2 and $PGF_{2\alpha}$), the thromboxanes (TxA_2) and prostacyclin (PGI_2).

The isolation and identification of PGE_2 and $PGF_{2\alpha}$ from rabbit renal medulla was first reported by Lee et al.[7]. Although $PGF_{2\alpha}$ is a potent venoconstrictor in other organs, it has no effect on blood flow in the kidney, and no renal role has been found for it to date. The major haemodynamic action of PGE_2 in the renal medulla arises from its profound vasodilatation of blood vessels and its ability to modulate the effect of vasoconstrictor stimuli[8]. Prostaglandin E_2 is also involved in the regulation of sodium and chloride excretion, and in the modulation of water excretion[8,9]. The two major sites of medullary synthesis of PGE_2 are the interstitial cells and the collecting tubules, both of which synthesize very large quantities of this stable prostaglandin. In addition, the medullary microvasculature synthesizes much smaller quantities of prostacyclin[10].

The pattern of synthesis of eicosanoids in the cortex is different both qualitatively and quantitatively. Depending on the species the cortex produces between 1 and 10% of the quantities of PGE_2 and $PGF_{2\alpha}$ synthesized by the medulla. The most important difference involves the cortical glomeruli. Human glomeruli synthesize PGI_2 predominantly, in contrast to rat glomeruli which produce more PGE_2 than prostacyclin. The most important role of this glomerular prostacyclin is the stimulation of renin secretion by the juxtaglomerular cells[10-12]. The cortical collecting duct produces mainly PGE_2 and the arterioles produce prostacyclin. These smaller quantities of PGE_2 and PGI_2 probably contribute to the control of cortical blood flow and glomerular filtration rate.

EFFECT OF NSAIs ON RENAL FUNCTION

Experiments in anaesthetized dogs[13] showed a relationship between renal blood flow and synthesis of renal of PGE_2 as measured in the renal venous blood, but Zins[14] did not observe changed renal blood flow in indomethacin-treated, conscious dogs. Neither indomethacin nor sodium meclofenamate (two structurally unrelated NSAIs) altered renal blood flow in conscious dogs in which renal arterial flow probes had been implanted 7 days earlier, despite a 75% decrease in prostaglandin synthesis[15]. These data and other experiments have indicated that the renal prostaglandins do not play a major role in the control of renal blood flow or glomerular filtration rate in healthy animals.

The results obtained by Lonigro et al.[13] suggest that activation of the sympathetic nervous system, and the renin-angiotensin system in their surgically stressed anaesthetized dogs, resulted in an increased renal release of PGE_2. McGiff and co-workers[8,9,16] had previously shown that vasoconstrictor interventions such as renal artery constriction, renal nerve stimulation, and intra-arterial infusions of norepinephrine or angiotensin II, all resulted in the release of renal PGE_2.

Inhibition of renal prostaglandin synthesis in the presence of such vasoconstrictor stimuli substantially increases the vaso-constrictor responses to the stimuli. It is reasonable to assume that the increased vasoconstrictor response is due to the removal of PGE_2 which normally has a defensive function. This concept was first proposed by Collier[3], who suggested that the function of prostaglandins is to mediate defensive reactions to noxious in-fluences and described aspirin and other NSAIs as "anti-defensive agents". Recent studies by Nadler et al.[17] have confirmed that these vasoconstrictor agents (e.g. angiotensin II) can also release renal prostaglandin E_2 in man. Both PGE_2 and PGI_2 were released by infusions of norepinephrine, although this release did not al-ways occur in parallel.

INVOLVEMENT OF RENAL EICOSANOIDS IN ANALGESIC NEPHROPATHY

There is no single convincing explanation for analgesic neph-ropathy in man[18]. It has been suggested[19] that NSAIs decrease renal production of PGE_2 (and PGI_2) which would allow local vasoconstrictor influences to progress unopposed. However, this increased renal vasoconstriction may only be one factor in the sub-sequent development of nephropathy. Normally the arachidonic acid cyclo-oxygenase forms PGG_2, which is then a substrate for the en-zyme prostaglandin hydroperoxidase. The product PGH_2, which is a 15-OH endoperoxide of arachidonic acid, can then be converted to other prostaglandins, PGI_2 and TxA_2. An increased formation of toxic metabolites of NSAIs or of analgesics could be produced by peroxidative enzymes in the kidney. This concept has been ex-plored in detail[20], and has led to a working hypothesis to explain the pathogenesis of renal papillary necrosis and urothelial car-cinoma. The basis of this hypothesis is that a number of reactive intermediates formed by hydroperoxides could generate other biologically reactive oxygen species. There could also be increased free radical formation from prostaglandin and fatty acid hydroperoxidases. The medullary interstitial cells contain very large quantities of polyunsaturated fatty acids which could them-selves be enzymatically converted to lipid peroxides, eicosanoids

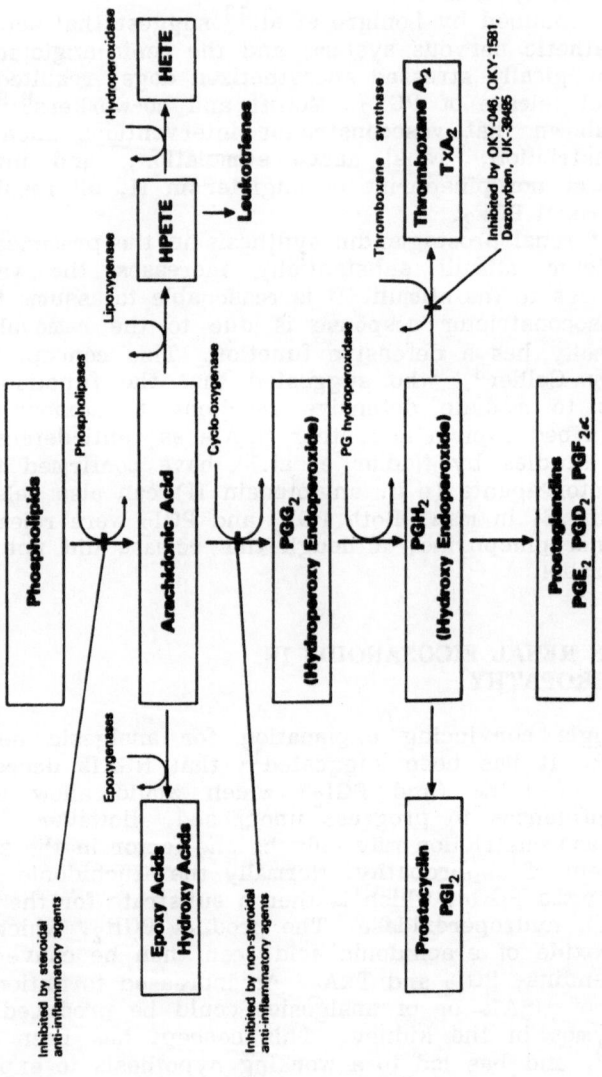

Figure 1 The arachidonic cascade. This scheme shows the synthesis of eicosanoids from arachidonic acid. Drugs which are capable of inhibiting enzymes participating in this cascade process are shown. PG = prostaglandin; HPETE = hydroperoxyeicosatetraenoic acid; HETE = hydroxyeicosatetraenoic acid.

produced by the lipoxygenase pathway shown in Figure 1. The role of such intermediates in the generation of free radicals is well documentated and known to produce injurious effects in the surrounding tissue.

However, in patients treated with a NSAI agent the enzyme cyclo-oxygenase is inhibited (in the case of aspirin it is an irreversible inhibition), but the hydroperoxidase is much more resistant to inhibition, and can accept other hydroperoxides as substrate. An alternative substrate could be 15-hydroperoxyeicosatetraenoic acid (15-HPETE) which is known to be generated in renal tissue[21]. Two drugs which are known to be activated to highly electrophilic products by such lipid hydroperoxides are phenacetin and acetaminophen (paracetamol). These intermediates could be the toxic agents responsible for the drug-induced medullary cell necrosis and cause damage to the urothelial cell nuclear material and initiate genotoxic changes. This hypothesis is attractive for two reasons. It accounts for the observation that the incidence of renal damage by high doses of aspirin alone in animals and patients is very small. Kerr[22] concluded that arthritic patients taking large doses of aspirin had no serious impairment of renal function. This suggested that if aspirin alone did cause analgesic nephropathy, it was "a sufficiently rare event that the risk need not weigh heavily in the choice of anti-rheumatic drug".

However, the incidence of analgesic nephropathy is much higher when a combination of NSAI agent and phenacetin is administered, both in animals and in man[18-20,22]. There has been considerable debate about the involvement of phenacetin when present as a mixture with other NSAI agents, as the cause of analgesic nephropathy[23]. However, one convincing piece of evidence which does incriminate phenacetin is the observed reduction in the incidence of analgesic nephropathy following the restrictions in its use in a number of countries[22]. It is inevitable that patients who have to take large doses of a NSAI drug for long periods may also have to take a number of different medicines for other diseases, some of which may have nephrotoxic potential. The kidneys of these patients may be subjected to various circulating vasoconstrictors, the effects of which cannot be prevented by renal prostaglandins (due to inhibition by the NSAI drug). Under these circumstances the decreased medullary perfusion could accentuate the toxic effects of these drugs. Increasing clinical interest in this area of multiple interactions will help to identify those drugs which could cause renal toxicity when given with analgesics and/or NSAI drugs.

Lipoxygenase products may be implicated in the renal lesion following puromycin aminonucleoside[24] (single i.p. dose of 100 mg/kg) which induces a model nephrotic syndrome in the rat. The i.p. administration of a 5-lipoxygenase inhibitor (AA-861) 6 days later decreased the urinary excretion of protein and elevated serum albumin. The enzyme 5-lipoxygenase is responsible for the conversion of arachidonic acid to LTB_4 and the leukotrienes (Figure 1). Thus it can be concluded that these lipoxygenase products may have been increased and caused some of the toxic effects of puromycin.

There have been numerous reports suggesting that NSAI

drugs can affect established kidney disease in man, such as chronic renal insufficiency[25], lupus erythematosus[26], and nephrotic syndrome[27,28]. Many investigators have interpreted these data as proof that prostaglandins (presumably PGE_2 or PGI_2) help to protect the kidney from the effects of the disease. This interpretation may be correct, but it has not been proven directly by clinical trials or experiments in animals. The recent report[29] that long-term intravenous infusions of PGE_1 in patients with chronic glomerulonephritis improved renal function does, however, support this suggestion.

IMMUNOLOGICAL CAUSES OF RENAL TOXICITY

Immune glomerulonephritis is associated with cellular infiltration and proliferation, changes in renal function and proteinuria. Numerous mediators have been shown to be involved in the progression of the lesions, including the renin-angiotensin system, prostaglandins and thromboxanes, and the complement system[11,30,31]. Glomerular immune injury can be induced in rats by the injection of basement membrane antibodies. The resulting nephrotoxic serum nephritis (NSN) is an established model of immune glomerular nephritis and has been reviewed by Thomson et al.[32]. The initial stages of the disease result in a complement-dependent infiltration of polymorphonuclear cells lasting for up to 3 days. The next stage results from the production and deposition of antibodies against the injected antibodies and there is considerable mononuclear cell infiltration. Dunn and co-worker measured cyclo-oxygenase and lipoxygenase products in glomeruli isolated from controls and rats with NSN to follow the progression of the lesion[11,30,33]. The major product was $PGF_{2\alpha}$ (400 pg/mg) and small quantities of PGE_2, PGI_2 (measured as 6-keto $PGF_{1\alpha}$) and TxA_2 (measured as TxB_2) were also synthesized. Two days after injection of nephrotoxic serum there was a 4-fold increase in $PGF_{2\alpha}$ and a 10-fold increase in TxA_2.

Within 2 hours of injecting basement membrane antibodies both glomerular filtration rate (GFR) and renal blood flow (RBF) were reduced, and it was thought that these decreases could be due to glomerular TxA_2 production. When two different thromboxane synthetase inhibitors (OKY-1581 and UK-38485) were administered, the glomerular TxA_2 synthesis was reduced by over 95% and this was accompanied by increased GFR and RBF. Interestingly only TxA_2 remained elevated on days 8, 11 and 14 of the disease[33].

Recently Stork and Dunn[34] were able to show marked elevations of glomerular PGE_2 in addition to increased TxA_2 over the 14 days studied using a more potent titre of antisera. These investigators concluded that TxA_2 has no pathophysiological action in the course of the disease. Increased PGE_2 was, on the other hand, thought to augment RBF and consequently maintain a normal GFR. It was concluded that increased PGE_2 may be a general adaptive mechanism in glomerular disease. This mechanism would agree with the earlier suggestions of Collier that prostaglandins play a defensive role in renal disease[3].

RENAL DISEASE ASSOCIATED WITH ALTERED EICOSANOID PRODUCTION

There are a number of diseases which are clearly not caused by elevated renal eicosanoid production, but which do result in their increased renal synthesis[8]. Such diseases include renal ischaemia[8,9,16,35], volume depletion due to non-renal salt loss and diuretic drug action[36], surgery and essential hypertension[11]. It is now generally accepted that most renal diseases, including immune glomerular disease[31], systemic lupus erythematosus with glomerular involvement and nephrotic syndrome[26] are associated with increased renal eicosanoid production (see reviews 10, 11, 32, 33). However, it is useful to consider the role of renal eicosanoids in Bartter's syndrome, because it is one of the more intensively studied diseases, the many controversial aspects of which illustrate the problems interpreting the role of renal prostaglandin changes in clinical conditions[37]. Bartter's syndrome is a relatively rare condition with an unusual form of secondary hyperaldosteronism in children, but retardation of growth and development are seen less frequently in young adults. Most of the symptoms (muscle weakness, cramping, nocturia and polyuria) are a result of electrolyte disorders which include hypokalaemia (due to excessive renal potassium excretion) and hypochloraemia alkalosis. There is increased plasma renin activity and elevated angiotensin II and aldosterone plasma levels. In keeping with this hyperreninaemic state, kidney biopsies indicate hyperplasia and hypertrophy of the juxtaglomerular apparatus. Despite these abnormalities, patients are normotensive and free from oedema[37]. The first indication that renal eicosanoids may be involved in this syndrome arose from the therapeutic use of indomethacin. Serum aldosterone levels and plasma renin activity were decreased by indomethacin, and the hypokalaemic alkalosis was suppressed. Further studies showed that renal PGE synthesis was indeed increased in patients with Bartter's syndrome, but whole-body PGE production was normal. Later it was shown that excretion of PGD_2, PGE_2 and the main metabolite of PGI_2, 6-keto-$PGF_{1\alpha}$, was markedly increased. These findings led some investigators to claim that this increased prostaglandin production by the kidney is the primary event in Bartter's syndrome[37,38]. This has been challenged by Dunn[39], who raised the following points:

1.   Urinary PG excretion is normal is some patients.

2.   Treatment with NSAI drugs generally only resulted in partial improvement in the electrolyte disturbance, even though the clinical condition of most patients improved markedly.

3.   Although PGE_2 can inhibit tubular chloride reabsorption, treatment with a NSAI drug does not cure the defect.

4.   There is a difficulty in assessing the reason for increased PG, angiotensin II and bradykinin levels, because experimentally these peptides can both stimulate PG production and be stimulated by PGs.

5.   The relationship between potassium depletion and renal prostaglandin synthesis is equally complex. Reports from experimental studies in animals and with isolated medullary interstitial cells suggest that hypokalaemia may stimulate renal PG synthesis. However, experimentally induced potassium depletion in humans and rats has failed to demonstrate increased PG biosynthesis. Moreover, patients with Bartter's syndrome receiving potassium repletion respond with an increased urinary PGE_2 excretion[39].

Although it would seem reasonable to assume that some of the elevated renal prostaglandins which arise in this condition do contribute to some of the clinical defects, it is impossible to assess the cause of the syndrome or the mechanism responsible for the renal damage[39]. Not only is the case against increased synthesis of eicosanoids "not proven"; there is not a case to be made for the presumption of a primary role of renal eicosanoids as toxic agents in this disease.

THE RENAL TOXICITY OF THROMBOXANE A_2 (TxA_2)

The effects of the renal generation of TxA_2 in nephrotoxic serum nephritis[11,30,33] have been discussed above. The first reports of exaggerated TxA_2 production by the kidney arose from work of Needleman and co-workers[40,41], who studied the effects of uretal obstruction in rabbits, and demonstrated increased PGE_2 release from the cortex, together with large quantities of TxA_2. However it was not possible to explain how the cortex could produce these quantities of PGE_2 and TxA_2 based on the biosynthetic capacity of the glomeruli alone[33]. The discovery of large quantities of infiltrating mononuclear cells in the cortex suggested[42] that these cells were responsible for the increased quantities of TxA_2 and PGE_2. Dunn et al.[11] have also suggested that the TxA_2 generated during nephrotoxic serum nephritis in rats may in part arise from infiltrating leukocytes and monocytes. These investigators have demonstrated that the increased intraglomerular levels of TxA_2 can lead to arteriolar constriction and mesangial contraction with subsequent reduction of glomerular filtration surface area. TxA_2-stimulated platelet and leukocyte adhesiveness and aggregation may also accelerate the glomerular immune injury. The administration of two different TxA_2 synthetase inhibitors during the acute phase (at 3 hours) of the disease improved RBF and GFR, although they were less effective at later periods[34].

Renal TxA_2 has been shown to be generated at an early stage of rejection of renal transplants in rats[43,44] and in man[45,46]. Again the major source of this TxA_2 has been proposed to arise from invading inflammatory cells[46]. Although renal TxA_2 is an accurate signal of early rejection, TxA_2 synthetase inhibitors delayed, but did not prevent, rejection of the transplanted kidney. This suggests that it arises as a consequence of changes associated with rejection rather than playing a direct role in the process. The complex role of renal prostaglandins in maintaining renal function in patients with chronic renal disease has been reviewed[10,47]. In addition to the increased levels of PGE_2 and PGI_2 which maintain renal blood flow, there is also considerable production of TxA_2. Gentillini and co-workers[47] have administered the TxA_2-synthetase inhibitor OKY-046 in an acute study in six patients with cirrhosis, ascites and avid sodium retention. They found that a single dose of 400 mg of this drug lowered the urinary TxB_2 levels by a half, which reflects a reduction in the renal production of TxA_2. At the same time there was a 50% increase in urinary PGE_2 excretion. These investigators suggested that these results justify a further study to evaluate the possible beneficial effects of this type of drug in this disease. Similar changes were confirmed by Zipser et al.[48], who reported that a different thromboxane inhibitor, dazoxiben, also produced a 50% reduction of urinary TxB_2 excretion, but without improving renal function in patients with hepatorenal syndrome. It seems that additional clinical studies of TxA_2 synthetase inhibitors in a variety of renal diseases may lead to some important clinical applications for this interesting class of drugs.

CONCLUSION

The three most abundant renal eicosanoids PGE_2, $PGF_{2\alpha}$ and PGI_2 are all available as pharmaceutical products[49], none of which have been reported to produce toxic effects in the kidney[50]. In the clinical situation these products are used at doses ranging from nanogram to milligram quantities for short periods of time only, exposure levels which are unlikely to result in renal toxicity. A number of diseases associated with increased eicosanoid production have been reported, but the available evidence suggests that over-production of PGE_2 or PGI_2 is a defensive response to maintain renal function in the face of adverse vasoconstrictor influences. TxA_2 is too unstable to synthesize in large quantities for toxicology studies. However in human renal transplant patients[46] and in animal models of immune glomerular nephritis[33,34], increased levels of TxA_2 have a deleterious effect on renal function, but this TxA_2 could not be shown to have direct toxic effects or cause organ rejection.

There is only one indirect reason to suspect that the leukotrienes may contribute to renal toxicity. NSAI drugs are potent prostaglandin synthase inhibitors, but are relatively inactive against the lipoxygenase pathway. Lipoxygenase products of arachidonic acid metabolism such as leukotrienes could contribute to the side effects seen in analgesic abusers. There is circumstantial evidence to support the involvement of lipid peroxides (including arachidonic acid hydroperoxides) and the lipid and prostaglandin hydroperoxidases in analgesic nephropathy[20].

Further studies of the effects of active oxygen species and free radicals on the production of reactive intermediates in the kidney are required before we can assess their role in the development of renal papillary necrosis and urothelial carcinoma. Similarly, it will be interesting to study the levels of lipoxygenase products produced by the kidney in animal models of nephrotoxicity and in patients with confirmed renal disease. Until such data become available it will not be possible to assess the full role of these arachidonic acid metabolites in renal disease, nor develop rational strategies to modulate these changes to a therapeutic advantage.

REFERENCES

1. Vane, J.R., Inhibition of prostaglandin synthesis as a mechanism of action for aspirin-like drugs, Nature (New Biology), 231, 232, 1971.
2. Smith, J.B. and Willis, A.L., Aspirin selectively inhibits prostaglandin production in human platelets, Nature (New Biology), 231, 235, 1971.
3. Collier, H.O.J., Prostaglandins and aspirin, Nature, 232, 17, 1971.
4. Moncada, S. and Vane, J.R., Pharmacology and endogenous roles of prostaglandin endoperoxides, thromboxane A_2 and prostacyclin, Pharm. Reviews, 293, 30, 1971.
5. Samuelsson, B. and Paoletti, R., Eds., Leukotrienes and other lipoxygenase products, Advances in Prostaglandin, Thromboxane and Leukotriene Research, Volume 9, Raven Press, New York, 1982.
6. McGiff, J.C., Schwartzman, M. and Ferreri, R., Renal prostaglandins and hypertension, in Platelets, Prostaglandins and the Cardiovascular System, Advances in Prostaglandin, Thromboxane and Leukotriene Research, Volume 13, Born, G.V.R., McGiff, J.C., Serneri, G.G.N. and Paoletti, R., Eds., Raven Press, New York, 1985, 161.
7. Lee, J.B., Crowshaw, K., Takman, B.H., Attrep, K.A. and Gougoutas, J.Z., The identification of prostaglandins E_2, $F_{2\alpha}$ and A_2 from rabbit kidney medulla, Biochem. J., 105, 1251, 1967.
8. Crowshaw, K. and McGiff, J.C., Prostaglandins in the kidney: A correlative study of their biochemistry and renal function, in Mechanisms of Hypertension, Sambhi, M.P., Ed., Excerpta Medica, Amsterdam, 1973, 254.
9. McGiff, J.C., Crowshaw, K. and Itskovitz, H.D., Prostaglandins and renal function, Fed. Proc. 33, 39, 1974.
10. Dunn, M.J., Renal prostaglandins, in Renal Endocrinology, Dunn, M.J., Ed., Williams and Wilkins, Baltimore, 1983, chap. 1.
11. Dunn, M.J., Scharschmidt, L.A., Lianos, E.A. and Konieczkowski, M., Renal cyclo-oxygenase and lipoxygenase products in health and disease, Clin. Physiol. Biochem., 2, 91, 1984.
12. Whorton, A.R., Smigel, M., Oates, J.A. and Frolich, J.C., Regional differences in prostacyclin formation by the kidney: Prostacyclin is a major prostaglandin of renal cortex, Biochim. Biophys. Acta, 529, 176, 1978.
13. Lonigro, A.J., Itskovitz, H.D., Crowshaw, K. and McGiff, J.C., Dependency of renal blood flow on prostaglandin synthesis in the dog, Circ. Res., 32, 712, 1973.
14. Zins, G.R., Renal prostaglandins, Am. J. Med., 58, 14, 1975.
15. Zambraski, E.J. and Dunn, M.J., Renal prostaglandin E_2 secretion and excretion in conscious dogs, Am. J. Physiol., 236, F552, 1979.
16. McGiff, J.C., Crowshaw, K., Terragno, N.A. and Lonigro, A.J., Renal prostaglandins: Possible regulators of the renal actions of pressor hormones, Nature, 227, 1255, 1970.
17. Nadler, J.L., Coleman, R., Zipser, R.D. and Horton, R., Stimulation of renal prostaglandins by vasoactive hormones in man: Comparison of PGE_2 and 6-keto-$PGE_{1\alpha}$. Presented at the V International Conference on Prostaglandins, Florence, May 18-21, 1982.
18. Winchester, J.F., Ed., Aspirin and acetaminophen: Georgetown University

symposium on analgesics, Arch. Intern. Med., 141, 1981.

19. Crowshaw, K., Role of inhibition of prostaglandin biosynthesis by anti-inflammatory drugs in the pathogenesis of renal damage, in Advances in Inflammation Research, Volume 6, Rainsford, K.D. and Velo, G.P., Eds., Raven Press, New York, 1984, 149.

20. Bach, P.H. and Bridges, J.W., The role of metabolic activation of analgesics and non-steroidal anti-inflammatory drugs in the development of renal papillary necrosis and upper urothelial carcinoma, Prostaglandins, Leukotrienes and Medicine, 15, 251, 1984.

21. Jim, K., Hassid, A., Sun, F. and Dunn, M.J., Lipoxygenase activity in rat glomeruli, glomerular epithelial cells, and cortical tubules, J. Biol. Chem., 257, 10294, 1982.

22. Kerr, D.N.S., Renal function after acute or prolonged consumption of aspirin, in Aspirin Symposium 1983: International Congress of Symposium Series Number 71, Hallam, J., Goldman, L. and Fryers, G.R., Eds., Royal Society of Medicine, London, 1984, 43.

23. Prescott, L.F., Analgesic nephropathy: A reassessment of the role of phenacetin and other analgesics, Drugs, 23, 75, 1982.

24. Mune, M., Gotoh, T., Morishita, S., Kimura, K., Yakuwa, S. and Nomoto, N., Effect of a 5-lipoxygenase inhibitor AA-861 on proteinuria of aminonucleoside induced nephrotic rat. Presented at the Kyoto Conference on Prostaglandins, November 26-28, 1984.

25. Berg, K.J., Acute effects of acetylsalicylic acid in patients with chronic renal insufficiency, Eur. J. Clin. Pharm., 11, 111, 1977.

26. Kimberly, R.P., Gill, J.R., Bowden, R.E. Keiser, H.R. and Platz, P.H., Elevated urinary prostaglandins and the effects of aspirin on renal function in lupus erythematosus, Ann. Intern. Med., 89, 336, 1978.

27. Arisz, L., Donker, A.J., Brentjens, J.R. and van der Hem, G.K., The effect of indomethacin on proteinuria and kidney function in the nephrotic syndrome, Acta Med. Scand., 199, 121, 1976.

28. Donker, A.J., Arisz, L., Brentjens, J.R.H., van der Hem, G.K. and Hollermans, H.J.G., The effect of indomethacin on kidney function and plasma renin activity in man, Nephron, 17, 288, 1976.

29. Niwa, T., Asada, H., Maeda, K., Shibata, M. and Yamada, K., PGE_1 infusion therapy of chronic glomerulonephritis. Presented at the Kyoto Conference on Prostaglandins, November 26-28, 1984.

30. Scharschmidt, L.A., Lianos, E. and Dunn, M.J., Arachidonate metabolites and the control of glomerular function, Fed. Proc., 3058, 42, 1983.

31. Cummings, N.B., Michael, A.F. and Wilson, C.B., Eds., Immune Mechanisms in Renal Disease, Plenum, New York and London, 1983.

32. Thomson, N.M., Holdsworth, S.R., Glasgow, E.F., Peters, D.K. and Atkins, R.C., Mechanism of injury in experimental glomerulonephritis, in Progress in Glomerulonephritis, Kincaid-Smith, P., d'Apice, A.J.F. and Atkins, R.C., Eds., John Wiley and Sons, New York, 1979, 51.

33. Lianos, E.A., Andres, G.A. and Dunn, M.J., Glomerular prostaglandin and thromboxane synthesis in rat nephrotoxic serum nephritis, J. Clin. Invest., 72, 1439, 1983.

34. Stork, J.E. and Dunn, M.J., The hemodynamic roles of thromboxane A_2 and prostaglandin E_2 in glomerulonephritis (in preparation).

35. Morrison, A.R., Benabe, J.E. and Taylor, A., The role of thromboxanes in renal disease, in Prostaglandins and the Kidney, Dunn, M.J., Patrono, C. and Cinotti, G.A., Eds., Plenum, New York and London, 1983, 309.

36. Olsen, U.B., Diuretics and kidney prostaglandins, in Prostaglandins and the Kidney, Dunn, M.J., Patrono, C. and Cinotti, G.A., Eds., Plenum, New York

and London, 1983, 205.

37.   Stoff, J.S., Clive, D.M., Leone, D., MacIntyre, D.E., Brown, R.S. and Salzman, E., The role of arachidonic acid metabolites in the pathophysiology of Bartter's syndrome, in Prostaglandins and the Kidney, Dunn, M.J., Patrono, C. and Cinotti, G.A., Eds., Plenum, New York and London, 1983, 353.

38.   Gill, J.R., Frolich, J.C. and Bowden, R.E., Bartter's syndrome: A disorder characterised by high urinary prostaglandins and a dependence of hyper-reninemia on prostaglandin synthesis, Am. J. Med., 61, 43, 1976.

39.   Dunn, M.J., Prostaglandins and Bartter's syndrome, Kidney Int., 19, 86, 1981.

40.   Morrison, A.R., Nishikawa, K. and Needleman, P., Unmasking of thromboxane A_2 synthesis by uretal obstruction in the rabbit kidney, Nature, 267, 259, 1977.

41.   Currie, M., Kawasaki, A., Jonas, P., Davis, B. and Needleman, P., The mechanism and site of the enhanced arachidonic metabolism in ureter obstruction, in Prostaglandins and the Kidney, Dunn, M.J., Patrono, C. and Cinotti, G.A., Eds., Plenum, New York and London, 1983, 299.

42.   Okegawa, T., Jonas, P.E., De Schryvner, K., Kawasaki, A. and Needleman, P., Metabolic and cellular alterations underlying the exaggerated renal prosta-glandin and thromboxane synthesis in ureter obstruction in rabbits, J. Clin. Invest., 71, 81, 1983.

43.   Foegh, M., Winchester, J.F., Zmudka, M., Helfrich, G.B. and Ramwell, P.W., Factors affecting immunoreactive thromboxane B_2 in kidney transplant patients, in Prostaglandins and the Kidney, Dunn, M.J., Patrono, C. and Cinotti, G.A., Eds., Plenum, New York and London, 1983, 399.

44.   Coffman, T.M., Yarger, W.E. and Klotman, P.E., Functional role of throm-boxane production in acutely rejecting renal allografts in rats, J. Clin. Invest., 75, 1242, 1985.

45.   Foegh, M.L., Zmudka, M., Cooley, C., Winchester, J.F., Helfrich, G.B. and Ramwell, P.W., Urine i-TxB_2 in renal allograft rejection, Lancet, 2, 431, 1981.

46.   Foegh, M.L., Alijani, M.R., Helfrich, G.B., Khirabadi, B.S., Goldman, M.H., Lower, R.R. and Ramwell, P.W., Thromboxane and leukotrienes in clinical and experimental transplant rejection, in Platelets, Prostaglandins and the Car-diovascular System; Advances in Prostaglandin, Thromboxane and Leukotriene Research, Volume 13, Born, G.V.R., McGiff, J.C., Serneri, G.G.N. and Paoletti, R., Eds., Raven Press, New York, 1985, 209.

47.   Gentilini, P., La Villa, G., Laffi, G., Buzzelli, G., Pinzani, M., Com-inelli, F., Moscarella, S. and Birardi, A., Sodium retention in cirrhosis: Aspects of pathophysiology and treatment, in Frontiers in Gastrointestinal Research, Karger, Basel (in press).

48.   Zipser, R.D., Kronborg, I., Rector, W., Reynolds, T.B. and Daskalupoulos, G., Therapeutic trial of thromboxane synthesis inhibition in the hepatorenal syndrome, Gastroenterology, 87, 1228, 1984.

49.   Caton, M.P.L. and Crowshaw, K., Pharmaceutical exploitation, in Handbook of Prostaglandins and Related Compounds, Curtis-Prior, P.B., Ed., Churchill Livingstone, Edinburgh (in press).

50.   Smith, E.R. and Mason, M.M., Toxicology of the prostaglandins, Prostaglan-dins, 7, 247, 1974.

12

XENOBIOTIC METABOLISM IN THE MAMMALIAN KIDNEY

J.B. TARLOFF, R.S. GOLDSTEIN AND J.B. HOOK

INTRODUCTION

The kidneys have a clearly defined role as excretory organs for xenobiotics and their polar metabolites. Less well understood is the involvement of the kidneys in the metabolism of xenobiotics, a function usually ascribed to the liver. The primary function of xenobiotic metabolism is to convert non-polar compounds to polar products that will not be reabsorbed from urine or bile. Although xenobiotic metabolism has been considered as a detoxification process, in certain instances, the products of metabolism may be potent toxicants. Recent investigations have shown significant catalytic activities of enzymes involved in xenobiotic metabolism in the kidney. Intrarenal xenobiotic metabolism may be a prerequisite for nephrotoxicity induced by some chemicals. Since an understanding of xenobiotic metabolizing enzymes is important in evaluating the biochemical mechanisms of nephrotoxicity, this chapter will focus on identification, localization, and activity of several renal enzymes involved in xenobiotic metabolism.

BALANCE BETWEEN ENZYMATIC ACTIVATION AND DETOXIFICATION

The intracellular concentration of toxic chemicals can be influenced by xenobiotic metabolism. For most chemicals, metabolic processes are not one-step events but occur via multiple competing and sequential pathways. Formation of toxicants is only one possible result of these pathways. The relative rates of metabolism of xenobiotics to toxic or non-toxic products represent a balance between enzymatic activation and detoxification and may determine, to a large extent, the response of an organ to toxicant exposure. Alterations in the relative activities of bioactivation and detoxification pathways could alter the generation of toxic metabolites in the tissue, and therefore the degree of injury produced[1,2]. Bioactivation reactions are generally catalysed by cytochrome P-450-dependent mixed function oxidases, whereas detoxification reactions are catalysed by mixed function oxidases, non-oxidative cytosolic enzymes, and enzymes involved in conjugation (glucuronidases, sulphotransferases and glutathione transferases) and hydration (epoxide hydrase). However, there are exceptions to these generalities which will be discussed below.

ENZYMES RESPONSIBLE FOR XENOBIOTIC METABOLISM

Three major classes of enzymes involved in xenobiotic metabolism include: (1) cytochrome P-450-dependent mixed function oxidases (Phase I reactions); (2) enzymes involved in conjugation reactions (glucuronidation, sulphation and glutathione conjugation, Phase II reactions); and (3) enzymes that do not belong to either of the first two groups.

1.   Cytochrome P-450-dependent mixed function oxidases

The oxidative and reductive metabolism of many xenobiotics is mediated by enzymes located in the microsomal fraction of mammalian tissues. The microsomal fraction consists of fragments of smooth endoplasmic reticulum and contains a family of closely related haemoproteins known as cytochrome P-450s, which act as terminal oxidases for a variety of oxidative reactions. The term P-450 refers to the ability of the reduced form of the haemoprotein to react with carbon monoxide, yielding a complex with an absorption peak at 450 nm.

Catalytic mechanism of cytochrome P-450.   The mixed function oxidases catalyse numerous hydroxylation reactions (termed Phase I reactions) including aromatic and aliphatic hydroxylation; N-, O-, and S-dealkylations, sulphoxidation, N-oxidation and epoxidation.   Substrates for renal cytochrome P-450 include steroids, fat-soluble vitamins, fatty acids[3], prostaglandins[4], and numerous xenobiotics[5].

The microsomal mixed function oxidase system is composed of three components: a haemoprotein, cytochrome P-450; a flavoprotein, NADPH-cytochrome P-450 reductase; and a lipid factor. Two electron flow pathways have been suggested (Figure 1). One consists of cytochrome P-450 and NADPH-cytochrome P-450 reductase; the other is composed of a haemoprotein, cytochrome b_5, and a flavoprotein, NADH-dependent cytochrome b_5 reductase. The mixed function oxidase system utilizes cytochrome P-450 to bind and activate molecular oxygen. Information in this area is based largely on studies of hepatic cytochrome P-450, but considerable evidence indicates that renal cytochrome P-450 systems contain the same two electron flow pathways[6-8].

The flavoprotein component, NADPH-cytochrome P-450 reductase, can catalyse single electron reductions, such as the reduction of quinones to semiquinone radicals[9]. Under aerobic conditions, reoxidation of the radical results in formation of superoxide anion

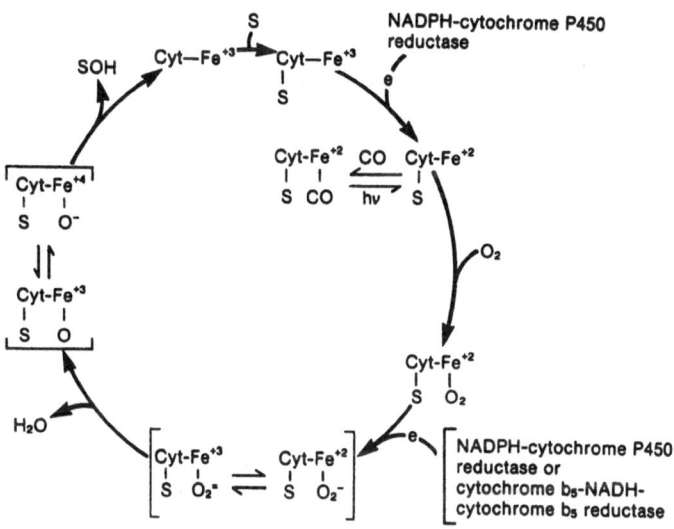

Figure 1   Electron flow diagram for cytochrome P-450-dependent oxidation of xenobiotics. Cyt = cytochrome P-450, S = substrate, SOH = oxidized substrate. From Anders[6].

radical and regeneration of the parent compound[10,11]. Enzyme-mediated redox cycling has been suggested as a fundamental mechanism underlying the toxicity of xenobiotics containing quaternary bipyridyl (paraquat), quinone (adriamycin) or nitro (nitrofurantoin) moieties.

<u>Multiplicity of renal cytochrome P-450 isozymes.</u>   Multiple forms of cytochrome P-450 have been identified in both hepatic and renal tissue. Hepatic isozymes of cytochrome P-450 have been characterized by substrate specificity and responses to inducing agents. Two broad classes of cytochromes P-450 may be distinguished by their response to inducing agents:

(1)   Phenobarbital-inducible cytochrome P-450. Phenobarbital increases the metabolism of a wide variety of substrates and the appearance of several isozymes of hepatic cytochrome P-450. Hepatic benzphetamine N-demethylation and ethoxycoumarin-O-deethylation are preferentially induced following phenobarbital pretreatment.

(2)   3-Methylcholanthrene (3-MC) and β-naphthoflavone (B-NF) inducible cytochrome P-450. A more limited number of substrates are involved with this form of hepatic cytochrome P-450. Hepatic ethoxyresorufin-O-deethylation and aromatic hydrocarbon hydroxylation are examples of reactions preferentially induced by 3-MC and B-NF.

Mixtures of polychlorinated and polybrominated biphenyls (PCBs and PBBs) produce a complex hepatic induction profile resembling the combined activities of phenobarbital and 3-MC.

Table 1 Induction of renal mixed function oxidase activities[a]

Inducer	Species	Phenobarbital inducible		3-MC, B-NF inducible	
		BPND	ECOD	EROD	BP
Phenobarbital	Mouse				0.9[12]
	Rat	ND[13,14]	0.9[14]	0.8[13]	1.2[15]
	Rabbit	5.6[13,14]	14.0[14,16]	1.2[13,15]	
	Hamster	1.8[17]	1.1[17]	1.0[17]	1.3[17]
	Guinea pig	ND[17]	0.7[17]	1.0[17]	1.0[17]
	Mini-pig	3.9[18]		9.5[18]	
3-MC	Mouse				2.9[19]
	Rat				200.0[15]
B-NF	Rat	ND[13]		80.0[13]	
	Rabbit	1.0[13]		120.0[13]	
	Hamster	0.8[17]	0.9[17]	15.0[17]	2.5[17]
	Guinea pig	ND[17]	0.7[17]	5.7[17]	5.7[17]
TCDD	Mouse				55.6[12]
	Rat		23.3[20]		60.4[22]
PCB/PBB	Mouse				2.1[12]
	Rat		6.4[21]		
	Hamster	0.9[17]	0.8[17]	0.7[17]	1.5[17]
	Guinea pig	ND[17]	1.3[17]	13.2[17]	10.3[17]

[a] Data are presented as the ratio of induced/control activity (moles product formed/min/mg protein) for the following mixed function oxidase activities: benzphetamine N-demethylation (BPND), ethoxycoumarin O-deethylation (ECOD), ethoxyresorufin O-deethylation (EROD), and benzo(a)pyrene hydroxylation (BP). ND = non-detectable activity

The ability to induce renal cytochrome P-450 activity varies widely among species (Table 1). Rat renal mixed function oxidases are induced by polycyclic aromatic hydrocarbons (3-MC, B-NF) but not by phenobarbital. In contrast, rabbit renal mixed function oxidases are induced by both polycyclic aromatic hydrocarbons and phenobarbital[13]. Renal cytochrome P-450 is induced by polycyclic aromatic hydrocarbons in most species; renal cytochrome P-450 is induced by phenobarbital in hamsters and rabbits but not in guinea pigs, rats and mice[17].

Inhibitors of mixed function oxidases have also been employed in order to differentiate multiple forms of cytochrome P-450. For example, SKF-525A and metyrapone inhibit phenobarbital-induced hepatic cytochrome P-450, whereas α-naphthoflavone (A-NF) inhibits reactions catalysed by 3-MC and B-NF-induced hepatic cytochrome P-450s. The effects of inhibitors on renal cytochrome P-450s are not as clear. A-NF inhibits renal cytochrome P-450 activity in rabbits and rats pretreated with B-NF and PBBs but not phenobarbital[13]. Metyrapone does not inhibit renal cytochrome P-450 activity in rats, consistent with the lack of phenobarbital-inducible renal cytochrome P-450 in this species[13]. In contrast, metyrapone inhibits rabbit renal cytochrome P-450 following B-NF, PBB or phenobarbital induction[13]. Inhibition of renal B-NF inducible-cytochrome P-450 by metyrapone is unexpected, since metyrapone is an inhibitor of phenobarbital-induced cytochrome P-450. Thus, the effects of inhibitors of cytochrome P-450 are not as clearly defined in kidney as in liver. Complicating the interpretation of inhibitor data is the observation that SKF-525A and piperonyl butoxide, inhibitors of phenobarbital-induced hepatic cytochrome P-450, reduce the renal cortical accumulation of phenobarbital in rats and rabbits[14]. Thus, inhibitors may have multiple effects on renal metabolism by altering transport, intracellular binding at non-catalytic sites, and cytochrome P-450-dependent biotransformation.

Renal cytochrome P-450 isozymes have also been distinguished immunologically. For example, in rabbit liver four major cytochrome P-450s have been characterized: form 2, induced by phenobarbital; form 3, constitutive form; form 4, induced in adult by B-NF or 2,3,7,8-tetrachlorodibenzo-p-dioxin (TCDD); and form 6, induced in neonates by TCDD[23]. Based on staining properties and autoradiography, rabbit kidney contains at least these four isozymes of cytochrome P-450[24]. Following TCDD pretreatment there is intense staining in the kidney for hepatic forms 4 and 6 with negligible staining for forms 2 and 3. Phenobarbital pretreatment increases staining in the kidney for hepatic form 2[24]. Similar distributions of renal cytochrome P-450s have been observed in other species[23-26]. At least three distinct forms of cytochrome P-450 have been isolated and purified from rabbit kidney[27,28]. The renal cytochrome P-450 induced by 3-MC pretreatment of rabbits is immunologically distinct from the hepatic form of the enzyme. Thus there are multiple forms of renal cytochrome P-450 based on responses to inducing agents, inhibitors, and antibodies.

Mixed function oxidase concentrations and intrarenal localization. The specific activities of the renal mixed function oxidases vary widely with species (Table 2). In general, renal cytochrome P-450 concentration is about 10% of hepatic cytochrome P-450. For example, rabbit hepatocytes contain 1.3 nmol cytochrome P-450/mg protein[32] compared to rabbit renal proximal tubules, which contain 0.15 nmol cytochrome P-450/mg protein[33]. Renal NADPH-cytochrome P-450 reductase activity is also about 10% of the hepatic activity in rabbits[32,33].

The low cytochrome P-450 concentration in the kidney compared to that of the liver has led to the suggestion that the kidney plays a relatively small role in overall xenobiotic metabolism. However, with certain substrates, the metabolic activity of renal cytochrome P-450 may exceed that of the liver. For example, chloroform metabolism (measured as covalent binding or CO_2 production) by renal microsomes from male mice is about half that observed with hepatic microsomes when expressed in terms of total protein. However, when chloroform metabolism is expressed as a

Table 2 Concentration of cytochrome P-450 mixed function oxidase components in renal tissue of various species

Species	Cyt P-450[a]	NADPH cyt c reductase[b]	Cyt b5[a]	Ref.
Mouse (Alderly Park Swiss-derived)				
male			0.146 ± 0.030	29
female			0.059 ± 0.006	29
Mouse (C57 B1/6N)				
male	0.200 ± 0.010			30
female	0.080 ± 0.003			30
Mouse (ICR)				
male	0.290 ± 0.060	32.3 ± 3.90	0.290 ± 0.040	31
female	0.060 ± 0.010	33.3 ± 7.10	0.150 ± 0.020	31
Rat (F344)	0.067 ± 0.002	9.38 ± 1.70	0.030 ± 0.003	13
Rat (Wistar)				
male	0.104 ± 0.012	48.8 ± 2.40	0.052 ± 0.011	29
female	0.127 ± 0.008	35.6 ± 5.60	0.072 ± 0.005	29
Rabbit	0.120 ± 0.010	8.62 ± 1.70	0.170 ± 0.010	13
	0.180 ± 0.100	21.0 ± 2.00		23
Hamster	0.250 ± 0.010	60.4 ± 12.2	0.180 ± 0.010	17
Guinea pig	0.130 ± 0.050	37.9 ± 13.4	0.110 ± 0.030	17
Mini-pig	0.53	28.25		26

[a] nmol/mg protein
[b] nmol cytochrome c reduced/min per mg protein

function of cytochrome P-450 concentration, renal activity is two-fold higher than hepatic activity[34].

In contrast to the well-established sex differences in hepatic cytochrome P-450 (males have higher concentration and activity than females), renal cytochrome P-450 concentration and activity in male and female rats[29,35] and rabbits[35] is not different. However, male mice have considerably higher renal cytochrome P-450 concentrations and higher catalytic activities than female mice[30,31,36], although these sex differences appear to be strain-dependent[29].

Mixed function oxidase activity is not distributed uniformly throughout the kidney. Cytochrome P-450 and NADPH-cytochrome P-450 reductase are in highest concentrations in renal cortex; the concentration of each enzyme declines within the outer and inner medulla in rats[37] and rabbits[32,33]. Within the renal cortex the greatest activity of cytochrome P-450 is localized within the proximal tubules; distal tubules have negligible cytochrome P-450 activity[33,38].

Morphologically, the proximal tubule is divided into three segments in rats[39] and rabbits[40,41]. The S$_1$ segment is the initial 1-1.5 mm of the proximal convoluted tubule, the S$_2$ segment is a transitional 1-2 mm segment comprising the terminal proximal convoluted tubule and the initial proximal straight tubule, and the S$_3$

segment is the terminal 1-2 mm of the proximal straight tubule extending from the corticomedullary junction through the outer medulla[40,41]. In rabbits, the S_2 segment is the portion most active in organic anion secretion (e.g. para-aminohippurate)[40,42] while the S_1 segment is the portion most active in organic cation secretion (e.g. tetraethylammonium, procainamide)[43,44]. In microdissected rabbit proximal tubules, cytochrome P-450 concentration is two to three times higher in the S_2 segment than in the S_1 or S_3 segments while the distal and cortical collecting tubules contain no measurable cytochrome P-450 (Figure 2)[33]. NADPH-cytochrome P-450 reductase is also located in highest concentration in the proximal tubule, primarily the S_2 and S_3 segments. In contrast to the lack of cytochrome P-450 in the rest of the nephron, NADPH-cytochrome P-450 reductase is also located in the distal tubule and medullary structures (Figure 2).

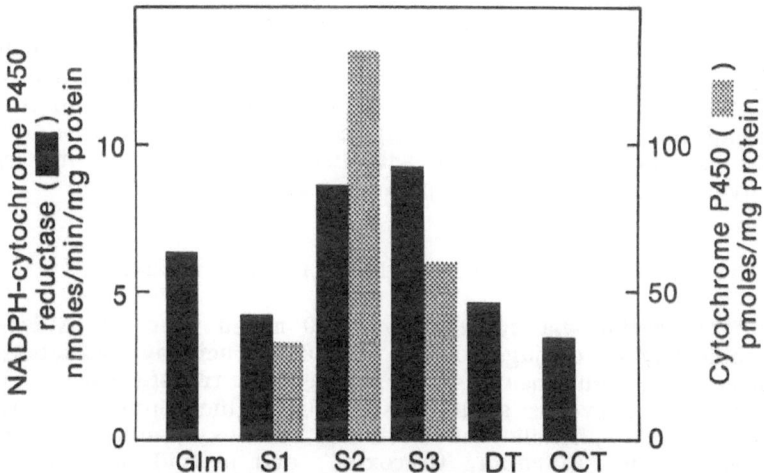

Figure 2 Segmental distribution of cytochrome P-450 and NADPH-cytochrome P-450 reductase in rabbit kidney. Glm = glomerulus, S1 = S_1 segment of proximal tubule, S2 = S_2 segment of proximal tubule, S3 = S_3 segment of proximal tubule, DT = distal tubule, CCT = cortical collecting tubule. Modified from Endou[33].

In rabbit kidney, smooth endoplasmic reticulum (SER), the site of mixed function oxidase activity, is located primarily in the S_3 segment and is absent from S_1 and S_2 segments[16]. There is generally a close correlation between induction of renal cytochrome P-450 concentration and activity and proliferation of SER. Following pretreatment of rabbits with phenobarbital, an inducer of cytochrome P-450 in rabbit kidney[35], there is an increase in SER in only S_3 segment[16]. In rats, proliferation of SER in S_3 segments results following pretreatment with TCDD[45], dieldrin[37], B-NF, and PBBs[46] but not phenobarbital. In mice, SER is found in both S_2 and S_3 segments; however, proliferation following B-NF or PBB pretreatment is difficult to detect[46].

In summary, the activities of renal cytochrome P-450 mixed

function oxidases are low in renal homogenates compared to liver. However, since cytochrome P-450 appears to be localized in S_2 and S_3 segments, renal cytochrome P-450 may have high cell-specific activity. Many compounds suspected or known to undergo bioactivation by cytochrome P-450-dependent mixed function oxidase reactions produce selective injury to the renal proximal tubules, the site of highest monooxygenase activity. The capability to concentrate xenobiotics within the proximal tubule epithelium via organic anion and cation transport pathways, coupled with the relatively high concentration of cytochrome P-450, predisposes this nephron segment to toxic injury due to mixed function oxidase-dependent metabolic bioactivation.

2. Conjugation reactions (Phase II metabolism)

Following oxidation by cytochrome P-450 mixed function oxidase, xenobiotics may undergo conjugation (Phase II) reactions to produce polar compounds that are rapidly eliminated. Additionally, conjugation reactions generally terminate the pharmacological activity of drug substrates. Some xenobiotics are primary substrates for conjugation enzymes, bypassing the cytochrome P-450 catalysed Phase I reactions. This section will discuss the renal enzyme systems involved in xenobiotic conjugation reactions.

a. Uridine diphosphate (UDP) glucuronyl transferase

Following oxidation via cytochrome P-450 mixed function oxidases, compounds may be conjugated with glucuronic acid by the action of the microsomal enzymes, UDP-glucuronyl transferases. The aglycones that serve as substrates for UDP-glucuronyl transferase include hydroxy (phenolic and alcoholic), carboxyl, sulphydryl and amino compounds. Bilirubin, thyroxine, and steroid hormones are important endogenous substrates for UDP-glucuronyl transferases[6]. Although for most compounds, glucuronide conjugation represents a pathway towards more rapid elimination and loss of biological activity, some glucuronide conjugates may be reactive compounds. In particular, glucuronides of certain N-hydroxy compounds, such as N-hydroxy-2-acetylaminofluorene and N-hydroxyphenacetin, are more reactive than the parent compound.

UDP-glucuronic acid (UDPGA) is synthesized from glucose-1-phosphate (G1P) as follows:

$$\text{(1) uridine triphosphate (UTP) + G1P} \xrightarrow{\text{pyrophosphorylase}} \text{UDP-glucose(UDPG) + pyrophosphate}$$

$$\text{(2) UDPG + 2NAD}^+ + H_2O \xrightarrow{\text{UDPG-dehydrogenase}} \text{UDP-glucuronic acid (UDPGA) + 2NADH + 2H}^+$$

                              glucuronyl
                              transferase
(3) UDPGA + substrate (S)   ─────────────> S-glucuronic acid + uridine diphosphate

UDP-glucuronic acid has an α configuration at the glucuronic acid-phosphate linkage, rendering it resistant to hydrolysis by β-glucuronidase, a lysosomal enzyme. Glucuronide conjugates have the β configuration at the glucuronic acid-substrate linkage, making these conjugates susceptible to β-glucuronidase hydrolysis.

Multiple UDP-glucuronyl transferase isozymes. Hepatic UDP-glucuronyl transferases have been partially purified and characterized with respect to substrate specificity[47],[48]. There are at least three distinct UDP-glucuronyl transferase isozymes: (1) GT_1 substrates include planar compounds such as 1-naphthol, 4-nitrophenol, N-hydroxy-2-naphthylamine and 3-hydroxybenzo(a)-pyrene; (2) GT_2 substrates include compounds where the substituent at the para position is non-planar and bulky, such as 4-hydroxybiphenyl, chloramphenicol, bilirubin and morphine; (3) GT_3 substrates include steroids such as testosterone and oestrone. GT_1 and GT_2 are altered differently by inducing agents. Specifically, 3-MC increases GT_1 activity with no alteration of GT_2 activity; phenobarbital induces GT_2 with no effect on GT_1. Neither 3-MC nor phenobarbital has an appreciable effect on the glucuronidation of GT_3 substrates[47]. Aroclor 1254 (a mixture of polychlorinated biphenyls) is a mixed-type inducer of cytochrome P-450 activity, resembling both 3-MC and phenobarbital[49]. Aroclor 1254 also acts as a mixed-type inducer of glucuronyl transferases in the liver, increasing both GT_1 and GT_2 activities[48].

In contrast to the three forms of glucuronyl transferases present in the liver, rat kidney contains primarily GT_1 with low to negligible levels of GT_2 and GT_3 activity. Species differences in renal glucuronyl transferase activities exist; human kidneys have high glucuronyl transferase activity toward 4-hydroxybiphenyl and morphine, both of which are GT_2 substrates[48]. Rabbit kidneys also have high glucuronyl transferase activity toward 4-hydroxy-biphenyl and low, but detectable activity toward chloramphenicol[50]. Additionally, rabbit kidneys glucuronidate oestrone, diethylstil-boestrol and acetaminophen (paracetamol), GT_2 and GT_3 substrates[50]. Considering the low GT_2 activity in rat kidneys, it is not surprising that phenobarbital fails to induce renal UDP-glucuronyl transferase activity[51-53]. Conflicting results have been reported in the inducibility of GT_1 activity in renal tissue following 3-MC pretreatment, with some investigators reporting a stimulation of activity[54],[55] and others reporting no effect[51-53]. Several other compounds have been found to increase renal and hepatic GT_1 activity: cincophen induces both hepatic and renal GT_1 and UDP-glucose dehydrogenase[51]; trans-stilbene oxide[53],[56], TCDD[20],[37], Aroclor 1254[48], and B-NF[53] all increase renal and hepatic GT_1 activities. Salicylic acid specifically increases the activity of rat renal GT_1 with no effect on hepatic glucuronyl transferase activities[51].

Intrarenal localization of UDP-glucuronyl transferases. UDP-glucuronyl transferase activity is not uniformly distributed throughout renal tissue but follows the gradient established for mixed function oxidase activity, i.e. highest activity in cortex and lowest in medulla[37],[50]. Although mixed function oxidase activity is not detectable in the medulla, measurable p-nitrophenol glucuronyl transferase activity (GT_1) is present in rat kidney medulla[37]. In rat kidney, UDP-glucuronyl transferase activity is found in both proximal and distal tubules, with glucuronidation capacity of the distal tubule about 50% that of proximal tubule[38]. Glucuronyl transferase activity may be limited by the availability of cosubstrate, UDP-glucuronic acid. UDP-glucuronic acid concentration in rabbit kidney cortex is twice as high as medulla[50].

In contrast to the relatively low renal cytochrome P-450 concentration and activity, glucuronidation capacity of the kidney is substantial and may make an important contribution to overall xenobiotic metabolism. In a direct comparison of isolated hepatocytes and renal tubular cells, rat renal cells catalyse cytochrome P-450-dependent O-de-ethylation of 7-ethoxycoumarin at a rate of 3% of the hepatic activity. In contrast, hepatocytes and renal cells both convert 50% of 7-hydroxycoumarin to the glucuronide conjugate[21]. Isolated renal cells, largely originating from the proximal tubule, produce only 5% of acetaminophen-glucuronide compared to liver[55]. Glucuronidation of o-aminophenol by rat renal homogenates is only 30% of liver activity[51]. Renal glucuronyl transferase activity may even be higher than that of liver for some substrates. For example, with 4-methylumbelliferone, renal homogenates produce twice as much glucuronide conjugate as hepatic tissue[20],[52]. Conjugation of p-nitrophenol by renal homogenates is 2.5 times greater than by hepatic homogenates[56].

Hepatic glucuronide conjugation is sex-dependent in rats; males form considerably more glucuronide conjugates than females. This difference is dependent on steroid hormones; testosterone enhances glucuronidation in females while oestradiol reduces glucuronidation in males[57]. These sex-related differences are not apparent in humans[57]. Renal glucuronyl transferase activity is also sex-dependent but in the opposite direction, i.e., microsomes from female rats form considerably more of the glucuronide conjugates of 1-naphthol and 4-nitrophenol than microsomes prepared from male rat kidneys[58]. The increased glucuronidation in female renal microsomes appears to be related to a higher V_{max} for females (1.05 nmol/min/mg vs. 0.22 nmol/min/mg protein in males) with no effect on K_m (0.23 mM in males vs. 0.28 mM in females)[58].

b.   Sulphotransferases

A second type of conjugation reaction involves the addition of an active sulphate group to a substrate. Substrates for sulphate conjugation include phenols, alcohols, amines, steroids, bilirubin, and vitamin D. The sulphotransferases are involved primarily with the synthesis of sulphated polysaccharides such as chondroitin sulphate and heparin.

Sulphate conjugation occurs as follows:

(4) SO_4^{2-} + adenosine triphosphate (ATP) $\xrightarrow{\text{ATP-sulph-urylase}}$ adenosine 5'-phosphosulphate (APS) + pyrophosphate

(5) APS + ATP $\xrightarrow{\text{APS-phospho-kinase}}$ ADP + 3'-phosphoadenosine 5'-phosphosulphate (PAPS)

(6) PAPS + substrate $\xrightarrow{\text{sulpho-transferase}}$ substrate-SO_3H + 3'-phosphoadenosine-5'-phosphate

Sulphotransferases are located in cytosol, although some sulphotransferases have been identified bound to microsomes or the Golgi apparatus. Formation of sulphate esters is an important detoxification step, since sulphate conjugates are highly polar and rapidly excreted in urine or bile. The endogenous sulphate pool is limited and may be depleted by sulphate conjugation.

Renal tissue contains sulphotransferase activity but the formation of sulphate conjugates by renal tissue is markedly lower than that of the liver[5]. The concentrations of both sulphotransferase and PAPS are highest in renal cortex and decline through the medulla[50]. Cortical PAPS concentration in rabbit kidney is one-tenth of cortical UDP-glucuronic acid concentration[50].

Rat renal cells can synthesize sulphate conjugates of acetaminophen[55] and 7-hydroxycoumarin[21]. Morphine is another substrate for renal sulphotransferases[59]. Renal sulphotransferase activity is not increased by pretreatment with 3-MC[55] or PBBs[21]. The role of the kidney in sulphate conjugation and the role of sulphate conjugation in detoxification of nephrotoxicants has not been fully explored.

c.   Glutathione conjugation and mercapturate synthesis

In a complex series of reactions, electrophilic substrates are conjugated with glutathione (γ-glutamyl-cysteinylglycine), sequentially degraded to the cysteine conjugate and excreted as the N-acetyl-cysteine (mercapturic acid) conjugate. Xenobiotic substrates that form glutathione conjugates include alkyl and aryl halides, epoxides and alkenes.

Glutathione.   Glutathione is a tripeptide containing glutamate, cysteine and glycine. Glutathione is the most abundant thiol-containing compound in mammalian cells[60]. The presence of a free sulphydryl group in the cysteine residue makes glutathione an excellent scavenger for electrophilic radicals. The unusual γ-glutamyl linkage between glutamate and cysteine is resistant to hydrolysis by most peptidases[61].

Glutathione is synthesized by the sequential reactions of the enzymes γ-glutamylcysteine synthetase and glutathione synthetase. In most cells, glutathione synthesis is limited by the availability of intracellular cysteine[62]. Glutathione plays an important role in detoxification by neutralizing electrophilic radicals and by acting as a cofactor for glutathione peroxidase. In addition, glutathione may have ligand binding and transport properties, and may be involved in the transfer of amino acids from the extracellular to intracellular space[61].

Glutathione-S-transferases. The initial step in glutathione conjugation of xenobiotics is catalysed by a family of soluble enzymes, glutathione (GSH) S-transferases. In rat liver, microsomal GSH-S-transferases have been identified; microsomal GSH-S-transferase activity is lacking in rat kidney[63]. Substrates for GSH-S-transferases include halogenated aromatic compounds, epoxides, halogenated alkyl and aralkyl groups and α,β-unsaturated compounds[64]. Endogenous substrates for GSH-S-transferases include oestrogen[64], prostaglandin A and 15-keto-prostaglandins[65].

Glutathione-S-transferases account for about 10% of total cytoplasmic protein in hepatocytes. Catalytic activity is dependent upon (1) binding of substrate to enzyme, (2) presence of an electrophilic atom on the substrate to allow interaction with glutathione, and (3) increased nucleophilicity of the thiol group of glutathione. Substrates react with glutathione by (1) substitution reactions, such as halogen replacement by the thioether group of glutathione, and (2) addition reactions, such as glutathione attacking an epoxide or α,β-unsaturated site[65]. The transferase enzyme facilitates the conjugation reaction by lowering the pK (9.3) of glutathione resulting in ionization (GSH $\longrightarrow$ GS$^-$ + H$^+$) which promotes interaction with enzyme-bound substrate through nucleo-philic-electrophilic interactions[65].

There are multiple forms of GSH-S-transferases present in the liver; nomenclature is confusing and often conflicting. Traditionally, the transferases have been named based on substrate specificity. For example GSH-S-aryl transferase catalyses the conjugation of the aryl substrate, 1,2-dichloro-4-nitrobenzene; GSH-S-alkene transferase catalyses the conjugation of ethacrynic acid; GSH-S-aralkyl-transferase utilizes p-nitrobenzyl chloride; GSH-S-epoxide transferase conjugates 1,2-epoxy-(3-p-nitrophenoxy)-propane; and GSH-S-alkyl transferase utilizes methyl iodide as a substrate[66]. Purification of hepatic cytosolic GSH-S-transferase activities reveals at least six distinct proteins; these have been named GSH-S-transferases A, B, C, E, AA, and M, in order of elution during purification[67]. The purified proteins identified as GSH-S-transferases display overlapping activities with various substrates, so it is not possible to identify a distinct protein with a distinct catalytic activity.

Total renal GSH-S-transferase activity, expressed per gram of wet tissue, is considerably less than hepatic activity[68]. Isolated renal cells or proximal tubules synthesize the glutathione conjugates of acetaminophen[55,66] and 7-ethoxycoumarin[21]. GSH-S-transferase activity towards 1-chloro-2,4-dinitrobenzene (α,β-unsaturated) is present exclusively and to an equal extent in rabbit proximal convoluted and proximal straight tubule[69].

Sex differences are apparent in the hepatic GSH-S-transferase activities in rats. Male rats have higher hepatic transferase activities than females[70]. Sex differences exist in renal GSH-S-transferase activities as well, but generally in the opposite direction. Specifically, for renal aralkyl, epoxide, and alkyl transferase activities, males have lower conjugation rates than females. In contrast, male rats have slightly higher renal GSH-S-aryl-transferase activity than females[71].

Comparative differences in renal and hepatic GSH-S-transferase activity depend upon the particular substrate in question. For example, renal GSH-S-aryl-transferase activity in both male and female rats is less than 5% of the corresponding hepatic activity[70,71]. In male rats, renal GSH-S-transferase activities as a percentage of hepatic activities are: aryl transferase, 3%; aralkyl transferase, 17%; epoxide transferase, 68%; and alkyl transferase, 92%. For female rats, renal GSH-S-transferase activities as a percentage of hepatic activities are: aryl transferase, 5%; aralkyl transferase, 67%; epoxide transferase, 138%; and alkyl transferase, 121%[70,71].

Glutathione-S-transferases have been purified from rat kidney; activity corresponds to three distinct proteins. One renal transferase is identical to hepatic transferase B (ligandin), a second renal transferase is active in the conjugation of trans-4-phenylbut-3-en-2-one (α,β-unsaturated transferase activity displayed by hepatic GSH-S-transferases), while the third renal transferase is active with p-nitrobenzyl chloride and does not correspond chemically to any identified hepatic transferase[68]. Hepatic GSH-S-transferases A and C have low renal activity (with 1,2-dichloro-4-nitrobenzene as the substrate) and transferases AA, B and E (with methyl iodide as the substrate) are relatively active in the kidney[72].

For hepatic GSH-S-transferases, there is a close correlation between induction of conjugation activity and induction of mixed function oxidase activity. The traditional inducing agents, phenobarbital and 3-MC, both increase the activities of rat hepatic GSH-alkyl-, aryl-, aralkyl-, and epoxide-transferases[70,72]. The similarity of the responses of cytochrome P-450 and GSH-S-transferases to inducing agents suggests that the two systems are coupled, i.e., transferases may detoxify electrophilic intermediates produced by microsomal enzymes[65]. A more complex picture emerges for renal GSH-S-transferases. Although phenobarbital fails to induce cytochrome P-450-dependent mixed function oxidase activity in rat kidney, phenobarbital does specifically increase GSH-S-aralkyl transferase activity. GSH-S-alkyl-, aryl-, and epoxide-transferase activities are not induced by phenobarbital treatment of rats. 3-MC induces renal GSH-S-aryl- and aralkyl-transferase activities but not GSH-S-alkyl- or epoxide-transferases[71,72]. Trans-stilbene oxide increases rat hepatic and renal GSH-aryl-S-transferase (1-chloro-2,4-dinitrobenzene) but not epoxide-S-transferase (1,2-epoxy-3-(p-nitrophenoxy)propane) activity[56].

Hepatic and renal GSH-S-transferases are under complex hormonal control. Hypophysectomy in male rats significantly increases renal and hepatic GSH-S-aryl-, aralkyl-, and epoxide-transferase activities without altering GSH-S-alkyl and alkene activities. The hypophysectomy-induced increase in GSH-S-aryl-transferase activity in both kidney and liver is prevented by thyroxine replacement therapy. Thyroxine therapy does not prevent the hypophysectomy-induced increase in GSH-S-aralkyl- or epoxide-transferase activities, nor does thyroxine alone (without hypophysectomy) reduce control hepatic or renal GSH-S-transferase activities. In contrast to the effects of hypophysectomy, castration or adrenalectomy does not alter hepatic or renal GSH-S-transferase activities[73]. Thus, although GSH-S-transferase activities appear to be regulated by the hypothalamopituitary complex, the precise mechanisms of regulation are unclear.

A number of endogenous and exogenous ligands may bind to GSH-S-transferases without undergoing conjugation to glutathione. The specific transferase involved is thought to be GSH-S-transferase B, formerly called ligandin. Renal and hepatic ligandin are identical immunologically[65]. Endogenous compounds that bind to ligandin include bilirubin, steroids, thyroid hormones and heme. Xenobiotic ligands include furosemide, para-aminohippurate, probenecid and penicillin. GSH-S-transferases may serve as a storage or transport protein for such bound ligands[74]. Several organic anions, such as probenecid and penicillin, bind to renal GSH-S-transferases and competitively inhibit organic anion transport, suggesting that renal GSH-S-transferases may act as cytoplasmic anion receptors. However, renal GSH-S-transferase activity and organic anion transport may be dissociated by factors such as acidosis and 3-MC treatment, both of which increase renal GSH-S-transferase activity but not organic anion transport. Conversely, organic anion transport but not GSH-S-transferase activity is enhanced after penicillin treatment or uninephrectomy. Thus, the role of renal GSH-S-transferases in organic anion transport remains unclear.

Mercapturic acid synthesis. While the kidney may be active in the formation of glutathione conjugates, a more important role of the kidney is in degradation of preformed glutathione conjugates into the corresponding mercapturic acid (Figure 3). The kidney contains an enzyme, γ-glutamyl transpeptidase, capable of cleaving the γ-glutamyl linkage of glutathione to produce the cysteinylglycine conjugate. γ-Glutamyl transpeptidase is concentrated within the brush border of renal proximal tubule, hydrolysing substrates within the tubular lumen[60]. The cysteinylglycine conjugate formed by the action of γ-glutamyl transpeptidase is a substrate for numerous peptidases, including aminopeptidase M, located within the brush border of proximal tubules[75,76]. These peptidases will cleave the glycine-cysteine linkage, producing the cysteinyl conjugate of the xenobiotic. The xenobiotic-cysteine conjugate may be excreted or, more likely, be absorbed and converted to the corresponding mercapturic acid by the action of microsomal N-acetyltransferase[77]. This complex reaction scheme is illustrated in Figure 4. Oestradiol in trace amounts is an endogenous compound excreted as a mercapturic acid[78].

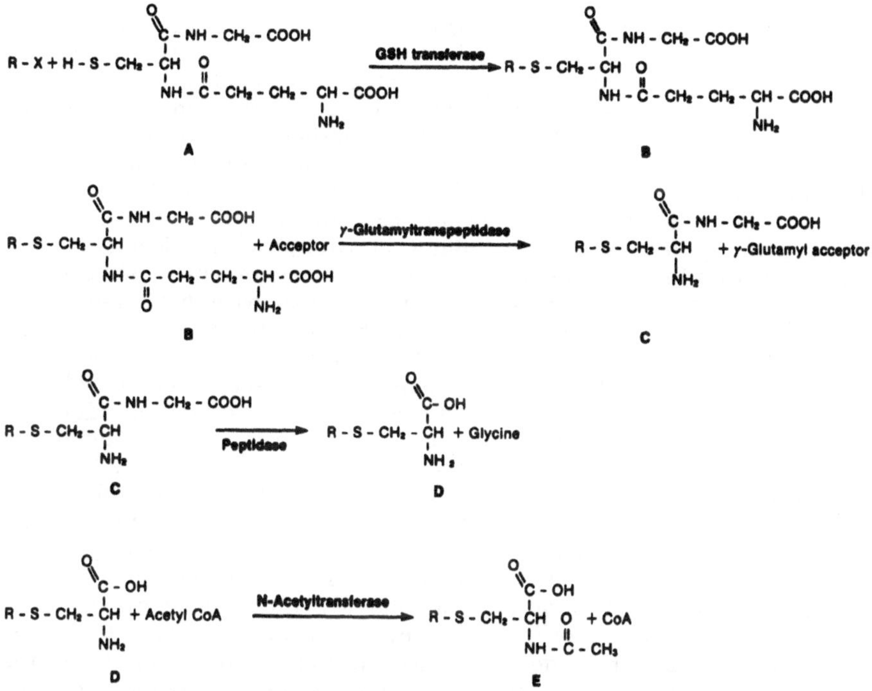

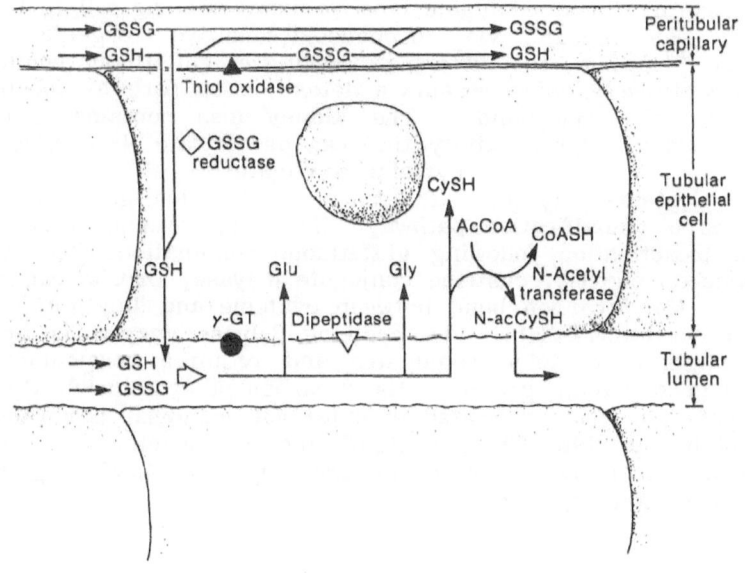

Figure 3 Enzymatic synthesis of glutathione conjugates and mercapturic acid conjugates. R-X = substrate, A = glutathione (GSH), B = glutathione conjugate, C = S-substituted cysteinylglycine, D = S-substituted cysteine, E = mercapturic acid conjugate. From Anders[6].

Figure 4 Processing of glutathione and glutathione conjugates by the renal proximal tubule. From Orrenius et al.[62].

The three enzymes primarily involved in mercapturic acid synthesis are concentrated within the outer stripe of the medulla in the rat kidney[79]. The N-acetylation step is rate-limiting for excretion of mercapturic acids[62,80]. The microsomal cysteine S-conjugate N-acetyltransferase is active with thioethers of L-cysteine and analogues such as O-benzyl-L-serine. Catalytic efficiency is a function of the lipophilicity of the sulphur substituent[81].

The role of the kidney in mercapturic acid synthesis has been investigated in studies using hepatocytes and isolated renal proximal tubule cells incubated with acetaminophen. Hepatocytes produce primarily glutathione-S-acetaminophen with little detectable cysteine or N-acetylcysteine conjugates[55]. Renal cells produce very little glutathione-S-acetaminophen but, rather, produce almost exclusively the N-acetylcysteine conjugate of acetaminophen[55]. If glutathione-S-acetaminophen produced by hepatocytes is added to medium containing isolated renal cells, the N-acetylcysteine-acetaminophen conjugate quickly accumulates[62]. Finally, when phenylalanylglycine, an inhibitor of cysteinylglycine dipeptidase, is included in the renal cell incubation medium, the cysteinylglycine-acetaminophen conjugate accumulates and N-acetylcysteine-acetaminophen disappears[62]. Isolated perfused rat kidneys excrete perfused acetaminophen or acetaminophen-S-glutathione as the mercapturic acid conjugate[80,82]. Thus, kidneys can form N-acetyl-cysteine-acetaminophen de novo from acetaminophen, or from the hepatic metabolite, glutathione-S-acetaminophen. Hepatocytes contain very little γ-glutamyl transpeptidase, the first enzyme in the reaction scheme. Once the glutathione conjugate is formed within the hepatocyte, it cannot undergo further metabolism but is released into the medium (or bile in vivo). Mercapturic acids are highly polar and will be readily excreted into the urine. Movement of mercapturic acid conjugate from proximal tubular cell to tubular lumen may occur via probenecid-sensitive organic anion secretion[80]. Thus, the further processing of glutathione conjugates to mercapturic acids represents a detoxification pathway for potentially reactive compounds. The kidney also contains a poorly characterized enzyme activity that can deacetylate N-acetylcysteine conjugates, reforming the cysteine conjugate[81].

Cysteine β-lyase. Glutathione conjugation generally functions as a detoxification pathway. However, compounds may undergo bioactivation following glutathione conjugation. The kidney contains an enzyme, cysteine conjugate β-lyase, that is capable of cleaving the β-carbon bond between cysteine and sulphur, leaving a reactive intermediate. The cysteine β-lyase enzyme is inactive with aliphatic cysteine conjugates and requires compounds that bear a good leaving group on the β-carbon of cysteine[83]. Cysteine conjugation β-lyase is located in outer mitochondrial membrane and cytosol in rat kidney[84]. The significance of cysteine conjugate β-lyase as an activator of protoxicants is only beginning to be recognized and explored.

d.   Glycine conjugation

A minor metabolic route involves condensation of a carboxylic acid-containing substrate with an amino acid such as glycine to form an amide (hippuric acid). The reaction involves activation of the carboxylic acid (e.g. salicylic acid) by binding coenzyme A. Salicyl-CoA and glycine are cosubstrates for acyl-CoA-glycine-N-acetyltransferase, which catalyses the condensation to salicyluric acid.

Glycine N-acetyltransferase activity is present in kidneys of rabbits, monkeys and humans[85]. The kidney may be a major site of metabolism of benzoic acid to hippuric acid, p-aminobenzoic acid to p-aminohippuric acid and salicylate to salicyluric acid[86-88]. The isolated rat kidney perfused with glycine and salicylic acid excretes 3-4% of the salicylic acid as the glycine conjugate[85]. These reactions are reversible; about 20% of perfused salicyluric acid is converted to salicylic acid by the isolated rat kidney whereas the liver does not convert salicyluric acid back to salicylate. Biosynthesized salicylate is rapidly excreted while perfused salicylate is more slowly excreted, suggesting that diffusion of salicylate into the cell is the rate-limiting step in its renal elimination, and that conversion of salicyluric acid to salicylate occurs within renal tubular cells[85].

Glycine conjugation may be competitively inhibited by other substrates such as benzoic acid or p-aminobenzoic acid. The amount of glycine present within cells is limited; thus, glycine conjugation would be expected to saturate with increasing concentrations of substrate. Glycine conjugation has not been investigated thoroughly and its role in renal xenobiotic metabolism is unclear.

3.   Other enzymes involved in xenobiotic metabolism

There are pathways for xenobiotic metabolism in the kidney that cannot be classified as Phase I or II reactions. This section will discuss several alternative pathways of xenobiotic metabolism.

a.   Epoxide hydrase (epoxide hydrolase)

Epoxides are highly reactive electrophiles that may interact with tissue macromolecules, leading ultimately to mutagenic and carcinogenic effects. Along with cytosolic GSH S-transferases, microsomal epoxide hydrase serves to detoxify epoxides. Epoxide hydrase catalyses the conversion of aliphatic and aromatic epoxides to trans-hydrodiols[6].

Epoxide hydrase activity is frequently coupled to cytochrome P-450 mixed function activity, as in the case of benzo(a)pyrene metabolism (Figure 5). Both enzyme activities are localized in the microsomal fraction of cells, making coordinated reactions likely. The initial steps in benzo(a)pyrene metabolism are cytochrome P-450-dependent oxidations to benzo(a)pyrene-4,5-oxide and benzo(a)pyrene 7,8-oxide. Epoxide hydrase catalyses the hydration of both reaction products, forming 4,5-dihydroxy-4,5-

387

dihydrobenzo(a)pyrene, a non-toxic product, and 7,8-dihydroxy-7,8-dihydrobenzo(a)pyrene, thought to be the ultimate carcinogen[89]. Thus, epoxide hydrase may serve to either detoxify or activate a protoxicant.

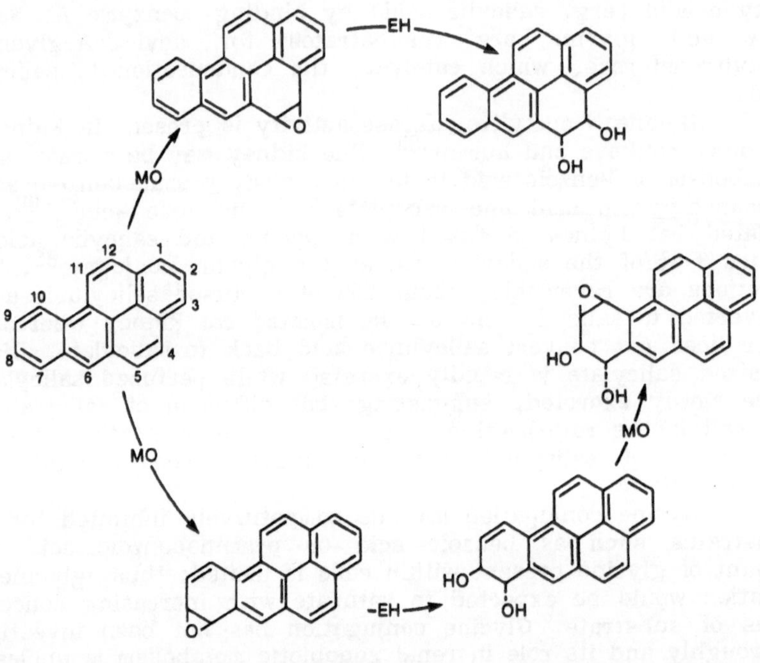

Figure 5 Interactions of cytochrome P-450 mixed function oxidases (MO) and epoxide hydrase (EH) in the metabolism of benzo(a)pyrene. From Schmassmann et al.[89].

The kidney contains epoxide hydrase activity that is approximately 10% of hepatic activity in rats, mice and hamsters[90]. Hepatic epoxide hydrase activity is enhanced by pretreatment of rats with phenobarbital, 16α-cyanopregnenolone and trans-stilbene oxide but is refractory to 3-MC or TCDD treatment[20,91,92]. In rats, renal epoxide hydrase activity is specifically increased by trans-stilbene oxide with no change in cytochrome P-450 aryl hydrocarbon hydroxylase activity[56,89], indicating that epoxide hydrase and cytochrome P-450 activities may be dissociated. Species differences exist in epoxide hydrase induction; epoxide hydrase activity is not induced by trans-stilbene oxide in mice and hamsters[90]. Hepatic epoxide hydrase activity is slightly higher in male compared to female rats; sex differences are not apparent in renal epoxide hydrase activity[90].

b. Aldehyde oxidation

The oxidation of aldehydes to ketones or carboxylic acids is catalysed by two groups of enzymes, aldehyde oxidase and aldehyde dehydrogenase. Both enzyme activities are present in the kidney[5].

Renal aldehyde oxidase activity is 40% of that in the liver with benzaldehyde as the substrate[6]. However, renal aldehyde oxidase activity is only 10% of renal aldehyde dehydrogenase activity, suggesting a minor role for renal aldehyde oxidase[6].

Aldehyde dehydrogenases are localized in the cytosol and mitochondria of cells and function to detoxify reactive aldehydes. Substrates for aldehyde dehydrogenases include formaldehyde, acetaldehyde, acrolein and malondialdehyde[93]. Within the kidney, two isozymes of aldehyde dehydrogenase have been identified in mitochondria and two in the cytosol. Using propionaldehyde as the substrate, the isozymes show different kinetic parameters, suggesting the presence of at least four separate isozymes[93].

Aldehyde dehydrogenases utilize NAD^+ or $NADP^+$, although activity with $NADP^+$ is only 30% of that observed with NAD^+[94]. In the kidney, aldehyde dehydrogenase activity is greatest in proximal tubule cells[93]. Although renal homogenate activity of aldehyde dehydrogenase is only 20% of hepatic activity[94], specific activity in proximal tubule cells is higher than hepatic activity[93].

c. Prostaglandin H synthase (prostaglandin endoperoxide synthetase)

The enzymatic processes discussed thus far are localized primarily in the renal cortex and proximal tubule. It has long been recognized that the renal medulla and papilla are also targets for toxicity. Specifically, the chronic abuse of analgesics (phenacetin, aspirin, acetaminophen) and non-steroidal anti-inflammatory agents (NSAIDs) is associated with renal papillary necrosis[95,96]. One mechanism by which these lesions occur is thought to involve xenobiotic cooxidation catalysed by prostaglandin H synthase (formerly prostaglandin endoperoxide synthetase).

Prostaglandin H synthase is a haemoprotein involved in biosynthesis of prostaglandins, thromboxanes and prostacyclins. Two enzymes are involved in the conversion of arachidonic acid to hydroxyendoperoxide PGH_2: fatty acid cyclooxygenase and prostaglandin hydroperoxidase activities. Fatty acid cyclooxygenase catalyses the initial bis-oxidation of unsaturated fatty acids, converting arachidonic acid to hydroperoxyendo-peroxide PGG_2. Two molecules of molecular oxygen are inserted into arachidonic acid to form a 15-hydroperoxy prostaglandin cyclic epoxide intermediate. Prostaglandin hydroperoxidase catalyses the cleavage of the 15-hydroperoxy group and acts as an electron donor, reducing PGG_2 to PGH_2, a 15-hydroxy cyclic endoperoxide. Prostaglandin hydroperoxidase is re-reduced, resulting in (co-)oxidation of the xenobiotic. PGH_2 undergoes further biotransformation to produce prostaglandins and thromboxanes[97]. The two enzyme activities may be distinguished by several criteria: (1) substrate requirement (fatty acid cyclooxygenase specifically requires polyunsaturated fatty acids while prostaglandin hydroperoxidase activity is supported by cumene hydroperoxide or tert-butyl hydroperoxide); (2) inhibitors (aspirin and NSAIDs are specific inhibitors of fatty acid cyclooxygenase activity without affecting prostaglandin hydroperoxidase activity); (3) heme requirement (prostaglandin hydroperoxidase specifically requires a ferric heme component; fatty acid cyclooxygenase does not); (4) oxygen requirement (fatty acid cyclooxygenase requires oxygen whereas prostaglandin hydroperoxidase will function under anaerobic conditions); and (5) production of radical intermediates (fatty acid cyclooxygenase does not produce free radicals, prostaglandin hydroperoxidase does)[97].

Xenobiotic cooxidation catalysed by prostaglandin H synthase. Prostaglandin H synthase from ram seminal vesicular microsomes metabolizes a variety of organic compounds by cooxidation[98]. Xenobiotic substrates include phenylbutazone and acetaminophen[99], compounds implicated in renal papillary necrosis. Other xenobiotic substrates for cooxidation include phenobarbital, sulindac sulphate, oxyphenylbutazone and benzo(a)pyrene[99]. One consequence of xenobiotic cooxidation is covalent binding of the activated xenobiotic metabolite to cellular macromolecules, DNA or RNA[97].

In rabbit kidney, prostaglandin H synthase activity is not distributed uniformly but follows a concentration gradient opposite that described for cytochrome P-450 mixed function oxidase activity. Specifically, prostaglandin H synthase activity is highest in inner medulla, intermediate in outer medulla and barely detectable in cortex[100,101]. Within cells, prostaglandin H synthase activity is localized in endoplasmic reticulum and nuclear membrane[102]. Hepatocytes contain relatively low prostaglandin H synthase activity[99].

Xenobiotic cooxidation is supported by the prostaglandin hydroperoxidase activity and may be independent of fatty acid cyclooxygenase activity of prostaglandin H synthase. Fatty acid cyclooxygenase activity is necessary for xenobiotic cooxidation when arachidonic acid is a co-substrate. Coincubation of acetaminophen and arachidonic acid with rabbit renal medullary microsomes results in covalent binding of an acetaminophen metabolite to trichloroacetic acid-precipitable protein. Inhibition of microsomal binding occurs with in vitro addition of, or in vivo pretreatment with, aspirin, an inhibitor of fatty acid cyclooxygenase[103]. Glutathione also inhibits covalent binding of acetaminophen during arachidonic acid-stimulated cooxidation, consistent with the notion that an electrophilic intermediate is generated by cooxidation[103]. When 15-HPETE (a substrate for prostaglandin hydroperoxidase that does not require prior metabolism by fatty acid cyclooxygenase) and acetaminophen are coincubated with medullary microsomes, covalent binding of acetaminophen still occurs but is no longer inhibited by aspirin. Covalent binding also occurs in aspirin-treated microsomes when 15-HPETE is supplied[103]. Thus, acetaminophen cooxidation and the resultant covalent binding require prostaglandin peroxidase activity but does not necessarily depend on cyclooxygenase activity.

A major criticism of the cooxidation theory of analgesic-induced renal papillary necrosis is the observation that most analgesics are fatty acid cyclooxygenase inhibitors[104]. Although some degree of cyclooxygenase inhibition may occur with analgesics, endogenous lipid peroxides may serve as cosubstrates for prostaglandin hydroperoxidase[105,106]. Thus, the ability of analgesics to inhibit cyclooxygenase activity does not preclude their activation via the separate prostaglandin hydroperoxidase activity.

Prostaglandin hydroperoxidase is not unique in supporting xenobiotic cooxidation. Other peroxidases (lactoperoxidase, chloroperoxidase, horseradish peroxidase) support the cooxidation of benzidine, as assessed by covalent binding of radiolabel derived from benzidine to protein[106]. Cumene hydroperoxide and tert-butyl hydroperoxide will support prostaglandin hydroperoxidase cooxidation in the absence of fatty acid substrates[105].

Xenobiotics that undergo cooxidation include compounds known to produce renal and bladder cancer, such as N-[4-(5-nitro-2-furyl)-2-thiazolyl]formamide (FANFT)[107], benzidine[108], and 2-amino-4-(5-nitro-2-furyl)thiazole formamide[109]. Reactive intermediates produced by cooxidation may be conjugated with glucuronic acid, catalysed by medullary UDP-glucuronyl transferases[37]. Generally, conjugation would serve to detoxify a reactive intermediate. However, N-glucuronides, as produced from some procarcinogens, are unstable at acidic pH. In the urinary bladder, these conjugates may be hydrolysed to release the free aryl hydroxylamines which are capable of covalent binding to tissue macromolecules[97].

Prostaglandin H synthase catalysed xenobiotic cooxidation is believed to be a mechanism whereby compounds produce specific medullary or papillary damage. In addition, renal cooxidation probably accounts for activation of some bladder carcinogens. Cooxidation produces reactive intermediates that are thought to ultimately produce tissue damage. It is possible that antioxidants or scavenger radicals (glutathione, N-acetyl cysteine) may prevent this type of tissue damage[97].

d.   DT-diaphorase

Among the reactive intermediates produced by prostaglandin H synthase-dependent cooxidation are quinones and quinonimines. As previously discussed, quinones may undergo redox cycling catalysed by NADPH cytochrome P-450 reductase. DT-diaphorase (NAD(P)H:quinone oxidoreductase) catalyses a two-electron reduction of quinones to produce the less reactive hydroquinones, thereby interrupting redox cycling and generation of superoxide anion radicals[110].

DT-diaphorase, a cytosolic enzyme, is present in the kidney and follows the distribution of prostaglandin H synthase, i.e. highest in inner medulla and lowest in cortex[111]. DT-diaphorase represents a major route of quinone detoxification in the kidney; renal DT-diaphorase in outer medulla is three-fold higher than in liver homogenates from rabbits[111].

METABOLIC FORMATION OF NEPHROTOXIC COMPOUNDS

The preceding section has described various pathways in the kidney for xenobiotic metabolism. While many of these pathways serve to detoxify reactive intermediates, some of these reactions may actually activate a protoxicant. Generation of a toxicant may occur in situ in the kidney following intracellular accumulation of parent compound or non-nephrotoxic metabolite formed in extrarenal tissue. This section will briefly discuss several examples of compounds that are activated to toxicants by renal metabolism.

1.   Nephrotoxic metabolites generated within the kidney

Reactive intermediates are likely to bind covalently to tissue macromolecules in close proximity to the site of their formation. It is unlikely that a highly reactive and unstable species could be transported in blood or bile to the site of toxicity. Some nephrotoxicants produce highly selective damage, injuring exclusively the proximal straight tubule or renal medulla. The presence of specific enzyme systems of xenobiotic metabolism in such discrete areas of the kidneys suggests that the kidneys are involved in bioactivation of protoxicants.

Chloroform. An example of a chemical that is metabolically activated within the kidney is chloroform[34,112,113]. Chloroform ($CHCl_3$), a common organic solvent that has been used widely in the chemical industry, is capable of producing hepatic and renal injury in humans and experimental animals. It has been suggested that tissue injury by chloroform is probably not due to $CHCl_3$ per se, but is produced by a $CHCl_3$ metabolite[114]. The initial step leading to $CHCl_3$-induced tissue injury is believed to be the biotransformation of $CHCl_3$ to a reactive intermediate, phosgene ($COCl_2$), by cytochrome P-450-dependent mixed function oxidases. Formation of $COCl_2$ has been postulated to proceed through an oxidative dechlorination mechanism involving oxidation of the C-H bond of $CHCl_3$, producing the trichloromethanol (CCl_3-OH) intermediate, a highly unstable species that would spontaneously dechlorinate to $COCl_2$. Phosgene may subsequently react with intracellular macromolecules to induce cell damage.

Since kidneys have relatively low xenobiotic-metabolizing enzyme activities, chemically induced nephrotoxicity has been assumed to be produced by toxic intermediates generated in the liver and transported to the kidney. If a single hepatic metabolite of $CHCl_3$ produced both kidney and liver injury, species, strain and sex differences in susceptibility to $CHCl_3$ nephro- and hepatotoxicity would be expected to be the same. However, species, strain and sex differences in susceptibility to $CHCl_3$ nephrotoxicity are not consistent with those of $CHCl_3$ hepatotoxicity. Furthermore, several modulators of tissue xenobiotic-metabolizing activities alter $CHCl_3$ nephrotoxicity and hepatotoxicity differently[112]. Since $CHCl_3$-induced kidney injury does not parallel liver damage, it is unlikely that hepatic metabolism of $CHCl_3$ is responsible for renal toxicity.

The concept that kidney injury is produced by a $CHCl_3$ metabolite generated in the kidney has been demonstrated directly using in vitro techniques. In order to avoid hepatic metabolism of $CHCl_3$, renal cortical slices from naive animals were incubated with $CHCl_3$ in vitro[34]. Under these conditions, the only site of metabolism of $CHCl_3$ is the kidney. In vitro exposure to $CHCl_3$ produced toxicity in kidney slices from male but not from female mice[34]. Furthermore, $^{14}CHCl_3$ was metabolized to $^{14}CO_2$ and covalently bound radioactivity by male, but not female, renal cortical microsomes. The in vitro metabolism of $CHCl_3$ by male but not female renal slices is consistent with reduced susceptibility of female mice to in vivo $CHCl_3$ nephrotoxicity[31,115]. Metabolism required oxygen, an NADPH regenerating system, was dependent on incubation time, microsomal protein concentration, and substrate concentration and was inhibited by carbon monoxide[34]. The negligible degree of $CHCl_3$ metabolism and toxicity in female mice is consistent with lower renal cytochrome P-450 concentration and activity in female versus male mice (Table 2)[34]. Pretreatment of rabbits with phenobarbital, a renal cytochrome P-450 inducer in this species, enhanced the toxic response of renal cortical slices to chloroform in vitro[116].

$CDCl_3$ is metabolized by the liver to phosgene ($COCl_2$) at approximately half the rate of $CHCl_3$ metabolism to $COCl_2$. $CDCl_3$ is also less hepatotoxic that $CHCl_3$. Since the C-D bond is stronger than the C-H bond, these data suggest that cleavage of the C-H bond is the rate-limiting step in the activation of $CHCl_3$. $CDCl_3$ is also less toxic to the kidney than $CHCl_3$[117,118]. This deuterium isotope effect on $CHCl_3$-induced nephrotoxicity suggests that the kidney metabolizes $CHCl_3$ in the same manner as the liver, e.g. by oxidation to $COCl_2$. Indeed, rabbit renal cortical microsomes incubated in media supplemented with L-cysteine metabolized $^{14}CHCl_3$ to radioactive phosgene-cysteine 2-oxothiazolidine-4-carboxylic acid[116]. These in vitro data collectively support the hypothesis that mouse and rabbit kidneys biotransform chloroform to a metabolite ($COCl_2$) that mediates nephrotoxicity.

Acetaminophen. Large overdoses of acetaminophen can produce massive centrilobular necrosis and acute renal failure. Acetaminophen-induced acute nephrotoxicity (proximal tubular necrosis) in laboratory animals is species- and strain-dependent. Large dosages of acetaminophen do not produce detectable histopathological changes in kidneys of Sprague-Dawley rats, mice, or rabbits but do produce renal proximal tubular necrosis in male Fischer-344 rats[119-122].

Metabolism of acetaminophen by microsomal cytochrome P-450 to a reactive, arylating intermediate is thought to be an obligatory biochemical event in acetaminophen-induced hepatic necrosis[123,124]. Similarly, acetaminophen-induced renal tubular necrosis is also thought to occur following metabolic activation. However, the exact mechanism of renal metabolic activation is not entirely clear.

Administration of nephrotoxic dosages of acetaminophen to Fischer-344 rats results in covalent binding to renal protein[119,121,124]. Acetaminophen can be metabolically activated in renal cortical microsomes from Fischer-344 rats by an NADPH-dependent, cytochrome P-450-mediated process[121,122,125]. However, renal cortical concentrations of cytochrome P-450 are approximately one-tenth of that in liver, yet in vivo arylation of hepatic and renal macromolecules by acetaminophen is almost identical[121], suggesting that some mechanism other than cytochrome P-450 activation may be involved in acetaminophen nephrotoxicity.

An alternative mechanism to cytochrome P-450-dependent activation of acetaminophen is enzymatic deacetylation to p-aminophenol (PAP). PAP is a potent, selective nephrotoxicant that damages the latter third of the proximal tubule[126]. Both acetaminophen and PAP deplete renal cortical reduced glutathione concentrations and arylate renal macromolecules[121,127]. The functional and histopathological lesions produced by PAP are indistinguishable from the renal lesions produced by acetaminophen administration[122]. Mouse renal cortical slices and homogenates are capable of deacetylating acetaminophen to PAP[128]. PAP has also been identified as a urinary metabolite of acetaminophen in both hamster[129] and Fischer-344 rat[122]. These data demonstrate that the rat is capable of deacetylating acetaminophen to PAP. In renal cortex, acetaminophen deacetylation occurs primarily in the cytosolic fraction[122]. Similarly, metabolic activation of acetaminophen to an arylating intermediate is dependent on the presence of a cytosolic deacetylase[125]. Furthermore, both PAP and bis-(p-nitro-phenyl)-phosphate (a carboxylesterase/amidase inhibi-tor) inhibit the covalent binding of acetaminophen to renal macromolecules[125]. Conclusive evidence that acetaminophen binds to renal macromolecules subsequent to deacetylation and metabolic activation to PAP was demonstrated by the covalent binding of [ring-^{14}C]acetaminophen but not [acetyl-^{14}C]acetaminophen to renal protein[125].

Acetaminophen activation by renal cortical tissue, therefore, can occur by two different mechanisms. One mechanism is dependent upon microsomal cytochrome P-450 as indicated by the requirement for NADPH. Another mechanism is dependent upon deacetylation of acetaminophen and subsequent metabolic activation of PAP. Formation of reactive intermediates from each pathway, by implication, indicates that both mechanisms may be involved in the pathogenesis of acetaminophen-induced renal cortical necrosis.

2. Non-nephrotoxic metabolites generated in extrarenal tissues with subsequent intrarenal conversion to nephrotoxicants

In certain instances, xenobiotics may be metabolized in extrarenal tissue, e.g. liver, to products that may be substrates for renal enzymes. These non-nephrotoxic metabolites are converted to toxic intermediates and produce kidney damage in situ. For instance, nephrotoxicity produced by hexachloro-1,3-butadiene (HCBD) appears to occur via sequential hepatic and renal metabolism.

Hexachloro-1,3-butadiene. Hexachloro-1,3-butadiene (HCBD) is a widespread environmetal pollutant that is a relatively potent nephrotoxicant in rats, mice, and other mammalian species. The kidneys appear to be the primary target of HCBD toxicity[130]. In rats the compound produces a well-defined lesion in the S_3 segment of the proximal tubule, characterized by a loss of brush border[130-133]. Functional changes at large dosages include decreased urinary concentrating ability[131,132,134,135], glucosuria and proteinuria[132,134], increased urinary excretion of alkaline phosphatase and N-acetyl-β-D-glucosaminidase[132], and reduction of the renal clearances of inulin, para-aminohippurate and tetraethyl-ammonium[132,135].

A time-dependent loss of renal, but not hepatic, cytochrome

P-450 is observed during the first 12 hours following HCBD administration to rats[136]. Neither cytochrome b_5 nor NADPH-cytochrome c-reductase are significantly affected. The metabolism of several cytochrome P-450 substrates is decreased in HCBD-treated female rats and male mice.

Reports on the effects of HCBD following pretreatment of animals with inducers and/or inhibitors of drug-metabolizing enzymes are conflicting. Early studies indicated that pretreatment of rats with inhibitors and inducers of cytochrome P-450 had little or no effect on the toxicity of HCBD, suggesting that HCBD may not be metabolically activated[133]. In more recent studies, however, isosafrole or B-NF reduced the nephrotoxicity of HCBD[136,137]. A systemically administered dose of HCBD is extensively metabolized; it appears that the majority of metabolites may originate from hepatic GSH conjugation with HCBD[130,135]. In adult male rats, HCBD causes depletion of hepatic but not renal GSH content[130,133,138,139], whereas, in female rats, a significant depletion of GSH occurs in the kidney at much lower doses than in the liver[130].

The formation of a GSH conjugate of HCBD has been demonstrated in rat liver microsomes and occurs under N_2 and CO in the absence of NADPH[140]. This suggests that the reaction is a substitution of the halogen catalysed by GSH S-transferase, rather than by cytochrome P-450. Once formed, the GSH conjugate of HCBD may be transported to bile, returned to the bloodstream via intestinal reabsorption, and excreted via the kidneys[141]. Rats fitted with biliary cannulae are completely protected from nephrotoxicity following HCBD administration, demonstrating that hepatic metabolites mediate HCBD nephrotoxicity[141]. In vivo and in vitro exposure to the cysteine conjugate of HCBD, S-pentachlorobuta-1,3-dienyl cysteine, causes dose-dependent nephrotoxicity localized in the proximal straight tubule[142]. Hepatic metabolism of HCBD-GSH may enable the production of a nephrotoxic intermediate via renal C-S lyase. A C-S lyase capable of activating such conjugates is present in the liver as well as the kidney; it is possible that the unique renal susceptibility to HCBD is related to the kidney's ability to accumulate these ionic conjugates. Probenecid, an inhibitor of organic anion transport, blocks both the renal accumulation of HCBD metabolites and nephrotoxicity[143], suggesting that organic anion transport is required for HCBD nephrotoxicity.

THE SIGNIFICANCE OF RENAL XENOBIOTIC METABOLISM

It has become apparent that the kidney possesses unique biochemical characteristics that may predispose it to the harmful effects of some chemicals. The activities of renal cytochrome P-450-dependent mixed function oxidases are low in renal homogenates when compared to liver. However, since mixed function oxidases appear to be concentrated within the S_2 and S_3 segments of proximal tubules, it is likely that these cells have very high specific activities. This would render the cortex vulnerable to compounds requiring metabolic activation by cytochrome P-450-mediated systems for toxicity. In the inner medulla and papilla, prostaglandin H synthase may bioactivate xenobiotics via cooxidation during synthesis of prostaglandins. This pathway may be of particular importance in the metabolism of bladder carcinogens. In addition, prostaglandin H synthase may contribute to the aetiology of papillary necrosis resulting from chronic analgesic abuse.

The precise biochemical mechanisms of nephrotoxicants have not been well defined. However, increasing evidence indicates that xenobiotics may be metabolically activated to toxic species within the kidney. A clearer understanding of biochemical protoxicant activation will require more complete information concerning the various enzymes involved in renal xenobiotic bioactivation, including the precise localization of such enzymes along the nephron and a thorough understanding of how those enzymes may be modulated.

REFERENCES

1. Kluwe, W.M. and Hook, J.B., Effects of environmental chemicals on kidney metabolism and function, Kidney Int., 18, 648, 1980.
2. Rush, G.F., Smith, J.H., Newton, J.F. and Hook, J.B., Chemically induced nephrotoxicity: role of metabolic activation, CRC Crit. Rev. Toxicol., 13, 99, 1984.
3. Ellin, A., Jakobsson, S.W., Schenkman, J.B., and Orrenius, S., Cytochrome P-450 of rat kidney cortex microsomes: its involvement in fatty acid ω-and (ω-1) hydroxylation, Arch. Biochem. Biophys., 150, 64, 1972.
4. Okita, R.T., Yasukochi, Y., Masters, B.S.S., Theoharides, A.D. and Kupfer, D., Prostaglandin ω- and (ω-1)-hydroxylation by pig kidney cortex cytochrome P-450, Prog. Lipid Res., 20, 283, 1981.
5. Goldberg, J.P. and Anderson, R.J., Renal metabolism and excretion of drugs, in The Kidney: Physiology and Pathophysiology, Seldin, D.W. and Giebisch, G., Eds., Raven Press, New York, 1985, 2097.
6. Anders, M.W., Metabolism of drugs by the kidney, Kidney Int., 18, 636, 1980.
7. Connelly, J.C. and Bridges, J.W., The distribution and role of cytochrome P-450 in extrahepatic organs, in Reviews in Biochemical Toxicology, Vol. 1, Bridges, J.W. and Chasseaud, L.F., Eds., John Wiley and Sons, New York, 1980, 1.
8. Jones, D.P., Orrenius, S. and Jakobsson, S.W., Cytochrome P-450-linked monooxygenase systems in the kidney, in Extrahepatic Metabolism of Drugs and other Foreign Compounds, Gram, T.E., Ed., Spectrum Publications, New York, 123, 1980.
9. Bachur, N.R., Gordon, S.L., Gee, M.V. and Kon, H., NADPH cytochrome P-450 reductase activation of quinone anticancer agents to free radicals., Proc. Natl. Acad. Sci., 76, 954, 1979.
10. Berlin, V. and Haseltine, W.A., Reduction of adriamycin to a semiquinone-free radical by NADPH cytochrome P-450 reductase produces DNA cleavage in a reaction mediated by molecular oxygen., J. Biol. Chem., 256, 4747, 1981.
11. Kappus, H. and Sies, H., Toxic drug effects associated with oxygen metabolism: Redox cycling and lipid peroxidation, Experientia, 37, 1233, 1981.
12. Kluwe, W.M., McCormack, K.M. and Hook, J.B., Selective modification of the renal and hepatic toxicities of chloroform by induction of drug metabolizing enzyme systems in kidney and liver, J. Pharmacol. Exp. Ther., 207, 566,

1978.

13.   Rush, G.F., Wilson, D.M. and Hook, J.B., Selective induction and inhibition of renal mixed function oxidases in the rat and rabbit, Fund. Appl. Toxicol., 3, 161, 1983.

14.   Kuo, C.-H., Rush, G.F. and Hook, J.B., Renal cortical accumulation of phenobarbital in rats and rabbits: lack of correlation with induction of renal microsomal monooxygenases, J. Pharmacol. Exp. Ther., 220, 547, 1982.

15.   Lake, B.G., Hopkins, R., Chakraborty, J., Bridges, J.W. and Parke, D.V.W., The influence of some hepatic enzyme inducers and inhibitors on extrahepatic drug metabolism, Drug Metab. Disp., 1, 342, 1973.

16.   Rush, G.F., Maita, K., Sleight, S.D. and Hook, J.B., Induction of rabbit renal mixed function oxidases by phenobabital: cell specific ultrastructural changes in the proximal tubule, Proc. Soc. Exp. Biol. Med., 172, 430, 1983.

17.   Smith, J.H., Rush, G.F. and Hook, J.B., Induction of renal and hepatic mixed function oxidases in the hamster and guinea pig, Toxicology, 38, 209, 1986.

18.   Masters, B.S.S., Okita, R.T., Yasukochi, Y., Parkhill, L.K. and Dees, J.H., Properties, function, and localization of two cytochromes P-450 from liver and kidney, in Proteins in Biology and Medicine, Bradshaw, R.A., ed.,Academic Press, New York, 1982, 183.

19.   Poland, A., Glover, E. and Kende, A.S., Stereospecific high affinity binding of 2,3,7,8-tetrachlorodibenzo-p-dioxin by hepatic cytosol, J. Biol. Chem., 251, 4936, 1976.

20.   Aitio, A. and Parkki, M.G., Organ specific induction of drug metabolizing enzymes by 2,3,7,8-tetrachlorodibenzo-p-dioxin in the rat, Toxicol. Appl. Pharmacol., 44, 107, 1978.

21.   Fry, J.R. and Perry, N.K., The effect of Aroclor 1254 pretreatment on the phase I and phase II metabolism of 7-ethoxycoumarin in isolated viable rat kidney cells, Biochem. Pharmacol., 30, 1197, 1981.

22.   Uotila, P., Parkki, M.G. and Aitio, A., Quantitative and qualitative changes in the metabolism of benzo(a)pyrene in rat tissues after intragastric administration of TCDD, Toxicol. Appl. Pharmacol., 46, 671, 1978.

23.   Liem, H.H., Muller-Eberhard, U. and Johnson, E.F., Differential induction by 2,3,7,8-tetrachlorodibenzo-p-dioxin of multiple forms of rabbit microsomal cytochrome P-450: evidence for tissue specificity, Mol. Pharmacol., 18, 565, 1980.

24.   Dees. J.H., Masters, B.S.S., Muller-Eberhard, U. and Johnson, E.F., Effect of 2,3,7,8-tetrachlorodibenzo-p-dioxin and phenobarbital on the occurrence and distribution of four cytochrome P-450 isozymes in rabbit kidney, lung, and liver, Cancer Res., 42, 1423, 1982.

25.   Dees, J.H., Coe, L.D., Yasukochi, Y. and Masters, B.S.S., Immunofluorescence of NADPH-cytochrome c (P-450) reductase in rat and minipig tissues injected with phenobarbital, Science, 208, 1473, 1980.

26.   Dees, J.H., Parkhill, L.K., Okita, R.T., Yasukochi, Y. and Masters, B.S.S., Localization of NADPH-cytochrome P-450 reductase and cytochrome P-450 in animal kidneys, in Nephrotoxicity: Assessment and Pathogenesis, Bach, P.H., Boner, F.W., Bridges, J.W., and Lock, E.A., eds., John Wiley & Sons, New York, 1982, 246.

27.   Ogita, K., Kusunose, E., Ichihara, K. and Kusunose, M., Multiple forms of cytochrome P-450 in kidney cortex microsomes of rabbits treated with 3-methylcholanthrene, J. Biochem., 92, 921, 1982.

28.   Ogita, K., Kusunose, E., Yamamoto, S., Ichihara, K. and Kusunose, M., Multiple forms of cytochrome P-450 from kidney cortex microsomes of rabbits treated with phenobarbital, Biochem. Int., 6, 191, 1983.

29.   Hook, J.B., Elcombe, C.R., Rose, M.S. and Lock, E.A., Characterization of

the effects of known hepatic monooxygenase inducers on male and female rat and mouse kidneys, Life Sci., 31, 1077, 1982.

30. Krijsheld, K.R. and Gram, T.E., Selective induction of renal microsomal cytochrome P-450-linked monooxygenases by 1,1-dichloroethylene in mice, Biochem. Pharmacol., 33, 1951, 1984.

31. Smith, J.H., Maita, K., Sleight, S.D. and Hook, J.B., Effect of sex hormone status on chloroform nephrotoxicity and renal mixed function oxidases in mice, Toxicology, 30, 305, 1984.

32. Zenser, T.V., Mattammal, M.B. and Davis, B.B., Differential distribution of the mixed function oxidase in rabbit kidney, J. Pharmacol. Exp. Ther., 207, 719, 1978.

33. Endou, H., Cytochrome P-450 monooxygenase system in the kidney: its intranephron localization and its induction, Jpn. J. Pharmacol., 33, 423, 1983.

34. Smith, J.H. and Hook, J.B., Mechanism of chloroform nephrotoxicity. III. Renal and hepatic microsomal metabolism of chloroform in mice, Toxicol. Appl. Pharmacol., 73, 511, 1984.

35. Litterst, C.L., Mimnaugh, E.G. and Gram, T.E., Alterations in extrahepatic drug metabolism by factors known to affect hepatic activity, Biochem. Pharmacol., 26, 749, 1977.

36. Hawke, R.L. and Welch, R.M., Major differences in the specificity and regulation of mouse renal cytochrome P-450 dependent monooxygenases, Molec. Pharmacol., 27, 283, 1985.

37. Fowler, B.A., Hook, G.E.R. and Lucier, G.W., 2,3,7,8-Tetrachlorodibenzo-p-dioxin induction of renal microsomal enzyme systems: ultrastructural effects on pars recta (S_3) proximal tubule cells of rat kidney, J. Pharmacol. Exp. Ther., 203, 712, 1977.

38. Cojocel, C., Maita, K., Pasino, D.A., Kuo, C.-H. and Hook, J.B., Metabolic heterogeneity of the proximal and distal kidney tubules, Life Sci., 33, 855, 1983.

39. Maunsbach, A.B., Observations on the segmentation of the proximal tubule in the rat kidney. Comparison of results from phase contrast, fluorescence and electron microscopy, J. Ultrastruct. Res., 16, 239, 1966.

40. Woodhall, P.B., Tisher, C.C., Simonton, C.A. and Robinson, R.R., Relationship between para-aminohippurate secretion and cellular morphology in rabbit proximal tubules, J. Clin. Invest., 51, 1320, 1978.

41. Kaissling, B. and Kriz, W., Structural analysis of the rabbit kidney, in Advances in Anatomy, Embryology and Cell Biology, Vol. 56 ,Brodal, A., Hild, W., van Limborgh, J., Ortmannm, R., Schievler, T.H., Tondury, G. and Wolff, E., eds., Springer-Verlag, New York, 1979, 123.

42. Shimomura, A., Chonko, A.M. and Grantham, J.J., Basis for heterogeneity of para-aminohippurate secretion in rabbit proximal tubules, Am. J. Physiol., 240, F430, 1981.

43. McKinney, T.D., Heterogeneity of organic base secretion by proximal tubules, Am. J. Physiol., 243, F404, 1982.

44. Schali, C., Schild, L, Overney, J. and Roch-Ramel, F., Secretion of tetraethylammonium by proximal tubules of rabbit kidney, Am. J. Physiol., 245, F238, 1983.

45. Fowler, B.A., The morphological effects of dieldrin and methyl mercuric chloride on pars recta segments in rat kidney proximal tubules, Am. J. Pathol., 69, 163, 1972.

46. Rush, G.F., Pratt, I.S., Lock, E.A. and Hook, J.B., Induction of renal mixed function oxidases in the rat and mouse: correlation with ultrastructural changes in the proximal tubule, Fund. Appl. Toxicol., 6, 307, 1986.

47. Bock, K.W., Josting, D., Lilienblum, W. and Pfeil, H., Purification of rat-liver microsomal UDP-glucuronyltransferase. Separation of two enzyme forms inducible by 3-methylcholanthrene or phenobarbital, Eur. J. Biochem., 98, 19, 1979.

48. Bock, K.W., Clausbruch, U.C.V., Kaufmann, R., Lilienblum, W., Oesch, F., Pfeil, H. and Platt, K.L., Functional heterogeneity of UDP-glucuronyltransferase in rat tissues, Biochem. Pharmacol., 29, 495, 1980.

49. Kluwe, W.M. and Hook, J.B., Comparative induction of xenobiotic metabolism in rodent kidney, testis and liver by commercial mixtures of polybrominated biphenyls and polychlorinated biphenyls, phenobarbital and 3-methylcholanthrene: absolute and temporal effects, Toxicology, 20, 259, 1981.

50. Hjelle, J.T., Hazelton, G.A., Klaassen, C.D. and Hjelle, J.J., Glucuronidation and sulphation in rabbit kidney, J. Pharmacol. Exp. Ther., 236, 150, 1986.

51. Hanninen, O. and Aitio, A., Enhanced glucuronide formation in different tissues following drug administration, Biochem. Pharmacol., 17, 2307, 1968.

52. Aitio, A., Induction of UDP glucuronyltransferase in the liver and extrahepatic organs of the rat, Life Sci., 13, 1705, 1973.

53. Rush, G.F. and Hook, J.B., Characteristics of renal UDP-glucuronyltransferase, Life Sci., 35, 145, 1984.

54. Aitio, A., Vainio, H. and Hanninen, O., Enhancement of drug oxidation and conjugation by carcinogens in different rat tissue, FEBS Lett., 24, 237, 1972.

55. Jones, D.P., Sundby, G.-B., Ormstad, K. and Orrenius, S., Use of isolated kidney cells for study of drug metabolism, Biochem. Pharmacol., 28, 929, 1979.

56. Kuo, C.-H., Hook, J.B. and Bernstein, J., Induction of drug-metabolizing enzymes and toxicity of trans-stilbene oxide in rat liver and kidney, Toxicology, 22, 149, 1981.

57. Mandel, H.G., Pathways of drug biotransformation: biochemical conjugations, in Fundamentals of Drug Metabolism and Drug Disposition, LaDu, B.N., Mandel, H.G. and Way, E.L., eds., Williams & Wilkins Co., Baltimore, 1971, 149.

58. Rush, G.F., Newton, J.F. and Hook, J.B., Sex differences in the excretion of glucuronide conjugates: the role of intrarenal glucuronidation, J. Pharmacol. Exp. Ther., 227, 658, 1983.

59. Rennick, B.R., Renal tubule transport of organic cations, Am. J. Physiol., 240, F83, 1981.

60. Meister, A. and Tate, S.S., Glutathione and related gamma-glutamyl compounds: biosynthesis and utilization, Ann. Rev. Biochem., 45, 559, 1976.

61. Meister, A., Selective modification of glutathione metabolism, Science, 220, 472, 1983.

62. Orrenius, S., Ormstad, K., Thor, H. and Jewell, S.A., Turnover and functions of glutathione studied with isolated hepatic and renal cells, Fed. Proc., 42, 3177, 1983.

63. Morgenstern, R., Lundqvist, G., Andersson, G., Balk, L. and DePierre, J.W., The distribution of microsomal glutathione transferase among different organelles, different organs, and different organisms, Biochem. Pharmacol., 33, 3609, 1984.

64. Reed, D.J. and Beatty, P.W., Biosynthesis and regulation of glutathione: toxicological implications, in Reviews in Biochemical Toxicology, Vol 2., Hodgson, E., Bend, J.R. and Philpot, R.M., eds., Elsevier/North-Holland, New York, 1980, 213.

65. Kaplowitz, N., Physiological significance of glutathione-S-transferases, Am.

J. Physiol., 239, G439, 1980.

66. Moldeus, P., Jones, D.P., Ormstad, K and Orrenius, S., Formation and metabo-
     lism of a glutathione-S-conjugate in isolated rat liver and kidney cells,
     Biochem. Biophys. Res. Commun., 83, 195, 1978.

67. Ahokas, J.T., Davies, C., Ravenscroft, P.J. and Emmerson, B.T., Inhibition
     of soluble glutathione-S-transferase by diuretic drugs, Biochem. Pharmacol.,
     33, 1929, 1984.

68. Hales, B.F., Jaeger, V. and Neims, A.H., Isoelectric focusing of
     glutathione-S-transferases from rat liver and kidney, Biochem. J., 175, 937,
     1978.

69. Fine, L.G., Goldstein, E.J., Trizna, W., Rozmaryn, L. and Arias, I.M.,
     Glutathione-S-transferase activity in the rabbit nephron: segmental
     localization in isolated tubules and formation of thiol adducts of
     ethacrynic acid, Proc. Soc. Exp. Biol. Med., 157, 189, 1978.

70. Kaplowitz, N., Kuhlenkamp, J. and Clifton, G., Drug induction of hepatic
     glutathione-S-transferases in male and female rats, Biochem. J., 146, 351,
     1975.

71. Clifton, G., Kaplowitz, N., Wallin, J.D. and Kuhlenkamp, J., Drug induction
     and sex differences of renal glutathione-S-transferases in the rat, Biochem.
     J., 150, 259, 1975.

72. Chasseaud, L.F., Extrahepatic conjugation with glutathione, in Extrahepatic
     Metabolism of Drugs and Other Foreign Compounds Gram, T.E., ed., Spectrum
     Publications, New York, 1980, 427.

73. Kaplowitz, N., Clifton, G., Kuhlenkamp, J. and Wallin, J.D., Comparison of
     renal and hepatic glutathione-S-transferases in the rat, Biochem. J., 158,
     243, 1976.

74. Kuo, C.-H., Braselton, W.E. and Hook, J.B., Effect of phenobarbital on
     cephaloridine toxicity and accumulation in rabbit and rat kidneys, Toxicol.
     Appl. Pharmacol., 64, 244, 1982.

75. Rankin, B.B., McIntyre, T.M. and Curthoys, N.P., Brush border membrane
     hydrolysis of S-benzyl-cysteine-p-nitroaniline, an activity of aminopep-
     tidase M, Biochem. Biophys. Res. Commun., 96, 991, 1980.

76. McIntyre, T.M. and Curthoys, N.P., The interorgan metabolism of glutathione,
     Int. J. Biochem., 12, 545, 1980.

77. Green, R.M. and Elce, J.S., Acetylation of S-substituted cysteines by a rat
     liver and kidney microsomal N-acetyltransferase, Biochem. J., 147, 283,
     1975.

78. Elce, J.S., Metabolism of a glutathione conjugate of 2-hydroxyoestradiol by
     rat liver and kidney microsomal N-acetyltransferase, Biochem. J., 116, 913,
     1970.

79. Hughey, R.P., Rankin, B.B., Elce, J.S. and Curthoys, N.P., Specificity of a
     particulate rat renal peptidase and its localization along with other en-
     zymes of mercapturic acid synthesis, Arch. Biochem. Biophys., 186, 211,
     1978.

80. Newton, J.F., Hoefle, D., Gemborys, M.W., Mudge, G.H. and Hook, J.B., Meta-
     bolism and excretion of a glutathione conjugate of acetaminophen in the iso-
     lated perfused rat kidney, J. Pharmacol. Exp. Ther., 237, 519, 1986.

81. Duffel, M.W. and Jakoby, W.B., Cysteine S-conjugate N-acetyltransferase from
     rat kidney microsomes, Molec. Pharmacol., 21, 444, 1982.

82. Newton, J.F., Braselton, W.E., Kuo, C.-H., Kluwe, W.M., Gemborys, M.W.,
     Mudge, G.H. and Hook, J.B., Metabolism of acetaminophen by the isolated per-
     fused kidney, J. Pharmacol. Exp. Ther., 221, 76, 1982.

83. Stevens, J. and Jakoby, W.B., Cysteine conjugate β-lyase, Molec. Pharmacol.,
     23, 761, 1983.

84. Lash, L.H., Elfarra, A.A. and Anders, M.W., Renal cysteine conjugate β-lyase. Bioactivation of nephrotoxic cysteine S-conjugates in mitochondrial outer membrane, J. Biol. Chem., 261, 5930, 1986.

85. Bekersky, I., Colburn, W.A., Fishman, L. and Kaplan, S.A., Metabolism of salicylic acid in the isolated perfused rat kidney. Interconversion of salicyluric and salicylic acids, Drug Metab. Disp., 8, 319, 1980.

86. Wan, S.H. and Riegelman, S., Renal contribution to overall metabolism of drug. I: Conversion of benzoic acid to hippuric acid, J. Pharm. Sci., 61, 1278, 1972.

87. Wan, S.H. and Riegelman, S., Renal contribution to overall metabolism of drugs. II: Biotransformation of salicylic acid to salicyluric acid, J. Pharm. Sci., 61, 1284, 1972.

88. Wan, S.H. and Riegelman, S., Renal contribution to overall metabolism of drugs. III: Metabolism of p-aminobenzoic acid, J. Pharm. Sci., 61, 1288, 1972.

89. Schmassmann, H., Sparrow, A., Platt, K. and Oesch, F., Epoxide hydratase and benzo(a)pyrene monooxygenase activities in liver, kidney and lung after treatment of rats with epoxides of widely varying structures, Biochem. Pharmacol., 27, 2237, 1978.

90. Oesch, F. and Schmassmann, H., Species and organ specificity of the trans-stilbene oxide induced effects on epoxide hydratase and benzo(a)pyrene monooxygenase activity in rodents, Biochem. Pharmacol., 28, 171, 1979.

91. VanCantfort, J., Manil, L., Gielin, J.E., Glatt, H.R. and Oesch, F., A new assay for glutathione-S-transferase using [^{3}H]-benzo(a)pyrene 4,5-oxide as substrate, Biochem. Pharmacol., 28, 455, 1979.

92. DePierre, J.W., Seidegard, J. Morgenstern, R., Balk, L., Meijer, J., Astrom, A., Norelius, I. and Ernster, L., Induction of cytosolic glutathione trans-ferase and microsomal epoxide hydrolase activities in extrahepatic organs of the rat by phenobarbital, 3-methylcholanthrene and trans-stilbene oxide, Xenobiotica, 14, 295, 1984.

93. Hjelle, J.T., Peterson, D.R. and Hjelle, J.J., Drug metabolism in isolated proximal tubule cells: aldehyde dehydrogenase, J. Pharmacol. Exp. Ther., 224, 699, 1983.

94. Dietrich, R.A., Tissue and subcellular distribution of mammalian aldehyde-oxidizing capacity, Biochem. Pharmacol., 15, 1911, 1966.

95. Duggin, G.G., Mechanisms in the development of analgesic nephropathy, Kidney Int., 18, 553, 1980.

96. Bach, P.H. and Bridges, J.W., Chemically induced renal papillary necrosis and upper urothelial carcinoma, CRC Crit. Rev. Toxicol., 15, 217, 1985.

97. Davis, B.B., Mattammal, M.B. and Zenser, T.V., Renal metabolism of drugs and xenobiotics, Nephron, 27, 187, 1981.

98. Marnett, L., Wlodawer, P. and Samuelsson, B., Co-oxygenation of organic sub-strates by the prostaglandin synthetase of sheep vesicular gland, J. Biol. Chem., 250, 8510, 1975.

99. Eling, T., Boyd, J., Reed, G., Mason, R. and Sivarajah, K., Xenobiotic meta-bolism by prostaglandin endoperoxide synthetase, Drug Metab. Rev., 14, 1023, 1983.

100. Zenser, T.V., Levitt, M. and Davis, B., Effect of oxygen and solute on PGE and PGF production by rat kidney slices, Prostaglandins, 13, 143, 1977.

101. Zenser, T.V., Mattammal, M. and Davis, B., Demonstration of separate path-ways for the metabolism of organic compounds in rabbit kidney, J. Pharmacol. Exp. Ther., 208, 418, 1979.

102. Rollins, T. and Smith, W., Subcellular localization of prostaglandin-forming cyclooxygenase in Swiss Mouse 313 fibroblasts by electron microscopi

immmunocytochemistry, J. Biol. Chem., 255, 4872, 1980.

103.   Zenser, T.V., Mattammal, M.B., Rapp, N.S. and Davis, B.B., Effect of aspirin on metabolism of acetaminophen and benzidine by renal inner medulla prostaglandin hydroperoxidase, J. Lab. Clin. Med., 101, 58, 1983.

104.   Flower, R.J., Drugs which inhibit prostaglandin biosynthesis, Pharmacol. Rev., 26, 33, 1974.

105.   Mohandas, J., Duggin, G.G., Horvath, J.S. and Tiller, D.J., Regional differences in peroxidative activation of paracetamol (acetaminophen) mediated by cytochrome P450 and prostaglandin endoperoxide synthetase in rabbit kidney, Res. Commun. Chem. Pathol. Pharmacol., 34, 69, 1981.

106.   Zenser, T.V. and Davis, B.B., Enzyme systems involved in the formation of reactive metabolites in the renal medulla: cooxidation via prostaglandin H synthase, Fund. Appl. Toxicol., 4, 922, 1984.

107.   Zenser, T.V., Mattammal, M. and Davis, B., Metabolism of N-[4-(5-nitro-2-furyl)-2-thiazolyl]formamide by prostaglandin endoperoxide synthetase, Cancer Res., 40, 114, 1980.

108.   Zenser, T., Mattammal, M., Armbrecht, H. and Davis, B., Benzidine binding to nucleic acids mediated by the peroxidative activity of prostaglandin endoperoxide synthetase, Cancer Res., 40, 2839, 1980.

109.   Mattammal, M.B., Zenser, T.V. and Davis, B.B., Prostaglandin hydroperoxidase-mediated 2-amino-4-(5-nitro-2-furyl)-^{14}C-thiazole metabolism and nucleic acid binding, Cancer Res., 41, 4961, 1981.

110.   Lind, C., Vadi, H. and Ernster, L., Metabolism of benzo(a)pyrene-3,6-quinone and 3-hydroxybenzo(a)pyrene in liver microsomes from 3-methylcholanthrene-treated rats, Arch. Biochem. Biophys., 190, 97, 1978.

111.   Mohandas, J., Chennell, A.F., Duggin, G.G., Horvath, J.S. and Tiller, D.J., DT-diaphorase: differential distribution in rabbit kidney and possible protection against quinone toxicity in the inner medulla, Res. Commun. Chem. Pathol. Pharmacol., 43, 463, 1984.

112.   Hook, J.B. and Serbia, V.C., Potentiation of the action of nephrotoxic agents by environmental contaminants, in Nephrotoxic Mechanisms of Drugs and Environmental Toxins, Porter, G.A., ed., Plenum, New York, 1982, 345.

113.   Smith, J.H. and Hook, J.B., Mechanism of chloroform toxicity. II. In vitro evidence for renal metabolism in mice, Toxicol. Appl. Pharmacol., 70, 480, 1983.

114.   Pohl, L.R., Biochemical toxicology of chloroform, in Reviews in Biochemcial Toxicology, Vol. 1, Hodgson, E., Bend, J.R. and Philpot, R.M., eds., Elsevier/North-Holland, New York, 1979, 79.

115.   Smith, J.H., Maita, K., Sleight, S.D. and Hook, J.B., Mechanism of chloroform nephrotoxicity. I. Time course of chloroform toxicity in male and female mice, Toxicol. Appl. Pharmacol., 70, 467, 1983.

116.   Bailie, M.B., Smith, J.H., Newton, J.F. and Hook, J.B., Mechanism of chloroform nephrotoxicity. IV. Phenobarbital potentiation of in vitro chloroform metabolism and toxicity in rabbit kidneys, Toxicol. Appl. Pharmacol., 74, 285, 1984.

117.   Ahmadizadeh, M., Kuo, C.-H. and Hook, J.B., Nephrotoxicity and hepatotoxicity of chloroform in mice: effect of deuterium substitution, J. Toxicol. Environ. Health, 8, 105, 1981.

118.   Branchflower, R.V., Nunn, D.S., Highet, R.H., Smith, J.H., Hook, J.B. and Pohl, L.R., Nephrotoxicity of chloroform: metabolism to phosgene by the mouse kidney, Toxicol. Appl. Pharmacol., 72, 159, 1984.

119.   Mitchell, J.R., McMurtry, R.J., Statham, C.N., and Nelson, S.D., Molecular basis for several drug-induced nephropathies, Am. J. Med., 62, 518, 1977.

120.   Hennis, H.L., Allen, R.C., Hennigar, G.R. and Simmons, M.A., A sensitiv

method for determinining the nephrotoxic effects of the analgesic acetaminophen upon esterases using isoelectric focusing, Electrophoresis, 2, 187, 1981.

121. McMurtry, R.J., Snodgrass, W.R. and Mitchell, J.R., Renal necrosis, glutathione depletion and covalent binding after acetaminophen, Toxicol. Appl. Pharmacol., 46, 87, 1978.

122. Newton, J.F., Yoshimoto, J., Bernstein, J., Rush, G.F. and Hook, J.B., Acetaminophen nephrotoxicity in the rat. I. Strain differences in nephrotoxicity and metabolism, Toxicol. Appl. Pharmacol., 69, 291, 1983.

123. Mitchell, J.R., Jollow, D.J., Potter, W.Z., Davis, D.C., Gillette, J.R. and Brodie, B.B., Acetaminophen-induced hepatic necrosis. I. Role of drug metabolism, J. Pharmacol. Exp. Ther. 187, 185, 1973.

124. Nelson, S.D., Metabolic activation and drug toxicity, J. Med. Chem., 19, 140, 1982.

125. Newton, J.F., Bailie, M.B. and Hook, J.B., Acetaminophen nephrotoxicity in the rat. Renal metabolic activation in vitro, Toxicol. Appl. Pharmacol., 70, 433, 1983.

126. Calder, I.C., Yong, A.C., Woods, R.A., Crown, C.A., Ham, K.N. and Tange, J.D., The nephrotoxicity of p-aminophenol. II. The effect of metabolic inhibitors and inducers, Chem.-Biol. Interact., 27, 245, 1979.

127. Crowe, C.A., Yong, A.C., Calder, I.C., Ham, K.N. and Tange, J.D., The nephrotoxicity of p-aminophenol. I. The effect of microsomal cytochromes, glutathione and covalent binding in kidney and liver, Chem. Biol. Interact., 27, 235, 1979.

128. Carpenter, H.M. and Mudge, G.H., Acetaminophen nephrotoxicity. Studies on renal acetylation and deacetylation, J. Pharmacol. Exp. Ther., 218, 161, 1981.

129. Gemborys, M.W. and Mudge, G.H., Formation and disposition of the minor metabolites of acetaminophen in the hamster, Drug Metab. Disp., 9, 340, 1981.

130. Lock, E.A. and Ishmael, J., The hepatotoxicity and nephrotoxicity of hexachlorobutadiene, in Advances in Pharmacology and Therapeutics, Vol. 5., II., Toxicology and Experimental Models, Yoshida, Y., Hagihara, Y., and Ebashi, S., eds., Permagon Press, New York, 1982, 87.

131. Harleman, J.H. and Seinen, W., Short-term toxicity and reproduction studies in rats with hexachloro-(1,3)-butadiene, Toxicol. Appl. Pharmacol., 47, 1, 1979.

132. Lock, E.A. and Ishmael, J., The acute toxic effects of hexachloro-1,3 butadiene on the rat kidney, Arch. Toxicol., 43, 47, 1979.

133. Lock, E.A. and Ishmael, J., Hepatic and renal non-protein sulfhydryl concentration following toxic doses of hexachloro-1,3-butadiene in the rat: effect of Aroclor 1254, phenobarbitone, or SKF-525A treatment, Toxicol. Appl. Pharmacol., 57, 79, 1981.

134. Berndt, W.O. and Mehendale, H.M., Effects of hexachlorobutadiene (HCBD) on renal function and renal organic ion transport in the rat, Toxicology, 14, 55, 1979.

135. Davis, M.E., Berndt, W.O. and Mehendale, H.M., Disposition and nephrotoxicity of hexachloro-1,3-butadiene, Toxicology, 16, 179, 1980.

136. Wolf, C.R., Hook, J.B. and Lock, E.A., Differential destruction of cytochrome P-450-dependent monooxygenases in rat and mouse kidney following hexachloro-1,3-butadiene administration, Mol. Pharmacol., 23, 206, 1983.

137. Hook, J.B., Rose, M.S. and Lock, E.A., The nephrotoxicity of hexachloro-1,3-butadiene in the rat: studies of organic anion and cation transport in renal slices and the effect of monooxygenase inducers, Toxicol. Appl. Pharmacol., 65, 373, 1982

138.   Kluwe, W.M., Harrington, F.W. and Cooper, S.E., Toxic effects of or-
        ganohalide compounds on renal tubular cells in vivo and in vitro, J. Phar-
        macol. Exp. Ther., 220, 597, 1982.
139.   Kluwe, W.M., McNish, M.R., Smithson, K. and Hook, J.B., Depletion by 1,2-
        dibromoethane, 1,2-dibromo-3-chloropropane, tris(2,3-dibromopropyl)-
        phosphate, and hexachloro-1,3-butadiene of reduced non-protein sulfhydryl
        groups in target and non-target organs, Biochem. Pharmacol., 30, 2265, 1981.
140.   Wolf, C.R., Berry, P.N., Nash, J.A., Green, T. and Lock, E.A., Role of
        microsomal and cytosolic glutathione-S-transferases in the conjugation of
        hexachloro-1:3-butadiene and its possible relevance to toxicity, J. Phar-
        macol. Exp. Ther., 228, 202, 1984.
141.   Nash, J.A., King, L.J., Lock, E.A. and Green, T., The metabolism and dis-
        position of hexachloro-1:3-butadiene in the rat and its relevance to nephro-
        toxicity, Toxicol. Appl. Pharmacol., 73, 124, 1984.
142.   Jaffe, D., Hassall, C.D., Brendel, K. and Gandolfi, A.J., In vivo and in
        vitro nephrotoxicity of the cysteine conjugate of hexachlorobutadiene, J.
        Toxicol. Environ. Health, 11, 57, 1983.
143.   Lock, E.A. and Ishmael, J., Effect of the organic anion transport inhibitor
        probenecid on renal cortical uptake and proximal tubular toxicity of
        hexachloro-1,3-butadiene and its conjugates, Toxicol. Appl. Pharmacol., 81,
        32, 1985.

13

METABOLISM OF GLUTATHIONE IN THE KIDNEY

K. ORMSTAD

INTRODUCTION

Glutathione (GSH) is a tripeptide, gamma-glutamylcysteinylglycine, which has been demonstrated in several types of mammalian cells at concentrations ranging from <0.05 to >4 mmol/l. The highest concentrations are found in the liver, but the kidney also contains considerable amounts. Extracellular concentrations of glutathione, however, are extremely low, usually stated to be in the micromolar range even including oxidized forms, thioether conjugates and mixed disulphides. Invariably sythesized intracellularly, plasma and urinary glutathione must be regarded as an export product used for further metabolism or excretion.

The current concepts on glutathione turnover can be summarized as follows: GSH is synthesized in the cytosolic fraction of cells by a two-step, two-enzyme-catalysed reaction sequence which requires 2 moles of ATP per mole of GSH. Within cells the thiol group of GSH is predominantly maintained in a reduced state. The abundance of the reduced form, as well as the presence of specific transhydrogenases, gives GSH a major role as a reductant of cellular thiol groups. Furthermore, it may act as a reductant of aldehydes and α-ketoaldehydes[1], as a cofactor in the glutathione redoxin system[2] and as a hydrogen donor in the glutathione peroxidase-catalysed reduction of potentially toxic hydroperoxides[3]. Another important function of cellular glutathione is to act as a nucleophile and to scavenge reactive electrophiles formed during biotransformation of xenobiotics[4]. This reaction may proceed spontaneously or be catalysed by glutathione-S-transferases[5]. Lastly, GSH seems to serve as a major reserve for cysteine in the organism[6].

In contrast to its synthesis, degradation of the tripeptide is initiated extracellularly. The initial step is release from the cells of origin, followed by transport via the circulating plasma to cells which possess gamma-glutamyltransferase (gamma-GT) and thus can split the gamma-glutamylcysteine peptide bond which otherwise protects GSH from attack by peptidases. The remaining cysteinyl-glycine bond is less resistant and can be split by a number of enzymes. Reuptake of the constituent amino acids and re-utilization in protein synthesis, transamination or synthesis of GSH completes the inter-organ metabolism of glutathione.

The plasma half-life of glutathione is extremely short; in the range of a few minutes, according to Wendel and Cikryt[7] about 2.6 min in man, even when glutathione is added exogenously up to concentrations of 0.6 mmol/l, which is approximately 1000-fold the normal level. Within the vascular bed the capacity for glutathione degradation is very low[7], which is why the contribution of other tissues to the catabolism of plasma glutathione has been extensively investigated. This research has shown that the kidneys play a predominant role in the catabolism of plasma glutathione.

Nephrectomy increases the half-life[8] of externally added plasma glutathione by a factor of 2, and increases endogenous plasma glutathione dramatically from 10- to 100-fold in rats[9]. It has been estimated that in the rat the kidneys contribute at least 50% of the total degradative capacity for plasma glutathione[8,9], whereas other organs take care of the rest. In man, however, it is likely that the liver plays a more central role with its comparatively high activity of gamma-GT.

The turnover of endogenous cellular glutathione is very rapid in the kidney. This can be considered an intra-organ process, because of the intra-renal localization of the enzymes responsible for glutathione degradation. The initial step is translocation from the epithelial cells to the tubular lumen. On the brush border surface endogenous renal glutathione is effectively broken down and the resulting free amino acids enter the same pool as those derived from the catabolism of non-renal glutathione.

A thorough understanding of renal metabolism of glutathione is of central importance for the knowledge of whole-body handling of this biochemically versatile tripeptide. The present chapter therefore aims to review the current knowledge on renal synthesis, utilization, transport, and degradation of glutathione.

SYNTHESIS

The bulk of an organism's glutathione content is localized intracellularly; mainly in the cytoplasm. This partly reflects the fact that synthesis occurs in the cytosolic fraction, and partly that most of the reactions in which glutathione is involved take place intracellularly.

It is generally agreed that all cells that contain glutathione have the necessary enzymatic/synthetic equipment to maintain their optimal glutathione level under normal conditions - i.e. to take up the relevant precursor amino acids and link them together to form the complete tripeptide. Early studies demonstrated that glutamate, cysteine and glycine are incorporated into hepatic glutathione in vivo[10] and in liver slices[11]. However, even though the different steps in this complex sequence of events may develop differently between cell types, as may the requirement for precursor amino acids, the general principles for the synthesis are assumed to be the same in all cells. Extensive work has been done to elucidate the pathway of GSH synthesis in various organs and cell types and they have been comprehensively reviewed[12,13].

The two enzymes required for glutathione biosynthesis occur at high activity in the cytosolic fraction of renal tubular epithelium. Gamma-glutamylcysteine synthetase (EC 6.3.2.2; L-glutamate: L-cysteine gamma-ligase (ADP-forming)) and glutathione synthetase (EC 6.3.2.3; gamma-L-glutamyl-L-cysteine-glycine ligase (ADP-forming)) catalyse the following reactions, respectively:

1. L-glutamate + L-cysteine $\xrightarrow{\text{Mg}^{2+}}$ L-gamma-glutamyl-L-cysteine

    ATP $\quad$ ADP + P_i

2. L-gamma-glutamyl/cysteine + glycine $\xrightarrow{\text{Mg}^{2+}}$ glutathione

    ATP $\quad$ ADP + P_i

In both reactions the cations Mg^{2+} (or Mn^{2+}) are necessary cofactors and neither of the enzymes are entirely specific for the above substrates.

In experiments with purified gamma-glutamyl cysteine synthetase from rat kidney[14] it was demonstrated that the activity of the enzyme was strongly inhibited by glutathione. The inhibition was competitive with respect to L-glutamate, and no change was observed upon addition of cysteine. Studies with a variety of compounds chemically related to GSH have proved that both the gamma-glutamyl and the SH groups are necessary for inhibition to occur - e.g. is ophthalmic acid, where the GSH cysteine is substituted with L-aminobutyrate, a weak inhibitor. The reported observations suggest that GSH binds to the glutamate site of the enzyme and also to another site, where binding seems to require an SH group - and this may be the cysteine site.

Glutathione synthetase has been purified from a variety of sources including rat kidney[12]. The enzyme is specific for glycine, but in addition to gamma-glutamylcysteine it is active towards gamma-glutamyl L-aminobutyrate and L-gamma-glutamylalanine, and thereby catalyses the formation of ophthalmic acid and norophthalmic acid, both of which occur normally in vivo, in addition to glutathione. Most of the other gamma-glutamyl amino acids are, however, neither substrates nor inhibitors[15].

Regulation of glutathione biosynthesis

Two factors are of central importance in the in vivo regulation of glutathione biosynthesis: the intracellular availability of cysteine and the concentration of glutathione. Intracellular concentrations of cysteine are probably lower than the apparent K_m of gamma-glutamylcysteine synthetase for cysteine (0.3 mmol/l)[14], and under experimental conditions where cellular GSH is depleted, supplementation with sulphur-containing amino acids will support replenishment of GSH[16,17].

The observation that purified gamma-glutamylcysteine synthetase is substantially inhibited by glutathione under conditions similar to those present in vivo strongly indicates a physiologically significant feedback control mechanism for glutathione synthesis. The apparent K_i for glutathione[14] is 2.3 mmol/l, which is close to the normal steady-state concentration in rat kidney. Feedback inhibition exerted by glutathione on its own synthesis fits well with the observation that patients suffering from the metabolic abnormality called S-oxoprolinuria, who are deficient in glutathione, exhibit an overproduction of gamma-glutamylcysteine[18]. Available data thus indicate that gammma-glutamylcysteine synthetase does not function at a maximal rate in the presence of normal steady-state concentrations of glutathione within the cells. But under conditions of cellular GSH depletion - such as under oxidative stress, or in the presence of electrophilic compounds - this feedback inhibition may be alleviated and the synthesis allowed to proceed at a faster rate until normal GSH levels are restored.

The rate of GSH synthesis is further dependent upon a sufficient supply of the necessary substrates. Normally, glutamate and glycine are present intracellularly at concentrations well above the K_m of the synthesizing enzymes, whereas cysteine occurs at considerably lower concentrations and constitutes the rate-limiting factor in the kidney[14], liver[16] and erythrocytes[19].

The turnover of renal tissue glutathione has been extensively studied by Meister and co-workers[20], and under normal in vivo conditions a half-life of 30 min has been observed, which apart from plasma GSH turnover $(t\frac{1}{2}=2-3 \text{ min})$[7] is the most rapid rate found in any tissue.

Freshly isolated tubular epithelial cells from rat kidney cortex have been employed as a model system for investigating renal GSH metabolism[17,21]. Incubations have been performed with cells from control animals as well as from rats pretreated with diethylmaleate to achieve a partial depletion of renal cellular glutathione in order to overcome the normally occurring feedback inhibition of synthesis. These studies have demonstrated that renal epithelial cells have a considerable capacity for GSH synthesis and under optimal conditions can restore their GSH content in 45 min when starting from 30% of control level (Figure 1). This is a rate of replenishment comparable to that of isolated hepatocytes[22], but the renal cellular requirements for precursors are obviously at variance. As previously mentioned the availability of intracellular cysteine is usually rate-limiting for GSH biosynthesis. In the liver, external addition of either cysteine, N-acetylcysteine or methionine efficiently supports GSH replenishment, whereas cystine - which is taken up at a very slow rate - does not. In the kidney, however, methionine has been reported to decrease cellular GSH content rather than support it[23,24], which has been confirmed in isolated renal cells[17]. This is most likely due to the ability of methionine to act as a gamma-glutamyl group acceptor in the gamma-GT-mediated transpeptidation reaction in combination with an inability of the kidney to convert methionine to cysteine via the so-called cysta-thionine pathway which is also found in the liver[25].

Cysteine is rapidly taken up into isolated kidney cells and is an efficient GSH precursor. This function is, however, concen-tration-dependent, i.e. at low extracellular concentrations of cys-teine ($\leq$0.2 mmol/l) supports the synthesis, whereas at 1 mmol/l it

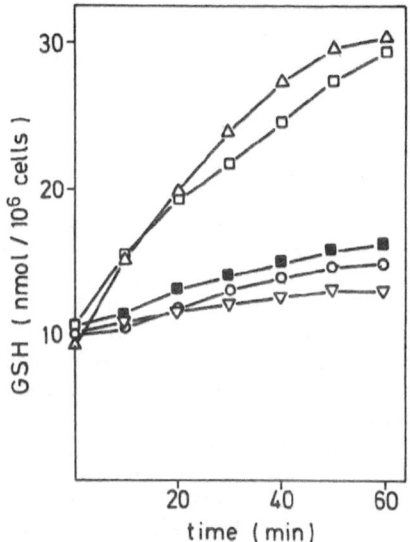

Figure 1 Resynthesis of glutathione by cells isolated from kidneys preperfused with 4 μmol diethylmaleate to lower cellular glutathione concentration. Cells were in-cubated at 37 °C under continuous gassing with 95% O_2 + 5% CO_2 in a Krebs-Henseleit buffer supplemented with glutamate and glycine at 1 mmol each. Additional sulphur containing amino acids as indicated by symbols: O: none; ▽: methionine, 1 mmol; △: cystine, 0.2 mmol; □: cysteine, 0.3 mmol; ■: cysteine, 1 mmol. One typical ex-periment.

retards cellular GSH reaccumulation. Krebs et al.[26] observed the same phenomenon in kidney homogenate, and also discovered that high concentrations of cysteine were toxic to liver cells. They suggested that this was due to a rapid formation of mixed disul-phides between cysteine and GSH, with a subsequent excretion of the mixed disulphides. Another explanation which may be more relevant in the kidney is that cysteine - like methionine - acts as a gamma-glutamyl group acceptor in the gamma-GT-mediated transpeptidation reaction. However, if according to the concept of the gamma-glutamyl cycle[27] cysteine were to be translocated into the cells at the expense of equimolar amounts of GSH as a gamma-glutamyl group donor, it would not supply any net sulphur.

The preferred sulphur source for GSH synthesis in kidney cells is obviously cystine. Most of plasma cysteine exists in disul-phide form[28], and in contrast to the liver, the kidney has an effi-cient uptake mechanism for disulphides. However, cystine is normally not accumulated in renal tissue, and incubation of isolated kidney cells with ^{35}S-cystine leads to an intracellular accumulation of ^{35}S-cysteine and ^{35}S-GSH only. Apparently cystine undergoes reduction during or immediately after uptake into the cells, and this occurs whether it is incorporated into GSH or not[17]. A two-step reaction mechanism catalysed by cytoplasmic thioltransferase (equations 3 and 4) and oxidized glutathione (GSSG) reductase (equation 5) has been suggested[29].

3.   CySGCys + GSH $\rightleftharpoons$ Cys + GS-CySH

4.   GS-Cys + GSH $\rightleftharpoons$ Cys + GSSG

5.   GSSG + NADPH + H$^+$ $\rightleftharpoons$ 2 GSH + NADP$^+$

This mechanism is further supported by the fact that cystine is also reduced when incubated in vitro with the cytosolic fraction from rat liver. The two relevant enzymes are present in liver cells, but since cystine is taken up in hepatocytes at a very limited rate, it does not act as a substrate with intact cells or in vivo. Moreover, we have shown that the above reduction mechanism also works for synthetic low molecular disulphides, e.g. dimesna (disodium-2-2'-dithiobis-ethane sulphonate[29]).

In partly GSH-depleted cells, normal GSH content is re-established after 30-45 min incubation in the presence of precursor amino acids. However, this does not reflect the true GSH-synthesizing capacity of the cells, since glutathione also accumulates in the incubation medium - either in the form of GSSG or as mixed disulphides between GSH and cysteine. Both these compounds are excellent substrates for gamma-GT; thus in order to quantitate them the incubation medium must be supplemented with a gamma-GT inhibitor, such as AT 125[30] or anthglutin[31]. In the presence of anthglutin 0.5 mmol/l a maximal GSH synthesis rate of about 1 nmol/10^6 cells per min has been observed (Ormstad, unpublished results).

Whether starting from a depleted or a normal level, renal cellular GSH never exceeds 120-130% of the normal concentration. The excess seems to be excreted from the cells where it is subjected to degradation by gamma-GT and cysteinylglycine dipeptidase.

INTRACELLULAR UTILIZATION

It seems likely that cellular GSH may take part in the same kinds of reactions in the kidney as in other organs, e.g. as a reductant, a cofactor or a scavenger of electrophiles. Qualitatively the majority of enzymes relevant for these reactions are found in both the kidney and the liver, e.g. GSH peroxidase, GSSG reductase, and GSH-S-transferases. We have previously reported[32] that during incubation of paracetamol (acetaminophen) with isolated renal epithelial cells sulphate, glucuronide and glutathione conjugates are formed (Figure 2). In as much as these conjugates, as well as GSSG formed during the action of glutathione as an intracellular reductant, seem to be actively extruded from the

410

cells, these reactions contribute to the rapid turnover of renal cellular glutathione.

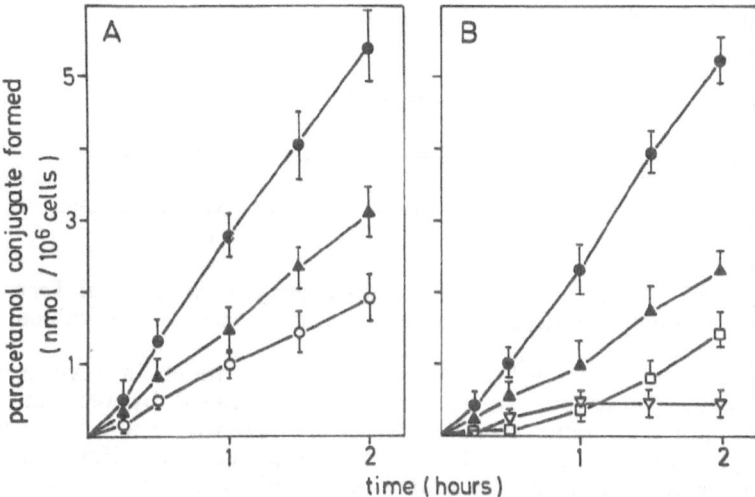

Figure 2 Formation of paracetamol conjugates during incubation of isolated kidney cells (10^6 cells/ml) with 5 mmol paracetamol. Panel A: gamma-GT inhibitor anthglutin (0.5 mmol) added. Panel B: without inhibitor. ●: glucuronide; ▲: sulphate; ○: glutathione-S-paracetamol; ▽: cysteine-S-paracetamol; □: N-acetylcysteine-S-paracetamol. Metabolites assayed by HPLC analysis of aliquots from total incubate (cells + medium). Results denote mean ± S.D. of three experiments (panel A) respective six experiments (Panel B).

DEGRADATION

The gamma-glutamyl bond of glutathione protects the molecule against attack by most peptide-splitting enzymes. So far, gamma-glutamyltranspeptidase (EC 2.3.2.2; S-glutamyl-peptide: amino acid S-glutamyltransferase) is the only enzyme known which is capable of splitting the gamma-glutamyl peptide bond. This enzyme is a glycoprotein which is located in the plasma membranes of certain cells, and by far the highest activity is found in the kidney. The bulk of activity resides in the luminal brush border membrane of proximal tubular cells[33]; increasing distally, i.e. maximal activity is found in the pars recta[34]. Recent investigations employing sensitive histochemical techniques have, however, demonstrated the existence of gamma-GT activity on the contraluminal side of the proximal tubular epithelium[35]. Irrespective of membranal localization the active site seems to be facing the exterior of the cell and thus is only available to extracellular substrates; i.e. unless translocated across the plasma membrane, cellular GSH is inaccessible to enzymatic degradation. Gamma-GT has been purified from various mammalian sources and exhibits remarkably similar catalytic properties and substrate specificity. Unsubstituted glutathione, as well as glutathione disulphide, mixed disulphides and S-substituted compounds, such as thioether conjugates of xenobiotics or

411

endogenous substances (e.g. leukotrienes) are all substrates. The reactions catalysed by gamma-GT are of three types: hydrolysis (equation 6), transpeptidation (equation 7) and autotranspeptidation (equation 8).

6. γ-Glu-Cys-Gly + H_2O $\longrightarrow$ Glu + HCys-Gly

7. γ-Glu-Cys-Gly + acceptor $\longrightarrow$ γ-Glu - acceptor + HCys-Gly

8. γ-Glu-Cys-Gly + γ-Glu-Cys-Gly $\longrightarrow$ γ-Glu-γ-Glu-Cys-Gly + HCys-Gly

The hydrolytic activity of the purified enzyme is maximal from pH 6 to 8, whereas maximal transpeptidation occurs at pH values between 8 and 9[36,37].

Sekura and Meister[20] have reported that under in vivo conditions renal glutathione turnover can be increased by feeding rats large amounts of amino acids or dipeptides known to act as gamma-glutamyl acceptors in the transpeptidation reaction. However, in studies employing isolated tubular epithelial cells, the presence of acceptor amino acids in the medium did not increase gamma-GT mediated catabolism of any glutathione compound studied[38,39], which indicates that under these conditions the dominating reaction was a hydrolytic cleavage of the gamma-glutamyl peptide bond, not a transpeptidation. This observation agrees with those of Curthoys et al.[40,41] and Elce and Broxmeyer[36].

The role of gamma-GT as the primary enzyme in glutathione degradation in vivo as well as in vitro is established beyond doubt. The identity of the enzyme(s) capable of cleaving the Cys-Gly peptide bond is less clear, and theoretically a wide variety of aminopeptidases have catalytic properties enabling them to cleave Cys-Gly derivatives. From human kidney tissue an enzyme has been purified which was called Cys-Gly dipeptidase[42]. In rat kidneys an aminopeptidase has been demonstrated in the brush border of proximal tubular epithelium[43], which closely resembles the aminopeptidase M that had already been isolated from rabbit renal brush borders[44]. This enzyme prefers substrates with a hydrophobic N-terminal residue, but has no activity towards glutathione. Furthermore, its localization is similar to that of gamma-GT, and the active site faces the luminal side of the brush border membrane[43]. Thus it seems reasonable that the two enzymes together may catalyse the conversion of GSH and glutathione-S-derivatives to cysteine or cysteine-S-derivatives. Recently, another renal brush border dipeptidase has been isolated from rat kidney. This enzyme contains zinc and is highly active against L-methyl-cysteinylglycine, cysteinyl-bis-glycine and leukotriene D4[45,46], but, like aminopeptidase M, less so with unsubstituted cysteinylglycine as a substrate. Other possibilities suggested by Meister[47] are that cysteinylglycine formed in the renal tubular lumen by gamma-GT-mediated transpeptidation may be translocated across the luminal brush border membrane (according to the theory of gamma-GT activity being involved in renal tubular reabsorption of amino acids and peptides) and subjected to cytosolic dipeptidases[48], or undergo auto-oxidation to cystinyl-bis-glycine extracellularly. None of these mechanisms can be totally refuted, but so far the in vivo operation of renal gamma-GT-mediated transport processes remains to be proven, and under the virtually anaerobic conditions of renal tubular fluid, auto-oxidation seems unlikely to be quantitatively significant.

During the sequential actions of gamma-GT and brush border dipeptidase(s) the three amino acids constituting glutathione are released to the tubular fluid. The bulk is probably reabsorbed in the proximal tubule or further down the nephron, to enter various pathways within the tubular epithelium or to be transferred to plasma. Several studies employing various in vivo and in vitro experimental model systems have demonstrated that the same pathways are involved in the degradation of unsubstituted glutathione, glutathione disulphide and glutathione-S-conjugates of xenobiotics as well as endogenous substances (e.g. the leukotrienes).

In a microperfusion study in rats Silbernagl et al.[49] demonstrated that during passage along the proximal convoluted tubule GSH as well as two S-substituted glutathione derivatives, S-methylglutathione and S-sulphobromophthalyl-GSH, underwent a two-step cleavage to the S-cysteinyl-glycyl and the S-cysteinyl derivatives, respectively.

These results are further confirmed by data[38] obtained by incubating renal epithelial cells and plasma membranes with a glutathione-S-conjugate of paracetamol (Figure 3). In the presence of intact cells (panel A) the glutathione-S-paracetamol rapidly disappeared from the incubate, simultaneously with a gradual (and stoichiometric) accumulation of the corresponding cysteine and N-acetylcysteine conjugates. The observation that the intermediary cysteinylglycine-S-paracetamol is only recovered in trace amounts, is consistent with high activity of cysteinylglycine dipeptidase relative to gamma-GT[43]. This was further substantiated by adding phenylalanylglycine, a competitive inhibitor of the relevant dipeptidase, to the incubate, which led to a substantial increase in the accumulation of the cysteinylglycine derivative.

During incubation with a suspension of isolated renal cortical plasma membranes (panel B) the same pattern of metabolites occurred, except from the accumulation of the N-acetylcysteine derivative. Addition of acetyl CoA had no effect, which confirms the localization of gamma-GT and dipeptidase to the plasma membrane, whereas N-acetyltransferases are intracellular enzymes.

Addition of gamma-GT inhibitors (anthglutin, 0.5 mmol/l or AT 125, 0.25 mmol/l) to incubates of renal cells or membranes and glutathione-S-paracetamol almost completely blocks the conjugate degradation. Furthermore, addition of unsubstituted GSH or GSSG exerts a dose-dependent competitive inhibition of conjugate metabolism, which demonstrates that this reaction pathway is similar for unsubstituted, oxidized and S-substituted glutathione[38].

The in vivo significance of gamma-GT-mediated degradation of glutathione is illustrated by the observation that a gamma-GT-deficient patient exhibited massive glutathionuria - a daily urinary output of 850 mg glutathione[50]. Furthermore, rats fed the synthetic gamma-GT inhibitior AT 125 excrete large amounts of glutathione in urine[51].

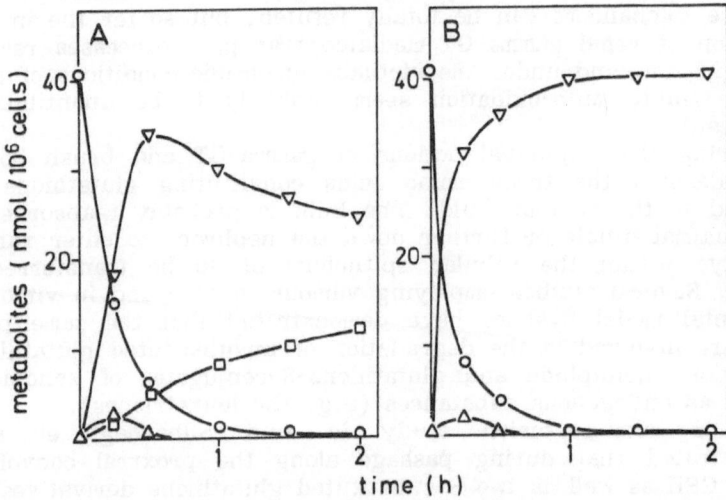

Figure 3 Metabolism of a glutathione-S-conjugate of paracetamol by isolated renal epithelial cells (A) and isolated renal cortical plasma membranes (B). Incubations were performed at 37 °C, pH 7.4 in an oxygen-saturated medium. Incubation (A) contained 10^6 cells/ml and incubation (B) 100 μg membrane protein/ml.

RENAL TRANSPORT OF GLUTATHIONE

According to Häberle et al.[8] the kidney accounts for about 50% of the total glutathione-degrading capacity of the organism, and up to 80% of renal arterial glutathione is extracted during one passage of the renal vascular bed. GSH as well as S-substituted glutathione derivatives are water-soluble at concentrations pertinent to the in vivo situation, and the molecular weight of these components is far below the limit for glomerular filtration. Thus, plasma glutathione is filtered in proportion to the glomerular filtration fraction which is 20-30%, and is subsequently subjected to stepwise degradation in the tubular lumen by the brush border enzymes as previously mentioned. However, other mechanisms must operate to account for the remaining 50% arteriovenous difference. It has been suggested[47] that even this glutathione degradation may be due to gamma-GT (which is also present, albeit at a very low activity, in glomerular capillaries and at the contraluminal side of tubular epithelium). Rankin and Curthoys[52] have, however, shown that when 98% of total renal gamma-GT activity was inhibited, the kidney still extracted 39% of renal arterial glutathione. Thus, it seems that renal glutathione extraction must also occur by a paratubular mechanism that is independent of gamma-GT. The existence of such a mechanism was suggested by experiments using isolated perfused rat kidneys, where single-pass arteriovenous extraction of glutathione was found to be independent of anthglutin-mediated gamma-GT inhibition and decreased by merely 20-30% upon cessation of glomerular filtration (Figure 4). Furthermore, renal

414

glutathione extraction was efficiently inhibited by probenecid, which is a competitive inhibitior of active renal secretion of a variety of organic acids. This observation suggests that the slightly acidic nature of the glutathione molecule is of relevance to the renal transtubular transport process.

A closer in vitro investigation of glutathione transport in renal tubular epithelium has been performed by Lash and Jones[53,54]. Using a purified preparation of basolateral membrane vesicles they were able to characterize a Na^+-dependent system transferring GSH, GSSG and gamma-glutamylglutamate across the vesicular wall against a massive concentration gradient. The transport system exhibited saturation kinetics with an apparent K_m for GSH of 3.0 mmol/l and a V_{max} of 19.5 nmol/mg protein per min. Lithium, but not potassium, could substitute for sodium. Transport was electrogenic; it was stimulated by negative and inhibited by positive vancomycin-induced K^+ diffusion potentials and thus was coupled to an Na^+-gradient as well as to the membrane potential. The GSH:Na^+ stoichiometry was estimated to be 2:1. Na^+-dependent glutathione transport was also independent of gamma-GT activity and NH_4^+ ions, but could be inhibited in a competitive fashion by probenecid and by other gamma-glutamyl compounds such as GSSG, gamma-glutamylglutamate and ophthalmic acid. Cysteinylglycine, on the other hand, did not inhibit GSH transport; thus it appears that inhibitory specificity is associated with the gamma-glutamyl moiety and that inhibition may be due to competition for the same carrier. Both gamma-glutamylglutamate and GSSG were transported

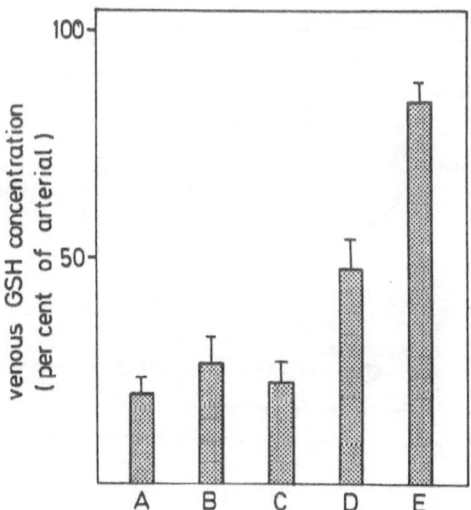

Figure 4 Glutathione extraction during single-pass perfusion of isolated rat kidneys with a medium containing 100 µmol GSH, supplemented with 50 µmol bathocuproine sulphonate to inhibit enzymatic oxidation of GSH. A: Control conditions; B: non-filtering kidney; C: gamma-GT inhibited (0.5 mmol anthglutin added to medium); D: medium supplemented with probenecid, 25 µmol; E: medium supplemented with probenecid, 100 µmol. Results given as mean ± SD of four separate perfusion experiments.

by the same mechanism as GSH, but at different rates: GSH transport was five times faster than that of GSSG.

Although important information was gained by this study, there are several more questions awaiting answers. The Na^+-dependent transport system for gamma-glutamyl compounds has so far been investigated only in vitro. Whether it also operates in vivo is still unknown, but if it does it may explain the mechanism responsible for the renal extraction of glutathione from the vascular bed. Moreover, it is still not clear what happens to glutathione after it has been taken across the contraluminal plasma membrane surface. Renal epithelial cells do not accumulate GSH to any significant degree above its normal steady-state level, and in order for a true clearance of glutathione to occur it must be brought into contact with the luminally facing enzymes gamma-GT and dipeptidase(s). Whether it is sequestered inside the cells or by some continuous pathway transferred across the tubular epithelial lining is still unknown. In the case of GSSG being taken up from the peritubular plasma it seems likely that the disulphide will undergo reduction to thiol from inside the epithelial cells since accumulation of GSSG does not seem to be "allowed" - at least not in vitro. Any reaction leading to intracellular glutathione oxidation is rapidly followed by either excretion of the disulphide or NADPH-dependent, glutathione reductase-catalysed reduction. Current knowledge concerning renal handling of unsubstituted glutathione is schematically outlined in Figure 5.

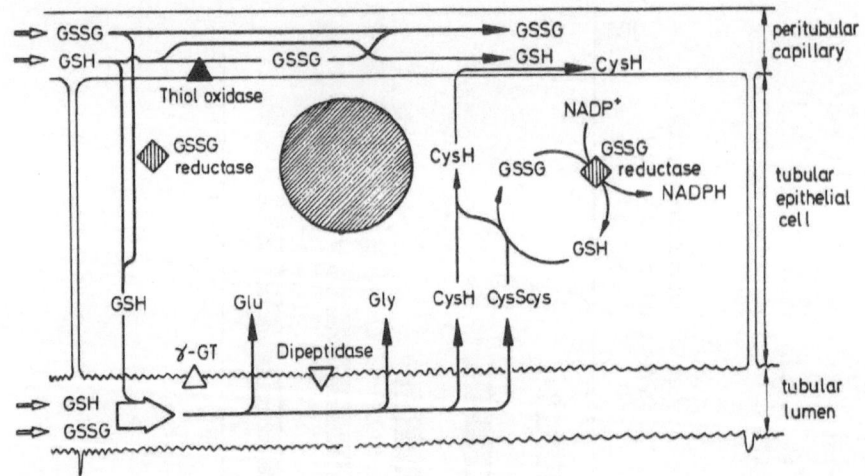

Figure 5 Schematic outline of tubular transport and catabolism of un-substituted glutathione in the kidney. ▲ : Thiol oxidase; △ : gamma-glutamyltransferase; ▽ : cysteinylglycine dipeptidase; ◈ : GSSG reductase.

Yet another mechanism for the translocation of glutathione into kidney tissue, and thus for the support of renal cellular glutathione, has recently been reported by Puri and Meister[55]. In an in vivo study on mice they found that administration of gamma-glutamylcysteinylglycyl monomethyl or -ethyl ester led to substantial increases in the levels of glutathione in liver and kidney. Even under conditions of inhibited glutathione synthesis glutathione-depleted animals responded to ester administration, which indicates that cellular glutathione repletion is not secondary to extracellular breakdown of the glutathionyl moiety of the ester and subsequent uptake and resynthesis. On the contrary it appears that intact ester molecules are absorbed and subjected to intracellular hydrolytic cleavage to liberate the tripeptide. The exact mechanism of this transport process remains to be established. At any rate it seems unlikely that it is identical to the Na^+-dependent glutathione uptake mechanism since the latter does not exist in the liver[54].

Cellular uptake of glutathione in the ester form may not have any physiological significance, since glutathionyl esters hardly occur under in vivo conditions. It may, however, be exploited as an experimental model system and possibly also have a therapeutic application in cases where hepatic or renal cellular GSH contents need to be replenished, e.g. in paracetamol overdosage.

EXTRACELLULAR GLUTATHIONE OXIDATION IN THE KIDNEY

A capability of renal tissue to oxidize GSH to GSSG has been known for 40 years[56,57], but the nature of this oxidation reaction has not been investigated until recently. Isolated renal cells incubated with GSH gave the same pattern of metabolites irrespective of whether glutathione was added in reduced (GSH) or oxidized (GSSG) form - i.e. they all contained a cystine moiety, which suggested that the initial step in the handling of GSH was an oxidation to GSSG. Moreover, upon inhibition of gamma-GT an accumulation of GSSG in the incubate was observed which was stoichiometric to GSH loss[38].

The GSH-oxidizing activity was further studied in purified subcellular fractions from a rat kidney homogenate[58,59] and in isolated perfused kidneys[60], and shown to reside in the basolateral part of the plasma membrane. Investigations have demonstrated that the GSH-oxidizing activity is due to a membrane-bound enzyme with its active site facing the capillaries; which is active with cysteine, N-acetylcysteine, and dithiothreitol (in addition to GSH) and is therefore denoted thiol oxidase[61,62]. However, it is not an entirely non-specific thiol oxidase since neither mercaptoethanol nor mercaptoethane sulphonate are substrates. Ashkar et al.[63] have purified the enzyme, and confirmed the suggestion that it contains copper[59] and that its activity exhibits Michaelis Menten kinetics (K_m for GSH 2.2 mmol/l, V_{max} 33 $nmol^{-1}$ mg $protein^{-1}$ in the purified enzyme preparation[63]).

A similar thiol oxidizing activity has also been demonstrated in bovine milk[64,65], in rat seminal vesicles[66] and in jejunal epithelium[64]. In none of these organs or secretions is the physiological function of the enzyme known, and one may also speculate on the identity of the natural substrate. Taking into consideration the high K_m of the enzyme for the naturally occurring substrates cysteine, N-acetylcysteine and GSH in comparison to the low concentrations of these compounds in extracellular fluids, it seems justifiable to postulate that the physiological substrate for thiol oxidase is some other compound, possibly a thiol-containing hormone or enzyme. However, based on the recent observation[54] that the transport of GSH occurred at a rate five times that of GSSG across the renal basolateral plasma membranes it may be speculated that the oxidase in some way is functionally involved in the transport system - e.g. in a regulatory fashion by oxidizing plasma GSH to GSSG and thus decrease the rate of renal glutathione extraction.

RENAL PROCESSING OF GLUTATHIONE-S-CONJUGATES

The formation of glutathione-S-conjugates is catalysed by a group of enzymes called glutathione-S-transferases or ligandins, which are present in microsomes, mitochondria and in the cytosolic fraction of several tissues[68]. The bulk of this enzyme activity resides in the cytosol but for hexachlorobutadiene, for example, the microsomal enzyme has been reported to be more effective[69]. The activity of glutathione-S-transferases is far higher in the liver than in the kidney[70], which suggests that conjugates formed in the liver may even have the main responsibility for extrahepatic effects. On the other hand, the enzymes responsible for degradation of glutathione-S-conjugates and formation of the final metabolites, mercapturic acids (gamma-GT, cysteinylglycine dipeptidase(s) and cysteine conjugate N-acetyltransferase) are more active in the kidney than in the liver.

The unsubstituted glutathione and glutathione-S-acetaminophen compete for the tripeptide-splitting enzymes in isolated renal epithelial cells[38]. However, whereas the final step in GSH degradation was cysteine or cystine, in incubations containing glutathione-S-paracetamol there was a gradual accumulation of N-acetyl-S-paracetamol (cf. Figure 3). This agrees with the observation that urinary excretion of paracetamol in the thioether form occurs as the mercapturate rather than as cysteine-S-conjugate[71]. Using styrene oxide as a substrate the same pattern of thioether metabolites is found in urine in vivo[72], but notably the capacity for N-acetylation of this conjugate is difficult to retain in the isolated perfused kidney. Steele et al.[72] reported that about 30% of urinary radioactivity appeared as a mercapturate, whereas 63% was as the cysteine-S-conjugate from the isolated perfused rat kidneys with [^{14}C]styrene-oxide-S-glutathione. This may be due to suboptimal effectivity of transport functions in the isolated kidney rather than to a lack of N-acetyltransferase activity.

Several N-acetyltransferases have been described in various tissues, but incomplete knowledge was available on the enzyme activity responsible for N-acetylation of S-substituted cysteines until Green and Elce[73] reported on a study of hepatic and renal subcellular fractions and described a cysteine-S-conjugate N-acetyltransferase which was associated with the endoplasmic reticular membranes of both liver and kidneys. The activity was higher in kidney than in liver, and within the nephron the bulk of this enzyme activity was found in the proximal convoluted tubule, which corresponds to the distribution of gamma-GT and the peptide-splitting activity for cysteinyl dipeptides[34,43]. The enzyme is specific for acetyl CoA as an acetyl group donor; the acceptor specificity shows a preference for S-substituted cysteine deriva-tives, although a somewhat broader spectrum of substrates appears to exist. The microsomal localization, as well as the substrate specificity, distinguish this N-acetyltransferase from those enzymes which catalyse acetylation of various endogenous and xenobiotic amines. The latter are confined to the cytosolic fraction and, moreover, are soluble, whereas the cysteine-S-conjugate N-acetyltransferase is relatively unstable and so far has not been solubilized.

METABOLIC COORDINATION OF LIVER, INTESTINE AND KIDNEY IN MERCAPTURATE SYNETHESIS

The renal epithelial cells possess all the enzymatic activities required for synthesis as well as for degradation of glutathione and glutathione-S-conjugates[32,38]. However, most cells are not that well equipped, and recent data on the compartmentalization of enzymes involved in glutathione metabolism strongly indicate trans-location of intracellularly synthesized glutathione derivatives to ex-tracellular sites and also inter-organ cooperation. Thus, glutathiones synthesized in cells which have gamma-GT activity may be transported across the plasma membrane and subjected to degradation by the membrane-bound enzyme, whereas glutathione and glutathione-S-conjugates formed in cells devoid of gamma-GT activity may enter the extracellular fluids and be transported by circulating plasma to gamma-GT located on the surface of other cells. Apart from renal epithelial cells the former situation may also exist in jejunal mucosal cells which possess a high gamma-GT ac-tivity. Inter-organ transport and cooperation is relevant for cells such as hepatocytes, which exhibit a high capacity for synthesis of glutathione and corresponding S-conjugates, but - at least in the rat - are virtually devoid of gamma-GT activity. Glutathione-containing compounds from these cells must be carried either by the bile to gamma-GT sites on jejunal brush border surfaces or by plasma via the hepatic vein to the kidneys. These metabolic relationships have been studied in in vivo systems, in isolated per-fused organs and with suspensions of isolated cells from liver jejunum and kidney[38,72,74-76].

The partition of hepatic glutathione-S-conjugates to bile or hepatic venous plasma seems to depend on the chemical nature of the adduct rather than on the glutathione moiety. Steele et al.[72] reported that only 8% of a styrene oxide-S-glutathione conjugate was found in bile, whereas paracetamol-S-glutathione was mainly recovered from the bile in an isolated perfused rat liver[75]. A predominant excretion of glutathione-S-conjugates to bile is also suggested by the work of Wahlländer and Sies[77], which showed that the glutathione-S-conjugate of 1-chloro-2,4-dinitrobenzene formed in the perfused liver is exclusively excreted via bile.

The fate of biliary glutathione-S-conjugates has been studied using paracetamol[38,75,77,78] and leukotriene C_3[79] as substrates and combining results from in vitro incubation of intestinal and renal epithelial cells with isolated liver perfusions and experiments performed on intact animals.

Freshly isolated jejunal mucosal epithelium rapidly converted paracetamol-S-glutathione to paracetamol-S-cysteine, which was slowly acetylated to the corresponding mercapturate. Addition of a gamma-GT inhibitor blocked this reaction and thus indicated an involvement of gamma-GT as an initiating enzyme. Biliary paracetamol-S-glutathione was metabolized similarly by the small intestine in situ; the subsequent appearance of the cysteine conjugate in portal venous plasma proved that the conversion occurred before or during transport of the conjugate across the intestinal wall. Direct absorption of paracetamol-S-cysteine from the jejunal lumen to portal blood was verified by instillation of this derivative in the intestinal lumen in situ. Hepatic extraction of paracetamol-S-thioether conjugates could not be observed; thus there is no transfer of circulating conjugates from plasma to bile.

Paracetamol-S-cysteine absorbed from the gut therefore seems to pass unnoticed through the liver and subsequently be transported by the systemic circulation to the kidney for excretion, partly preceded by N-acetylation.

Using leukotriene C_3 (an endogenous glutathione-S-conjugate) as a substrate, a different pattern was found. Most of the dose instilled in the intestinal lumen was recovered intact in the portal plasma. During incubation with isolated intestinal cells uptake was not affected by gamma-GT-inhibitors; nor was there any gamma-GT-mediated degradation. Moreover, leukotriene C_3 was actively extracted from hepatic arterial and renal arterial plasma, which was also confirmed in experiments using isolated perfused organs. Leukotriene C_3 taken up in the liver was rapidly metabolized and excreted in the bile, whereas during kidney perfusion the bulk of radioactivity accumulated in the renal tissue and only lesser amounts could be recovered from the perfusate - mostly in the form of leukotriene E_3 (cysteine-S-conjugate).

Obviously there are differences in the affinity of the various transport and biotransformation systems for different glutathione-S-based conjugates. Inoue et al.[74] injected S-carbamido-[^{14}C]methyl-glutathione i.v. into mice and reported a transitory renal accumulation of radioactivity within 1-2 min followed by a redistribution to the liver. The bulk of hepatic radioactivity was accounted for by S-carbamidomethylcysteine and its corresponding mercapturate. The cysteine derivative (given i.v.) selectively accumulated in the liver. In both cases urinary radioactivity was fully accounted for by N-acetyl-S-carbaminomethylcysteine, and when this mercapturate was injected i.v., radioactivity preferentially accumulated in the kidneys and was rapidly excreted.

Based on these observations the following sequence of events was suggested: The glutathione conjugate (the bulk of which derives from the liver) accumulates in the kidneys and undergoes degradative metabolism to the corresponding cysteine-S-conjugate in the tubular lumen. The cysteine-S-conjugate is reabsorbed and transferred to the liver, acetylated to form mercapturate and subsequently, after translocation to hepatic venous plasma, carried to the kidney for final excretion. Such an inter-organ cooperation in xenobiotic transport and processing may be termed hepatorenal circulation in analogy with the concept of enterohepatic circulation which is operating for conjugates released from liver tissue to bile.

Whereas considerable evidence suggests that glutathione-S-conjugates are taken up into renal tubular epithelial cells from the luminal side, a topographically different transport mechanism is described for N-acetylcysteine conjugates. Inoue et al.[80] administered S-benzyl-N-acetyl-L-[^{14}C]cysteine intravenously to rats and observed a rapid renal accumulation and subsequent urinary excretion of the compound in essentially unchanged form. Whereas bilateral ureter ligation only slightly affected the rate of excretion, nephrectomy completely blocked plasma clearance of the conjugate. Furthermore, probenecid significantly inhibited urinary excretion of the basolateral side of the tubular epithelium. Such a translocation mechanism fits in with a well-organized coordination of hepatic and S-benzyl-N-acetyl-L-[^{14}C]cysteine, and the results were inter-

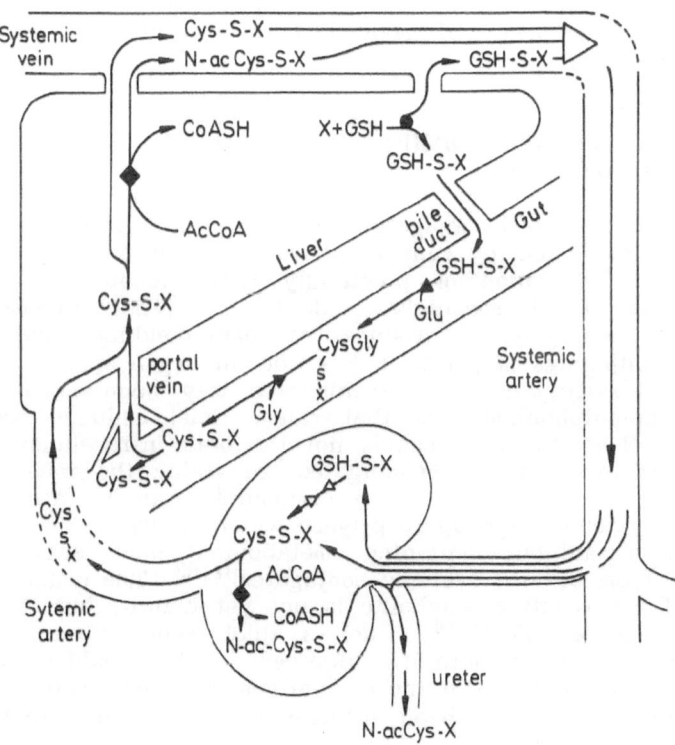

Figure 6 Schematic outline of interorgan transport and handling of glutathione-derived thioether conjugates. The relevance of various pathways differs among conjugates, depending on the chemical nature of the adduct (X). ● : Glutathione-S-transferase; △ : gamma-glutamyltransferase; ▽ : cysteinylglycine dipeptidase; ◆ : microsomal N-acetyltransferase.

preted as evidence for an active transport process operating from renal participation in whole-body handling of glutathione-derived thioether conjugates. It may or may not be identical to the mechanism reponsible for paratubular renal extraction of un-substituted GSH or GSSG.

Inoue et al.[74] did not rule out the possibility that N-acetylation of the cysteine-S-conjugate may take place in the kidney directly after reabsorption from the tubular lumen. Incubations of microsomal preparations from mouse liver and kidney with S-carbamidomethylcysteine showed similar kinetics for mercapturate formation; K_m was identical (8.0 mmol/l) and V_{max} somewhat higher in renal than in hepatic microsomes (0.63 and 0.31 µmol/min per mg protein, respectively). This is in line with our observation of N-acetylcysteine-S-acetominophen during in vitro incubation of the corresponding glutathione-S-conjugate with isolated kidney cells[38]; and it seems likely that the relative organ specificity for N-acetylation of cysteine-S-conjugates is dependent on the chemical properties of the S-substituents. The schematic representation in Figure 6 depicts the proposed possibilities for inter-organ coordination of transport and metabolism of glutathione-derived thioether conjugates.

ROLE OF THIOETHER CONJUGATE METABOLISM IN NEPHROTOXICITY

Whereas glutathione-S-conjugation and subsequent transformation to mercapturates is usually considered an important pathway for inactivation and excretion of potentially toxic xenobiotics, it has recently become increasingly evident that renal processing of glutathione conjugates to produce the corresponding S-substituted cysteine conjugates may play a key role in organ-specific nephrotoxicity. Firstly, cysteine-S-conjugates may spontaneously form reactive episulphonium ions that cause renal cellular damage[81]. Secondly, N-acetyltransferase is not the only intracellular enzyme responsible for cysteine-S-conjugates traversing the renal tubular epithelium. Alternatively, these compounds may be attacked by cytosolic cysteine-S-conjugate β-lyase which catalyses the formation of reactive sulphur-containing metabolites plus ammonia and pyruvate from several cysteine conjugates[82,83]. The exact chemical nature of the reactive metabolite is not yet known, but it is suggested to be a thiol[82,84]. Such a thiol could subsequently be methylated by thiol-S-methyltransferase[85], which would explain the in vivo formation of methylthio derivatives of several xenobiotics[86].

So far β-lyase has been implicated in the nephrotoxicity of halogenated hydrocarbons such as hexachlorobutadiene[84], tetra-fluoroethylene[87] and S-(1,2-dichlorovinylcysteine)[87]. β-lyase activity is also found in liver[82] and in intestinal microflora[88], but its contribution to local toxicity may be dependent on the presence of relevant substrates as well as on inter-organ differences in catalytic activity. The nature of the renal enzyme is still not completely defined, and it is possible that the "β-lyase activity" is due to more than one enzyme.

Neither glutathione, cysteinylglycine nor N-acetylcysteine conjugates are substrates for renal β-lyase[82]. Thus intratubular hydrolysis of the glutathione moiety is a prerequisite for β-lyase-catalysed nephrotoxicity to occur, and N-acetylation protects against it. However, the kidney also possesses deacetylase activity[89], which may lead to a recycling of mercapturates - unless rapidly translocated out of the cells - to the non-acetylated form. Such a reaction mechanism has been suggested to account for the nephrotoxicity of N-acetyl-S-(1,1,2,3,4-pentachloro-1,3-buta-dienyl)-L-cysteine[84].

Thus, although glutathione is usually regarded as a reliable intracellular scavenger, one does well to remember that it may also lend itself to a lethal synthesis. A schematic outline of various transport functions and biotransformation pathways involved in renal handling of thioether conjugates is given in Figure 7. Investigations concerning the nature of the thiol intermediate and cellular mechanism of toxicity are being conducted by several groups, and this new knowledge will increase our understanding of nephrotoxicity and the full roles of glutathione metabolism in the kidney.

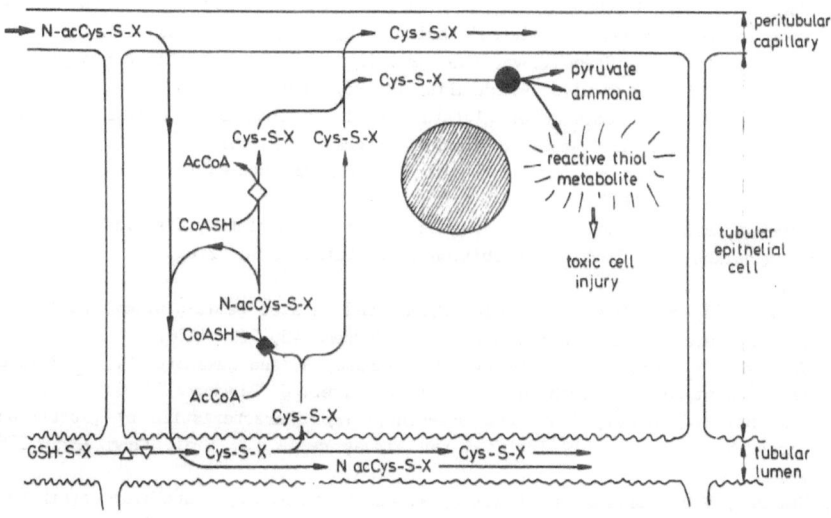

Figure 7 Schematic outline of tubular transport and metabolism of glutathione-derived thioether conjugates in the kidney. The relevance of various pathways differ among conjugates, depending on the chemical nature of the adduct (X). △ : gamma-Glutamyltransferase; ▽ : cysteinylglycine dipeptidase; ◆ : microsomal N-acetyltransferase; ◇ : cytosolic deacetylase; ● : cysteine-S-conjugate beta-lyase.

REFERENCES

1. Grafström, R.C., Willey, J., Sundqvist, K., Saladino, A.J. and Harris, C.C., Cytotoxicity of tobacco-related aldehydes in cultured human bronchial epithelial cells. US Air Force Technical Report, in press, 1985.

2. Holmgren, A., Glutathione-dependent synthesis of deoxyribonucleotides, J. Biol. Chem. 254, 3664, 1979.

3. Sies, H. and Summer, K.H., Hydroperoxide metabolizing systems in rat liver. Eur. J. Biochem. 57, 503, 1975.

4. Boyland, E. and Chasseaud, L.F., The role of glutathione and glutathione-S-transferases in mercapturic acid biosynthesis, Adv. Enzymol. 32, 173, 1969.

5. Habig, W.H., Pabst, M.J. and Jakoby, W.B., Glutathione-S-transferases. The first enzymatic step in mercapturic acid formation. J. Biol. Chem. 249, 7130, 1974.

6. Tateishi, N. and Higashi, T., Turnover of glutathione in rat liver. In Functions of Glutathione in Liver and Kidney, Sies, H. and Wendel, A., Eds., Springer-Verlag, Heidelberg, 1978, 3.

7. Wendel, A. and Cikryt, P., Level and half-life of glutathione in human plasma. FEBS Lett. 120, 209, 1980.

8. Häberle, D., Wahlländer, A. and Sies, H., Assessment of kidney function in maintenance of plasma glutathione concentration and redox state in anaesthetized rats. FEBS Lett. 108, 335, 1979.

9. Griffith, O.W. and Meister, A., Glutathione: inter-organ translocation, turnover and metabolism. Proc. Natl. Acad. Sci. USA, 76, 5606, 1979

10. Waelsh, H. and Rittenberg, D., Glutathione; metabolism of glutathione studied with isotopic ammonia and glutamic acid. J. Biol. Chem. 144, 53, 1942.

11. Braunstein, A.E., Shamshikova, G.A. and Ioffe, A.L., Glutathione biosynthesis in animal tissues in vivo. Biokhimija, 13, 95, 1948.

12. Meister, A., Biochemistry of glutathione. In Metabolism of Sulfur Compounds, Greenberg, D.M., Ed., Academic Press, New York, 1975, 101.

13. Kosower, N.S. and Kosower, E.M., The glutathione status of cells. Int. Rev. Cytol. 54, 109, 1978.

14. Richman, P.G. and Meister, A., Regulation of gamma-glutamylcysteine synthetase by nonallosteric feedback inhibition of glutathione. J. Biol. Chem. 250, 1422, 1974.

15. Meister, A. and Tate, S.S., Glutathione and related gamma-glutamyl compounds: biosynthesis and utilization. Ann. Rev. Biochem. 45, 559, 1976.

16. Tateishi, N., Higashi, T., Shinya, S., Naruse, A. and Sakamoto, Y., Studies on the regulation of glutathione level in rat liver. J. Biochem. 75, 93, 1974.

17. Ormstad, K., Jones, D.P. and Orrenius, S., Characteristics of glutathione biosynthesis by freshly isolated rat kidney cells. J. Biol. Chem. 255, 175, 1980.

18. Wellner, V.P., Sekura, R., Meister, A. and Larsson, A., Glutathione synthetase deficiency, an inborn error of metabolism involving the gamma-glutamyl cycle in patients with 5-oxo-prolinuria (pyroglutamic aciduria). Proc. Natl. Acad. Sci. USA, 71, 2505, 1974.

19. Heinle, H., Sawatski, G. and Wendel, A., Glutathionbiosynthese VII (1-3): Die Biosynthese von Glutathion in Human Erythrozyten. Hoppe-Zeyler's Z. Physiol. Chem. 357, 1451, 1976.

20. Sekura, R. and Meister, A., Glutathione turnover in the kidney; considerations relating to the gamma-glutamyl cycle and the transport of amino acids. Proc. Natl. Acad. Sci. USA, 71, 2969, 1974.

21. Moldéus, P., Ormstad, K. and Reed, D.J., Turnover of glutathione in isolated rat kidney cells. Eur. J. Biochem. 116, 13, 1981.

22. Högberg, J. and Kristoferson, A., Glutathione turnover in isolated hepatocytes. Acta Pharmacol. Toxicol. 42, 271, 1978.

23. Richardson, R.J., Wilder, A.C. and Murphy, S.D., Maintenance of glutathione levels in renal cortex slices of the rat. Proc. Soc. Exp. Biol. Med. 154, 360, 1977.

24. Griffith, O.W., Bridges, R.J. and Meister, A., Evidence that the gamma-glutamyl cycle functions in vivo using intracellular glutathione: effects of amino acids and selective inhibition of enzymes. Proc. Natl. Acad. Sci. USA, 75, 5405, 1978.

25. Reed, D.J. and Orrenius, S., The role of methionine in glutathione biosynthesis by isolated hepatocytes. Biochem. Biophys. Res. Commun. 77, 1257, 1977.

26. Krebs, H.A., Hems, R. and Viña, J., Regulation of the hepatic concentration of reduced glutathione. In Functions of Glutathione in Liver and Kidney, Sies, H. and Wendel, A., Eds., Springer-Verlag, Heidelberg, 1978, 8.

27. Meister, A., On the enzymology of amino acid transport. Science, 180, 33, 1973.

28. Crawhall, J.C. and Segal, S., The extracellular ratio of cysteine and cystine in various tissues. Biochem. J. 105, 891, 1967.

29. Ormstad, K., Orrenius, S., Låstbom, T., Uehara, N., Pohl, J., Stekar, J. and Brock, N., Pharmacokinetics and metabolism of sodium-2-mercaptoethane sulfonate in the rat. Cancer Res. 43, 333, 1983

30. Kozak, E.M. and Tate, S.S., Interaction of the antitumor drug, L-(α-S-5S)-α-amino-3-chloro-4,5-dihydro-5-isoxazole acetic acid (AT-125) with renal brush border membranes. Specific labeling of gamma-glutamyl transpeptidase. FEBS Lett. 122, 175, 1980.

31. Minato, S., Isolation of anthglutin, an inhibitor of gamma-glutamyl-transpeptidase from Penicillum oxalicum. Arch. Biochem. Biophys. 192, 235, 1979.

32. Jones, D.P., Sundby, G.-B., Ormstad, K. and Orrenius, S., Use of isolated kidney cells for study of drug metabolism. Biochem. Pharmacol. 28, 929, 1979.

33. Albert, Z., Orlowski, M. and Szewczuk, A., Histochemical demonstration of gamma-glutamyltranspeptidase. Nature 191, 767, 1961.

34. Heinle, H., Wendel, A. and Schmidt, U., The activities of the key enzymes of the gamma-glutamyl cycle in microdissected segments of the rat nephron. FEBS Lett. 73, 220, 1977.

35. Spater, H.W., Poruchynsky, M.S., Quintana, N., Inoue, M. and Novikoff, A.B., Immunocytochemical localization of gamma-glutamyltransferase in rat kidney with protein A - horseradish peroxidase. Proc. Natl. Acad. Sci. USA, 79, 3547, 1982.

36. Elce, J.S. and Broxmeyer, B., Gamma-glutamyltransferase of rat kidney. Simultaneous assay of the hydrolysis and transfer reactions with (glutamate⁻ ^{14}C)glutathione. Biochem. J. 153, 223 1976.

37. Voletti, A.M., de Burlet, G. and Sudaka, P., Human renal gamma-glutamyltransferase hydrolysis and transfer reactions with glutathione as substrate. Arch. Int. Physiol. Biochem. 88, 117, 1980.

38. Jones, D.P., Moldéus, P., Stead, A.H., Ormstad, K., Jörnvall, H. and Orrenius, S., Metabolism of glutathione and a glutathione conjugate by isolated kidney cells. J. Biol. Chem. 271, 2787, 1979.

39. Ormstad, K., Tanaka, M. and Orrenius, S., Functions of gamma-glutamyltransferase in the kidney. In Gamma glutamyltransferases; Advances in Biochemical Pharmacology, 3rd Series, Siest, G. and Heusghem, S., Eds., Masson, Paris, 1982, 7.

40. Curthoys, N.P. and Hughey, R.P., Characterization and physiological function of rat renal gamma-glutamyltranspeptidase. Enzyme, 24, 383, 1979.

41. McIntyre, T.C. and Curthoys, N.P., Comparison of the hydrolytic and transfer activities of rat renal gamma-glutamyltranspeptidase. J. Biol. Chem. 254, 6499, 1979.

42. Stetson, P., Isolation and properties of L-cysteinylglycine dipeptidase from human kidney cortex. Fed. Proc., Fed. Am. Soc. Exp. Biol. 34, 557, 1975.

43. Hughey, R.P., Rankin, B.B., Elce, J.S. and Curthoys, N.P., Specificity of a particulate rat renal peptidase and its localization along with other enzymes

of mercapturic acid synthesis. Arch. Biochem. Biophys. 186, 211, 1978.

44. George, S.G. and Kenny, A.J., Studies on the enzymology of purified preparations of brush border from rabbit kidney. Biochem. J. 134, 43, 1973.

45. Kazok, E.M. and Tate, S.S., Glutathione-degrading enzymes of microvillus membranes. J. Biol. Chem. 257, 6322, 1982.

46. Andersson, M.E., Allison, R.D. and Meister, A., Interconversion of leukotriene catalyzed by purified gamma-glutamyltranspeptidase: concomitant formation of leukotriene D4 and gamma-glutamyl amino acids. Proc. Natl. Acad. Sci. USA, 79, 1088, 1982.

47. Meister, A. and Anderson, M.E., Glutathione. Ann. Rev. Biochem. 52, 711, 1983.

48. Meister, A., New aspects of glutathione biochemistry and transport: selective alteration of glutathione metabolism. Fed. Proc. 43, 3031, 1984.

49. Silbernagl, S., Pfaller, W., Heinle, H. and Wendel, A., Topology and function of renal gamma-glutamyltranspeptidase. In Functions of Glutathione in Liver and Kidney, Sies, H. and Wendel, A., Eds. Springer-Verlag, Heidelberg, 1978, 60.

50. Schulman, J.D., Goodman, S.J., Mace, J.W., Patrick, A.D., Tietze, F. and Butler, E.J., Glutathionuria: inborn error of metabolism due to tissue deficiency of gamma-glutamyltranspeptidase. Biochem. Biophys. Res. Commun. 65, 68, 1975.

51. Griffith, O.W. and Meister, A., Excretion of cysteine and gamma-glutamylcysteine moieties in human and experimental animal gamma-glutamyl transpeptidase deficiency. Proc. Natl. Acad. Sci. USA, 77, 3384, 1980.

52. Rankin, B.B. and Curthoys, N.P., Evidence for the renal paratubular transport of glutathione. FEBS Lett. 147, 193, 1982.

53. Lash, L.H. and Jones, D.P., Transport of glutathione by renal basal-lateral membrane vesicles. Biochem. Biophys. Res. Commun. 112, 55, 1983.

54. Lash, L.H. and Jones, D.P., Renal glutathione transport. Characteristics of the sodium-dependent system in the basal-lateral membrane. J. Biol. Chem. 259, 14508, 1984.

55. Puri, R.N. and Meister, A., Transport of glutathione, as gamma-glutamyl-cysteinylglycyl ester, into liver and kidney. Proc. Natl. Acad. Sci. USA, 80, 5258, 1983.

56. Ames, S.R. and Elvehjem, C.A., Enzymatic oxidation of glutathione. J. Biol. Chem. 159, 549, 1945.

57. Ziegenhagen, A.J., Ames, S.R. and Elvehjem, C.A., Enzymatic oxidation and hydrolysis of glutathione by different tissues. J. Biol. Chem. 167, 129, 1947.

58. Ormstad, K., Moldéus, P. and Orrenius, S., Partial characterization of a glutathione oxidase present in rat kidney plasma membrane fraction. Biochem. Biophys. Res. Commun. 89, 497, 1979.

59. Ormstad, K., Låstbom, T. and Orrenius, S., Characteristics of renal glutathione oxidase activity. FEBS Lett. 130, 239, 1981.

60. Ormstad, K., Låstbom, T. and Orrenius, S., Evidence for different localization of glutathione oxidase and gamma-glutamyltransferase activities during extracellular glutathione metabolism in isolated perfused rat kidney. Biochem. Biophys. Acta, 700, 148, 1982.

61. Schmelzer, C.H., Swaisgood, H.E. and Horton, H.R., Resolution of renal sulfhydryl oxidase from gamma-glutamyltransferase by covalent chromatography on cysteinylsuccinamidopropyl glass. Biochem. Biophys. Res. Commun. 107, 196, 1982.

62. Lash, L.H. and Jones, D.P., Localization of the membrane-associated thiol oxidase of rat kidney to the basal-lateral plasma membrane. Biochem. J. 203, 371, 1982.

63. Ashkar, S., Binkley, F. and Jones, D.P., Resolution of a renal sulfhydryl (glutathione) oxidase from gamma-glutamyltransferase. FEBS Lett. 124, 166, 1981.

64. Janolino, V.G. and Swaisgood, H.E., Isolation and characterization of sulfhydryl oxidase in bovine milk. J. Biol. Chem. 250, 2532, 1975.

65. Schmelzer, G.H., Phillips, C., Swaisgood, H.E. and Horton, H.R., Immunological similarity of milk sulfhydryl oxidase and kidney glutathione oxidase. Arch. Biochem. Biophys. 228, 681, 1984.

66. Ostrowski, M.C. and Kistler, W.S., Properties of a flavoprotein sulfhydryl oxidase from rat seminal vesicle secretion. Biochemistry, 19, 2639, 1980.

67. Grafström, R.C., Stead, A.H. and Orrenius, S., Metabolism of extracellular glutathione in rat small intestinal mucosa. Eur. J. Biochem. 106, 571, 1979.

68. Jakoby, W.B., The glutathione-S-transferases: a group of multifunctional detoxification proteins. Adv. Enzymol. 46, 383, 1978.

69. Wolf, C.R., Berry, P.N., Nash, J.A., Green, T. and Lock, E.A., Role of microsomal and cytosolic glutathione-S-transferases in the conjugation of hexachloro-1,3-butadiene and its possible relevance to toxicity. J. Pharmacol. Exp. Ther. 228, 202, 1984.

70. Chasseaud, L.F., The nature and distribution of enzymes catalyzing the conjugation of glutathione with foreign compounds. Drug Metab. Rev. 2, 185, 1973.

71. Mitchell, J.R., Thorgeirsson, S.S., Potter, W.Z., Jollow, D.J. and Keiser, H., Acetaminophen-induced hepatic injury: protective role of glutathione in man and rationale for therapy. Clin. Pharmacol. Ther. 16, 676, 1974.

72. Steele, J.W., Yagen, B., Hernandez, O., Cox, R.H., Smith, B.R. and Bend, J.R., The metabolism and excretion of styrene oxide-glutathione conjugates in the rat and by isolated perfused liver, lung and kidney preparations. J. Pharmacol. Exp. Ther. 219, 35, 1981.

73. Green, R.M. and Elce, J.S., Acetylation of S-substituted cysteines by a rat liver and kidney microsomal N-acetyltransferase. Biochem. J. 147, 283, 1975.

74. Inoue, M., Okajima, K. and Morino, Y., Metabolic coordination of liver and kidney in mercapturic acid biosynthesis in vivo. Hepatology, 2, 311, 1982.

75. Grafström, R., Ormstad, K., Moldéus, P. and Orrenius, S., Paracetamol metabolism in the isolated perfused rat liver with further metabolism of a biliary paracetamol conjugate by the small intestine. Biochem. Pharmacol. 28, 3573, 1979.

76. Okajima, K., Inoue, M., Itoh, K., Horiuchi, S. and Morino, Y., Inter-organ cooperation in enzymic processing and membrane transport of glutathione-S-conjugates. In Glutathione - Storage, Transport and Turnover in Mammals, Sakamoto, Y., Higashi, T. and Tateishi, N., Eds., Jap. Sci. Soc. Press, Tokyo, 1982, 131.

77. Wahlländer, A. and Sies, H., Glutathione-S-conjugate formation from 1-chloro-2,4-dinitrobenzene and biliary S-conjugate excretion in the perfused rat liver. Eur. J. Biochem. 96, 441, 1979.

78. Moldéus, P., Jones, D.P., Ormstad, K. and Orrenius, S., Formation and metabolism of a glutathione-S-conjugate in isolated rat liver and kidney cells, Biochem. Biophys. Res. Commun. 83, 195, 1978.

79. Ormstad, K., Uehara, N., Orrenius, S., Örning, L. and Hammarström, S., Uptake and metabolism of leukotriene C_3 by isolated rat organs and cells. Biochem. Biophys. Res. Commun. 104, 1434, 1982.

80. Inoue, M., Okajima, K. and Morino, Y., Renal transtubular transport of mercapturic acid in vivo. Biochem. Biophys. Acta, 641, 122, 1981.

81. Schasteen, C. and Reed, D.J., The hydrolysis and activities of S-2(2-haloethyl)-L-cysteine analogs - evidence for extended half-life. Toxicol. Appl. Pharmacol. 70, 423, 1983.

82. Tateishi, M., Suzuki, S. and Shimizu, H., Cysteine conjugate β-lyase in rat liver: a novel enzyme catalyzing formation of thiol-containing metabolites of drugs. J. Biol. Chem. 253, 8854, 1978.

83. Dohn, D.R. and Anders, M.W., Assay of cysteine conjugate β-lyase with S-2(2-benzothiazolyl)cysteine as the substrate. Anal. Biochem. 120, 379, 1982.

84. Nash, J.A., King, L.J., Lock, E.A. and Green, T., The metabolism and disposition of hexachloro-1:3-butadiene in the rat and its relevance to nephrotoxicity. Toxicol. Appl. Pharmacol. 73, 124, 1984.

85. Weisiger, R.A. and Jakoby, W.B., Thiol-S-methyltransferase from rat liver. Arch. Biochem. Biophys. 196, 631, 1979.

86. Jakoby, W.B. and Stevens, J.L., Cysteine conjugate β-lyase and the thiomethyl shunt. Biochem. Soc. Trans. 12, 33, 1984.

87. Elfarra, A.A. and Anders, M.W., Renal processing of glutathione conjugates. Role in nephrotoxicity. Biochem. Pharmacol. 33, 3729, 1984.

88. Tomisawa, H., Suzuki, S., Shigeyasu, I., Fukazawa, H. and Tateishi, M., Purification and characterization of C-S lyase from Fusobacterium varium. J. Biol. Chem. 259, 2588, 1984.

89. Tateishi, M. and Shimizu, H., Cysteine conjugate β-lyase. In Enzymatic Basis of Detoxication II. Jakoby, W.B., Ed., Academic Press, London, 1980, 121.

14

METABOLIC ACTIVATION OF HALOGENATED CHEMICALS AND ITS RELEVANCE TO NEPHROTOXICITY

E.A. LOCK

INTRODUCTION

A number of chlorine-, bromine- and fluorine-containing organic molecules cause nephrotoxicity in experimental animals and in some cases in man. Many of these chemicals are used as industrial solvents, chemical intermediates or pesticides, while others have had a more direct clinical application as anticancer chemotherapeutic agents or anaesthetics. Several reviews on the effect of these chemicals on the kidney are available[1-5]. This chapter will therefore not discuss all halogenated chemicals which produce renal necrosis, but instead will review selected examples of the types of mechanism(s) whereby halogenated chemicals can be activated by renal tissue and thereby cause toxicity.

The chapter has been divided into three parts: one, a brief discussion on the anatomy and physiology of the kidney with particular regard to cellular heterogeneity and toxicity; two, the enzyme systems present in the kidney which are capable of activating halogenated chemicals, and three, some examples of the mechanisms whereby certain halogenated nephrotoxic chemicals are thought to undergo metabolic activation to their proximate toxins.

1. THE KIDNEY AS A TARGET ORGAN FOR CHEMICAL INJURY

The kidney, lung and liver are frequently targets for a wide variety of chemical toxicity because these organs represent the primary routes of secretion or elimination. The kidneys are often more susceptible to toxic effects for the following reasons. They represent less than 1% of the body weight, but receive about 25% of the resting cardiac output. Thus large quantities of chemicals will be delivered to the renal cortex, which receives 80-85% of the total renal blood flow. Solutes filtered at the glomerulus are reab-

429

sorbed by both passive and active mechanisms, where they may pass through or concentrate in tubular cells. Both protein-bound chemicals and those in free solution may undergo active secretion into the tubular lumen via the organic acid or base transport systems, thereby exposing those cells to very high concentrations. This, together with the ability of the kidney to concentrate chemicals within the lumen, may greatly enhance proximal tubular toxicity.

The kidney is composed of cortex and medulla. The cortex contains the glomeruli, proximal and distal tubules and receives the majority of the renal blood flow. There are morphologically and functionally discrete cell types within the proximal tubule which have been designated the S_1, S_2 and S_3 segments[6,7]. The cortex has a high oxygen consumption and is particularly susceptible to those agents that produce cellular anoxia, especially to the S_3 segment[7]. In contrast the renal medulla receives less blood flow, is more anaerobic in its metabolism and is the site of the countercurrent mechanism which is responsible for concentrating the urine. This mechanism concentrates compounds in the medulla to many times those present in plasma[8,9].

The high concentration of a chemical in a kidney cell may act directly or it may require further intrarenal metabolism to produce a toxic response. Direct-acting chemicals could interfere with an important metabolic event, such as inhibiting mitochondrial function leading to anoxia or impairing other key functional enzymes. Alternatively, the chemical may be metabolized to a reactive intermediate that may bind covalently to protein, or initiate lipid peroxidation, resulting in cellular damage. In the latter case the chemical may have already undergone metabolism by extrarenal enzymes, to give a stable metabolite which can enter the kidney via the systemic circulation.

Most of the common enzymes involved in the metabolism of foreign compounds, e.g. cytochrome P-450 mixed-function oxidases and glutathione-S-transferases, are present in the kidney, although the specific activities of these enzymes are generally lower than those found in the liver[10-12]. However, in the kidney there are marked regional differences in the relative amounts of certain enzymes in specific regions of the nephron. Thus the use of the whole kidney as opposed to renal cortical or papillary regions can grossly underestimate the metabolic activity of certain regions of the kidney. Frequently the intrarenal site of necrosis represents the site of accumulation of the chemical, and the location of the activation enzymes which are responsible for producing the reactive moiety.

2. RENAL ENZYMES CAPABLE OF METABOLISM AND ACTIVATION OF HALOGENATED CHEMICALS

Many chlorinated solvents undergo metabolism in vivo to reactive intermediates which are the proximate toxins. Metabolic activation was first proposed as a mechanism of renal carcinogenesis for dimethylnitrosamine, where the reactive intermediate methylated DNA and protein[13,14]. The mechanism of metabolic activation has now been extended to include other chemically induced acute tissue injury, a topic which has been widely reviewed[15-18]. Frequently, marked species, sex or strain differences are seen in chemically induced nephrotoxicity. Many of these differences can be accounted for by differences in the activity of those enzymes involved in metabolic activation or detoxification.

(A)   Cytochrome P-450

Cytochrome P-450 catalyses a variety of reactions including aliphatic and aromatic hydroxylations, epoxidation, N-oxidation and sulphoxidation and N-, O- and S-dealkylation. Further metabolism may then occur by conjugation (e.g. glucuronidation or sulphation) to give usually a more water soluble metabolite which may be excreted by the kidney. However, cytochrome P-450 mediated metabolism does not always result in detoxification, as highly electrophilic intermediates may be formed which can bind to important macromolecules leading to cellular damage[19].

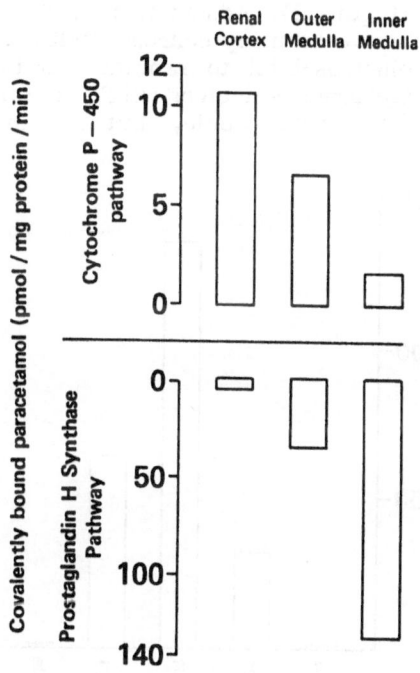

Figure 1 Intrarenal differences in distribution of cytochrome P-450 and prostaglandin H synthase involved in the activation of acetaminophen. (Modified from Mohandes et al.[48].)

Renal mono-oxygenases are capable of metabolizing a variety of foreign chemicals (for a review see ref. 20). Generally, renal cytochrome P-450 content and enzyme activities, with the exception of lauric acid hydroxylation, are much lower than in the liver. Renal cytochrome P-450 content is only about 10-20% of that in liver, the renal concentration being in the range of 0.1-0.3 nmol/mg microsomal protein for the rat and mouse[20]. Rat renal mixed function oxidases are induced by polycyclic aromatic hydrocarbons, e.g. (3-methylcholanthrene and β-naphthoflavone), non-planar polychlorinated biphenyls and polybrominated biphenyl compounds, 2,3,7,8-tetrachlorodibenzo-p-dioxin (TCDD), isosafrole and hydrocarbon solvents, but are refractory to phenobarbital and planar polychlorinated biphenyls[21-26]. In contrast, renal mono-oxygenases are induced in the rabbit by polycyclic aromatic hydrocarbons, TCDD and phenobarbital[27-30]. The reason for this species difference is not clear.

Renal mixed function oxidases are not uniformly distributed along the nephron. The highest concentration is in the cortex with a decreasing concentration in the outer medulla and little in the inner medulla[29,31] (Figure 1). Even within the cortex, mixed function oxidases are not distributed evenly along the proximal tubule. Endou[32], using isolated rabbit kidney nephron segments, showed the highest concentration was localized in the S_2 segment in untreated rabbits (Figure 2). Administration of 3,4-benzo(a)pyrene induced a two-fold increase in cytochrome P-450 in the S_1 segment. Administration of phenobarbital to rabbits resulted in a proliferation of smooth endoplasmic reticulum (SER) localized specifically to the S_3 segment of proximal tubule, but not in the adjacent S_2

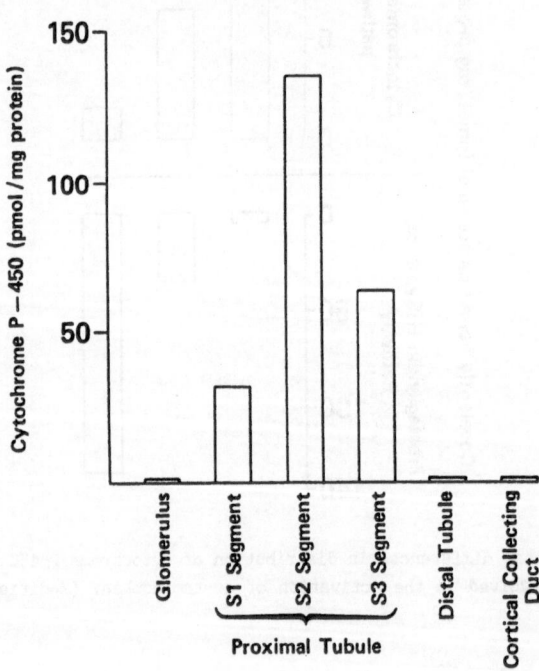

Figure 2 Localization of cytochrome P-450 along the rabbit nephron. (Modified from Endou[32].)

segment[33]. TCDD, β-naphthoflavone and polybrominated biphenyls produce a similar distribution of SER in rat kidney[29,33,34]. Immunocytochemical localization using antibodies to four forms of hepatic cytochrome P-450 (forms 2, 3, 4 and 6) which cross-reacted with renal tissue have been studied in rabbit kidney[35]. In untreated kidney, form 2 (phenobarbital-inducible) was found in the S_3 and lower portion of the S_2 segment, while form 3 (constitutive) was localized in the S_2 and S_3 segments. Very little cross-reactivity occurred with forms 4 and 6 (TCDD-inducible). Prior treatment with phenobarbital did not alter the location of the cytochrome isoenzymes, although a slight increase in intensity was seen with form 2 in the S_3 segment.

In contrast, TCDD treatment decreased the cross-reactivity to forms 2 and 3, but forms 4 and 6 gave an intense response in the S_2 and S_3 segments of the proximal tubule. These results, together with those of others[36,37], suggest that there are at least four forms of cytochrome P-450 which may exist in rabbit kidney, and that they are not evenly distributed along the nephron. Thus chemicals can increase renal cytochrome P-450 in certain selected cell types, which may explain in some cases the location of the injury caused by a nephrotoxin.

(B) Prostaglandin H synthase

Prostaglandin H synthase (PHS) is a haemoprotein consisting of two separate activities: fatty acid cyclo-oxygenase and prostaglandin hydroperoxidase[38]. Fatty acid cyclo-oxygenase is responsible for the initial bis-dioxygenation of the unsaturated fatty acid (primarily arachidonic acid). The hydroperoxidase is then responsible for the subsequent reduction of the lipid peroxide, prostaglandin G_2. During this reduction a suitable electron donor becomes oxidized, which is shown on Figure 3 by the conversion of A to B. For example, acetaminophen (paracetamol), benzidine and diphenylbenzofuran have been shown to be co-oxygenated by this mechanism[39-41]. Arachidonic acid co-oxidation is inhibited by indomethacin and aspirin[42].

In the absence of arachidonic acid, co-oxidation can occur following the addition of a substrate for the hydroperoxidase enzyme such as cumene hydroperoxide or tertiary-butyl hydroperoxide[42]. During the co-oxidation step, oxygen from atmospheric oxygen is directly incorporated into the donor chemical[43]. As certain radical scavengers (ethoxyquin, butylated hydroxytoluene, vitamin E) are inhibitors of co-oxidation, it has been suggested that co-oxidation probably occurs via a free radical pathway[43].

Renal PHS is primarily located in the inner medulla with significantly less activity in the outer medulla (Figure 1). Little or no PHS activity is detected in the cortex[44]. This localization contrasts sharply with the renal mixed function oxidases[44] (Figure 1). Cyclo-oxygenase has been localized by immunocytochemical techniques to medullary intestitial cells, collecting tubules and renal vascular endothelium[45].

Several carcinogens or toxic chemicals have been shown to be

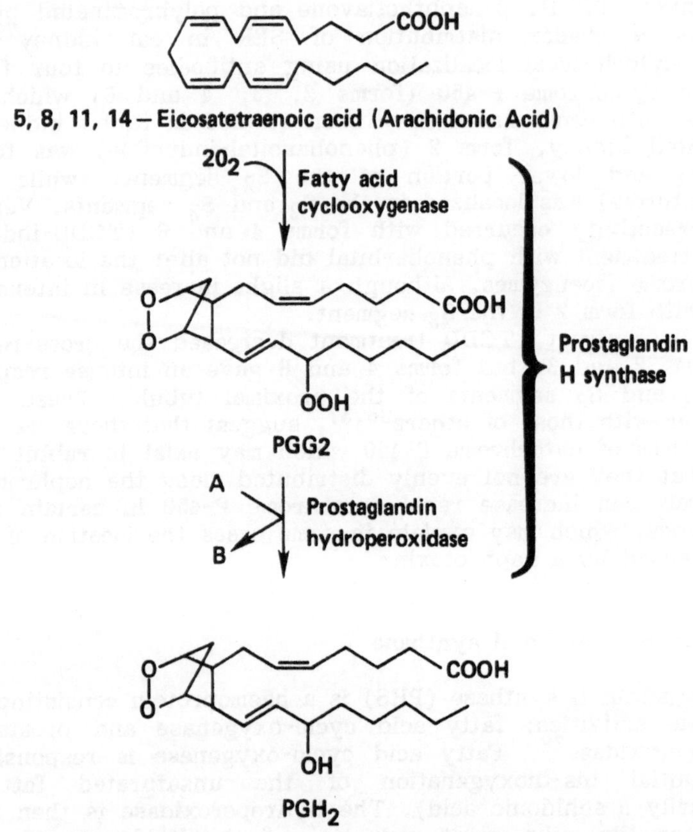

5, 8, 11, 14 — Eicosatetraenoic acid (Arachidonic Acid)

PGG2

PGH$_2$

Prostaglandin
H synthase

Fatty acid
cyclooxygenase

Prostaglandin
hydroperoxidase

Figure 3 Reaction catalysed by prostaglandin H synthase.

oxidized by the hydroperoxidase activity of PHS to reactive intermediates which can bind to macromolecules (for a review see ref.
46). For example acetaminophen undergoes metabolism with PHS
from rat seminal vesicles or rabbit renal medulla to give a protein
bound metabolite which is inhibited by indomethacin and supported
by hydroperoxy fatty acids[47,49]. The nature of the reactive intermediate is unknown, but several workers have suggested it is N-
acetyl-p-benzoquinone imine[47-48]. In addition, PHS can activate
benzo(a)pyrene-7,8-diol, benzidine, β-naphthylamine and certain
other polycyclic aromatic hydrocarbons and aromatic amines to
cause bacterial mutation in strains of Salmonella typhimurium[46].

Thus PHS co-oxidation may play a similar role to cytochrome
P-450 in the metabolic activation of foreign chemicals in selective
regions of the kidney.

(C) Glutathione conjugation as a route of metabolic activation

Conjugation with glutathione (GSH) is generally regarded as a
route of detoxification. However, there is now evidence that

glutathione conjugation of certain halogenated chemicals can result in the formation of reactive intermediates. In the kidney at least two different mechanisms have been reported for GSH-dependent generation of reactive intermediates. The first mechanism involves

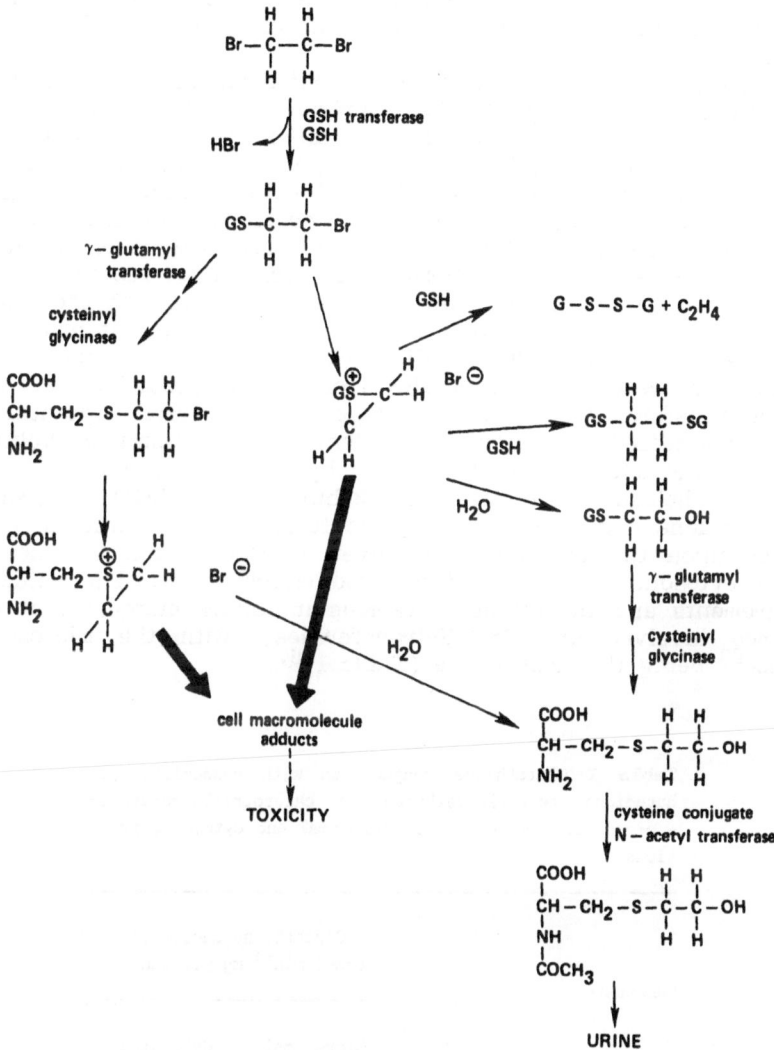

Figure 4 The metabolic activation of 1,2-dibromoethane.

the conjugation of 1,2-dihaloethanes with GSH. The S-(2-haloethyl)-glutathione formed may then rearrange to give the highly reactive ethylene-S-glutathionylepisulphonium ion[50-52] or undergo degradation to S-(2-haloethyl)-L-cysteine prior to rearranging to give the reactive episulphonium ion[53,54] (Figure 4). The second mechanism for GSH-dependent metabolic activation involves the formation of stable GSH conjugates which are subsequently degraded to cysteine conjugates, concentrated in renal cells and activated by the renal enzyme cysteine conjugate β-lyase[55]. The glutathione conjugates of hexachloro-1,3-butadiene[56], chlorotrifluoroethylene[57] and tetrafluoroethylene[58] produce their nephrotoxicity via such a mechanism. The mechanism whereby these reactive intermediates derived from GSH are formed will be discussed below.

Both these mechanisms require GSH-S-transferase(s) to form the initial GSH conjugate. 1,2-Dibromo- and 1,2-dichloroethane form mutagenic metabolites upon the addition of liver cytosolic fractions and reduced GSH[50-52,59-61]. The subcellular distribution, cofactor requirements and the effect of various inhibitors suggest that the enzymes involved in the formation of reactive intermediates are GSH-S-transferase(s)[50-52,59-61]. Studies with purified cytosolic GSH-S-transferases confirmed the formation of reactive intermediates from 1,2-dichloro- and 1,2-dibromo-ethane with the isoenzyme Ya Yc (or B) being the most active[59,62]. There is also some evidence that a microsomal GSH-S-transferase[63] can catalyse the formation of reactive intermediates from 1,2-dichloroethane[61]. The GSH-S-transferases and their endogenous substrate, glutathione are both localized to a significant extent in the proximal convoluted tubule[64], the site of necrosis, caused by these chemicals.

The haloalkenes hexachloro-1,3-butadiene (HCBD), chlorotrifluoroethylene and tetrafluoroethylene form stable glutathione conjugates upon the addition of rat liver microsomal and to a lesser extent cytosolic fractions and reduced GSH[58,65,66]. The cofactor requirements and the effect of various inhibitors suggest that the enzymes involved are GSH-S-transferases, with the microsomal enzyme[63] being the most active (Table 1)[67].

Table 1 Glutathione conjugation with hexachloro-1,3-butadiene, tetrafluroethylene and chlorotrifluoro-ethylene-mediated by rat liver microsomal and cytosolic fractions

Substrate	Glutathione depletion ($nmol\ min^{-1}\ mg\ protein^{-1}$)	
	Microsomal	Cytosolic
Hexachloro,1,3-butadiene	1.4	0.35
Tetrafluoroethylene	3.0	0.7
Chlorotrifluoroethylene	35-70	5-15

Data from refs. 58, 65, 67.

Rat liver cytosol[66], isolated hepatocytes[68] and purified GSH-S-transferases A, B, and in addition to forming a single conjugate also appear to form a double conjugate with 2 moles of glutathione per mol of HCBD. Both the microsomal and cytosolic GSH-S-transferases for HCBD are present in the liver of a number of species including man[67]; in fact, man has the highest ratio of microsomal:cytosolic enzyme activity for HCBD at 38:1, while in the rat and mouse it is 4:1 and 1.5:1 respectively[67].

Following the formation of these GSH conjugates, they are then degraded to cysteine conjugates and subsequently bioactivated to a reactive metabolite by renal cysteine conjugate β-lyase (or C-S lyase). The cysteine conjugate of trichloroethylene, dichlorovinyl-L-cysteine (DCVC) appears to produce its nephrotoxicity by this mechanism. Studies in the 1960s showed that DCVC is cleaved by a renal C-S lyase enzyme at the thioether link to produce pyruvate, ammonia and chloride in a stoichiometric relationship of 1:1:2[69], and an unidentified metabolite containing sulphur and carbon from the vinyl moiety which can combine with proteins and GSH[69]. The substrate specificity for the renal enzyme was examined using a wide range of sulphur- and non-sulphur-containing amino acids; significant pyruvate production was only detected with L-DCVC and L-DCVC-sulphoxide as substrates[69]. The mercapturate, N-acetyl DCVC, the D-isomer of DCVC, and the methylester of L-DCVC were not substrates for the enzyme. GSH, dithiothreitol, L-cysteine and N-acetylcysteine increased the activity of renal DCVC-lyase in vitro, probably by trapping the reactive thiovinyl moiety and preventing alkylation of the enzyme. Both hydroxylamine and isobutylamine, which inhibit pyridoxal phosphate-catalysed reactions, inhibited the DCVC-lyase activity. Subsequent addition of pyridoxal phosphate did not restore the enzyme activity[69]. The enzyme responsible for the cleavage of DCVC is present in renal and hepatic cytosol and hepatic mitochondria[71,72,75].

Recent studies by Tateishi et al.[73] and Stevens and Jakoby[74] have described the purification to homogeneity of the enzyme cysteine conjugate β-lyase from rat liver, which is believed to be responsible for the formation of thiomethyl-containing metabolites. This enzyme will cleave DCVC and appears to have a substrate specificity and cofactor requirements similar to that described by Anderson and Schultze[70]. However, the enzyme will also cleave aromatic substrates such as S-(2,4-dinitrophenyl)-L-cysteine, S-(p-bromophenyl)-L-cysteine and S-(2-benzothiazolyl)-L-cysteine[73-75], and the aliphatic amino acid β-chloro-L-alanine[74].

Thus a rather broad spectrum of substrates can be accommodated by the hepatic cysteine conjugate β-lyase enzyme. In addition, Stevens[76] has reported that rat liver cysteine conjugate β-lyase possesses kynureninase activity (Figure 5) and has concluded from his studies that kynureninase and cysteine conjugate β-lyase are the same enzyme. Purified cysteine conjugate β-lyase cleaves kynurenine and 3-hydroxykynurenine and both these substrates inhibit the cleavage of S-(2-benzothiazolyl)-L-cysteine (Figure 5). Similarly, purified kynureninase can be inhibited by β-chloro-L-alanine and S-(2-benzothiazolyl)-L-cysteine[76] (Figure 5). These studies using various substrates with the liver and kidney

437

enzymes[72,75,77], indicate that the renal and hepatic cysteine conjugate β-lyase may be different. This is supported by the finding that an antibody prepared against the purified liver enzyme did not cross react with an extract containing the enzyme from rat kidney[74,76]. The liver antibody was, however, able to remove kynureninase activity from rat kidney cytosol without affecting the activities with DCVC or S-(2-benzothiazolyl)-L-cysteine. These findings suggest the presence of multiple forms of cysteine conjugate β-lyase activities in both kidney and liver, with a different distribution of the forms in the two organs.

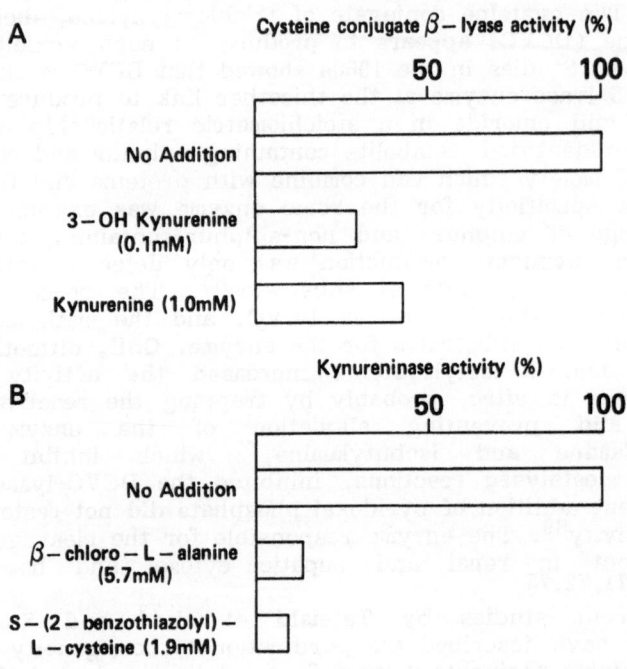

Figure 5 Inhibition of rat liver. (A) cysteine conjugate β-lyase by kynurenine and (B) inhibition of kynureninase activity by substrates which undergo β-elimination. (Modified from Stevens[76].)

The precise location of cysteine conjugate β-lyase in the nephron is not currently known, although studies with the nephrotoxin HCBD, which requires activation via this enzyme, suggest it is present in the pars recta of the proximal tubule of the rat kidney[78]. Similarly, it is not known whether various physiological conditions or treatments with xenobiotics can induce different forms of this enzyme in the kidney or liver.

3. HALOGENATED CHEMICALS CAUSING NEPHROTOXICITY AFTER METABOLIC ACTIVATION

(A) Metabolic activation of chloroform by cytochrome P-450 as a probable route of nephrotoxicity

Administration of chloroform either by injection, ingestion, inhalation or dermal absorption can produce hepatic and renal damage in most species including man (for a review see ref. 79). Primarily, chloroform induces hepatic damage where it causes centrilobular necrosis as a result of hepatic metabolism via cytochrome P-450 to produce the reactive intermediate phosgene which is thought to be the ultimate hepatotoxin[80]. Renal necrosis produced by chloroform is mainly seen in mice where the lesion is sex-dependent, only the males being susceptible[81,82]. The lesion is primarily localized in the proximal tubule and characterized by a marked increase in kidney weight and swelling of tubular epithelium associated with marked necrosis and tubular casts[81,83,84]. Changes in renal function include glucosuria, proteinuria and an increase in blood urea nitrogen[85,86]. In vitro accumulation of organic ions by renal cortical slices was also decreased by in vivo administration of chloroform[86-88].

Renal metabolism of chloroform

The mechanism of chloroform-induced nephrotoxicity has been assumed to be similar to that established in the liver, namely the generation of phosgene directly in the kidney. Studies in vitro have established that kidney cortex slices from rats[89] and male, but not female, mice[90] can metabolize chloroform to CO_2, which is a known degradation product of phosgene (Figure 6). Ilett and co-workers[91] reported the generation of a chemically reactive metabolite of chloroform which in vivo became covalently bound to renal protein in male mice. Autoradiographic studies showed that radioactivity accumulated in proximal convoluted tubular cells, which are the site of necrosis, strongly suggesting that the covalent binding and necrosis were related events[91,92]. The activation of chloroform to a reactive intermediate by male mice renal microsomes appears to be cytochrome P-450 dependent as the covalent binding to microsomal protein: (1) requires NADPH and O_2 and (2) can be inhibited by carbon monoxide and metyrapone[93]. Direct evidence that a metabolite of chloroform is probably involved comes from studies showing that male mice kidney homogenates can metabolize chloroform to phosgene which is trapped by two molecules of GSH to form diglutathionyldithiocarbonate (GS-CO-SG)[94,95]. This metabolite then undergoes further metabolism to 2-oxothiazolidine-4-carboxylic acid (OTZ)[94,95] (Figure 6). The renal metabolism of chloroform to phosgene (trapped as OTZ) requires the presence of O_2 and NADPH and can be inhibited by carbon monoxide, further supporting a role for cytochrome P-450[95]. Administration of chloroform to male mice produces a depletion of renal GSH[88,94,96]. This suggests that phosgene is also formed in vivo as a metabolite in mouse kidney, and further that GSH is scavenging this reactive

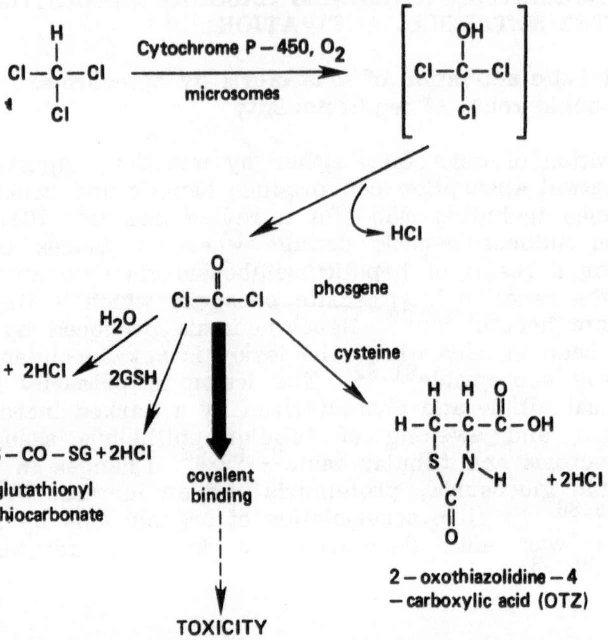

Figure 6 Metabolism and activation of chloroform by the male mouse kidney.

electrophile and thereby reducing the extent of reaction with tissue macromolecules and hence tissue damage. The finding that $CDCl_3$ is less nephrotoxic than $CHCl_3$ to mice in vivo and to kidney slices from mice also supports the idea that a metabolite of chloroform is involved in the nephrotoxicity. These findings also strongly suggest that the metabolism of chloroform to phosgene by the kidney is the rate-limiting step in the process which leads to nephrotoxicity.

Table 2 Cytochrome P-450 dependent metabolism of chloroform to phosgene by mouse kidney homogenates

Conditions	Phosgene trapped as OTZ ($pmol\ min^{-1}\ mg\ protein^{-1}$)
Complete system in air	959 ± 80
- NADPH	45 ± 2
+ CO:O_2 (80/20)	279 ± 25
$CDCl_3$	180 ± 9
+ N_2	not detectable

Modified from Pohl et al.[95]

440

Findings consistent with this hypothesis are that: (1) kidney homogenates metabolize $CDCl_3$ to OTZ less rapidly than they do $CHCl_3$[95] (Table 2), and (2) $CDCl_3$ produces a smaller decrease in renal GSH than does $CHCl_3$.

Thus chloroform undergoes oxidative dechlorination to trichloromethanol in the kidney catalysed by a phenobarbitone-inducible cytochrome P-450[98]. Trichloromethanol is unstable and spontaneously dechlorinates to give phosgene. Phosgene is extremely electrophilic and will react readily with nucleophiles in cellular macromolecules at or near the site of generation, and thereby causes renal tubular necrosis. In addition it can react with GSH to form GS-CO-SG which can then undergo rapid metabolism by renal enzymes to OTZ. The major route for chloroform metabolism is, however, to CO_2 (Figure 6).

Sex and strain differences in renal metabolism

It has been known for many years that the sensitivity to $CHCl_3$-induced nephrotoxicity varies depending on the strain and sex of mouse. Eschenbrenner[81] first described the marked sex difference in renal tubular necrosis, showing that males had extensive necrosis after oral administration, whereas no necrosis was seen in female mice. Eschenbrenner and Miller[99] then reported that castration of male mice abolished their susceptibility to renal necrosis, while treatment with testosterone could restore their susceptibility. These original observations have been confirmed and extended[100-103]. Chloroform nephrotoxicity also shows a marked strain variation, for example male DBA/2J mice are more susceptible to chloroform toxicity than are male C57BL/6J mice, whereas the male F_1 hybrids of these two strains are of intermediate sensitivity[103,104].

The findings from several investigations have indicated that variations in the rate of metabolism of chloroform to a reactive and toxic metabolite form the basis of the genetic and sex differences in sensitivity to chloroform. For example, when radiolabelled chloroform was dosed to male DBA/2J and C57BL/6J mice, more of the radioactivity became bound to kidney tissue of the DBA/2J mice[103,104]. Similarly, more of the radiolabel was bound to the kidney of male mice than to that of female mice[91,92]. Testosterone treatment of the female mice, however, increased the amount of radioactivity bound to the kidney[92]. In addition, when radiolabelled chloroform was added to renal cortical slices from male and female mice more radioactivity was converted to CO_2 and became bound to protein in the tissue from male mice[93].

The metabolism of chloroform to phosgene via the enzyme cytochrome P-450 is the rate limiting step in the metabolism, and findings consistent with the sex and strain difference in chloroform nephrotoxicity are that kidney homogenates from DBA/2J (susceptible) mice metabolized chloroform to phosgene, trapped as OTZ, more rapidly than did homogenates from male C57BL/6J (less susceptible) mice[95] (Table 3). Similarly kidney homogenates from male mice metabolized chloroform to phosgene about ten times more rapidly than female mice[95] (Table 3).

441

Table 3 Sex and strain difference in the metabolism of chloroform to phosgene by mouse kidney homogenates

Source of kidney homogenate	Phosgene trapped as OTZ (pmol min^{-1} mg protein^{-1})
Male ICR mice	307 ± 6
Female ICR mice	35 ± 1
Female ICR pretreated with testosterone	223 ± 14
Male DBA/2J mice	413
Male C57BL/6J mice	226

Modified from Pohl et al.[95]

Testosterone treatment of female mice, however, increased the amount of phosgene trapped as OTZ, produced by kidney homogenates[95] (Table 3). Consistent with these observations is the finding that kidneys from female mice possess a lower cytochrome P-450 content than kidneys from male mice[105]. Castration of male mice reduced the renal cytochrome P-450 content to that found in the female, while testosterone treatment of female mice increased the cytochrome P-450 content to the same level as that in the normal male kidney[105]. These latter findings indicate that renal cytochrome P-450 content is under hormonal control.

Testosterone-induced chloroform nephrotoxicity in female mice can be blocked by treatment with the anti-androgenic compound flutamide[103]. Clemens[103] also reported that the Tfm/Y strain of mice which lack androgen receptors are not responsive to chloroform-induced renal damage even when androgen treated. These findings, together with others, suggest that the androgen-induced renal susceptibility to chloroform is mediated via the androgen receptor. This is located in the proximal tubular cells, and appears to control the concentration of cytochrome P-450, which modulates the metabolism of chloroform to phosgene.

(B) Metabolic activation via conjugation with glutathione as a route of nephrotoxicity

1,2-Dihaloethanes

1,2-Dibromoethane and 1,2-dichloroethane have been reported to produce kidney damage, in addition to damaging other organs such as the liver, in experimental animals[106,107] and man[108]. Lifetime studies in animals given 1,2-dibromoethane by either inhalation or gavage[109-111] have shown tumour induction in a number of organs including the kidney. 1,2-Dichloroethane also produces tumours in animals following lifetime oral administration[112].

Very few studies have dealt specifically with the question of renal metabolism and activation of dihaloethanes and its relevance

442

to nephrotoxicity. However, hepatic metabolism has been extensively studied and may be important in determining the extent of renal damage. 1,2-Dichloroethane lowers hepatic glutathione levels in the rat[113] while 1,2-dibromoethane lowers both hepatic and renal glutathione content[114,115]. Subsequent work has shown that 1,2-dibromoethane is excreted primarily in urine as 2-hydroxy-ethylmercapturic acid, which is formed by further metabolism of the glutathione conjugate[52,116] (Figure 4). The involvement of glutathione in the metabolism of this compound was investigated by Nachtomi[117], who showed that S-(2-hydroxyethyl)glutathione and S,S'-ethylene-bis-glutathione, the conjugation products of 1,2-dibromoethane with one and two molecules of glutathione, respectively, were present in hepatic and renal tissues of rats dosed with 1,2-dibromoethane. Rannug and co-workers[59] have implicated glutathione and cytosolic glutathione S-transferses in the activation of 1,2-dichloro- and 1,2-dibromoethane to metabolites, presumably S-(2-haloethyl)-glutathione derivatives, which were mutagenic to Salmonella typhimurium TA 1535. S-(2-haloethyl) glutathione conjugates are thought to form electrophilic episulphonium ions, by the internal displacement of the second halogen atom by the sulphur atom (Figure 4), which can then react with macromolecules[52,59]. An interesting finding was the alkylation of nucleic acids in preference to proteins by 1,2-dihaloethanes[51,61,118,119]. This binding is dependent on cytosolic enzymes and glutathione, but not on microsomal proteins[119,120].

Recently, irreversible binding to DNA by a 1,2-dibromoethane-glutathione adduct formed by a glutathione-S-transferase catalysed reaction has been reported[62,121]. In this case equimolar amounts of [^{35}S]-glutathione and 1,2-dibromo[1,2^{14}C]ethane were bound to DNA in the presence of glutathione-S-transferase or isolated hepatocytes. An S-[2-(N^7-guanyl)ethyl]glutathione adduct was identified after enzymatic degradation of the DNA[121]. Vadi and co-workers[122] have recently reported a marked difference between the interaction of S-(2-chloroethyl)-L-cysteine and S-(2-chloroethyl)glutathione with supercoiled plasmid DNA in vitro. Extensive binding of ^{35}S from labelled [^{35}S](2-chloro- or bromoethyl)-L-cysteine was found on DNA, whereas ^{35}S from S-(2-chloroethyl)-glutathione did not bind, suggesting a major difference in reactivity of the corresponding episulphonium ions of the conjugates.

Twenty-four hours after the administration of 1,2-dibromo[1,2^{14}C]ethane renal protein, DNA and RNA exhibited the highest concentration of covalently bound radioactivity compared to other organs[51]. The renal cortex contains substantial quantities of glutathione-S-transferases[64] and displays a high activity with dibromoethane as substrate[51]. It is therefore likely that reactive episulphonium ions can be generated within renal cells, alkylate protein and DNA and cause necrosis and carcinogenesis respectively. S-(2-chloroethyl)-L-cysteine, a putative metabolite of 1,2-dichloroethane formed via glutathione conjugation is nephrotoxic in the rat[54]. Whereas analogues of S-(2-chloroethyl)-L-cysteine in which the chlorine atom has been replaced by a hydrogen atom, a hydroxy group or a chloromethylene group were not nephrotoxic[54]. These findings strongly implicate episulphonium ion formation in S-(2-chloroethyl)-L-cysteine-induced nephrotoxicity. S-(2-chloroethyl)-L-cysteine is not a substrate for the hepatic or renal enzyme cysteine conjugate β-lyase[54] (see below).

Hepatic glutathione dependent metabolism of 1,2-dichloroethanes may account for some of the 1,2-dihaloethane-induced nephrotoxicity in vivo. The half sulphur mustard formed subsequent to glutathione conjugation may be secreted into bile in sufficient concentration to be reabsorbed from the intestines and reach the kidney. It could then be further degraded in the kidney to the cysteine conjugate and rearrange to form the reactive episulphonium ion[54]. Evidence for biliary secretion is supported by the demonstration of increased mutagenicity of rat and mouse bile, produced by perfused livers, when 1,2-dibromoethane is included in the perfusion medium[123]. In addition, Schasteen and Reed[53] have suggested that S-(2-chloroethyl)glutathione may have a significantly longer half-life than S-(2-chloroethyl)-L-cysteine, thus S-(2-chloroethyl)glutathione formed in the liver may be transported to the kidney.

The organ selectivity of S-(2-haloethyl)-L-cysteine conjugates may be related to selective accumulation by renal tissue via a probenecid-sensitive transport system. Elfarra and co-workers[54] have shown that probenecid administration can partially protect against the nephrotoxicity produced by S-(2-chloroethyl)-L-cysteine in the rat.

Hexachloro-1,3-butadiene

Administration of hexachloro-1,3-butadiene (HCBD), either by injection, ingestion, inhalation or to the skin, produces renal necrosis[124-129]. In contrast to many other nephrotoxins, HCBD produces mild liver injury, the main changes being a reversible hydropic swelling and some proliferation of smooth endoplasmic reticulum in periportal hepatocytes[130,131].

Renal necrosis produced by HCBD in the rat is restricted to the straight portion of the proximal tubules (S_3 segment) where it causes a distinct band of damage in the outer stripe of the outer medulla[127,129,132]. The earliest morphological changes detected in the electron microscope were mitochondrial swelling in the S_1 and S_2 segments of the proximal tubule 2 h after HCBD administration (300 mg/kg i.p.). By 4 and 8 h the major pathological changes were confined to the S_3 segment and consisted of mitochondrial swelling and cellular necrosis. Although extensive necrosis of the S_3 segment was present for 1-4 days, by day 5 active tubular regeneration was apparent and by day 14 substantial recovery of morphology had occurred[132]. Female rats are more sensitive to HCBD-induced renal necrosis than are males[127,133]. In the mouse HCBD (50 mg/kg) produces renal necrosis of both the S_2 and S_3 segments of the proximal tubule, this pattern of injury being different from that in the rat[132]. Mice do not show a marked sex difference in nephrotoxicity and have a sensitivity of the same order as female rats[134].

Changes in renal function following HCBD administration to male rats at doses of 100 mg/kg and above include decreased urine concentrating ability[127-129,135], glucosuria and proteinuria[56,128,129], increased urinary excretion of alkaline phosphatase, N-acetyl-β-D-glucosaminidase, alanine aminopeptidase and gamma-glutamyltransferase[56,129] and significant reductions in the renal clearances of inulin, urea, p-aminohippurate (PAH) and tetraethylammonium (TEA) with a concomitant increase in plasma urea[129,135]. In vitro accumulation of PAH, but not TEA, by renal cortical slices was decreased by in vivo administration of HCBD[128,129,136]. This discrepancy between the in vitro and in vivo ability to transport TEA may be related to the haemodynamic effect of HCBD in vivo, since both inulin clearance (glomerular filtration rate) and PAH clearance (renal blood flow) are reduced[129,135]. In addition, the reduction in PAH accumulation in vitro is probably a reflection of the selective accumulation HCBD of or a metabolite[78] into the cells, which leads to necrosis.

Chronic administration of HCBD to rats results in renal tubular adenomas and adenocarcinomas and an increase in renal tubular epithelial hyperplasia[137].

Metabolism of hexachloro-1,3-butadiene

Following i.p. or oral administration of a nephrotoxic dose of radiolabelled HCBD, radioactivity appears primarily in the faeces (being eliminated via the bile) with about 10% appearing in urine[56,135,138]. The tissues containing the highest concentrations of radioactivity are initially fat and then the kidneys where the radioactivity persists[55,135,138]. Within the kidney, autoradiography showed accumulation of radioactivity in the outer stripe of the outer medulla, the site of necrosis, suggesting that retention or binding and necrosis were related events[56,78].

Administration of HCBD to adult male rats produces a depletion of hepatic, but not renal, non-protein sulphydryl (GSH) content, even at doses which greatly exceed the lethal dose[115,133,139,140]. In contrast, renal GSH was decreased at very high doses, whereas hepatic GSH was virtually unaffected in female rats, which are more susceptible to HCBD-induced renal damage[133]. The mechanism of GSH depletion may have been due to: (1) GSH conjugation with a reactive metabolite (such as an epoxide) formed via cytochrome P-450 mediated metabolism; or (2) direct substitution of one of the halogens mediated by glutathione-S-transferase. Treatment of rats in vivo with a number of inhibitors or inducers of both hepatic and renal mixed function oxidases, had little or no effect on the toxicity of HCBD, suggesting that HCBD is not activated by the cytochrome P-450 monooxygenase enzymes[136,139,140]. Administration of glutathione[128] or cysteine[141] was also without effect, although diethylmaleate treatment markedly increased the HCBD-induced impairment of renal function[136,142]. In fact HCBD conjugation with glutathione by rat hepatic microsomes and cytosol appears to be independent of cytochrome P-450 as the conjugate is formed: (1) in the presence of CO; (2) does not require NADPH or O_2; and (3) can be inhibited by 1-chloro-2,4-dinitrobenzene, but requires reduced GSH[66]. Direct evidence for a substitution followed by halogen elimination was provided by the isolation and identification of the conjugate as S-(1,2,3,4,4-pentachloro-1,3-butadienyl)glutathione (HCBD-GSH) from rat liver microsomes[66]. The rate of formation of HCBD-GSH in rat liver microsomal fraction is about twice that found in the cytosol[66] and appears to be a good substrate for the microsomal transferase. This initial observation has been confirmed and HCBD appears to be a model substrate for hepatic microsomal GSH-S-transferase in a number of species including man[67]. In rat liver cytosolic fraction, HCBD forms an additonal glutathione conjugate with 2 mol of GSH per mol of HCBD[66],[67]. These observations on the formation of mono- or di-glutathionyl conjugates have been confirmed in studies with isolated hepatocytes[68].

Analysis of bile from HCBD-treated animals showed HCBD-GSH was the major metabolite[56]. The finding that cannulation of the bile duct of HCBD-treated animals prevents the nephrotoxicity, while the administration of lyophilized bile, collected from HCBD-treated rats, to untreated rats produced renal necrosis analogous to that caused by the parent compound, supported the idea that a glutathione-derived metabolite of HCBD is involved in the nephrotoxicity[56]. These findings are strongly supported by the findings that chemically synthesized HCBD-GSH, its cysteine conjugate (HCBD-CYS) and mercapturate (HCBD-NAC) damage the outer stripe of the outer medulla of the kidney[56,78,134,143]. Thus HCBD undergoes conjugation in the liver and then elimination via the bile. In addition, further metabolism occurs in bile where the cysteinyl-glycine conjugate has been identified[144], presumably following cleavage by the enzyme gamma-glutamyltransferase. Rapid hydrolysis of the biliary derived glutathione conjugates to their corresponding cysteine conjugates would be anticipated within the intestine[145,146]. Reabsorption of these conjugates will allow them to reach the kidney in significant amounts. The sensitivity of the kidney to metabolites of HCBD is related to the kidney's ability to accumulate organic anions[78]. Mercapturic acids (like HCBD-NAC) are readily accumulated by the kidney, probably within the proximal tubule where HCBD-NAC can reach concentrations within the cortex many times that present in plasma[78]. This accumulation can be prevented by the organic anion transport inhibitor probenecid, which also gives protection against the nephrotoxicity[78]. HCBD-NAC undergoes rapid deacetylation by rat kidney cytosol to HCBD-CYS and results in covalent binding of radioactivity to renal protein[147]. Radioactivity from HCBD-NAC also becomes covalently bound to renal protein in vivo, in a dose related manner which can be prevented by probenecid[78]. These findings indicate that further metabolism and activation of HCBD-CYS in proximal renal tubular cells is necessary to produce toxicity. A structurally similar compound, dichlorovinyl-L-cysteine (DCVC), has been reported to undergo activation via cysteine conjugate β-lyase which cleaves the C-S bond generating 1 mol of pyruvate, 1 mol of ammonia, 2 mol of chloride ions and a reactive mercaptan moiety[69]. HCBD-CYS, but not HCBD-NAC, is a substrate for this enzyme from rat kidney which generates 1 mol of pyruvate, 1 mol of ammonia and a reactive moiety which inhibits the transport of PAH and TEA into renal cortical slices[55,148]. The reactive thiobutadienyl moiety presumably reacts with: (1) GSH, which may account for the decrease in renal GSH seen under some conditions[115,133,134]; (2) protein, where it binds covalently[78,138] perhaps to cysteine residues or across disulphide links in proteins; and (3) DNA, where it is mutagenic in the Ames Salmonella typhimurium bacterial assay[148]. HCBD binding to DNA could not be detected in vitro when incubated with glutathione-S-transferase and [^{35}S]GSH, whereas 1,2-dibromoethane showed extensive binding under the same conditions[62]. These findings indicate that HCBD does not produce its toxicity by forming a reactive episulphonium ion analogous to 1,2-dibromoethane. Three metabolites have so far been identified in rat urine from HCBD-treated animals: pentachloro-1,3-butadienyl sulphenic acid[56], pentachloro-1-methylthio-1,3-butadiene and pentachlorocarboxymethylthio-1,3-butadiene[138]. Two of these metabolites support the in vitro data, indicating that C-S bond cleavage has occurred followed by subsequent methylation or oxidation. A summary of the pathways of HCBD metabolism is shown in Figure 7.

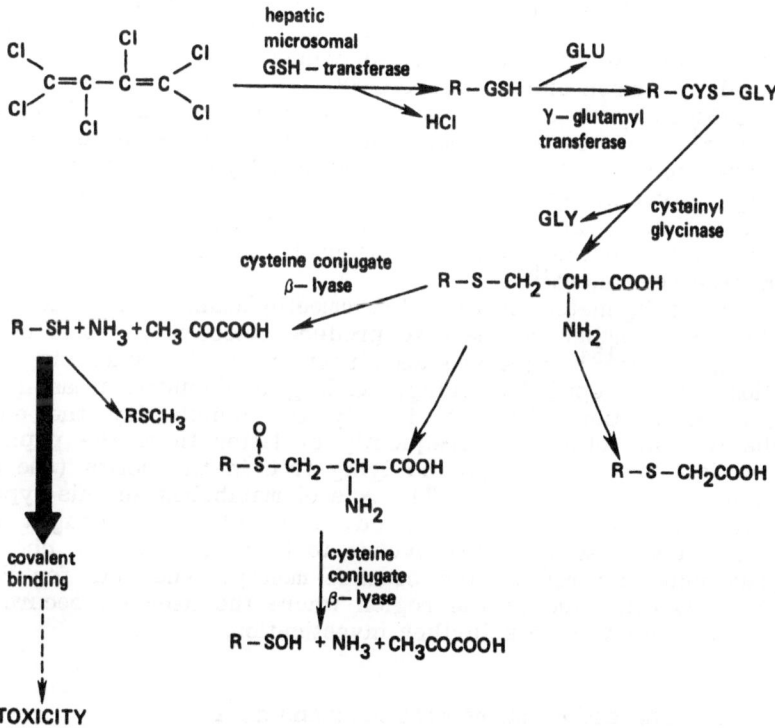

Figure 7 Metabolism and activation of hexachloro-1,3-butadiene by the rat.

(C) Metabolic activation by prostaglandin H synthase as a possible route of nephrotoxicity

The toxicological implications of the arachidonic acid-dependent pathway are as yet unclear, however the localization of prostaglandin H synthase (PHS) to the inner medulla suggests it may play a role in the onset of analgesic nephropathy. Recently, acetaminophen (APAP) has been demonstrated to be metabolized to an acylating metabolite in vitro by PHS[47,48]. Arachidonic acid-dependent in vitro covalent binding of APAP was greatest in the papilla and lowest in the cortex, whereas cytochrome P-450 dependent binding was entirely confined to the cortex and could not be detected in the papilla[48]. PHS-dependent covalent binding of APAP to rabbit medullary microsomes was reduced by aspirin, indomethacin and ethoxyquin, inhibitors of prostaglandin synthase and by antioxidants (ascorbic acid and butylated hydroxy-anisole)[41,47,48,149]. Glutathione also reduced PHS-dependent covalent binding of APAP, forming a glutathione conjugate[149]. The precise mechanism of PHS-dependent activation of APAP is not understood, but it probably involves a one-electron oxidation, which would result in hydrogen abstraction and formation of the phenoxyradical of APAP[149]. The APAP radical may be conjugated directly with glutathione, or after further oxidation to the N-acetylquinoneimine[149]. This mechanism of APAP oxidation is similar to the horseradish peroxidase-dependent oxidation of APAP reported by Nelson and co-workers[150].

2-Bromohydroquinone, a nephrotoxic metabolite of bromo-benzene[151], has recently been reported to undergo arachidonic acid-dependent covalent binding to rat renal papillary tissue, suggesting activation by PHS[152]. The covalent binding was reduced by indomethacin, an inhibitor of the cyclo-oxygenase component, and by propylthiouracil and methimidazole inhibitors of the hydroperoxidase component[152].

The halogenated chemical 2-bromoethylamine (BEA) has been known for a number of years to produce selective necrosis of the renal papilla[153,154]. BEA produced necrosis of the collecting ducts and loss of the epithelial lining, leading to denuded areas in the most distal portion within 24 h. By the fourth day the entire papilla was necrotic, and frequently at latter times the papillary tip was lost and could be found lying free in the pelvis (see also Sabatini and co-workers[155]). The role of metabolism in this type of selective toxicity is not understood, although it is thought that BEA in aqueous solution can cyclize to form the reactive chemical ethyleneimine and release the bromine moiety. The role for PHS, which is concentrated in the region where the necrosis occurs, is not known, but warrants further investigations.

(D) Metabolic activation of bromobenzene as a possible route of nephrotoxicity

Some halogenated chemicals may undergo activation by more than one metabolic pathway to produce reactive metabolites, which may be responsible for the nephrotoxicity. An example of current interest is bromobenzene. Administration of bromobenzene to mice or rats produces necrosis of the proximal convoluted renal tubules between 24 and 48 h after dosing[156]. The renal necrosis is associated with the covalent binding of radiolabelled material to kidney protein. Studies in mice on the metabolism and covalent binding of

[^{14}C]bromobenzene in vitro suggest that renal necrosis is caused by a metabolite formed extrarenally and transported to the renal tubules, since prior treatment of mice with phenobarbital which induces hepatic, but not renal, cytochromes P-450 increases the in vivo covalent binding to both tissues[156]. The postulated hepatotoxic metabolite of bromobenzene, bromobenzene-3,4-oxide, (Figure 8) is sufficiently stable to escape from hepatocytes in vitro[157] and can be detected in retro-orbital sinus blood[158]. It is possible that this epoxide may be sufficiently stable to reach the kidney and elicit toxicity. However, the kidney possesses a greater capacity to detoxify the epoxide than the liver[159]. Thus the role of this epoxide in renal toxicity may be very limited.

A major bromobenzene metabolite, 4-bromophenol (Figure 8), gives rise to covalently bound material in the kidney in vivo[160], and is nephrotoxic[161]. Similarly other metabolites of bromobenzene, 3-bromophenol and 4-bromocatechol (Figure 8), are also nephrotoxic[161,162]. 3-Bromophenol reduces renal but not hepatic glutathione content[162], and radiolabel from 3-bromophenol becomes covalently bound to renal protein but not liver protein in vivo[162]. Monks and co-workers[151] have recently identified 2-bromo-hydroquinone as a metabolite of bromobenzene (Figure 8) formed from rat liver microsomes. 2-Bromohydroquinone is the major metabolite formed in rat liver microsomes from 3-bromophenol[151]. 2-Bromohydroquinone is also a potent nephrotoxin in rats, causing histopathological changes indistinguishable from bromobenzene[163]. However, covalent binding and 2-bromohydroquinone formation from 3-bromophenol only occurs with hepatic but not renal microsomes in vitro, suggesting that 2-bromohydroquinone or a metabolite may be transported from the liver to the kidney. Incubation of rat liver microsomes with 2-bromohydroquinone and [^{35}S]glutathione, leads to the formation of glutathione-derived conjugates, which when incubated with rat kidney cytosol gave rise to covalently bound material[164,165].

Administration of the chemically synthesized glutathione and cysteine conjugates of 2-bromohydroquinone produced marked renal necrosis similar to that seen with bromobenzene itself[165]. These data strongly suggest that the cysteine conjugate of bromobenzene may undergo activation by the renal enzyme cysteine conjugate β-lyase to produce nephrotoxicity.

The mechanism of oxidation of 2-bromohydroquinone to reactive intermediates which combine with glutathione to form the glutathione conjugates is not known, although it appears to be by a mechanism other than cytochrome P-450. Lau and co-workers[152] have recently reported that PHS from the renal medulla can metabolize radiolabelled 2-bromohydroquinone to covalently bound material in the presence of arachidonic acid. Glutathione and inhibitors of PHS, indomethacin, propylthiouracil and methimidazole all significantly reduce the arachidonic acid-dependent covalent binding[152]. These studies suggest PHS may play a role in the oxidation of 2-bromohydroquinone to intermediates which can react readily with glutathione to form conjugates.

449

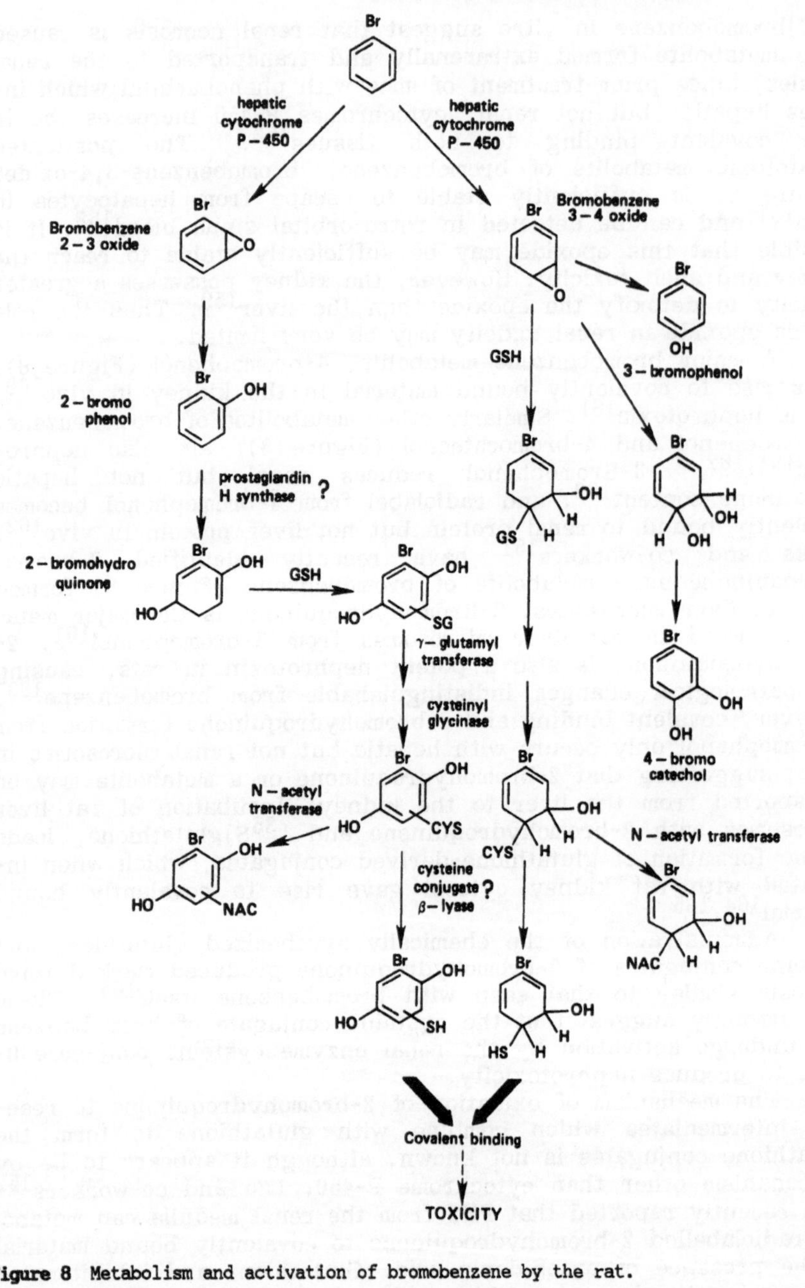

Figure 8 Metabolism and activation of bromobenzene by the rat.

This last example, although not fully elucidated, indicates that bromobenzene-mediated toxicity may involve a combination of metabolic pathways (Figure 8) which include activation by cytochrome P-450, a possible role for PHS, conjugation with glutathione and possible activation by renal cysteine conjugate β-lyase.

450

SUMMARY

A few well-established examples have been selected to illustrate the mechanism(s) whereby halogenated chemicals undergo metabolic activation and produce nephrotoxicity. Many of the chemicals illustrated are not selective for the kidney, but will also undergo metabolism, and produce toxicity in the liver and other extrahepatic tissues. For example, the mechanism of chloroform activation by cytochrome P-450 was initially established in the liver[80], and was only demonstrated later to occur in the kidney. The generation of highly reactive episulphonium ions from dihaloethane glutathione conjugates will occur in a number of tissues, but especially at the site of application, for example the gastric mucosa following oral administration[110]. PHS is present in high concentrations in rat seminal vesicles and will activate APAP[49,149] in an analogous manner to renal medullary microsomes[48]. However, the nephrotoxic substrates of renal cysteine conjugate β-lyase appear to show considerable selectivity for the kidney, causing only mild hepatic injury at very high doses[130,131,166] although the liver contains the enzyme cysteine conjugate β-lyase[70,73,74,76]. The basis for this selectivity lies in the fact that glutathione conjugates formed in the liver are generally excreted via the bile, reabsorbed, and then transported to the kidney where they undergo further metabolism. The mercapturic acid conjugate of HCBD is actively transported into renal cortical slices in vitro[167] and into the renal cortex in vivo[78] by a probenecid-sensitive transport system. Once in the renal cell cytosol the balance between the two competing pathways of acetylation and deacetylation will determine the susceptibility to nephrotoxicity. Several recent studies have examined the renal accumulation and transport of glutathione conjugates of haloalkenes[168-171] and for further information readers are referred to a review by Elfarra and Anders[172].

All the chemicals discussed are activated by metabolites to a reactive metabolite which becomes covalently bound to protein and/or DNA. Further work is needed to identify the chemical species which alkylate renal proteins or DNA similar to that reported for dibromoethane[121]. It is also important to ascertain which are the critical site(s) on macromolecules that are alkylated, and the sequence of biochemical events which lead to renal tubular necrosis. Further studies are needed to determine the mechanism of nephrotoxicity of these chemicals at the biochemical and molecular level. Some studies suggest that mitochondria are a prime target for DCVC and HCBD where they interfere with oxygen consumption[173-176]. Pohl and co-workers[95] have suggested that the mitochondrial location of cytochrome P-450, which can activate chloroform to phosgene, may be a key site of activation.

Little is known about these enzyme steps in man. Studies in vitro with human tissue to determine the rates of hepatic conjugation and with renal tissue to determine enzyme activities of cysteine conjugate β-lyase are important future steps to help extrapolate these findings in experimental animals to man.

451

ACKNOWLEDGEMENTS

The author wishes to thank Drs. D.M. Stonard, G.J.A. Oliver and P.H. Bach for their constructive criticism of the draft manuscript. I am also indebted to Mrs B. Holroyd and Mrs C. Howard for their patience in typing the manuscript.

REFERENCES

1.   Maher, J.F., Toxic nephropathy, in The Kidney, Brenner, B.M. and Rector, F.C. Jr., Eds., Saunders, Philadelphia, 1976, 1355.

2.   Kluwe, W.M., The nephrotoxicity of low molecular weight halogenated alkane solvents, pesticides and chemical intermediates, in Toxicology of the Kidney, Hook, J.B., Ed., Raven Press, New York, 1981, 179.

3.   Hook, J.B., McCormack, K.M. and Kluwe, W.M., Biochemical mechanisms of nephrotoxicity, in Reviews in Biochemical Toxicology, Vol. 1, Hodgson, E., Bend, J.R. and Philpot, R.M., Eds., Elsevier, New York, 1979, 53.

4.   Lock, E.A., Renal necrosis produced by halogenated chemicals, in Nephrotoxicity: Assessment and Pathogenesis, Bach, P.H., Bonner, F.W., Bridges, J.W. and Lock, E.A., Eds., J. Wiley, Chichester, 1982, 396.

5.   Rush, G.F., Smith, J.H., Newton, J.F. and Hook, J.B., Chemically induced nephrotoxicity: role of metabolic activation, CRC Crit. Rev. Toxicol., 13, 99, 1984.

6.   Tisher C.A., Anatomy of the kidney, in The Kidney, Brenner, B.M. and Rector F.C. Jr., Eds., Saunders, Philadelphia, 1976, 3.

7.   Venkatchalam, M.A., Bernard D.B., Donohoe, J.F. and Levinsky, N.G., Ischemic damage and repair in the rat proximal tubule: differences among the S_1, S_2 and S_3 segments, Kidney Int., 14, 31, 1978.

8.   Valtin, H., Renal Function: mechanisms preserving fluid and solute balance in health, Little, Brown, Boston, 1973.

9.   Hook, J.B., Mechanisms of renal toxicity, in Organ-Directed Toxicity - Chemical Indices and Mechanisms, Brown, S.S. and Davies, D.S., Eds., Pergamon Press, Oxford, 1981, 45.

10.   Litterst, C.L., Mimnaugh, E.G., Reagan, R.L. and Gram, T.E., Comparison of in vitro drug metabolism by lung, liver and kidney of several common laboratory species, Drug. Metab. Dispos., 3, 259, 1975.

11.   Litterst, C.L., Mimnaugh, E.G., and Gram, T.E., Comparative alterations in extrahepatic drug metabolism by factors known to affect hepatic activity, Biochem. Pharmacol., 26, 749, 1977.

12.   Fry, J.R., Wiebkin, P., Kao, J., Jones, C.A., Gwynn, J. and Bridges, J.W., A comparison of drug-metabolising capability in isolated viable rat hepatocytes and renal tubule fragments, Xenobiotica, 8, 113, 1978.

13.   Magee, P.N. and Barnes, J.M., Carcinogenic nitroso compounds, Adv. Cancer Res., 10, 163, 1967.

14.   Swann, P.F. and McLean, A.E.M., Cellular injury and carcinogenesi; The effect of a protein-free high-carbohydrate diet on the metabolism of dimethylnitrosamine in the rat, Biochem. J., 124, 283, 1971.

15.   Gillette, J.R., A perspective on the role of chemically reactive metabolites of foreign compounds in toxicity. I. Correlation of changes in covalent binding of reactive metabolites with changes in incidence and severity of toxicity, Biochem. Pharmacol., 23, 2785, 1974.

16. Gillette, J.R., A perspective on the role of chemically reactive metabolites of foreign compounds in toxicity. II. Alterations in the kinetics of covalent binding, Biochem. Pharmacol., 23, 2427, 1974.

17. Bonse, G. and Henschler, D., Chemical reactivity, biotransformation and toxicity of polychlorinated aliphatic compounds, CRC Crit. Rev. Toxicol., 4, 395, 1976.

18. Nelson, S.D., Boyd, J.R. and Mitchell, J.R., Role of metabolic activation in chemical-induced tissue injury, in Drug Metabolism Concepts, Jerina, D.M., Ed., American Chemical Society, Washington DC, 1977, Chap. 8.

19. Gillette, J.R., Mitchell, J.R. and Brodie, B.B., Biochemical mechanisms of drug toxicity, Ann. Rev. Pharmacol., 14, 271, 1974.

20. Jones, D.P., Orrenius, S. and Jakobsson, S.W., Cytochrome P-450 linked monooxygenase system in kidney, in Extrahepatic Metabolism of Drugs and other Foreign Compounds, Gram, T.E., Ed., SP Medical and Scientific Books, New York, 1980, 123.

21. Lake, B.G., Hopkins, R., Chakaborty, J., Bridges, J.W. and Parke, D.V., The influence of some hepatic enzyme inducers and inhibitors on extrahepatic drug metabolism, Drug Metab. Dispos., 1, 342, 1973.

22. Hook, G.E.R., Haseman, J.K. and Lucier, J.W., Induction and suppression of hepatic and extrahepatic microsomal foreign compound-metabolising enzyme systems by 2,3,7,8-tetrachlorodibenzo-p-dioxin, Chem.-Biol. Interact., 10, 199, 1975.

23. Hook, J.B., Elcombe, C.R., Rose, M.S. and Lock E.A., Characterisation of the effects of known hepatic monooxygenase inducers on male and female rat and mouse kidneys, Life Sci., 31, 1077, 1982.

24. McCormack, K.M., Kluwe, W.M., Rickert, D.E., Sanger, V.L. and Hook, J.B., Renal and hepatic microsomal enzyme stimulation and renal function following three months of dietary exposure to polybrominated biphenyls, Toxicol. Appl. Pharmacol., 44, 539, 1978.

25. Kluwe, W.M. and Hook, J.B., Comparative induction of xenobiotic metabolism in rodent kidney, testis and liver by commercial mixtures of polybrominated biphenyls and polychlorinated biphenyls, phenobarbital and 3-methylcholanthrene: absolute and temporal effects, Toxicology, 20, 259, 1981.

26. Lock, E.A., Stonard, M.D. and Elcombe, C.R, The induction of w and β-oxidation of fatty acids and α_{2u}-globulin in the liver and kidney of rats administered 2,2,4-trimethylpentane, Xenobiotica, 17, 513, 1987.

27. Uehleke, H. and Griem, H., Stimulierung des oxydation von Fremdstoffen in nierenmikdrosomen durch phenobarbital, Naunyn-Schmiedebergs Arch. Pharmakol. Exp. Pathol., 261, 151, 1968.

28. Kuo, C-H, Rush, G.F. and Hook, J.B., Renal cortical accumulation of phenobarbital in rats and rabbits: lack of correlation with induction of renal microsomal mono-oxygenases, J. Pharmacol. Exp. Ther., 220, 547, 1982.

29. Fowler, B.A., Hook, G.E.R. and Lucier, G.W., Tetrachlorodibenzo-p-dioxin induction of renal microsomal enzyme systems. Ultrastructural effects on pars recta (S_3) proximal tubule cells of the rat kidney, J. Pharmacol. Exp. Ther., 203, 712, 1977.

30. Rush, G.F., Wilson, D.M. and Hook, J.B., Selective induction of renal mixed function oxidases in the rat and rabbit, Fundam. Appl. Toxicol., 3, 161, 1983.

31. Zenser, T.V., Mattammal, M.B. and Davis, B.B., Differential distribution of the mixed function oxidase activities in rabbit kidney, J. Pharmacol. Exp. Ther., 207, 719, 1978

32. Endou, H., Cytochrome P-450 monoxygenase system in the rabbit kidney, its

intranephron localisation and its induction, Japan. J. Pharmacol., 33, 423, 1983.

33.   Rush, G.F., Maita, K. Sleight, S.D. and Hook, J.B., Induction of rabbit renal mixed-function oxidases by phenobarbital: cell specific ultrastructural changes in the proximal tubule, Proc. Soc. Exp. Biol. Med., 172, 430, 1983.

34.   Pratt, I.S., Lock, E.A., Hook, J.B. and Rush, G.F., Effects of the monooxygenase inducers polybrominated biphenyl and α-naphthoflavone on renal morphology and biochemistry in rats and mice, in Renal Heterogeneity and Target Cell Toxicity, Bach, P.H. and Lock, E.A., Eds., J. Wiley, Chichester, 1985, 123.

35.   Dees, J.H., Masters, B.S.S., Muller-Eberhard, U and Johnson, E.F., Effect of 2,3,7,8-tetrachlorodibenzo-p-dioxin and phenobarbitone on the occurrence and distribution of four cytochrome P-450 isoenzymes in rabbit kidney, Cancer Res., 42, 1423, 1982.

36.   Ogita, K., Kusunose, E., Yamamoto, S., Ichihara, K. and Kusunose, M., Multiple forms of cytochrome P-450 from kidney cortex microsomes of rabbits treated with phenobarbital, Biochem. Int., 6, 191, 1983.

37.   Wolf, C.R., Hook, J.B. and Lock, E.A., Differential destruction of cytochrome P-450 dependent monooxygenases in rat and mouse kidney following hexachloro-1,3-butadiene administration, Mol. Pharmacol., 23, 206, 1983.

38.   Onki, S., Ogino, N., Yamamoto, S. and Hayaishi, O., Prostaglandin hydroperoxidase, an integral part of prostaglandin endoperoxide synthetase from bovine vesicular gland microsomes, J. Biol. Chem., 254, 829, 1979.

39.   Zenser, T.V., Mattammal, M.B., Brown, W.W. and Davies, B.B., Cooxygenation by prostaglandin cyclooxygenase from rabbit inner medulla. Kidney Int., 16, 688, 1979.

40.   Zenser, T.V., Mattammal, M.B. and Davis, B.B., Cooxidation of benzidine by renal medullary prostaglandin cyclooxygenase, J. Pharmacol. Exp. Ther., 211, 460, 1979.

41.   Mattammal, M.B., Zenser, T.V., Brown, W.W., Herman, C.A. and Davis, B.B., Mechanism of inhibition of renal prostaglandin production by acetaminophen, J. Pharmacol. Exp. Ther., 210, 405, 1979.

42.   Marnett, L.J. Wlodawer, P. and Samuelsson, B., Co-oxidation of organic substrates by the prostaglandin synthetase of sheep vesicular gland, J. Biol. Chem., 250, 8510, 1975.

43.   Marnett, L.J., Bienkowski, M.J. and Pagels, W.R., Oxygen 18 investigations of the prostaglandin synthetase-dependent co-oxidation of diphenylisobenzofuran, J. Biol. Chem., 254, 5077, 1979.

44.   Zenser, T.V., Mattammal, M.B. and Davis, B.B., Demonstration of separate pathways for the metabolism of organic compounds in rabbit kidney, J. Pharmacol. Exp. Ther., 208, 418, 1979.

45.   Smith, W.L. and Bell, T.G., Immunohistochemical localisation of the prostaglandin-formed cyclooxygenase in renal cortex, Am. J. Physiol., 235, F451, 1978.

46.   Marnett, L.J. and Eling, T.E., Cooxidation during prostaglandin biosynthesis: a pathway for the metabolic activation of xenobiotics, in Reviews in Biochemical Toxicology Vol. 5, Hodgson, E., Bend, J.R. and Philpot, R.M., Eds., Elsevier, New York, 1983, 135.

47.   Boyd, J.A. and Eling, T.E., Prostaglandin endoperoxide synthetase-dependent co-oxidation of acetaminophen to intermediates which covalently bind in vitro to rabbit renal medullary microsomes, J. Pharmacol. Exp. Ther., 219, 659, 1981.

48.   Mohandes, J., Duggin, G.G., Horvath, J.S. and Tiller, D.J., Metabolic

oxidation of acetaminophen (paracetamol) mediated by cytochrome P-450 mixed function oxidase and prostaglandin endoperoxide synthase in rabbit kidney, Toxicol. Appl. Pharmacol., 61, 552, 1981.

49. Moldeus, P. and Rahimtula, A., Metabolism of paracetamol to a glutathione conjugate catalysed by prostaglandin synthetase, Biochem. Biophys. Res. Commun., 96, 469, 1980.

50. Livesey, J.C. and Anders, M.W., In vitro metabolism of 1,2-dihaloethanes to ethylene, Drug. Metab. Dispos., 7, 199, 1979.

51. Hill, D.L., Shih, T.W., Johnston, T.P. and Struck, R.F., Macromolecular binding and metabolism of the carcinogen 1,2-dibromoethane, Cancer Res., 38, 2438, 1978.

52. Van Bladeren, P.J., Breimer, D.D., Rotteveel-Smijs, G.M.T., De Jong, R.A.W., Buijs, W., Van Der Gen, A. and Mohn, G.R., The role of glutathione conjugation in the mutagenicity of 1,2-dibromoethane, Biochem. Pharmacol., 29, 2975, 1980.

53. Schasteen, C.S. and Reed, D.J., The hydrolysis and alkylation activities of S-(2-haloethyl)-L-cysteine analogs - evidence for extended half-life, Toxicol. Appl. Pharmacol., 70, 423, 1983.

54. Elfarra, A.A., Baggs, R.B. and Anders, M.W., Structure-nephrotoxicity relationships of S-(2-chloroethyl)-DL-cysteine and analogs: role for an episulphonium ion, J. Pharmacol. Exp. Ther., 233, 512, 1985.

55. Lock, E.A. and Green, T., Selective activation of chemicals by the kidney: its relevance to toxicity and mutagenicity, in Proceeding 9th International Congress of Pharmacology, Vol. 1, Paton, W., Mitchell, J. and Turner, P., Eds., Macmillan, London, 1984, 197.

56. Nash, J.A., King, L.J., Lock, E.A. and Green T., The metabolism and disposition of hexachloro-1,3-butadiene in the rat and its relevance to nephrotoxicity, Toxicol. Appl. Pharmacol., 73, 124, 1984.

57. Gandolfi, A.J., Nagle, R.B., Soltis, J.J. and Plescia, F.H., Nephrotoxicity of halogenated vinyl cysteine compounds, Res. Comm. Pathol. Pharmacol., 33 249, 1981.

58. Odum, J. and Green T., The metabolism and nephrotoxicity of tetrafluoroethylene in the rat, Toxicol. Appl. Pharmacol., 76, 306, 1984.

59. Rannug, U., Sundvall, A. and Ramel, C., The mutagenic effect of 1,2-dichloroethane on Salmonella typhimurium I. Activation through conjugation with glutathione in vitro, Chem-Biol. Interact., 20, 1, 1978.

60. Van Bladeren, P.J., Breimer, D.D., Rotteveel-Smijs, G.M.T., De Knijff, P., Mohn, G.R., Van Meeteren-Walchi, B., Buijs, W. and Van Der Gen, A., The relation between the structure of vicinal dihalogen compounds and their mutagenic activation via conjugation to glutathione, Carcinogenesis, 2, 499, 1981.

61. Guengerich, F.P., Crawford, W.M., Domoradzki, J.Y., Macdonald, T.L. and Watanabe, P.G., In vitro activation of 1,2-dichloroethane by microsomal and cytosolic enzymes, Toxicol. Appl. Pharmacol., 55, 303, 1980.

62. Inskeep, P.B. and Guengerich, F.P., Glutathione-mediated binding of dibromoalkanes to DNA: specificity of rat glutathione-S-transferases and dibromoalkane structure, Carcinogenesis, 5, 805, 1984.

63. Morganstern, R., Guthenberg, C. and De Pierre, J.W., Microsomal glutathione S-transferase, Eur. J. Biochem., 128, 243, 1982.

64. Ross, B.D. and Guder, W.G., Heterogeneity and compartmentation in the kidney, in Metabolic Compartmentation, Sies, H., Ed., Academic Press, London-New York, 1982, 363.

65. Dohn, D.R. and Anders, M.W., The enzymatic reaction of chlorotrifluoroethylene with glutathione, Biochem. Biophys. Res. Commun., 109, 1339,

1982.

66.   Wolf, C.R., Berry, P.N., Nash, J.A., Green, T. and Lock, E.A., The role of microsomal and cytosolic glutathione-S-transferases in the conjugation of hexachloro-1,3-butadiene and its possible relevance to toxicity, J. Pharmacol. Exp. Ther., 228, 202, 1984.

67.   Oesch, F. and Wolf, C.R., Properties of the microsomal glutathione transferases involved in hexachlorobutadiene and chloro-2,4-dinitrobenzene conjugation, Mol. Pharmacol., in press.

68.   Gerdes, R.G., Jones, T.W., Ormstad, K and Orrenius, S., The formation of glutathione conjugates of hexachlorobutadiene by isolated liver cells, in Renal Heterogeneity and Target Cell Toxicity, Bach, P.H. and Lock E.A., Eds., J. Wiley, Chichester, 1985, 145.

69.   Bhattacharya, R.K. and Schultze, M.O., Enzymes in bovine and turkey kidneys which cleave S-(1,2-dichlorovinyl)-L-cysteine, Comp. Biochem. Physiol., 22, 723, 1967.

70.   Anderson, P.M. and Schultze, M.O., Cleavage of S-(1,2-dichlorovinyl)-L-cysteine by an enzyme of bovine origin, Arch. Biochem. Biophys., 111, 593, 1965.

71.   Stonard, M.D. and Parker, V.H., Metabolism of S-(1,2-dichlorovinyl)-L-cysteine by rat liver mitochondria, Biochem. Pharmacol., 20, 2429, 1971.

72.   Stevens, J.L., Cysteine conjugate β-lyase activities in rat kidney cortex: subcellular localisation and relationship to the hepatic enzyme, Biochem. Biophys. Res. Commun., 129, 499, 1985.

73.   Tateishi, M., Suzuki, S. and Shimizu, H., Cysteine conjugate β-lyase in rat liver, J. Biol. Chem., 253, 8854, 1978.

74.   Stevens, J. and Jakoby, W.B., Cysteine conjugate β-lyase, Mol. Pharmacol., 23, 761, 1983.

75.   Dohn, D.R. and Anders, M.W., A simple assay for cysteine conjugate β-lyase activity with S-(2-benzothiazolyl) cysteine as the substrate, Anal. Biochem., 120, 379, 1982.

76.   Stevens, J.L., Isolation and characterisation of a rat liver enzyme with both cysteine conjugate β-lyase and kynureninase activity, J. Biol. Chem., 260, 7945, 1985.

77.   Tateishi, M. and Shimizu, H., Cysteine conjugate β-lyase, in Enzymatic Basis of Detoxication Vol. 2, Jakoby, W.B., Ed., Academic Press, New York, 1980, 121.

78.   Lock, E.A., and Ishmael, J., Effect of the organic acid transport inhibitor probenecid on renal cortical uptake and proximal tubular toxicity of hexachloro-1,3-butadiene and its conjugates, Toxicol. Appl. Pharmacol, 81, 32, 1985.

79.   Davidson, I.W.F., Sumner, D.D. and Parker, J.C., Chloroform: a review of its metabolism, teratogenic, mutagenic and carcinogenic potential, Drug Chem. Toxicol., 5, 1, 1982.

80.   Pohl, L.R., Biochemical toxicology of chloroform, in Reviews in Biochemical Toxicology, Vol. 1, Hodgson, E., Bend, J.R. and Philpot, R.M., Eds., Elsevier, New York, 1979, 79.

81.   Eschenbrenner, A.B., Induction of hepatomas in mice by repeated oral administration of chloroform with observations on sex differences, J. Natl. Cancer Inst., 5, 251, 1945.

82.   Deringer, M.K., Dunn, T.B. and Heston, W.B., Results of exposure of strain C3H mice to chloroform, Proc. Soc. Exp. Biol. Med., 83, 474, 1953.

83.   Shubik, P. and Ritchie, A.C., Sensitivity of male DBA mice to the toxicity of chloroform as a laboratory hazard, Science, 117, 285, 1953.

84.   Hewitt, H.B., Renal necrosis in mice after accidental exposure to

chloroform, Brit. J. Exp. Pathol., 37, 32, 1956.

85. Plaa, G.L. and Larson, R.E., Relative nephrotoxic properties of chlorinated methane, ethane and ethylene derivatives in mice, Toxicol. Appl. Pharmacol., 7, 37, 1965.

86. Kluwe, W.M. and Hook, J.B., Polybrominated biphenyl-induced potentiation of chloroform toxicity, Toxicol. Appl. Pharmacol., 45, 861, 1978.

87. Watrous, W.M. and Plaa, G.L., Effects of halogenated hydrocarbons on organic ion accumulation by renal cortical studies of rats and mice, Toxicol. Appl. Pharmacol., 22, 528, 1972.

88. Smith, J.H., Maita, K., Sleight, S.D. and Hook, J.B., Mechanism of chloroform toxicity, I. Time course of chloroform toxicity in male and female mice, Toxicol. Appl. Pharmacol., 70, 467, 1983.

89. Paul, B.B. and Rubinstein, D., Metabolism of carbon tetrachloride and chloroform by the rat, J. Pharmacol. Exp. Ther., 141, 141, 1963.

90. Smith, J.H. and Hook, J.B., Mechanism of chloroform toxicity. II. In vitro evidence for renal metabolism in mice, Toxicol. Appl. Pharmacol., 70, 480, 1983.

91. Ilett, K.F., Reid, W.D., Sipes, I.G. and Krishna, G., Chloroform toxicity in mice: correlation of renal and hepatic necrosis with covalent binding of metabolites to tissue macromolecules, Exp. Mol. Pathol., 19, 215, 1973.

92. Taylor, D.C., Brown, D.M., Keeble, R. and Langley, P.F., Metabolism of Chloroform. II. A sex difference in the metabolism of (^{14}C)-chloroform in mice, Xenobiotica, 4, 165, 1974.

93. Smith, J.H. and Hook, J.B., Mechanism of chloroform nephrotoxicity. III. Renal and hepatic microsomal metabolism of chloroform in mice, Toxicol. Appl. Pharmacol., 73, 511, 1984.

94. Branchflower, R.V., Nunn, D.S., Highet, R.J., Smith, J.H., Hook, J.B. and Pohl, L.R., Nephrotoxicity of chloroform: metabolism to phosgene by the mouse kidney, Toxicol. Appl. Pharmacol., 72, 159, 1984.

95. Pohl, L.R., George, J.W. and Satoh, H., Strain differences in chloroform induced nephrotoxicity: different rates of metabolism of chloroform to phosgene by the mouse kidney, Drug Metab. Dispos., 12, 304, 1984.

96. Kluwe, W.M. and Hook, J.B., Potentiation of acute chloroform nephrotoxicity by the glutathione depletor diethylmaleate and protection by the microsomal enzyme inhibitor piperonyl butoxide, Toxicol. Appl. Pharmacol., 59, 457, 1981.

97. Ahmadizadeh, M., Kuo, C.-H. and Hook, J.B., Nephrotoxicity and hepatotoxicity of chloroform in mice: effect of deuterium substitution, J. Toxicol., Environ. Health, 8, 105, 1981.

98. Bailie, M.B., Smith, J.H., Newton, J.F. and Hook, J.B., Mechanism of chloroform nephrotoxicity. IV. Phenobarbital potentiation of in vitro chloroform metabolism and toxicity in rabbit kidneys, Toxicol. Appl. Pharmacol., 74, 285, 1984.

99. Eschenbrenner, A.B. and Miller, E., Sex differences in kidney morphology and chloroform necrosis, Science, 102, 302, 1945.

100. Culliford, D, and Hewitt, H.B., The influence of sex hormone status on the susceptibility of mice to chloroform-induced necrosis of the renal tubules, J. Endocrinol, 14, 381, 1957.

101. Jacobsen, L., Anderson, E.K. and Thorbery, J.V., Accidental chloroform nephrosis in mice, Acta. Pathol. Microbiol. Scand., 61, 503, 1964.

102. Krus, S., Starzynski, S., Zaleska-Rutczynska, Z. and Naciazek-Wieniawska, A., The role of testosterone in developing chloroform-induced renal tubular necrosis in mice, Nephron, 12, 275, 1974.

103. Clemens, T.L., Hill, R.N., Bullock, L.P., Johnson, W.D., Sultatos, L.G. and

457

Vesell, E.S., Chloroform toxicity in the mouse: role of genetic factors and steroids, Toxicol. Appl. Pharmacol., 48, 117, 1979.

104. Hill, R.N., Clemens, T.L., Liu, D.K., Vesell, E.S. and Johnson, W.D., Genetic control of chloroform toxicity in mice, Science, 190, 159, 1975.

105. Smith, J.H., Maita, K., Sleight, S.D. and Hook, J.B., Effect of sex hormone status on chloroform nephrotoxicity and renal mixed function oxidases in mice, Toxicology, 30, 305, 1984.

106. Rowe, V.K., Spencer, H.C., McCollister, D.D., Hollingsworth, R.L. and Adams, E.M., Toxicity of ethylene dibromide determined on experimental animals, Arch. Ind. Hyg. Occup. Med., 6, 158, 1952.

107. Spencer, H.C., Rowe, V.K., Adams, E.M., McCollister, D.D. and Irish, D.D., Vapour toxicity of ethylene dichloride determined by experiments on laboratory animals, Arch. Ind. Hyg. Occup. Med., 4, 482, 1951.

108. Olmstead, E.V., Pathological changes in ethylene dibromide poisoning, Arch. Ind. Health, 21, 525, 1960.

109. Weisburger, E.K., Carcinogenicity studies on halogenated hydrocarbons, Environ. Health Perspect., 21, 7, 1977.

110. Olson, W.A., Habermann, R.T. and Weisburger, E.K., Induction of stomach cancer in rats and mice by halogenated aliphatic fumigants, J. Natl. Cancer Inst., 51, 1993, 1972.

111. Wong, L.C.K., Winston, J.M., Hong, C.B. and Plotnick, H., Carcinogenicity and toxicity of 1,2-dibromoethane in the rat, Toxicol. Appl. Pharmacol., 63, 155, 1982.

112. National Cancer Institute, Technical background information report 55 on carcinogenesis bioassay of 1,2-dichloroethane (EDC), U.S. DHEW Publication (NIH), 78-136, Government Printing Office, Washington DC, 1978.

113. Johnson, M.K., The influence of some aliphatic compounds on rat liver glutathione levels, Biochem. Pharmacol., 14, 1383, 1965.

114. Nachtomi, E., Alumot, E. and Bondi, A., Biochemical changes in organs of chicks and rats poisoned with ethylene dibromide and carbon tetrachloride, Isr. J. Chem., 6, 803, 1968.

115. Kluwe, W.M., McNish, R., Smithson, K. and Hook, J.B., Depletion by 1,2-dibromoethane, 1,2-dibromo-3-chloropropane, tris(2,3-dibromopropyl) phosphate and hexachloro-1,3 butadiene of reduced non-protein sulphydryl groups in target and nontarget organs, Biochem. Pharmacol., 30, 2265, 1981.

116. Nachtomi, E., Alumot, E. and Bondi, A., The metabolism of ethylene dibromide in the rat. I Identification of detoxication products in urine, Isr. J. Chem., 4, 239, 1966.

117. Nachtomi, E., The metabolism of ethylene dibromide in the rat: the enzymic reaction with glutathione in vitro and in vivo, Biochem. Pharmacol., 19, 2853, 1970.

118. Banerjee, S. and Van Duuren, B.L., Binding of carcinogenic halogenated hydrocarbons to cell macromolecules, J. Natl. Cancer. Inst., 63, 707, 1979.

119. Shih, T-W and Hill, D.L., Metabolic activation of 1,2-dibromoethane by glutathione transferase and by microsomal mixed function oxidase: further evidence for formation of two reactive metabolites, Res. Commun. Chem. Pathol. Pharmacol., 33, 449, 1981.

120. Sundheimer, D.W., White, R.D., Brendel, K. and Sipes, I.G., The bioactivation of 1,2-dibromoethane in rat hepatocytes: covalent binding to nucleic acids, Carcinogenesis, 3, 1129, 1982.

121. Ozawa, N. and Guengerich, F.P, Evidence for formation of an S-[2-(N[7]-guanyl)ethyl]glutathione adduct in glutathione-mediated binding of the carcinogen 1,2-dibromoethane to DNA, Proc. Natl. Acad. Sci., 80, 5266, 1983.

122. Vadi, H.V., Schasteen, C.S. and Reed, D.J., Interactions of S-(2-haloethyl)

mercapturic acid analogs with plasmid DNA, Toxicol. Appl. Pharmacol., 80, 386, 1985.

123.   Rannug, U. and Beije, B., The mutagenic effect of 1,2-dichloroethane on Sal-monella typhimurium: II. Activation by the isolated perfused rat liver, Chem-Biol. Interact., 24, 265, 1979.

124.   Gradiski, D., Duprat, P., Magadur, J-L. and Fayein, E., Etude toxicologique experimentale de l'hexachlorobutadiene, Eur. J. Toxicol., 8, 180, 1975.

125.   Kociba, R.J., Schwetz, B.A., Keyes, D.G., Jersey, G.C., Ballard, J.J. Dit-tenber, D.A., Quast, J.F., Wade, C.E. and Humiston, C.G., Chronic toxicity and reproduction studies of hexachlorobutadiene in rats. Environ. Health Perspect., 21, 49, 1977.

126.   Duprat, P. and Gradiski, D., Percutaneous toxicity of hexachlorobutadiene, Acta Pharmacol. Toxicol., 43, 346, 1978.

127.   Harleman, J.H. and Seinen, W., Short-term toxicity and reproduction studies in rats with hexachloro-1,3-butadiene, Toxicol. Appl. Pharmacol., 47, 1, 1979.

128.   Berndt, W.O. and Mehendale, H.M., Effects of hexachlorobutadiene (HCBD) on renal function and renal organic ion transport in the rat, Toxicology, 14, 55, 1979.

129.   Lock, E.A. and Ishmael, J., The acute toxic effects of hexachloro-1,3-butadiene on the rat kidney, Arch. Toxicol., 43, 47, 1979.

130.   Lock, E.A., Ishmael, J. and Pratt, I.S., Hydropic change in rat liver in-duced by hexachloro-1,3-butadiene, J. Appl. Toxicol., 2, 315, 1982.

131.   Lock, E.A., Pratt, I.S. and Ishmael, J., Hexachloro-1,3-butadiene-induced hydropic change in mouse liver, J. Appl. Toxicol., 5, 74, 1985.

132.   Ishmael, J., Pratt, I.S. and Lock, E.A., Necrosis of the pars recta (S_3 segment) of the rat kidney produced by hexachloro-1,3-butadiene, J. Pathol., 138, 99, 1982.

133.   Hook, J.B., Ishmael, J. and Lock E.A., Nephrotoxicity of hexachloro-1,3-butadiene in the rat: the effect of age, sex and strain, Toxicol. Appl. Pharmacol., 67, 121, 1983.

134.   Lock, E.A., Ishmael, J. and Hook, J.B., Nephrotoxicity of hexachloro-1,3-butadiene in the mouse: the effect of age, sex, strain, monooxygenase modifiers, and the role of glutathione, Toxicol. Appl. Pharmacol., 72, 484, 1984.

135.   Davis, M.E., Berndt, W.O. and Mehendale, H.M., Disposition and neph-rotoxicity of hexachloro-1,3-butadiene, Toxicology, 16, 179, 1980.

136.   Hook, J.B., Rose, M.S. and Lock E.A., The nephrotoxicity of hexachloro-1,3-butadiene in the rat: studies of organic anion and cation transport in renal slices and the effect of monooxygenase inducers, Toxicol. Appl. Pharmacol., 65, 373, 1982.

137.   Kociba, R.J., Keyes, D.G., Jersey, G.C., Ballard, J.J., Dittenber, D.A., Quast, J.F., Wade, C.E., Humiston, C.G. and Schwetz, B.A., Results of a two year chronic toxicity with hexachlorobutadiene in rats, Am. Ind. Hyg. Assoc. J., 38, 589, 1977.

138.   Reichert, D., Schutz, S. and Metzler, M., Excretion pattern and metabolism of hexachlorobutadiene in rats: evidence for metabolic activation by con-jugation reactions, Biochem. Pharmacol., 34, 399, 1985.

139.   Lock, E.A. and Ishmael, J., Hepatic and renal non-protein sulphydryl con-centration following toxic doses of hexachloro-1,3-butadiene in the rat: the effect of Arochlor 1254, phenobarbitone or SKF 525A treatment, Toxicol. Appl. Pharmacol., 57, 79, 1981.

140.   Davis, M.E., Changes of hexachlorobutadiene nephrotoxicity after piperonyl butoxide treatment, Toxicology, 30, 217, 1984.

141. Davis, M.E., Berndt, W.O. and Mehendale, H.M., Diethylmaleate or cysteine pretreatment modifies hexachlorobutadiene nephrotoxicity, Toxicologist, 1, 9, 1981.

142. Bagget, J. McC. and Berndt, W.O., Renal and hepatic glutathione concentrations in rats after treatment with hexachloro-1,3-butadiene and citrinin, Arch. Toxicol., 56, 46, 1984.

143. Jaffe, D.R., Hassall, C.D., Brendel, K. and Gandolfi, A.J., In vivo and in vitro nephrotoxicity of the cysteine conjugate of hexachlorobutadiene, J. Toxicol. Environ. Health, 11, 857, 1983.

144. Nash, J.A., The metabolism and disposition of hexachloro-1,3-butadiene in the rat and its relevance to nephrotoxicity, M.Phil. thesis, University of Surrey, 1985.

145. Grafstrom, R., Ormstad, K., Moldeus, P. and Orrenius, S., Paracetamol metabolism in the isolated perfused rat liver with further metabolism of biliary conjugate by small intestines, Biochem. Pharmacol., 28, 3573, 1979.

146. Hirata, E. and Takahashi, H., Degradation of methyl mercury glutathione by the pancreatic enzymes in bile, Toxicol. Appl. Pharmacol., 58, 483, 1981.

147. Pratt, I.S., Ormond, T and Lock, E.A., Metabolism of the mercapturic acid of hexachloro-1,3-butadiene by rat kidney cytosol in vitro, Proc. 27th Congress Eur. Soc. Toxicol., Harrogate, UK., 27th-29th May 1986.

148. Green, T. and Odum J., Structure/activity studies of the nephrotoxic and mutagenic action of cysteine conjugates of chloro and fluoroalkenes, Chem.-Biol. Interact., 54, 15, 1985.

149. Moldeus, P., Andersson, B., Rahimtula, A. and Beggren, M., Prostaglandin synthetase catalysed activation of paracetamol, Biochem. Pharmacol., 31, 1363, 1982.

150. Nelson, S.D., Dahlin, D.C., Rauckman, E.J. and Rosen, G.M., Peroxidase-mediated formation of reactive metabolites of acetaminophen, Mol. Pharmacol., 20, 195, 1981.

151. Monks, T.J., Lau, S.S. and Gillette, J.R., Identification of 2-bromohydroquinone as a metabolite of bromobenzene, Pharmacologist, 25, 104, 1983.

152. Lau, S.S., Hubbard, W.C. and Monks, T.J., Metabolism of the nephrotoxin 2-bromohydroquinone by renal protaglandin synthetase, in Proceedings 6th International Symposium on Microsomes and Drug Oxidation, Brighton, Sussex, U.K., 5-10 August 1984, 80.

153. Murray, G., Wyllie, R.G., Hill, G.S., Ramsen, P.W. and Heptinstall, R.H., Experimental papillary necrosis I. Morphologic and functional data, Am. J. Pathol., 67, 285, 1972.

154. Hill, G.S., Wyllie, R.G., Miller, M. and Heptinstall, R.H., Experimental papillary necrosis of the kidney. II. Electron microscopic and histochemical studies, Amer. J. Pathol., 68, 213, 1972.

155. Sabatini, S., Alla, V., Wilson, A., Cruz-Soto, M., De White, A., Kurtzman, N.A. and Arrunda, J.A.L., The effects of chronic papillary necrosis on acid secretion, Pflugers Arch., 393, 262, 1982.

156. Reid, W.D., Mechanism of renal necrosis induced by bromobenzene or chlorobenzene, Exp. Mol. Pathol., 19, 197, 1973.

157. Monks, T.J., Lau, S.S. and Gillette, J.R., Diffusion of reactive metabolites out of hepatocytes, in 8th European Workshop on Drug Metabolism, 1982, 113.

158. Lau, S.S., Monks, T., Greene, K.E. and Gillette, J.R., Detection of bromobenzene-3,4-oxide in blood, in 1st International Symposium on Foreign Compound Metabolism, 1983, 41.

159. Monks, T.J., Lau, S.S. and Gillete, J.R., A dual role of glutathione transferase in the detoxification of bromobenzene-3,4-oxide, Fed. Proc., 42,

1137, 1983.

160. Monks, T.J., Hinson, J.A. and Gillette, J.R., Bromobenzene and p-bromophenol toxicity and covalent binding in vivo, Life Sci., 30, 841, 1982.

161. Rush, G.F., Newton, J.F., Maita, K., Kuo, C.-H. and Hook, J.B., Nephrotoxicity of phenolic bromobenzene metabolites in the mouse, Toxicology, 30, 259, 1984.

162. Lau, S.S., Monks, T.J., Greene, K.E. and Gillette, J.R., The role of ortho-bromophenol in the nephrotoxicity of bromobenzene in rats, Toxicol. Appl. Pharmacol., 72, 539, 1984.

163. Lau, S.S., Monks, T.J., Greene, K.E. and Gillette, J.R., Nephrotoxicity of o-bromophenol and 2-bromohydroquinone metabolites of bromobenzene in the rat, Pharmacologist, 25, 105, 1983.

164. Monks, T.J., Lau, S.S. and Gillette, J.R., Glutathione conjugates of 2-bromohydroquinone, a metabolite of bromobenzene are nephrotoxic, in 1st International Symposium on Foreign Compound Metabolism, 1983, 48.

165. Monks, T.J., Lau, S.S. and Gillette, J.R., The metabolism and nephrotoxicity of 2-bromohydroquinone glutathione conjugates, in 6th International Symposium on Microsomes and Drug Oxidation, Brighton, Sussex, U.K., 5-10 August 1984, 23.

166. Terracini, B. and Parker, V.H., A pathological study on the toxicity of S-Dichlorovinyl-L-cysteine, Fd. Cosmet. Toxicol., 3, 67, 1965.

167. Lock, E.A., Odum, J. and Ormond, P., Transport of N-acetyl-S-pentachloro-1,3-butadienylcysteine by rat renal cortex, Arch. Toxicol., 15, 12, 1986.

168. Hassall, C.D., Gandolfi, A.J. and Brendel, K., Effect of halogenated vinyl cysteine conjugates on renal tubular active transport, Toxicology, 26, 285, 1983.

169. Hassall, C.D., Gandolfi, A.J., Duhamel, R.C. and Brendel K., The formation and biotransformation of cysteine conjugates of halogenated ethylenes by rabbit renal tubules., Chem.-Biol. Interact., 49, 283, 1984.

170. Earl, L.K., McLean, A.E.M. and Lock, E.A., Use of isolated kidney cells for studying nephrotoxicity: hexachloro-1,3-butadiene as a model compound, Human Toxicol., 3, 332, 1984.

171. Lash, L.H. and Jones, D.P., Uptake of the glutathione conjugate S-(1,2-dichlorovinyl)glutathione by renal basal-lateral membrane vesicles and isolated kidney cells, Mol. Pharmacol., 28, 278, 1985.

172. Elfarra, A.A. and Anders, M.W., Renal processing of glutathione conjugates: role in nephrotoxicity, Biochem. Pharmacol., 33, 3729, 1984.

173. Parker, V.H., A biochemical study of the toxicity of S-dichlorovinyl-L-cysteine, Fd. Cosmet. Toxicol., 3, 75, 1965.

174. Stonard, M.D. and Parker, V.H., 2-oxoacid dehydrogenases of rat liver mitochondria as the site of action of S-(1,2-dichlorovinyl)-L-cysteine and S-(1,2-dichlorovinyl)-3-mercaptopropionic acid, Biochem. Pharmacol., 20, 2417, 1971.

175   Stonard, M.D., Further studies on the site and mechanism of action of S-(1,2-dichlorovinyl)-L-cysteine and S-(1,2-dichlorovinyl)-3-mercaptopropionic acid in rat liver, Biochem. Pharmacol., 22, 1329, 1973.

176. Schnellmann, R.G., Lock, E.A. and Mandel, L.J., A mechanism of S-(1,1,2,3,4-pentachloro-1,3-butadienyl)-L-cysteine (PCBC) toxicity to rabbit proximal tubules (RPT), Toxicologist, 6, 176, 1986.

INDEX

THIS INDEX COMBINES PARTS 1 AND 2